Scutchfield and Keck's

PRINCIPLES OF PUBLIC HEALTH PRACTICE

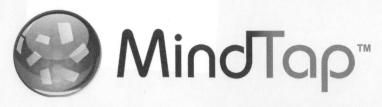

Tap into **engagement**

MindTap empowers you to produce your best work—consistently.

MindTap is designed to help you master the material. Interactive videos, animations, and activities create a learning path designed by your instructor to guide you through the course and focus on what's important.

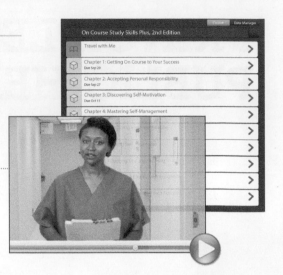

MindTap delivers real-world activities and assignments

that will help you in your academic life as well as your career.

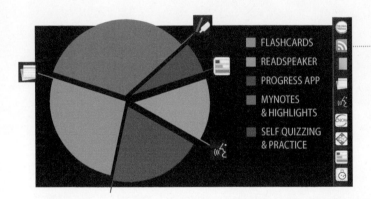

- FLASHCARDS
- READSPEAKER
- PROGRESS APP
- MYNOTES & HIGHLIGHTS
- SELF QUIZZING & PRACTICE

MindTap helps you stay organized and efficient

by giving you the study tools to master the material.

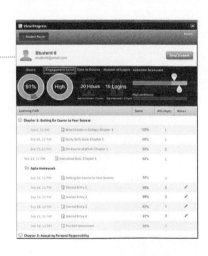

MindTap empowers and motivates

with information that shows where you stand at all times—both individually and compared to the highest performers in class.

"MindTap was very useful—it was easy to follow and everything was right there."
— Student, San Jose State University

"I'm definitely more engaged because of MindTap."
— Student, University of Central Florida

"MindTap puts practice questions in a format that works well for me."
— Student, Franciscan University of Steubenville

Tap into more info at: **www.cengage.com/mindtap**

Scutchfield and Keck's

PRINCIPLES OF PUBLIC HEALTH PRACTICE

Fourth Edition

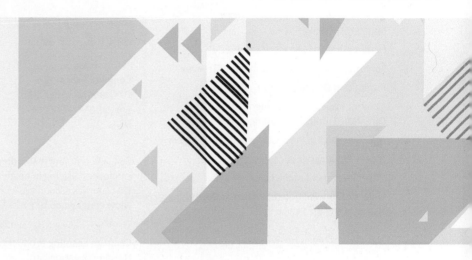

PAUL C. ERWIN, MD, DRPH

Professor and Head of the Department of
Public Health
University of Tennessee, Knoxville
Knoxville, TN

ROSS C. BROWNSON, PHD

Bernard Becker Professor of Public Health
The Brown School and Division of Public Health
Sciences, Alvin J Siteman Cancer Center,
Washington University School of Medicine
St. Louis, MO

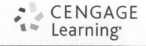

CENGAGE
Learning·

Australia • Brazil • Mexico • Singapore • United Kingdom • United States

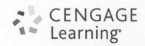

Scutchfield and Keck's Principles of Public Health Practice, Fourth Edition
Paul C. Erwin and Ross C. Brownson

SVP, GM Skills & Global Product Management: Dawn Gerrain

Product Director: Matthew Seeley

Product Manager: Jadin Kavanaugh

Senior Director, Development: Marah Bellegarde

Product Development Manager: Juliet Steiner

Senior Content Developer: Lauren Whalen

Product Assistant: Mark Turner

Vice President, Marketing Services: Jennifer Ann Baker

Marketing Manager: Jessica Cipperly

Senior Production Director: Wendy Troeger

Production Director: Andrew Crouth

Content Project Management and Art Direction: Lumina Datamatics, Inc.

Manager, Digital Production: Jamilynne Myers

Media Producer: Jessica Peragine

Cover image(s): Fotolia.com/Windyk

Unless otherwise noted, all items Copyright © 2017 Cengage Learning®.

Library of Congress Control Number: 2015949541

ISBN: 978-1-2851-8263-6

Cengage Learning
20 Channel Center Street
Boston, MA 02210
USA

Cengage Learning is a leading provider of customized learning solutions with employees residing in nearly 40 different countries and sales in more than 125 countries around the world. Find your local representative at: **www.cengage.com.**

Cengage Learning products are represented in Canada by Nelson Education, Ltd.

To learn more about Cengage Learning, visit **www.cengage.com.**

Purchase any of our products at your local college store or at our preferred online store **www.cengagebrain.com.**

Notice to the Reader

Publisher does not warrant or guarantee any of the products described herein or perform any independent analysis in connection with any of the product information contained herein. Publisher does not assume, and expressly disclaims, any obligation to obtain and include information other than that provided to it by the manufacturer. The reader is expressly warned to consider and adopt all safety precautions that might be indicated by the activities described herein and to avoid all potential hazards. By following the instructions contained herein, the reader willingly assumes all risks in connection with such instructions. The publisher makes no representations or warranties of any kind, including but not limited to, the warranties of fitness for particular purpose or merchantability, nor are any such representations implied with respect to the material set forth herein, and the publisher takes no responsibility with respect to such material. The publisher shall not be liable for any special, consequential, or exemplary damages resulting, in whole or part, from the readers' use of, or reliance upon, this material.

Printed in the United States of America
Print Number: 06   Print Year: 2022

DEDICATION

We dedicate this book to our wives, Renee' Hyatt and Carol Brownson, for their support, encouragement, and understanding while we were preparing this book. We know all too well that time given away can never be regained.

We also dedicate this book to our mentors—these individuals were outstanding teachers and public health practitioners with whom we have worked. They inspired us in many lasting ways. Paul is especially grateful to Dr. John H. Bryant and Ross to Drs. John Bagby and John Reif.

Finally, we dedicate this book to the hundreds of students who over the past few decades have energized us and will adeptly implement many of the concepts in this book.

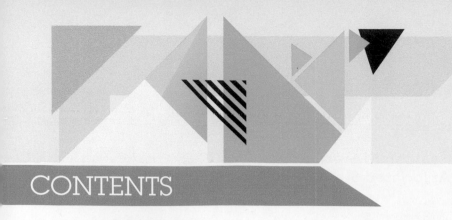

CONTENTS

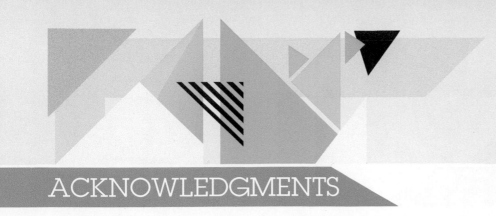

ACKNOWLEDGMENTS

First and foremost we wish to acknowledge our families, who are always the most directly impacted when work gets added to our plates. We are both blessed with families who are understanding and supportive, and from whom we have learned the meaning of the word forbearance. We were humbled by the invitation from Drs. Doug Scutchfield and Bill Keck to take on this fourth edition, and it is with both gratitude and respect that we requested their names as part of the title of the textbook—a public health legacy that must live on. We are deeply grateful to the many colleagues who gave of their time to actually write these chapters—if students will gain in knowledge what we have as we have edited this text, the book will be a success. We have benefited from the generous support of our academic leaders, Dean Bob Rider at the College of Education, Health, and Human Sciences at the University of Tennessee, and Dean Edward F. Lawlor at the Brown School, Washington University in St. Louis. To our academic colleagues and our students we are appreciative of what you have taught us, and to our partners in public health practice we are ever grateful for the opportunities you have provided us to learn, study, and help create the evidence-base for public health. Finally, we thank our editors at Cengage Learning, Lauren Whalen and Jadin Kavanaugh, who have provided significant support in the preparation of this textbook.

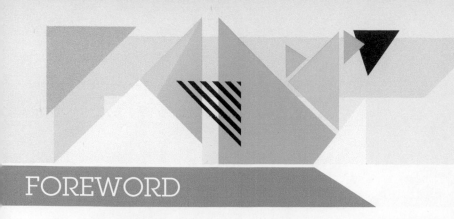

FOREWORD

When we began planning our first edition of the text you hold in your hands we were motivated by a number of events. The 1988 Institute of Medicine report on *The Future of Public Health* had been released and had created a stir in the public health community. We could see change occurring in response to that report in both the practice and teaching of public health. Efforts began to better connect public health practice to its academic bases. We witnessed the evolution of the core functions of public health into the 10 essential services and despaired as President Clinton's health care reform package, so full of positive proposals for public health practice, went down to defeat in Congress. The strengthening of existing national public health professional organizations and the development of new ones, however, gave us hope that the discipline might come to be better understood and supported in its efforts to improve the health of Americans.

We could not, at the time, find a good textbook that pulled together the knowledge required for students and practitioners to develop and improve skills required to function well in a rapidly evolving environment. We believed that, with the support of many of our expert colleagues across the country, we could use the editing perspective of both a public health academician and a practitioner to solicit and assemble a collection of chapters that would both document the public health philosophic renaissance under way and provide practical information of value to the practitioner facing a changing world.

The evolution of the discipline since that first edition appeared in 1997 has been substantial. Two subsequent editions of the text appearing in 2003 and 2009 contained our and our other contributors' attempts to chronicle the accelerating change that has become the new norm. The growing size of the book is an indication of how much new information was being generated and the need to place it in its appropriate context.

Schools and programs of public health have expanded dramatically; public health is now a career option discussed with students by high school counselors; funding for public health-related research has grown and helped to bring academicians and practitioners together forming academic health departments and practice-based research networks; competencies for public health practice underpin both training and work performance evaluation; there is now an accreditation process for state and local health departments and a certification process for public health workers; and a new era of national health reform offers exciting opportunities to better meld medicine and public health.

Some lessons remain unheeded, however. The economic recession that began in 2008 cut deeply into the resources available to public health practitioners. Dr. C. Everett Koop's reminders in his forewords to past editions hold true today: the work of public health goes unnoticed until a crisis occurs. The recent outbreak of ebola in Africa is a current indicator of the risks we assume when we allow public health systems to deteriorate.

Nevertheless, we believe the future of public health remains bright, although challenging. We have done our best to help our readers understand not only the current events of the discipline, but also to prepare for the opportunities likely to occur in the future. In that vein we have decided to plan for the future of this book by stepping aside. We are both at retirement age and less engaged in the daily give and take of practice and academia than we once were. Because we believe that engagement is critical for editing this text we would like to introduce you to your new editors, Paul C. Erwin and Ross Brownson. We are convinced they will provide the excellence required to make this text useful to you.

F. Douglas Scutchfield, MD and
C. William Keck, MD, MPH

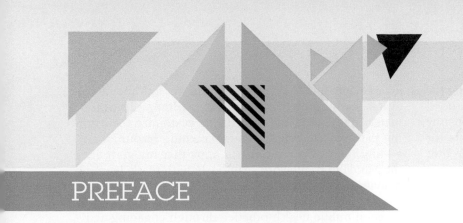

PREFACE

This fourth edition of *Scutchfield and Keck's Principles of Public Health Practice* is meant primarily, although by no means exclusively, for the graduate student in a public health academic program. Students and teachers in undergraduate public health programs may also find this textbook a valuable resource that bridges across the multiple disciplines within public health. Others who have used earlier editions include students in public policy, medicine, nursing, nutrition, and social work, and selected topics have been used by students in courses that range from environmental studies, to economics, to law and ethics. For those who recognize these disciplines as part and parcel of the social determinants of health, this should come as no surprise. With the recent movements to include "health in all policies," a comprehensive textbook on public health practice must, by its very nature, range across these various disciplines. This is also reflected in the growing number of dual degree programs that require both a broad and deep understanding of health as the product of multiple influences, e.g., the Master of Public Health (MPH) paired with degrees in social work, nutrition, business, law, and veterinary medicine.

It has been over seven years since the third edition of this textbook was published. In those intervening years there have been several major "forces of change" on the practice of public health, including: the Great Economic Recession of 2008 (with the loss of approximately 50,000 public health practice positions nationwide); the national voluntary public health accreditation program; the quickening pace of climate change; the exponential growth of public health informatics and reach of social media; and the 1,000-pound gorilla in the room, the Patient Protection and Affordable Care Act (ACA). Although the full impact of any of these recent forces has yet to be realized (as we describe more fully in the final chapter), it is critical for the public health student to understand how public health practice has been impacted, what it means for the nature of practice today, and where the path may be taking the public health practitioner of the future. This revision is meant to capture the dynamics of these forces as they impact what public health practice is all about, who the practitioner is, how the art and science of practice and

academe merge, and what the practitioner might anticipate in the coming years.

In our approach to bringing this fourth edition to life, we began with the framework that Doug Scutchfield and Bill Keck used so successfully in previous editions. We not only wanted to include most of those same basic elements, but we also sought to very purposively bring additional material to this revision that could reflect the growing collaborations between public health practice and academia. But the flavor and perspective is still largely from and for the practice of public health, primarily, but again, not exclusively, within the context of *governmental* public health. Both of us bring to this editorial task the perspectives of both the practitioner and the academician—the so-called pracademic—with both of us having worked in governmental public health and now in academic settings. It is a perspective, we hope, that understands the difference between statistical significance and public health importance. In that regard, we also bring to this revision our own current collaborative activities, with a strong practice-based research focus through evidence-based public health and the concept of the "Academic Health Department."

Organization of the Text

As we describe in Chapter 1, this textbook is organized by the *why, where, how, and what* of public health practice. Section 1—the *why*—includes chapters on the history of public health, the social determinants of health, public health law and ethics, and the policy basis of public health practice. Section 2—the *where*—describes the settings where public health practice takes place, including the federal, state, local, tribal, and territorial levels. Section 3—the *how*—includes chapters that focus on the skills, tools, and knowledge-base required for effective public health practice. Section 4—the *what*—covers the broad programmatic areas of public health practice, including *who* exactly is doing the work of public health practice. The final Section 5 considers the impact of the ACA on public health practice, a global health perspective, and a glimpse at what we believe are current forces of change shaping the future. At the end of each chapter, the chapter authors provide probing questions for students to consider, clearly indicating the specific topics of greatest importance from the authors' perspectives. These questions should stimulate healthy classroom discussion and can serve as the basis for additional exploration of topics covered in greater detail elsewhere.

New to this Edition

Users of previous editions will note several new chapters in this revision. It may simply reflect the nature and evolution of knowledge and learning, but the intent was to show the dynamism of the field and how public health practice moves with or is impacted by society at large. New to the fourth edition are chapters on tribal and territorial public health practice; evidence-based public health; evaluation; public health services and systems research; community development; and the ACA. Our appendices provide a listing of current major public health professional associations and an updated overview of public health practice competencies. In addition to these new chapters, there are new chapter authors—and thus new and revitalized content—on public health law, federal and state public health departments, the quantitative sciences (e.g., epidemiology and biostatistics), community health planning, performance management, workforce, leadership, infectious and communicable diseases, environmental health, primary care, oral health, public health laboratories, and global health. Thus, while the Scutchfield and Keck framework remains, there are only three chapters in the fourth edition that have the same exact authors and coauthors as in the third edition.

STUDENT ANCILLARY PACKAGE

The complete supplement package for *Scutchfield and Keck's Principles of Public Health Practice, Fourth Edition* was developed to achieve two goals:

1. To assist students in learning and applying the information presented in the text, and
2. To assist instructors in planning and implementing their courses in the most efficient manner and provide exceptional resources to enhance their students' experience.

MindTap to Accompany Scutchfield and Keck's Principles of Public Health Practice, Fourth Edition

MindTap is a fully online, interactive learning experience built upon authoritative Cengage Learning content. By combining readings, multimedia, activities, and assessments into a singular learning path, MindTap elevates learning by providing real-world application to better engage students. Instructors customize the learning path by selecting Cengage Learning resources and adding their own content via apps that integrate into the MindTap framework seamlessly with many learning management systems.

The guided learning path demonstrates the importance of public health practice through engaging activities and interactive exercises. These activities, such as case studies, quizzes, and research assignments, elevate the study of public health by challenging students to apply concepts to practice.

To learn more, visit www.cengage.com/mindtap

INSTRUCTOR ANCILLARY PACKAGE

Instructor Companion Website

ISBN 13: 978-1-285-18264-3

Spend less time planning and more time teaching with Cengage Learning's Instructor Resources to accompany *Scutchfield and Keck's Principles of Public Health Practice, Fourth Edition*. The Instructor Companion Website can be accessed by going to http://www.cengage.com/login to create a unique user log-in. The password-protected Instructor Resources include the following:

Instructor's Manual

An electronic Instructor's Manual provides instructors with invaluable tools for preparing class lectures and examinations. Following the text chapter-by-chapter, the Instructor's Manual reiterates objectives, provides a synthesized recap of each chapter's main points and goals, and houses the answers to each chapter's review questions.

Online Test Bank

An electronic test bank provides questions to generate quizzes. This test bank includes a rich bank of over 100 short answer and essay questions that test students on retention and application of what they have learned in the course. Answers are provided for all questions, so instructors can focus on teaching, not grading.

Instructor PowerPoint Slides

A comprehensive offering of more than 500 instructor support slides created in Microsoft® PowerPoint outlines concepts and objectives to assist instructors with lectures.

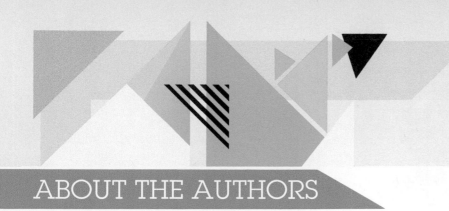

ABOUT THE AUTHORS

Paul C. Erwin, MD, DrPH, is currently Professor and Head of the Department of Public Health at the University of Tennessee, Knoxville. Prior to his academic appointment Dr. Erwin served with the Tennessee Department of Health for 16 years, with the last 12 as regional director for 15 county health departments, primarily in rural Appalachia. He is boarded in internal medicine as well as public health and preventive medicine. His research focus is in the larger arena of applied public health systems and services research, with a particular interest in the formal relationships between practice and academe known as Academic Health Departments.

Ross C. Brownson, PhD, is the Bernard Becker Professor of Public Health at the Brown School, the Division of Public Health Sciences within the Department of Surgery, and the Alvin J. Siteman Cancer Center, Washington University School of Medicine, Washington University in St. Louis. He is also the Co-Director of the Prevention Research Center in St. Louis. Prior to his academic career Dr. Brownson served with the Missouri Department of Health for eight years. He is the author or editor of several books, including *Chronic Disease Epidemiology and Control*, *Applied Epidemiology: Theory to Practice*, and *Evidence-Based Public Health*.

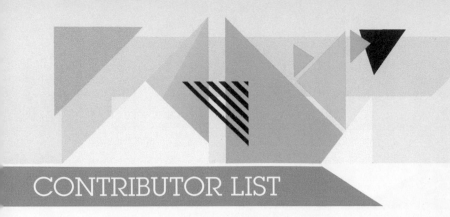

CONTRIBUTOR LIST

Susan M. Allan, MD, JD, MPH
Associate Professor, Department of Health Services
University of Washington
Seattle, WA

Edward L. Baker MD, MPH
Adjunct Professor
University of North Carolina at Chapel Hill
Chapel Hill, NC

Susan P. Baker, MPH, ScD (Hon)
Professor, Department of Health Policy and
    Management
Johns Hopkins University Bloomberg School of Public
    Health
Baltimore, MD

Angela J. Beck, PhD, MPH
Research Assistant Professor, Department of Health
    Management & Policy, School of Public Health
University of Michigan
Ann Arbor, MI

Scott J. Becker, MS
Executive Director
Association of Public Health Laboratories
Silver Spring, MD

Kyle T. Bernstein, PhD, ScM
Branch Chief, Epidemiology and Statistics Branch,
Division of STD Prevention
Centers for Disease Control and Prevention
Atlanta, GA

Eric C. Blank, DrPH
Senior Director, Public Health Systems
Association of Public Health Laboratories
Silver Spring, MD

Matthew L. Boulton, MD, MPH
Senior Associate Dean, Professor of
    Epidemiology & Preventive Medicine,
    Professor of Health Management & Policy,
    School of Public Health; and, Professor of

Internal Medicine, Infectious Disease
    Division, School of Medicine
University of Michigan
Ann Arbor, MI

Ross C. Brownson, PhD
Bernard Becker Professor of Public Health
Washington University in St. Louis
St. Louis, MO

Brian C. Castrucci, MA
Chief Program and Strategy Officer
de Beaumont Foundation
Bethesda, MD

Derek A. Chapman, PhD, MS
Associate Director for Research, Center on Society and
    Health
Virginia Commonwealth University
Richmond, VA

Emi Chutaro
Executive Director, Pacific Islands Health Officers
    Association
Honolulu, Hawaii

Vicki L. Collie-Akers, PhD, MPH
Associate Director, Work Group for Community
    Health and Development
University of Kansas
Lawrence, KS

Janet L. Collins, PhD
Director, Division of Nutrition, Physical Activity
    and Obesity
Centers for Disease Control and Prevention
Atlanta, GA

José F. Cordero, MD, MPH
Gordhan L. and Virginia B. "Jinx" Patel
Distinguished Professor in Public Health
University of Georgia College of Public Health
Athens, GA

Gregory Dever, MD
Regional Human Resources for Health Coordinator
Pacific Islands Health Officers Association
Honolulu, Hawaii

Cecile Dinh, MPH
Medical Student
Tulane University School of Medicine
New Orleans, LA

Maria C. Dolce, PhD
Associate Professor, School of Nursing
Northeastern University
Boston, MA

A. Mark Durand, MD, MPH
Performance & Health Information Systems
    Coordinator
Pacific Islands Health Officers Association
Honolulu, Hawaii

John P. Elder, PhD, MPH
Distinguished Professor of Public Health
San Diego State University
San Diego CA

Paul Campbell Erwin, MD, DrPH
Professor and Head, Department of Public Health
University of Tennessee
Knoxville, TN

Caswell A. Evans, DDS, MPH
Associate Dean, Division of Prevention and Public
    Health Sciences
University of Illinois at Chicago, College of Dentistry
Chicago, IL

Stephen B. Fawcett, PhD
Senior Advisor, Work Group for Community Health
    and Development
University of Kansas
Lawrence, KS

Elizabeth Fee, PhD
Chief Historian, National Library of Medicine
National Institutes of Health
Bethesda, MD

Joseph Seahquia Finkbonner, RPh, MHA
Executive Director
Northwest Portland Area Indian Health Board
Portland, OR

Antoine Flahault, MD, PhD
Professor Institute of Global Health/University of
    Geneva
Geneva, Switzerland

Douglas M. Frye, MD, MPH
Chief, Epidemiology Unit, Office of Health Assessment
    and Epidemiology
Los Angeles County Department of Public Health
Los Angeles, CA

Tracy Elizabeth Garland, BA, MUP
Founding Director
National Interprofessional Initiative on Oral Health
DentaQuest Foundation,
Boston, MA

Cassandra M. Gibbs Pickens, MPH
PhD Candidate, Department of Epidemiology
Emory University, Rollins School of Public Health
Atlanta, GA

Anita Duhl Glicken, MSW
Associate Dean and Professor Emerita, Department of
    Pediatrics
University of Colorado, School of Medicine
Denver, CO

Judith E. Haber, PhD, RN, FAAN
The Ursula Springer Leadership Professor in Nursing
New York University, College of Nursing
New York, NY

Amber Haley , MPH
Instructor, Division of Epidemiology, Department of
    Family Medicine and Population Health
Virginia Commonwealth University
Richmond, VA

Paul K. Halverson, DrPH
Dean, The Richard M. Fairbanks School of Public
    Health
The Indiana University
Indianapolis, IN

Michael T. Hatcher, DrPH
Chief, Environmental Medicine Branch*
Division of Toxicology and Human Health Sciences,
    Agency for Toxic Substances and Disease Registry
Atlanta, GA

Latoya T. Hill, MPH
Epidemiologist
Maryland Department of Mental Health and Hygiene
Baltimore, MD

Alan R. Hinman, MD, MPH
Director for Programs, Center for Vaccine Equity
Task Force for Global Health
Decatur, GA

Carol Jane Rowland Hogue, PhD, MPH
Terry Professor of Maternal and Child Health and
    Professor of Epidemiology
Emory University, Rollins School of Public Health
Atlanta, GA

Christina M. Holt, MA
Associate Director, Work Group for Community
    Health and Development
University of Kansas
Lawrence, KS

Susan Hyde, DDS, MPH, PhD
Associate Professor and Chair, Division of Oral
    Epidemiology and Dental Public Health
University of California, San Francisco
San Francisco, CA

Richard C. Ingram, DrPH
Assistant Professor
University of Kentucky
Lexington, KY

Paul E. Jarris, MD, MBA
Executive Director Association of State and Territorial
    Health Officials
Arlington, VA

C. William Keck, MD, MPH
Professor Emeritus, Department of Family and
    Community Medicine
Northeast Ohio Medical University
Rootstown, OH

Denise Koo, MD, MPH, CAPT, USPHS
Advisor to the Associate Director for Policy
Centers for Disease Control and Prevention
Atlanta, GA

Cynthia Lamberth, MPH, CPH
Co-director, Kentucky Population Health Institute
Frankfort, KY

Linda Young Landesman, DrPH, MSW
Visiting Lecturer
University of Massachusetts Amherst
Amherst, MA

Rice Leach, MD
Commissioner
Lexington-Fayette County Health Department
Lexington, KY

Carolyn J. Leep, MS, MPH
Senior Director, Research & Evaluation
National Association of County and City Health Officials
Washington, DC

Carl Leukefeld, DSW
Professor and Chair, Department of Behavioral Science
    and Center on Drug and Alcohol Research
University of Kentucky
Lexington, KY

Jeffrey Levi, PhD
Professor, Department of Health Policy and
    Management
Milken Institute School of Public Health, The George
    Washington University
Washington, DC

Laura C. Leviton, PhD
Special Adviser for Evaluation, Research, Evaluation
    and Learning
The Robert Wood Johnson Foundation
Princeton, NJ

Daniel F. López-Cevallos, PhD, MPH
Associate Director of Research, Center for Latino/a Studies
    and Engagement; Assistant Professor, Ethnic Studies
Oregon State University
Corvallis, OR

Mary-Beth Malcarney, JD, MPH
Assistant Research Professor, Department of Health
    Policy and Management
Milken Institute School of Public Health, The George
    Washington University
Washington, DC

Katherine R. Marks, PhD
Fellow, Department of Behavioral Science and Center
    on Drug and Alcohol Research
University of Kentucky
Lexington, KY

Samuel C. Matheny, MD, MPH
Professor of Family and Community Medicine
University of Kentucky
Lexington, KY

Leah Michele Maynard, PhD
Epidemiologist, Division of Nutrition, Physical Activity
    and Obesity
Centers for Disease Control and Prevention
Atlanta, GA

Kerry Anne McGeary, PhD
Senior Program Officer, Research, Evaluation and
Learning
The Robert Wood Johnson Foundation
Princeton, NJ

J. Lloyd Michener, MD
Professor & Chair, Department of Community &
Family Medicine
Duke University
Durham, NC

Christina A. Mikosz, MD, MPH
Acting Tuberculosis Controller and Medical Consultant
(TB/Acute Communicable Disease), Division of
Communicable Disease Control and Prevention
Alameda County Public Health Department
Oakland, CA

Judith A. Monroe, MD
Deputy Director, Centers for Disease Control and
Prevention, and Director, Office for State, Tribal,
Local and Territorial Support
Centers for Disease Control and Prevention
Atlanta, GA

Georgia A. Moore, MS
Associate Director for Policy, Office for State, Tribal,
Local and Territorial Support
Centers for Disease Control and Prevention
Atlanta, GA

Sarah Newman, MPH
Senior Research & Evaluation Specialist
National Association of County and City Health
Officials
Washington, DC

Kevin A. Pearce, MD, MPH
Chair of the Department of Family and Community
Medicine
University of Kentucky
Lexington, KY

Robert M. Pestronk, MPH
Trustee
Ruth Mott Foundation
Washington, DC

Robert L. Phillips, Jr., MD, MSPH
Vice President for Research and Policy
American Board of Family Medicine
Washington, DC

Keshia M. Pollack, PhD, MPH
Associate Professor, Department of Health Policy and
Management
Johns Hopkins University Bloomberg School of Public
Health
Baltimore, MD

Elizabeth R. Pulgarón, PhD
Assistant Professor, Division of Clinical Psychology
University of Miami
Miami, FL

Ana R. Quiñones, PhD, MS
Assistant Professor, School of Public Health
Oregon Health & Science University
Portland, OR

Thomas C. Ricketts, PhD, MPH
Professor Emeritus, Health Policy and Management
and Social Medicine
University of North Carolina at Chapel Hill
Chapel Hill, NC

William J. Riley, PhD
Professor, School for the Science of Health Care
Delivery
Arizona State University
Phoenix, AZ

Jerry A. Schultz, PhD
Co-Director, Work Group for Community Health and
Development
University of Kansas
Lawrence, KS

F. Douglas Scutchfield, MD
Bosomworth Professor of Health Services Research
and Policy
University of Kentucky
Lexington, KY

Maria Segui-Gomez, MD, ScD
Director General
Directorate General for Traffic, Spain
Madrid, Spain

Naomi K. Seiler, JD
Associate Research Professor, Department of Health
Policy and Management
Milken Institute School of Public Health, The George
Washington University
Washington, DC

Katie Sellers, DrPH, CPH
Chief Science and Strategy Officer
Association of State and Territorial Health Officials
Arlington, VA

Margaret Shih, MD, PhD
Medical Director
United Health Group
Minneapolis, MN

Mina Silberberg, PhD
Associate Professor, Vice-Chief for Research and
    Evaluation, Duke Division of Community Health
Duke University Medical Center
Durham, NC

Danelle Stevens-Watkins, PhD
Associate Professor, Department of Behavioral Science
    and Center on Drug and Alcohol Research
University of Kentucky
Lexington, KY

Siobhan L. Tarver, PhD
Physical Scientist, Office of Environmental Justice and
    Sustainability
U.S. Environmental Protection Agency
Atlanta, GA

George Wesley Taylor, DMD, DrPH
Professor, Department of Preventive and Restorative
    Dental Sciences and Associate Dean for Diversity
    and Inclusion
University of California San Francisco, School of
    Dentistry
San Francisco, CA

Steven M. Teutsch, MD, MPH
Leonard D. Schaeffer Center for Health Policy and
    Economics
University of Southern California
Los Angeles, CA

Craig W. Thomas, PhD
Director, Division of Public Health Performance
    Improvement, Office for State, Tribal, Local and
    Territorial Support
Centers for Disease Control and Prevention
Atlanta, GA

James Conley Thomas, MPH, PhD
Associate Professor of Epidemiology
University of North Carolina at Chapel Hill
Chapel Hill, NC

Ralph Timperi, MPH
Senior Advisor, Laboratory Practice and Management
Association of Public Health Laboratories
Silver Spring, MD

David Patrick Upjohn, MS
Quality Improvement Consulting Fellow
Mayo Clinic
Scottsdale, AZ

Jomella Watson-Thompson, PhD, MUP
Associate Director, Work Group for Community
    Health and Development
University of Kansas
Lawrence, KS

Darien J. Weatherspoon, DDS, MPH
Assistant Professor, Division of Prevention and Public
    Health Sciences
University of Illinois at Chicago, College of Dentistry
Chicago, IL

Isaac Weisfuse, MD, MPH
Associate Professor of Clinical Public Health
Mailman School of Public Health, Columbia University
New York, NY

Didier Wernli, MD, MA
Senior Research Associate, Deputy Director of the
    Master Programme in Global Health
Global Studies Institute, University of Geneva
Geneva, Switzerland

Ivey Wohlfeld, BA
Program Associate
Patient-Centered Outcomes Research Institute
Washington, DC

Steven H. Woolf, MD, MPH
Director, Center on Society and Health
Virginia Commonwealth University
Richmond, VA

April Young, PhD
Assistant Professor, Department of Behavioral Science
    and Center on Drug and Alcohol Research
University of Kentucky
Lexington, KY

Emily B. Zimmerman, PhD, MS
Associate Professor, Division of Epidemiology,
    Department of Family Medicine and Population
    Health
Virginia Commonwealth University
Richmond, VA

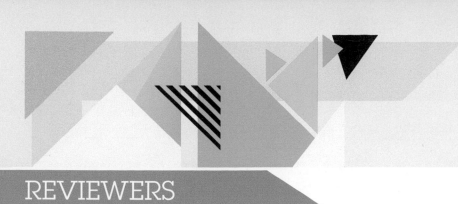

REVIEWERS

Edward Baker, MD, MPH
University of North Carolina at Chapel Hill
Chapel Hill, NC

Ken Johnson, PhD, FACHE
Weber State University
Ogden, UT

Ruth Metzger, BA, BSN, MBA
University of Southern Indiana
Evansville, IN

Miryam Pirnazar, MPH, CHES
Davenport University
Livonia, MI

Vicki Simpson, PhD, RN, CHES
Purdue University School of Nursing
West Lafayette, IN

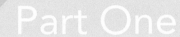

Part One

THE BASIS OF PUBLIC PUBLIC HEALTH

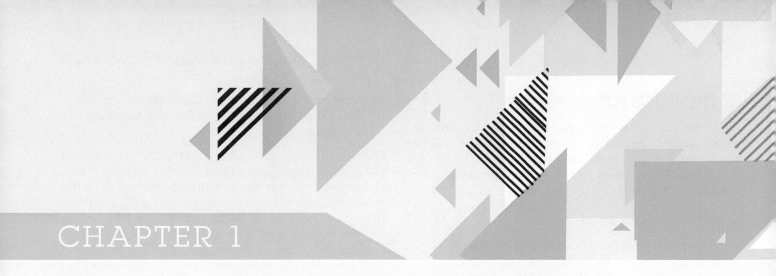

CHAPTER 1

The Why, Where, How, and What of Public Health Practice
An Introduction and Overview

Paul C. Erwin, MD, DrPH • Ross C. Brownson, PhD

LEARNING OBJECTIVES

Upon completion of this chapter, the reader will be able to:

1. Define public health and public health practice.

2. Recognize how the definitions of public health and public health practice provide a framework for this textbook.

3. Describe how this textbook is organized by the *why, where, how,* and *what* of public health practice.

KEY TERMS

evidence-based public health (EBPH)
public health
public health practice

INTRODUCTION

This book is about the practice of **public health**, which begs at least two questions: What is public health, and what do we mean by "practice"? In his *A Dictionary of Public Health*, John Last provides a definition of public health that is not only comprehensive, but one that can serve as a framework for this book. Public health is:

> An organized activity of society to promote, protect, improve, and, when necessary, restore the health of individuals, specified groups, or the entire population.[1]

As a *societal* activity that aims to prevent disease, public health has its own history, at times connected to and at times estranged from the history of medicine, but most often originating from a desire to prevent or control the spread of communicable diseases. But as the word implies, the health of populations is often determined by larger societal forces that go beyond the microbe or infectious agent. As an *organized* activity, public health is delivered through an array of governmental, nongovernmental, and private agencies, organizations, and institutions. While the primary focus of this book will be on governmental public health, we will examine public health practice writ large, building on the notion that public health is more than what governmental health departments do. Last continues:

> It is a combination of sciences, skills, and values that function through collective societal activities and involve programs, services, and institutions aimed at protecting and improving the health of all the people.

The ethics of public health are a reflection of the values we have as individuals and communities, and such values and ethics may become codified into law. The internal ethic of public health practice, ultimately, is a movement toward social justice. It is a movement that connects issues of fairness, inequities in the fundamental determinants of health, and community engagement in decision making. The public health skills disciplines of epidemiology and biostatistics are critical to understanding how disease and illness occur in populations, providing insights into how the public's health can be protected. The actual delivery of public health services through programs and institutions is a major focus of this book, but it is concerned with *all the people*, not just those who may avail themselves of such services and programs. And Last goes on to state:

> The term "public health" can describe a concept, a social institution, a set of scientific and professional disciplines and technologies, and a form of practice.... It is a way of thinking, a set of disciplines, an institution of society, and a manner of practice.

The *way of thinking* requires a population perspective where, for example, the public health physician places her stethoscope on the community rather than the individual. And to continue the analogy with medicine, just as we speak of the individual physician "practicing" medicine, the organized *activity* that takes place through *an institution of society* defines the practice of public health. The individual at work delivering public health services in this context is the *public health practitioner*.

CEA Winslow, a pioneer public health practitioner in the early twentieth century, included in his definition of public health the concepts of health as a human right: "[Public health is organized for] the development of the social machinery to insure everyone a standard of living adequate for the maintenance of health, so organizing these benefits as to enable every citizen to realize his/her birthright of health and longevity."[2] His definition presaged how the Institute of Medicine defined public health in its 1988 landmark report, *The Future of Public Health*: "Public Health is organized community efforts aimed at the prevention of disease and promotion of health. Its mission is the fulfilment of society's interest in assuring conditions in which people can be healthy."[3]

ACHIEVEMENTS OF PUBLIC HEALTH

The societal impact of public health initiatives is illustrated in the Centers for Disease Control and Prevention's (CDC's) "Ten Great Public Health Achievements of the 20th Century" (Table 1–1).[4] Many of the specific content areas are addressed in other chapters in this text. These public health approaches contributed in large part to the 30-year lengthening of the American life span from 1900–1999. It is also important to note that every one of these 10 achievements involved policy changes at national (workplace standards), state (laws requiring use of seatbelts), or local (ordinances requiring fluoridation of drinking water) levels.

Building on these definitions of public health, we ascribe to **public health practice** "The strategic, organized, and interdisciplinary application of knowledge, skills, and competencies necessary to perform essential public health services and other activities to improve the population's health."[5] Public health practice is about the art of *doing* public health, just as the practice of medicine is about the art of *doing* medicine.

TABLE 1–1   Ten Great Public Health Achievements—United States, 1900–1999

Achievement	Description
Vaccination	Programs of population-wide vaccinations resulted in the eradication of smallpox; elimination of polio in the Americas; and control of measles, rubella, tetanus, diphtheria, *Haemophilus influenzae* type b, and other infectious diseases in the United States and other parts of the world.
Motor-vehicle safety	Improvements in motor-vehicle safety have contributed to large reductions in motor-vehicle-related deaths. These improvements include engineering efforts to make both vehicles and highways safer and successful efforts to change personal behavior (e.g., increased use of safety belts, child safety seats).
Safer workplaces	Work-related health problems, such as coal workers' pneumoconiosis (black lung), and silicosis—common at the beginning of the century—have been significantly reduced. Severe injuries and deaths related to mining, manufacturing, construction, and transportation also have decreased.
Control of infectious diseases	Control of infectious diseases has resulted from clean water and better sanitation. Infections such as typhoid and cholera, major causes of illness and death early in the twentieth century, have been reduced dramatically by improved sanitation.
Decline in deaths from coronary heart disease and stroke	Decline in deaths from coronary heart disease and stroke have resulted from risk-factor modification, such as smoking cessation and blood pressure control coupled with improved access to early detection and better treatment.
Safer and healthier foods	Since 1900, safer and healthier foods have resulted from decreases in microbial contamination and increases in nutritional content. Identifying essential micronutrients and establishing food-fortification programs have almost eliminated major nutritional deficiency diseases such as rickets, goiter, and pellagra in the United States.
Healthier mothers and babies	Healthier mothers and babies are a result of better hygiene and nutrition, availability of antibiotics, greater access to health care, and technologic advances in maternal and neonatal medicine.
Family planning	Access to family planning and contraceptive services has altered social and economic roles of women. Family planning has provided health benefits such as smaller family size and longer interval between the birth of children; increased opportunities for preconceptional counseling and screening; fewer infant, child, and maternal deaths; and the use of barrier contraceptives to prevent pregnancy and transmission of human immunodeficiency virus and other STDs.
Fluoridation of drinking water	Fluoridation of drinking water began in 1945 and in 1999 reaches an estimated 144 million persons in the United States. Fluoridation safely and inexpensively benefits both children and adults by effectively preventing tooth decay, regardless of socioeconomic status or access to care.
Recognition of tobacco use as a health hazard	Recognition of tobacco use as a health hazard in 1964 has resulted in changes in the promotion of cessation of use, and reduction of exposure to environmental tobacco smoke. Since the initial Surgeon General's report on the health risks of smoking, the prevalence of smoking among adults has decreased, and millions of smoking-related deaths have been prevented.

SOURCE: Centers for Disease Control and Prevention. Ten great public health achievements—United States, 1900–1999. *MMWR. Morbidity and Mortality Weekly Report.* 1999;48(12):241.

THE TARGET AUDIENCE FOR THIS TEXTBOOK

This book is intended for students from a broad array of disciplines, but most especially for students in academic public health programs (i.e., students who have adequate time to cover the core disciplines of public health). The purpose of the book is to provide the student with a clear understanding of what is meant by *public health practice*, where practice takes place, the skills and tools used in practice, the activities by which practice is often defined in the public's eye, and how public health practice has developed and continues to evolve. This text is meant to show students how the core academic disciplines of public health—Biostatistics, Epidemiology, Environmental Health Science, Health Policy and Management, and Social and Behavioral Sciences—can be brought together when such disciplines are applied in the practice setting. The corollaries with clinical sciences, especially medicine and nursing, abound. The pathophysiology of, for example, diabetes, requires an understanding of the regulation of the Embden-Meyerhof pathway of glycolysis, learned by students in biochemistry and molecular biology. The application of that knowledge by the clinician, however, takes place at the bedside, where the student-clinician incorporates knowledge and skills from other disciplines, the values and beliefs of the patient, and the ethics of medical practice to treat disease, relieve suffering, and assure the best outcomes possible. So it is with public health practice, where the application of knowledge, skills, and competencies across multiple disciplines and in various settings is meant to promote and protect the public's health.

ORGANIZATION OF THIS TEXTBOOK

The textbook is organized through considerations of the *why, where, how,* and *what* of public health practice. In Part One (Chapters 1–6) we consider the *why* of public health practice by first describing the history of public health and the emergence of a new public health in the twenty-first century. An exploration of the social determinants of health provides the conceptual framework for public health practice and shows why issues of fairness, equity, and social justice are at the core of practice. The legal, ethical, and policy bases of public health practice provide the undergirding for not only why practice is necessary, but also why it must take place within codified value systems and structures.

In Part Two (Chapters 7–10) we provide an overview of the *where* of public health practice. In its most basic rendering, governmental public health practice most often takes place in local (county, city) health departments, in state-level health departments and related agencies, at the federal level through the (CDC) and other agencies within the U.S. Department of Health and Human Services, and through analogous structures and systems within Native American tribes and the U.S. Territories. While each setting has its unique attributes and concomitant responsibilities and purview, there is also overlap, intentional and unintentional redundancies, and even conflict and competition—particularly when it comes to addressing unmet needs with scarce resources. The practice of public health, more broadly speaking, takes place in many settings other than federal, state, and local

governmental public health agencies—such as schools (e.g., provision of healthy foods and policies on physical education), businesses (e.g., worksite wellness programs), nonprofit agencies (e.g., breast cancer education and screening through the Susan G. Komen Foundation), hospitals (e.g., community health assessments as a requirement of community benefit), and the faith community (e.g., influenza prevention information and vaccinations for minority populations). Attention to these nongovernmental settings of public health practice will be apparent throughout the textbook as they provide many of the critical threads that allow the whole tapestry of public health practice to be created.

In Part Three (Chapters 11–17) the focus shifts to the *how* of public health practice by considering the various tools and skill sets that are in use and needed for the effective delivery of the essential services of public health. The overarching framework for describing what goes in the public health practitioner's toolbox is **evidence-based public health (EBPH),** defined as the process of integrating science-based interventions with community preferences to improve population health.[6] Structured on a community and agency health planning cycle, EBPH requires certain data management and analytical skills in developing and identifying evidence; an understanding of methods of program development and prioritization; abilities to effectively translate and disseminate science and evidence on programs and policies; and the absolutely critical application of elements of evaluation—including economic evaluation—that allows the public health practitioner to determine the outcomes, impact, and effect of practice. These are the skill sets that often form the core of academic public health programs and are, unfortunately, most often the skill sets that practitioners themselves identify as most lacking in the practice setting.

Part Four (Chapters 18–29) of the textbook provides the *what* of public health practice by describing the major programs, services, and activities that are delivered or take place on a day-to-day basis in local, state, and federal public health practice settings. Describing the *what* of public health practice, however, cannot be effectively done without a full consideration of *who* is doing the practice—thus Part Four begins with an overview of the public health workforce. Some of the programs and activities described in the ensuing chapters have been a part of public health practice since the first organized efforts to establish federal, state, and local public health authority, e.g., control of communicable diseases and a focus on the well-being of infants, children, and mothers. The establishment and operation of other programs are more recent, at least within the public health practice settings, such as programs to address chronic diseases and emergency preparedness. Some of the programs directly correlate with one of the core academic public health disciplines (environmental health), while others cross disciplines with clinical nursing and medical care (primary care), and still others describe a unique niche of public health practice (public health labs).

Part Five (Chapters 30–32)—rounds out the textbook by first considering the known and potential impacts of health reform on public health practice, with a significant focus on the Patient Protection and Affordable Care Act (ACA). Given the partisan political efforts to oppose much or all of ACA, any textbook which attempts to define, delineate, and prognosticate about its impact runs a major risk of being out-of-date and off-the-mark by the time the student reads this chapter; yet no textbook on public health practice can safely ignore or leave out what is certainly one of the most important "forces of change" with which practitioners have had to grapple in over a decade. As a textbook focused on public health practice in the United States, we can only begin to scratch the surface in examining core public health functions around the world, but even such a basic rendering can be of value for the student or practitioner as international borders give way before the rapid transport of people, places, and ideas, and how we communicate through various electronic and wireless channels evolves faster than our public health systems can absorb. Finally we do our best as soothsayers by considering how public health practice might continue to evolve, given the paths it has already taken and current macrolevel forces (e.g., the Affordable Care Act, the explosion of information technologies).

SUMMARY

Public health is fulfilling society's interest in assuring conditions in which people can lead healthy lives. Public health practice is the application of knowledge, skills, and competencies necessary to perform essential public health services and other activities to improve the public's health. This fourth edition of Scutchfield and Keck's *Principles of Public Health Practice* is organized along the lines of the *why*, *where*, *how*, and *what* of public health practice.

REFERENCES

1. Last JM. *A Dictionary of Public Health.* Vol 13: Oxford University Press: Oxford/New York; 2007:306.

2. Winslow CEA. The Untilled Fields of Public Health. *Science.* 1920;51(1306):23–33.

3. Institute of Medicine. *The Future of Public Health.* Washington, DC: National Academy Press; 1988.

4. Centers for Disease Control and Prevention. Ten great public health achievements—United States, 1900–1999. *MMWR. Morbidity and Mortality Weekly Report.* 1999;48(12):241.

5. Association of Schools of Public Health: Demonstrating Excellence in Academic Public Health Practice. *Public Health Rep.* Sep 1999;114(5):480–483.

6. Kohatsu ND, Robinson JG, Torner JC. Evidence-based public health: an evolving concept. *Am J Prev Med.* Dec 2004;27(5):417–421.

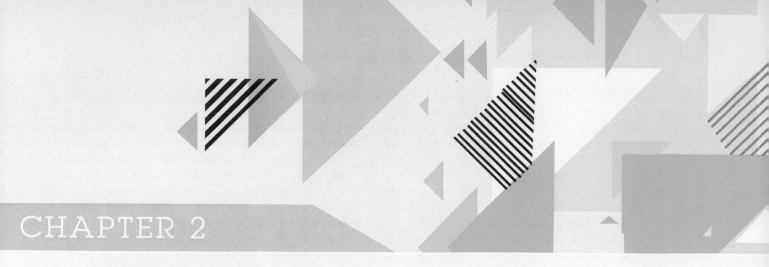

CHAPTER 2

The History and Emergence of a New Public Health

Elizabeth Fee, PhD • C. William Keck, MD, MPH

LEARNING OBJECTIVES

Upon completion of this chapter, the reader will be able to:

1. Outline the early development of public health institutions in the United States.

2. Discuss the contribution of social reformers, the U.S. Army, the Rockefeller philanthropies, and the U.S. Public Health Service.

3. Explain the problems, constraints, and accomplishments of public health practice.

4. Discuss the developments that have produced today's public health philosophic renaissance.

KEY TERMS

core functions
Local Public Health System (LPHS)
poverty
quarantine
social reform
10 Essential Services of Public Health
War on Poverty

INTRODUCTION

The history of public health in the United States coincides with the birth of the nation itself, with the first organized activities occurring in the late eighteenth century. In the roughly 200 years since, public health has evolved in both practice and as an academic discipline, through the bacteriological period, the sanitary period, the social reform movements, and through the Great Society era forward to the current landscape of health reform. This chapter on the history and development of public health in the United States is divided into two major sections: (1) public health in the eighteenth and nineteenth centuries and the professionalization of public health in the early-mid-twentieth century and (2) the emergence of a new public health, with the renaissance stimulated by a seminal report of the Institute of Medicine in 1988, *The Future of Public Health*. In many ways the second part of the chapter serves as an introduction for several chapters which follow.

PUBLIC HEALTH IN THE EIGHTEENTH AND NINETEENTH CENTURIES

Public health activities in the eighteenth and nineteenth centuries centered on large cities and their ports, because ships, their passengers, and crews could carry infectious diseases, of which the most feared were cholera and yellow fever. When careful inspection revealed illness in passengers or crew members, ships were placed in quarantine until all signs of disease had passed.

Large cities were also the focus of public health measures because they were increasingly crowded with immigrants and the poor who could only afford the dreadful housing conditions of the tenements. Cities also harbored the "nuisance trades"—the slaughterhouses, tanneries, skin dressers, glue boilers, and other trades that used animal parts and produced toxic wastes and noxious odors. The largest cities were the first to establish city health departments or boards of health (e.g., Baltimore in 1793, Boston in 1793, and New York in 1866). Public health officials did their best to guarantee the cleanliness of cities, water, food and milk supplies, farms, and factories, and to inspect the adequacy of housing and working conditions. They also hired men to clean the privies and to remove dead animals, horse manure, and decaying vegetable matter from the streets and public places.[1] Placards were fixed to the houses and tenements warning of any contagious disease within a family, and often indicating that houses were quarantined, residents were confined to houses, and no visitors were allowed. In some cases, sick family members were carried off and put into isolation hospitals.

Those taking responsibility for public health were generally the social elite who saw exerting control over disease as an imperative both for political reasons—to guard the social order—and also for humanitarian concerns. There were many theories of disease causation, including ignorance, filth, lack of godliness, and contagion which could be brought in from outside, typically by ships, and spread quickly through dense and impoverished areas.

In Great Britain, industrialization and its attendant social miseries had occurred earlier than in America and public health efforts were also organized somewhat earlier. Many of the most famous epidemiologists and statisticians of this period were English, for example, William Farr, John Snow, William Budd, and John Graunt. American public health officials could learn from their experiences and discoveries. France and Germany also experienced relatively early industrialization. In France, the most outstanding public health leader was Louis René Villermé, best known for his study of the health conditions of textile workers. Germany had a number of public health notables, of whom the best known is Rudolf Virchow, who argued that the central function of public health was to study the impact of social and economic conditions on health.

Early Public Health Programs, Activities, and Social Reformers

Serious endemic diseases of the time, including tuberculosis, smallpox, typhus, dysentery, diphtheria, typhoid fever, measles, influenza, malaria, and scarlet fever, were often met with an indifference born of familiarity and a sense of helplessness. Politicians tended to ignore the fate of the multitudes of the immigrant poor, unless compelled to action by the insistent demands of reform groups or the fear of popular unrest.[2,3] In some cities active and energetic reform groups helped to focus attention on the elimination of filthy and crowded conditions, but also expanded the conception of public health. The antislavery movement, the temperance movement, and the various organizations arrayed against child labor, agitated for a shorter working day and for better, safer working conditions that promoted a broadened public health agenda.[4,5]

In other parts of the country, a few farsighted men and women argued for the need to collect vital statistics, register births and deaths, and keep careful records on the health of the population. The most notable of these, Lemuel Shattuck, was largely responsible for implementing a system of vital statistics in Massachusetts. Shattuck's *Report of the Sanitary Commission of Massachusetts (1850)* advocated a decennial census and collection of data by age, sex, race, occupation, economic status, and locality. It also discussed the need for environmental sanitation, the regulation of food and drugs, and control of communicable disease. In addition, Shattuck recommended attention to well-child care, mental health, health education, smallpox vaccination, alcoholism, town planning, and the teaching of preventive medicine in medical schools.[2,6]

The Civil War helped enforce a national consciousness of epidemic disease. Appalling sanitary conditions on the battlefield as well as in prisoner of war camps resulted in two-thirds of the 360,000 Union soldier deaths caused by infectious diseases rather than by war wounds.[7,8] A voluntary organization, the U.S. Sanitary Commission, promoted sanitary measures and provided nursing care and supplies for the wounded.

Formation of the American Public Health Association

In 1872, 10 health reformers from various parts of the country met in New York City at the home of Stephen Smith and announced the creation of the American Public Health Association (APHA). Its purpose was to advance sanitary science and especially the "practical application of public hygiene."[9] Its members devoted themselves to the reform activities of citizens' sanitary associations and encouraged the formation and development of local and state health agencies. The APHA was notable in welcoming physicians, engineers, lawyers, municipal officials, and lay reformers to its membership, and in this respect, it helped shape the specific character of American public health practice as we know it today.[9]

The Marine Hospital Service

The origins of a federal organization of public health lie in the provision of medical and hospital care for merchant seamen and sailors. In 1798, Congress passed the Act for the Relief of Sick and Disabled Seamen to finance the construction and operation of public hospitals in port cities. In 1870, the Marine Hospital Service was reorganized as a national hospital system with centralized administration under a medical officer, the Supervising Surgeon, who was later given the title of Surgeon General. The first Supervising Physician, Dr. John Woodworth, was appointed in 1871; his title was subsequently changed to "Surgeon General of the Marine Hospital." In 1912, the Marine Hospital Service became the U.S. Public Health Service, which was specifically authorized to investigate the causes and spread of disease, provide health information to the public, examine the pollution and sanitation of navigable streams and lakes, inspect the health of immigrants arriving at Ellis Island, conduct field investigations of endemic rural diseases such as trachoma, and research diseases such as pellagra and Rocky Mountain spotted fever.[10]

National and International Health

Public health quickly grew to become a national and even international issue. Broadening control of trade routes, the building of the Panama Canal, and the establishment of strategic bases in the Caribbean and Western Pacific built up pressure for the United States to pay attention to public health abroad. In 1898, the United States entered the Spanish-American War and learned it could not afford military expansion overseas unless more attention was paid to sanitation and public health. When the U.S. Army in Cuba was threatened by yellow fever, an army commission under Walter Reed was sent to study the disease. The commission was able to confirm the hypothesis of Cuban physician Carlos Finlay that yellow fever was spread by mosquitoes. Surgeon Major William Gorgas was then able to eliminate yellow fever from Havana.[11]

In 1904 Gorgas campaigned against the malaria and yellow fever that had caused enormous mortality among workers attempting to dig the Panama Canal. In one of the great triumphs of practical public health, these diseases were brought under control, and the canal successfully completed in 1914.

U.S. industrialists brought some of the lessons of Cuba and the Panama Canal home to the southern United States. John D. Rockefeller had created the General Education Board to support "the general organization of rural communities for economic, social, and educational purposes."[12] Convinced that the real cause of misery and lack of productivity in the South was hookworm, the "germ of laziness," Rockefeller agreed to provide $1 million to create the Rockefeller Sanitary Commission for the Eradication of Hookworm Disease.[13] This was the first installment in Rockefeller's massive national and international investment in public health. Going beyond the task of attempting to control a single disease, the Rockefeller Sanitary Commission expanded the role of public health agencies in the Southern states; county appropriations for local public health work across the South increased from a total of $240 to $110,000 between 1910 and 1914.

By 1915, the Public Health Service, the U.S. Army, and the Rockefeller Foundation were the major agencies involved in public health activities, supplemented on a local level by a network of city and state health departments. In addition, it was during this same time that the first schools of public health were established – at Johns Hopkins University and Harvard University – both, also, with substantial support from the Rockefeller Foundation.

THE PROFESSIONALIZATION OF PUBLIC HEALTH

At the turn of the nineteenth century, existing health departments were often dominated by politics. Progressives wanted to insulate boards of health from local political control in order to make all forms of public administration more rational and efficient.[14] The goal was for well-trained professionals to conduct social reform along scientific lines. This led to a demand for people trained in public health to direct the new programs being created at the local, state, and national levels.

At the time, the main disciplines needed for public health training were defined as medical diagnosis, sanitary engineering, epidemiology, vital statistics, law, public health nursing, public health inspection and regulation, politics, sociology, economics, and, tying all these together, public health administration. However, in the period immediately following the brilliant experimental work of Louis Pasteur and Robert Koch, the bacteriological laboratory became the first and primary symbol of a new, scientific public health. The clarity and simplicity of bacteriological methods and discoveries gave them tremendous cultural importance: the agents of particular diseases had been made visible under the microscope.[15]

The powerful new methods of identifying diseases drew attention away from the larger and more diffuse problems of environmental hazards and the living conditions of the poor. The public health laboratory, by focusing on the diagnosis of infectious diseases, narrowed the distance between medicine and public health and brought public health into potential conflict with medical care practice. Physicians began to resent the public health officials' claim to diagnose, and often treat, infectious diseases.

Although the bacteriological view was dominant, there were competing models for public health research and practice. It is worth noting the broad and comprehensive definition of public health offered by Charles-Edward A. Winslow, professor of public health at Yale University, in 1920:

> Public health is the science and art of preventing disease, prolonging life, and promoting physical health and efficiency through organized community efforts for the sanitation of the environment, the control of community infections, the education of the individual in principles of personal hygiene, the organization of medical and nursing service for the early diagnosis and preventive treatment of disease, and the development of the social machinery which will ensure to every individual in the community a standard of living adequate for the maintenance of health.[16,17]

Public Health Organization and Practice

The practical importance of public health was well recognized by the early decades of the twentieth century. The incidence of tuberculosis, diphtheria, and other infectious diseases was falling dramatically, and many cities had established school health clinics and maternal and child health centers. The realization that a substantial proportion of the young men registered for the draft in World War I were either physically or mentally unfit for combat, along with the devastating 1916–1918 influenza epidemic, also led to increased support for public health activities.

In the 1920s, state and municipal health departments hired more public health personnel, especially public health nurses. Although bacteriological laboratories continued to be important, other health department divisions focused on maternal and child health, venereal diseases, public health administration, and, increasingly, health education.

At a national level, the medical profession had moved from a position of strong support for public health activities to a cautious and sometimes suspicious ambivalence.[18] For example, the Sheppard-Towner Maternity and Infancy Act of 1921, which provided grants to states to teach prenatal and infant care to mothers, was denounced by conservatives as socialistic, and by many physicians as interfering with the proper purview of medicine. This program was allowed to expire in 1929.

The most important federal organization in public health continued to be the U.S. Public Health Service, which aided the development of state health departments by giving grants-in-aid, loaning expert personnel, and providing advice and consultation on specific health problems.[19]

The Influence of the Great Depression

Sadly, most attention has been given to public health only in times of crisis. The depression demonstrated the hardships of vast numbers of people facing poverty, unemployment, sickness, and hunger. The Social Security Act of 1935 was America's first broad-based social welfare legislation, providing old-age benefits, unemployment insurance, and public health services.

From the public health point of view, the Social Security Act was a huge leap forward. Title V of the act established a program of grants to states for maternal and child health services, and Title VI of the act expanded financing of the Public Health Service and allotted federal grants to states to assist them in developing their public health services.

Public Health and World War II

Mobilization for World War II acted as a major force in the expansion and development of public health in the United States.[20] Previous experience had made it clear that public health was a national priority for the armed forces and for the civilian population engaged in military production. Selective Service examinations, however, found that 40 percent of the 16 million young men trying to register were physically or mentally unfit, with the leading causes of rejection being defective teeth, vision problems, orthopedic impairments (from polio, for example), diseases of the cardiovascular system, nervous and mental diseases, hernia, tuberculosis, and venereal diseases.[21,22]

With the war mobilization, hundreds of thousands of workers moved into defense industry areas, and the troops moved into army camps, some in malaria endemic areas.[23] In order to control malaria in the South, the Public Health Service established the Center for Controlling Malaria in the War Areas. After the war, this organization was gradually transformed into the Centers for Disease Control (CDC, now the Centers for Disease Control and Prevention).[24] Among its most important innovations was the Epidemic Intelligence Service created by Alexander Langmuir.

Postwar Reorganization

In the immediate postwar period, considerable optimism and energy were devoted to the possible reorganization of public health and medical care. Many discussions posited the potential unification of preventive and curative medicine. Some public health leaders advocated the direct administration of tax-supported medical care by health departments. Others opposed such a development, feeling that if public health and medical care administration were combined, preventive and educational efforts would be submerged by the demand for costly therapeutic services.[25]

In the postwar years, as a result of decades of improvements in sanitation, as well as the development of antibiotics and vaccines, it became clear that the major causes of death in the country had changed from infectious to chronic diseases, especially heart disease and cancer, as well as deaths from motor vehicle accidents. Health departments recognized that they must now deal with the problems and prevalence of chronic diseases as well as with issues such as mental illness, drug and cigarette addiction, environmental health, and occupational safety and health.

Postwar reconstruction, however, came to mean massive expenditures for biomedical research and hospital construction, the partial payment for medical care by expanding private insurance coverage, the relative neglect of public health services, and a refusal to pay attention to the social determinants of health and disease.

The New York Academy of Medicine's Committee on Medicine and the Changing Order recommended the extension of public health services in 1947, but argued that the quality of public health officers must be improved by better recruitment, training, assured tenure, and adequate salaries.[26] Some maintained that the problems of public health were largely political since state health officers were limited in their freedom to introduce new programs, too often accepted political constraints and bureaucratic barriers,[27] and too seldom were willing to risk their positions by appealing to a larger constituency.

The most significant accomplishment of the postwar years was the development of the polio vaccine and its implementation on a mass scale in the 1950s.[28-30] It was a huge popular success; however, despite the triumph over polio, the real expenditures of public health departments failed to keep pace with the increase in population.[31] Federal grants-in-aid to the states for public health programs steadily declined, falling from $45 million in 1950 to $33 million in 1959. At a time when public health officials were facing a whole series of new, poorly-understood health problems, they were also underbudgeted and understaffed.

The 1960s and the War on Poverty

The 1960s saw the growing power of the civil rights movement, riots in urban African-American ghettos, and federal support for the War on Poverty. The antipoverty effort and other Great Society programs soon became deeply involved with medical care.[32] Growing concern over access to medical care and hospitalization, especially for the elderly and poverty populations, culminated in Medicare and Medicaid legislation in 1965 to cover medical care costs for those on Social Security and for the poor. Other antipoverty programs, such as the neighborhood health centers, fared poorly because they were seen as competing with the interests of private (medical) care providers.[33]

Public Health in the 1970s and 1980s

In the 1970s, public health departments became providers of last resort for the poor and uninsured. By 1988, almost three-quarters of all state and local health department expenditures went for personal health services.[34] As Harry Mustard, then Commissioner of Health in New York City, had predicted some 40 years earlier, direct provision of medical care absorbed much of the limited resources—in personnel, money, energy, time, and attention—of public health departments, leading to a slow erosion of public health and preventive activities. The problem of caring for the uninsured and the indigent loomed so large that it eclipsed the need for a basic public health infrastructure in the minds of many legislators and the general public.

Battles raged over the Surgeon General's Report on Smoking and Health which had been released by Surgeon General Luther Terry in 1964 and was the first federal government report linking smoking to cancer and heart disease. The 1970s also brought increasing alarm over environmental pollution, perhaps best symbolized by the first Earth Day in 1970. These concerns led to the creation of the Environmental Protection Agency (EPA), also in 1970. Similarly, the Occupational Safety and Health Administration was established in 1971, as a result of horrific industrial and mining accidents.

In the Reagan revolution of the 1980s, federal funding for public health programs was decimated. Through the mechanism of the block grants, power was returned to state health agencies, but in the context of funding reductions this was the unpopular power to cut existing programs.[35] State health departments also had to deal with the problems of drug abuse, alcoholism, teenage pregnancy, family violence, and homelessness. Meanwhile, the AIDS epidemic and the resurgence of tuberculosis gave a new visibility and urgency to public health efforts.[36,37]

The most frequently cited genesis of what became a contemporary public health philosophic renaissance was the important work by the Institute of Medicine (IOM) in its study of the U.S. public health system described in *The Future of Public Health* (1988).[34] The report serves as a departure point for most, if not all, contemporary public health thinking. The institute's conclusion that public health in the United States is a system in disarray acted as a call to action for the public health profession, a call to which the public health community responded enthusiastically.

THE 1990S AND BEYOND: A PHILOSOPHIC RENAISSANCE

President Clinton promised comprehensive health care reform at the time of his election in 1992. The IOM description of a public health system in disarray and the president's health care reform initiative, coming relatively close together, acted as driving forces for the public health profession to better define its role and increase public understanding of its contributions to health. The resulting activities were far-ranging and productive. They were characterized by a renewed sense of

purpose, high productivity, and an unprecedented collaboration between agencies of the federal government, national public health organizations, academic institutions, local and state health departments, and many individuals.

Among the IOM's disturbing findings were the absence of a clear mission for public health, tension between professionals and politics, few strategies to demonstrate the worth of public health, an uneasy relationship with medicine, inadequate research resources, and a decoupling of public health practice from its academic base(s).[34] In the absence of an identifiable universal mission statement, the IOM suggested the following:

> "The mission of public health is to fulfil society's interest in assuring conditions in which people can be healthy."[34 (p7)]

Because the IOM was unable to identify universally accepted core functions for local health departments (LHDs), they proposed the following three core functions for every public health agency:[34 (pp7–8)]

Assessment: Regularly and systematically collect, assemble, analyze, and make available information on the health of the community.

Policy Development: Lead in the development of science-based public health policies.

Assurance: Encourage services necessary to achieve agreed-upon health goals by other entities (private or public sector), by requiring such action through regulation, or by providing services directly.

The 10 Essential Services

The CDC used the three core functions to develop an expanded list of 10 basic public health practices, i.e., if health departments were expected to operationalize these three core functions, these 10 practices (later, 10 essential services) would be a means for doing so.[38] A version of this list, termed the "Core Functions of Public Health," appeared in Title III of the Health Security Act forwarded by President Clinton to Congress in October 1993.[39] In 1994, shortly after this effort to reform health care was defeated, the CDC put together a working group to try to develop consensus on the "essential services of public health." The resulting statement provided a vision for public health in America: "Healthy People in Healthy Communities," and a nationally accepted list of the 10 Essential Services of Public Health:[40]

1. Monitor health status to identify community health problems.

2. Diagnose and investigate health problems and health hazards in the community.

3. Inform, educate, and empower people about health issues.

4. Mobilize community partnerships to identify and solve health problems.

5. Develop policies and plans that support individual and community health efforts.

6. Enforce laws and regulations that protect health and ensure safety.

7. Link people to needed personal health services and assure the provision of health care when otherwise unavailable.

8. Assure a competent public health and personal health care workforce.

9. Evaluate effectiveness, accessibility, and quality of personal and population-based health services.

10. Research for new insights and innovative solutions to health problems.

The Council on Linkages Between Academia and Public Health Practice

Funded by the Health Resources and Services Administration (HRSA) and CDC for two years, the Faculty/Agency Forum was established in 1988 to address the educational and academic dimensions of the findings of the IOM. The Forum's major accomplishment was the development and publication of the first compendium of competencies required for successful public health practice. Their report also proposed ways that public agencies and educational institutions could work together.[41]

The Council on Linkages (COL) was established in 1991 under a cooperative agreement between HRSA and the Association of Schools of Public Health (ASPH), as a sequel to the Faculty/Agency Forum. It brought representatives from national public health professional organizations and federal agencies together to "improve public health practice and education by refining and implementing recommendations of the Public Health Faculty/Agency Forum, establishing links between academia and the agencies of the public health community, and creating a process for continuing public health education throughout one's career."[42] The council's major contribution is its development of a modernized and regularly updated list of Core Competencies for Public Health Professionals (the latest in 2014, described further in Appendix B). This list represents over 25 years of work on this subject by the council and numerous other organizations and individuals in public health academia and practice settings. In addition, the COL began developing Community Public Health Practice Guidelines now carried out by the CDC, and a research agenda based on the 10 essential services, which became the

forerunner of public health systems research (see Chapter 17). The COL compiles and disseminates tools to foster academic/practice linkages, and promotes the development of academic health departments. Its newest program is the national Academic Health Department Learning Community begun in 2011.

Public Health Academic Programs

When the Council on Education for Public Health (CEPH) took over public health training program accreditation from the APHA in 1974, there were 18 accredited schools of public health, up from the original 10 accredited schools in 1946. That change has accelerated. The most notable difference in the public health professional preparation landscape now and 40 years ago is the sheer number of institutions of higher education offering graduate training in public health. As of 2014, CEPH accredits 52 schools and 108 programs, or 160 public health training sites in total.[43] This has been a remarkable period of growth that shows no sign of diminishing. Currently CEPH lists an additional 40 institutions that have taken the first steps toward accreditation (five are current accredited programs that are in the process of becoming full-fledged schools of public health).[44]

New Professional Associations

The capacity for local health departments to boost workforce competency, political sophistication, and public understanding was enhanced by two new professional associations, the National Association of Local Boards of Health (NALBOH) and the National Association of County and City Health Officials (NACCHO). The large majority of LHDs are governed by boards of health that serve as a link between local public health agencies and the communities they serve. Board members may be health professionals, but many have no training or experience in public health. Several states tried to fill this gap by forming statewide board of health associations in the 1980s. In November 1992, representatives of states and these kinds of organizations formed NALBOH to provide a national organization to help board of health members better understand their opportunities and responsibilities.

The combination in 1994 of the U.S. Conference of Local Health Officers and the National Association of County Health Officials into NACCHO, a single professional association representing directors of all LHDs, was a very significant occurrence. The organization has expanded beyond the traditional association roles of maintaining membership and facilitating communication and continuing education, to involvement in public policy, leadership training, defining and expanding the public health research agenda, and other activities. Staff and resources have grown dramatically and critical partnerships have been established with other professional organizations and federal agencies.

The CDC and Public Health Practice

The establishment of the Public Health Practice Program Office (PHPPO) at the CDC in 1988 meant, for the first time, there would be a locus in the CDC dedicated to strengthening the public health infrastructure in the United States. The involvement of the office was significant as it brought a strong federal presence to the evolution of the discipline during the 1990s and the early 2000s. Its efforts were focused on strengthening workforce competence (including leadership), developing public health information systems, building local health department organizational capacity, strengthening the science base for infrastructure development, and developing science-based public health performance standards. The latter led to a group of national performance standards based on the 10 essential services that communities could use to assess their capacity to deliver public health services effectively.[45] Separate standards for state and local systems were developed, and a continuum of performance levels was identified for each standard. In addition, PHPPO led the development of a Local Public Health Governance Assessment Instrument focusing on the governing body accountable for public health at the local level. These three standard measurement tools were then field tested and refined.[46] Many felt that the Local Public Health System (LPHS) performance standards would be a mechanism to measure LHD performance. They may indeed prove helpful in that regard, but it is clear that they really measure the capacity of a community, including all agencies, institutions, and individuals working in the area of health, to deliver those services. The standards will be useful in measuring the impact of the consortium of community services required, emphasizing the idea that partnerships remain key to the improvement of health status at the local level.

On April 21, 2005 the CDC underwent a major reorganization and PHPPO's functions were assigned to the Office of the Chief of Public Health Practice (OCPHP)[47] which served as the advocate, guardian, promoter, and conscience of public health practice throughout the CDC and in the larger public health community.[48] A second reorganization before the end of the decade saw the disappearance of the OCPHP and the transfer of its responsibilities to the newly formed Office for State, Tribal, Local and Territorial Support (OSTLTS), which was charged with improving health department capacity and performance, developing assessment and capacity-building tools, and engaging state, tribal, local and territorial health officials with CDC.[49]

Partnering Between Medicine and Public Health

The professions of medicine and public health have struggled over decades to find common ground in the work to improve the health of Americans. Hard-fought political campaigns about health care and growing awareness that the health status of Americans is less than it could be, have tended to highlight differences between the two groups and bolster the concept that partnering should be accelerated.

A joint effort of the American Medical Association (AMA) and the American Public Health Association (APHA), the Medicine/Public Health Initiative (MPHI) was established in 1994 as a formal attempt to develop stronger working relationships between these two disciplines. In 1997, the New York Academy of Medicine was asked to describe the current "state of the art" of collaboration between medicine and public health. The Academy's report, *Medicine and Public Health: The Power of Collaboration,* highlighted positive case studies from more than 400 collected.[50] In 1998, the Macy Foundation published proceedings from a meeting in Florida, "Education for More Synergistic Practice of Medicine and Public Health," which explored more effective ways to enhance the synergistic practice of medicine and public health through professional training.[51]

Another example of collaboration between medicine and public health was the cooperative agreement between the Association of American Medical Colleges and the CDC on the development of regional centers to introduce medical students to public health and population medicine. In order to obtain grant funding, medical schools had to partner with one or more public health agencies to enhance population health/public health education for all medical students. Seven schools were funded in 2003 and another 11 were added in 2006.[52]

The passage of the Patient Protection and Affordable Care Act in 2010 with its emphasis on prevention and improved outcomes for patients is a new opportunity to meld medicine and public health in meaningful ways (see below and Chapters 24 and 30).

Managed Care

The swing to managed care after the defeat of the Clinton health care proposal might have helped bring clinical care and public health together. The central theme of managed care was to approach clinical care from a population perspective and to emphasize those clinical preventive services likely to improve the length and quality of life for the enrolled population. Correctly done, this should meld with the broader health promotion and

In the intervening years, substantial attention was paid to the topic of preparedness in the form of legislation to help prevent, protect against, and respond to acts of terrorism, and to protect against natural disasters. State and local health departments, along with many other agencies and institutions, received significant funding and were included in regional planning and preparedness activities. This combination of resources and enhancement of working partnerships with other health and law enforcement organizations has improved surveillance and their response capabilities. (For a thorough discussion of these issues, see Chapter 26.) Unfortunately, at the same time that new federal funding for preparedness became available, federal support for many other areas of public health diminished. Concomitant revenue shortfalls in many states actually led to reductions in funding for population-based public health services across the country. Instead of building capacity overall, public health agencies had to fund their basic services and the new preparedness expectations with, in many cases, an overall reduction in funding.

The Affordable Care Act

The Patient Protection and Affordable Care Act (ACA) was signed into law by President Obama on March 23, 2010. The signing came only after bitter partisan debate in Congress, lobbying by special interests, and significant political compromises. As described by Benjamin, et al.:

> The Patient Protection and Affordable Care Act of March 2010 was the clearly recognizable product of the political process that created it. The long and very complicated legislation lacks a simple coherence and is, instead, a multi-layered composite of regulations, public insurance expansions, mandates, subsidies to help purchase private insurance, and incentives for system improvement that affect different groups of people at different times.[68]

Despite its complexity, the ACA has brought access to health care to millions of Americans and has begun to shift the culture of medical care in the United States to a stronger focus on health promotion, disease prevention, and positive outcomes of treatment. It has also provided opportunities for the public health community to enter into new partnerships with medical care providers focused on improving the health of whole communities. For further discussion of these issues, see Chapter 30.

Certification of Public Health Workers

Many health professionals working in public health are certified in their primary disciplines of medicine, nursing, health education, environmental health, and so on. Until recently, however, there was no process to certify that health professionals were well qualified to practice their particular discipline in public health settings. In 1999 APHA and the Association of Schools of Public Health (ASPH) began working together to develop a certificate process for public health workers. In September 2005 the National Board of Public Health Examiners was incorporated, and in 2008 the inaugural Certified in Public Health examination was offered. Those eligible to take the exam include public health professionals who have taken core courses in public health at CEPH-accredited institutions and also have five years' work experience or a relevant graduate degree.[69]

Health Department Accreditation

A long-held concern that public health facilities remained the only major providers of health services that did not have an accreditation process was addressed in earnest in 2004 and 2005 when the Robert Wood Johnson Foundation and the CDC supported the involvement of the major national public health professional organizations (APHA, ASTHO, NACCHO, and NALBOH) with others to explore the potential for accreditation of local, state, and tribal health departments. The group's conclusions and recommendations to develop a voluntary national accreditation effort were published in winter 2006–2007.[70]

Action soon followed with the incorporation of the Public Health Accreditation Board (PHAB) in May 2007. In February 2009 PHAB released a description of its initial accreditation process and a set of draft standards. A beta test utilizing 30 local, state, and tribal health departments followed during 2009–2010, and on September 14, 2011 a voluntary national public health department accreditation process was launched.[71] As of September 2015, a total of 80 health departments (local and state) had achieved accreditation through PHAB.

SUMMARY

Since the early 1990s, the country has been embroiled in debates over health care reform, illicit drugs, violence, environmental health, and women's reproductive health. These are all public health issues, yet public health as such is rarely mentioned. This is in part a failure of communications. Public health professionals need to be more effective in presenting their views and accomplishments to the media, the politicians, and the public.

The growth in the technical knowledge of public health in the past 100 years has been extraordinary—and insufficiently addressed in this brief account—but our ability to implement this knowledge in health and social reform has advanced little. The issues of public health today include and intersect with the great social issues of modern America: health care reform and the coverage of the uninsured; environmental health and safety; immigration; gun control; women's health, abortion, and fertility control; family violence and child abuse; AIDS, tuberculosis, and emerging epidemics; the continuing problems of chronic disease; and the need for home health services and long-term care for an aging population.

Public health is a vitally important field for the future well-being of America, its citizens, and its communities. Public health professionals must learn to communicate better the vital importance of their activities, mobilize public support, build a more effective public health infrastructure, and demonstrate clearly the benefits of prevention to the public at large by finding innovative ways of responding to endemic social problems and new crises.

REVIEW QUESTIONS

1. Before the germ theory, what were believed to be the causes of epidemic diseases?
2. How did social reformers begin to tackle the tasks of public health?
3. What disciplines contributed to public health work?
4. What are some of the lessons to be learned from the history of public health?
5. What was the major criticism of public health practice in the United States described in the 1988 Institute of Medicine report on *The Future of Public Health*?
6. List at least five key developments that have contributed to the "philosophic renaissance" of public health during the past 25 years.

REFERENCES

1. Baltimore City Ordinance 11, approved April 7, 1797. In: Howard WT. *Public Health Administration and the Natural History of Disease in Baltimore, Maryland, 1797–1920*. Washington, DC: Carnegie Institution; 1924.
2. Rosen G. *A History of Public Health*. Expanded ed. Baltimore, MD: Johns Hopkins University Press; 1993.
3. Duffy J. The *Sanitarians: A History of American Public Health*. Urbana: University of Illinois Press; 1990.
4. Rosner D, ed. *Epidemic! Public Health Crises in New York*. New Brunswick, NJ: Rutgers University Press; 1994.
5. Citizens' Association of New York. Report of the Council of Hygiene and Public Health of the Citizens' Association of New York upon the Sanitary Condition of the City. New York: Arno Press; 1970: xxi–xxxv.
6. Shattuck L. Report of a General Plan for the Promotion of Public and Personal Health, Devised, Prepared, and Recommended by the Commissioners Appointed under a Resolve of the Legislature of the State. Cambridge, MA: Harvard University Press; 1948.
7. Adams GW. *Doctors in Blue*. New York: Henry Schuman; 1952.
8. Woodward JJ. *Chief Camp Diseases of the United States Armies*. Philadelphia, PA: JB Lippencott; 1863.
9. Cavins HM. The national quarantine and sanitary conventions of 1857–1858 and the beginnings of the American Public Health Association. *Bull Hist Med*. 1943; 13: 419–425.
10. Williams RC. *The United States Public Health Service, 1798–1950*. Washington, DC: US Government Printing Office; 1951.
11. Kelley HA. *Walter Reed and Yellow Fever*. Baltimore, MD: Medical Standard Book Co; 1906.
12. Fosdick RB. *Adventure in Giving: The Story of the General Education Board*. New York: Harper & Row; 1962:57–58.
13. Ettling J. *The Germ of Laziness: Rockefeller Philanthropy and Public Health in the New South*. Cambridge, MA: Harvard University Press; 1981.
14. Schiesl MJ. *The Politics of Efficiency: Municipal Administration and Reform in America, 1880–1920*. Berkeley: University of California Press; 1980.
15. Jordan EO, Whipple GC, Winslow CEA. *A Pioneer of Public Health: William Thompson Sedgewick*. New Haven, CT: Yale University Press; 1924.
16. Winslow CEA. The untilled fields of public health. *Science*. 1920;51:23.
17. Winslow CEA. *The Evolution and Significance of the Modern Public Health Campaign*. New Haven, CT: Yale University Press; 1923.
18. Duffy J. The American medical profession and public health: from support to ambivalence. *Bull Hist Med*. 1979;53:1–22.

19. Mullan F. *Plagues and Politics: The Story of the United States Public Health Service*. New York: Basic Books; 1989.

20. Mustard HS, ed. Yesterday's school children are examined for the army. *Am J Public Health*. 1941; 31:1207.

21. Perrott G. StJ. Findings of selective service examinations. *Milbank Q*. 1944;22:358–366.

22. Perrott G. StJ. Selective service rejection statistics and some of their implications. *Am J Public Health*. 1946;36:336–342.

23. Maxcy KF. Epidemiologic implications of wartime population shifts. *Am J Public Health*. 1942;32:1089–1096.

24. Etheridge EW. *Sentinel for Health: A History of the Centers for Disease Control*. Berkeley: University of California Press; 1992.

25. Stern BJ. *Medical Services by Government: Local, State, and Federal*. New York: The Commonwealth Fund; 1946:31–32.

26. New York Academy of Medicine, Committee on Medicine in the Changing Order. *Medicine in the Changing Order*. New York: The Commonwealth Fund; 1947:109.

27. Mustard HS. *Government in Public Health*. New York: The Commonwealth Fund; 1945:112.

28. Benison S. *Tom Rivers: Reflections on a Life in Medicine and Science*. Cambridge, MA: MIT Press; 1967.

29. Klein AE. *Trial by Fury: The Polio Vaccine Controversy*. New York: Scribner's; 1972.

30. Paul JR. *A History of Poliomyelitis*. New Haven, CT: Yale University Press; 1971.

31. Sanders BS. Local health departments: Growth or illusion. *Public Health Rep*. 1959;74:13–20.

32. Davis K, Schoen C. *Health and the War on Poverty*. Washington, DC: Brookings Institution; 1978.

33. Sardell A. *The U.S. Experiment in Social Medicine: The Community Health Center Program, 1965–1986*. Pittsburgh, PA; University of Pittsburgh Press; 1988.

34. Institute of Medicine, Committee for the Study of the Future of Public Health. *The Future of Public Health*. Washington, DC: National Academy Press; 1988.

35. Omenn GS. What's behind those block grants in health? *New Eng J Med*. 1982;306:1057–1060.

36. Fee E, Fox DM, eds. *AIDS: The Making of a Chronic Disease*. Berkeley: University of California Press; 1992.

37. Krieger N, Margo G, eds. *AIDS: The Politics of Survival*. New York: Baywood; 1994.

38. Roper WL, Baker EL, Dial WW, Nicola RM. Strengthening the public health system. *Public Health Rep*. 1993;107(6):609–615.

39. *Health Security Act, Title III-Public Health Initiatives, HR3600*. Washington, DC: 103d Congress; 1993.

40. Public Health in America. Available at: http://www.health.gov/phfunctions/public.htm.

41. Sorensen AA, Bialek RG. *The Public Health Faculty Agency Forum: Linking Graduate Education and Practice, Final Report*. Gainesville: University Press of Florida; 1993.

42. Council on Linkages between Academia and Public Health Practice. Available at: http://www.phf.org/link/index.htm.

43. Council on Education for Public Health. Accredited Schools and Programs. Available at: http://ceph.org/accredited/

44. Council on Education for Public Health. Applicants. Available at: http://ceph.org/accredited/applicants/

45. Public Health Practice Program Office. Available at: http://www.answers.com/topic/public-health-practice-program-office.

46. National Public Health Performance Standards Program Local Public Health System Performance Assessment Instrument. Available at: http://www.cdc.gov/od/ocphp/nphpsp/TheInstruments.htm.

47. Notice to Readers: CDC Announces Landmark Reorganization. *MMWR*. 2005;54(15):387.

48. Centers for Disease Control and Prevention. *Office of Chief of Public Health Practice*. Atlanta, GA; 2005. Available at: http://www.cdc.gov/maso/pdf/OCPHPfs.pdf.

49. Centers for Disease Control and Prevention. *Office for State, Tribal, Local and Territorial Support*. Atlanta, GA; 2014. Available at: http://www.cdc.gov/stltpublichealth/docs/OSTLTS-Factsheet.pdf.

50. Lasker RD. *Medicine and Public Health: The Power of Collaboration*. New York: The New York Academy of Medicine; 1997.

51. Hager M. *Education for More Synergistic Practice of Medicine and Public Health*. New York: The Josiah Macy Jr. Foundation; 1999.

52. Association of American Medical Colleges. Development of regional centers to improve medical students' exposure to public health and population medicine. Washington, DC; 2007. Available at: http://www.aamc.org/members/cdc/aamcbased/regionalcenters.htm.

53. Robinson JC. The end of managed care. *JAMA*. 2001;285(20):2622–2628.

54. Scutchfield DS, Harris JR, Koplan JP, *et al.* Managed care and public health. *J Public Health Manage Pract.* 1998;4(1):1–11.

55. Holahan J, Ghosh A. Understanding the recent growth in Medicaid spending, 2000–2003. *Health Affairs.* 2005:25(1):52–62.

56. Turning Point. Collaborating for a New Century in Public Health. Available at: http://www.turning-pointprogram.org.

57. Lavizzo-Mourey R. Public Health Is for the Public Good. Gene Matthews Public Health Law Lecture. Atlanta, GA: CDC 4th Annual Partnership Conference; 2005.

58. Lloyd P, Bialek R, *et al. Practice Guidelines for Public Health: Assessment of Scientific Evidence, Feasibility and Benefits.* Washington, DC: Council on Linkages between Academia and Public Health; 1995.

59. McGinnis MJ, Foege W. Guide to community preventive services: Harnessing the science. *Am J Prev Med.* 2000;18(1S):1–2.

60. Zaza S, Briss PA, Harris KW. *The Guide to Community Preventive Services.* New York: Oxford University Press; 2005.

61. Council on Linkages Public Health Research Project. Available at: http://www.phf.org/link/ phsr/April99Concept.pdf.

62. Council on Linkages. Public Health Systems Research. Available at: http://www.phf.org.

63. Public Health Services and Systems Research. Practice-based Research Networks. Available at: http://www.publichealthsystems.org/

64. Green LW, Fielding J. The U.S. Healthy People Initiative: Its Genesis and its Sustainability. *Annual Rev Public Health.* 2011;(32):451-70.

65. *Healthy People 2020.* Washington, DC: US Depart of Health and Human Services; 2010. See: http://www.healthypeople.gov/2020/default.aspx.

66. American Public Health Association. *Code of Ethics. 2001.* Available at: http://www.apha.org/NR/rdonlyres/1CED3CEA-287E-4185-9CBD-BD405FC60856/0/ethicsbrochure.pdf.

67. *Chemical and Biological Terrorism: Research and Development to Improve Civilian Medical Response.* Institute of Medicine, National Research Council. Washington, DC: National Academy Press; 1999.

68. Benjamin GC, Brown TM, Ladwig S, Berkman E. *The Quest for Health Reform: A Cynical History.* Washington, DC: American Public Health Association; 2013.

69. National Board of Public Health Examiners. *History.* 2014. Available at: http://www.nbphe.org/history.cfm.

70. Public Health Accreditation Board. *Exploring Accreditation: Final Recommendations for a Voluntary National Accreditation Program for State and Local Health Departments.* Winter 2006–2007. Available at: http://www.phaboard.org/wp-content/uploads/ExploringAccreditation-FullReport1.pdf.

71. Public Health Accreditation Board. *Public Health Department Accreditation Background.* 2014. Available at: http://www.phaboard.org/about-phab/public-health-accreditation-background/

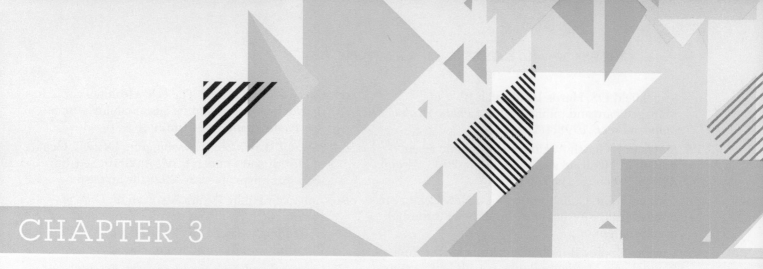

Social Determinants of Health: Their Influence on Personal Choice, Environmental Exposures, and Health Care

Derek A. Chapman, PhD • Latoya Hill, MPH • Emily B. Zimmerman, PhD • Amber Haley, MPH • Robert L. Phillips, MD, MSPH • Steven H. Woolf, MD, MPH

LEARNING OBJECTIVES

Upon completion of this chapter, the reader will be able to:

1. Describe the complexities of the relationship between social conditions and individual, environmental, and clinical determinants of health status.

2. Describe how social determinants affect personal health-related choices (e.g., health habits, seeking clinical attention, self-care of diseases), environmental exposures, and access to quality health care.

3. Describe the social conditions of the U.S. population with respect to education, income, race, ethnicity, homelessness, food insecurity, and access to health care.

4. Compare the relative importance of social conditions and advances in medical care in their relative influence on the health status of the population.

5. Describe the contextual policy circumstances and public attitudes that impede or facilitate progress in ameliorating adverse social conditions.

KEY TERMS

health disparities
health inequities
inequality
modifiable
nonmodifiable
social class
social determinants

> "...when it comes to health in this country your longevity and health are more determined by your ZIP code than they are by your genetic code."[1]
>
> --Thomas Frieden, MD MPH, Director Centers for Disease Control and Prevention

INTRODUCTION

The health of individuals and of populations is a product of multiple influences. Health status is affected by *individual* characteristics, which include both nonmodifiable host factors (e.g., age, race, genotype) and modifiable behaviors. Modifiable behaviors include choices about using health care services and lifestyle habits that affect health, such as diet, physical activity, smoking, substance abuse, sexual behavior, and injury-reducing practices. The influence of host factors is strong—age being the most powerful determinant of health and disease—but personal choices also play a major role. Smoking is responsible for an estimated 467,000 deaths per year in the United States, accounting for about one in five deaths, and overweight/obesity (216,000 deaths) and physical inactivity (191,000 deaths) also contribute substantially to chronic disease-related mortality.[2]

As noted, personal choices unrelated to lifestyle also influence health status, such as those made in relation to accessing health care. People choose whether and how promptly to obtain screening tests while healthy and how quickly to seek clinical attention when symptoms of illness emerge. Delays in diagnosis and treatment can affect health outcomes, as do patients' choices in how carefully to adhere to treatment and follow-up recommendations.

Health is also affected by *environmental* characteristics that exist apart from individual host factors and personal choices. An individual's health is affected by toxic pollutants in the air, water, and food supply. Such effects arise from exposure to environmental tobacco smoke produced by cigarette smokers, to infectious agents transmitted by humans or animals, to asbestos and lead released by old housing, to intentional injuries inflicted by others, and to workplace hazards. Exposure to stress—at home or work—affects both mental and physical health.[3] Children exposed to family and parental dysfunction are also more prone to health and developmental disorders.[4,5]

Finally, health is influenced by *health care*, which includes personal medical care and preventive services (e.g., immunizations). The degree to which health care improves health status is a function of the efficacy and effectiveness of interventions—e.g., screening, diagnosis, treatment—but these effects are dampened when individuals encounter barriers and delays in accessing care and when the care to which they have access is deficient in quality. The outcomes of health care are therefore mediated by both access and quality. Together, health care interacts with individual and environmental characteristics to influence health status. Health care has traditionally dealt better with the former than the latter, but there is increasing focus on population

health capacity to deal better with both. For example, Accountable Care Organizations in the United States,[6] Community Care Organizations in Oregon,[7] and Primary Health Networks in Australia[8] all seek to identify patterns of poor health and cost outcomes, including associated environmental clustering and characteristics. All three have increased focus on managing individual characteristics predictive of poor outcomes, but they are more strategic about population health, social determinants, and strategic placement of services. Social determinants of health are factors outside of health care and health behaviors that influence health outcomes. There is also an increasing effort to better integrate primary care and public health with the explicit goal of collaboration to reduce the impact of social determinants on health.[9]

THE MAGNITUDE OF THE PROBLEM

The notion that social conditions can affect health is easily understood, but it is equally easy to dismiss its relative impact on health—in comparison to medical care or biological and genetic determinants—as marginal. It is mistakenly assumed that ameliorating adverse social conditions would improve health on the margins but that more substantial health gains can be anticipated from biomedical research and technological advances in health care.

This assumption is problematic on two grounds. First, the magnitude (effect size) with which social conditions influence health is substantial—in some cases doubling or tripling the risk of death—whereas few biomedical advances affect health outcomes to this degree (see the following section). Second, the prevalence of adverse social conditions is high. Were either untrue—if adverse social conditions were uncommon or if they had minor impacts on health—it would be appropriate to make them less of a priority, but unfortunately the prevalence of societal distress in the United States is quite high despite the nation's overall affluence (Table 3–1).

The substantial prevalence of adverse social conditions, combined with their profound influence on health outcomes, creates the opportunity for social change to influence disease rates on a scale that rivals biomedical advances. As shown in Figure 3–1, age-adjusted mortality rates over the past century have declined at a mean rate of 1 percent per year.[21] Except for the influenza pandemic in 1918, neither the public health advances in the early century nor the technological advances in later decades did much to alter the pace of this decline. All the while, however, black mortality rates remained higher than those of whites.[22] The mortality rate for blacks was still 19 percent higher than that for whites in 2011.[23]

TABLE 3–1   Prevalence of Societal Influences on Health in the United States

Education

- As of 2009, 15 percent of U.S. adults age 25 and older had not graduated from high school, and only 28 percent had graduated from college.[10]
- Compared with other developed countries, American 15-year-old students score below average for proficiency in mathematics (32nd), science (27th), reading (23rd) and problem solving (20th).[11,12]
- Approximately 90 million adults in the United States have reading skills that test below high school level. Experts estimate that a similar number lack needed health literacy skills to effectively use the U.S. health system.[13]

Income

- As of 2012, 15 percent of the U.S. population (22 percent of children) lived in poverty (i.e., have incomes below the poverty threshold).[14]
- Income inequality has widened steadily in the United States. The Gini index,[15] a key measure of inequality, increased by 5.3 percent from its most recent low of 0.454 in 1993 to 0.477 in 2012.
- U.S. household income, adjusted for inflation, declined by 8.3 percent between 2007 and 2012, from a median of $55,627 to $51,017.

Race and Ethnicity

- Minorities, the subgroup at elevated risk for adverse health outcomes, represent a growing proportion of the U.S. population.
- Between 2012 and 2060, the proportion of the U.S. population represented by non-Hispanic whites is expected to decrease from 63 percent to 43 percent, whereas the Hispanic population is expected to grow from 17 percent to 31 percent.[16]
- Growth is also expected among blacks (from 13 percent to 15 percent), Asians (from 5 percent to 8 percent), and other races (from 4 percent to 8 percent), which include American Indian and Alaskan natives, native Hawaiians, other Pacific Islanders, and those of two or more races. By one estimate, Hispanics and people of color will constitute 57 percent of the U.S. population by 2060.

Homelessness

- On any given night in 2013 approximately 610,042 Americans (138,149 children) were in homeless shelters.[17]

Food Insecurity

- As of 2012, 14.5 percent of U.S. households were food insecure (uncertain of having or unable to acquire enough food for all household members because of insufficient money and other resources for food). In 10 percent of U.S. households, children were food insecure.[18]

Access to Health Care

- As of 2011–2012, 20 percent of U.S. adults and 4 percent of children had no usual source of health care.[19]
- As of 2012, 15 percent of the U.S. population (9 percent of children) lacked health insurance coverage. A survey the same year by the Commonwealth Fund reported that 46 percent of adults under age 65 were either uninsured or underinsured.[20]
- As of 2012, 80 million Americans (43 percent of adults) reported going without needed health care because of costs. By the time of the 2012 Commonwealth Fund survey, 30 percent of adults were reporting substantial problems paying their medical bills.

Eliminating the black-white mortality gap could save more lives than the year to year reductions achieved by biomedical advances. For example, from 1991 to 2000, such advances in medical care averted an estimated 176,633 deaths, but five times as many lives (886,202) would have been saved if blacks experienced the mortality rates of whites.[24]

Addressing the root cause of these disparities could rival medical breakthroughs as a strategy to improve health. For example, if all adults had the lower mortality rate of people who attend college, eight times as many lives would be saved as those saved by medical advances.[25] The ripple effects of such interventions extend beyond health, which makes a business case for social change. Education, for example, yields economic gains not only by improving health—for example, reduced medical spending—but also by providing access to better jobs that provide health insurance and higher earnings.[26] An educated workforce strengthens the economy and global competitiveness.[27] Crime and

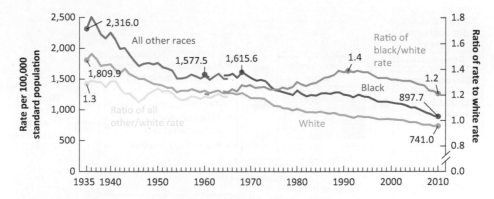

NOTE: 2010 data are preliminary. Age-adjusted rates are per 100,000 U.S. standard population.
Rates for 2001–2009 are revised and may differ from rates previously published.

FIGURE 3–1   Age adjusted death rates and ratio of rates by race: U.S., 1935–2010.

SOURCE: CDC/NCHS National Vital Statistics System, Mortality

incarceration rates may be lowered.[28,29] The higher incomes of educated workers boost tax returns to government and reduce demands for welfare assistance and Medicaid.[30] A study that took these broader societal benefits into consideration found that reducing class sizes in grade school would improve the health status of students' lives *and* generate net savings for society ($168,000 per high school graduate).[31] Medical advances cannot produce such sweeping effects, and they rarely save money.[32]

A strategy to reduce disease in America should emphasize the alleviation of societal distress at least as much as medical advances. As stated by Len Nichols, "It is entirely plausible (but not yet proved) that transferring some money from Medicaid to public housing or education could yield much greater return than would spending the extra dollars within Medicaid or on health care in general."[33] Compared to the United States, which spends more of its gross domestic product on health care, countries with better health outcomes spend proportionately more on social services.[34,35] Unfortunately, budget pressures fomented by rising health expenditures, along with political sentiments, have caused Congress and state legislatures to reduce funding for social programs, thereby undercutting an upstream strategy to curtail health spending.[36,37]

THE INFLUENCE OF SOCIAL DETERMINANTS OF HEALTH

Including the crew, the *Titanic* sailed with 2,223 persons aboard, of whom 1,517 were lost and 706 were saved. It will be noted in this connection that 60 percent of the first-class passengers were saved, 42 percent of the second-class

passengers were saved, 25 percent of the third-class passengers were saved, and 24 percent of the crew were saved.[38]

–U.S. Senate Commerce Committee Report on the Loss of the *S.S. Titanic*, 1912.

Since life boats were loaded by class and deck, despite the same "exposure," the *Titanic*'s first class passengers fared much better than their second and third class counterparts, providing an extreme example of how social determinants can influence health. Social determinants provide the context in which we live, and there is increasing recognition that individual, environmental, and medical determinants of health are each mediated by social determinants such as education, occupation, income, gender, race, and ethnicity. Some researchers suggest that behaviors, environmental factors, and health care are the intermediate or "proximal" pathways by which social determinants affect health.[39,40] But these social determinants are not randomly distributed in the population. Socioeconomic stratification and social class divisions are created and maintained by social and political mechanisms including: the labor market, the educational system, political institutions and other cultural and societal values (see Figure 3–2).[41]

Other chapters in this book delve more deeply into how population health is affected by lifestyle, the environment, and health care. This chapter focuses on how these factors are, in turn, influenced by social determinants. Due to space considerations, this chapter focuses on the relationship between disparities in social conditions and health status, delving less into the social justice of the existence of these disparities, a topic with deep ethical and historical roots that is examined in detail elsewhere.[42] Because we are not discussing the extent to which disparities are avoidable and unjust, we

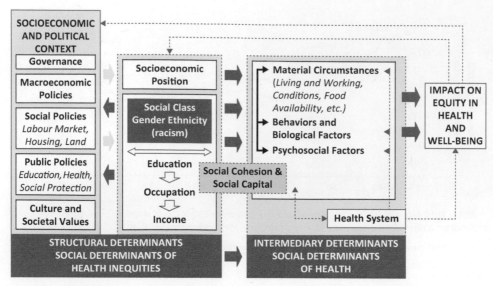

FIGURE 3–2   World Health Organization's Conceptual Model for Social Determinants of Health.

Reprinted from A Conceptual Framework for Action on the Social Determinants of Health: Social Determinations of Health Discussion Paper 2, World Health Organization, The CSDH Conceptual Framework, 5, 2010. Reprinted by permission.

will use the term **health disparities** instead of **health inequities** to refer to differences in health status.[43] See the works of Rawls[44] and Sen[45] to learn more about social justice.

Also because of space considerations, this chapter focuses on social determinants in the United States. Health status in developing countries is certainly more deeply influenced by social determinants, but the spectrum of problems extends well beyond the topics raised in this chapter to include more egregious social conditions such as civil wars, refugee displacements, and additional issues that are more characteristic of other regions of the globe. Fully 17 percent of the world's population (more than one billion people) live in extreme poverty (income less than $1.25 per day).[46] The prevalence of problems discussed in this chapter, such as food insecurity and poverty, is far more profound in the developing world than in the United States. Several excellent publications examine social determinants of health from an international perspective.[47,48] Chief among these is the work of the World Health Organization Commission on Social Determinants of Health, the establishment of which in 2005 signaled the vital importance of the topic to health status globally.

Although social determinants affecting health are more profound in the developing world, similar patterns of health inequality also exist in industrialized or "developed" countries.[49,50] Universal access to health care, as in the United Kingdom, and more egalitarian income distributions, as in Scandinavian countries, may ameliorate the effects of social determinants—but they do not change the common pattern of differential health outcomes related to socioeconomic or social class.[51,52]

This chapter cannot properly address the deep cross-cutting effects of social conditions on health without first acknowledging the role of confounding variables—the profound clustering of determinants that make it difficult to tease apart the causal effects.[53] The complex interrelationships between the social conditions of individuals, families, and communities complicate any discussion of social determinants of health.[51] People with limited education are more likely to be poor, and the poor have greater difficulty obtaining a good education. Lahelma *et al.* estimated, based on Finnish data, that at least one-third of health inequalities by education are mediated by occupational class and income.[54] Health inequalities are prominently associated with race and ethnicity; however, limited education and income are also more prevalent among blacks, Hispanics, and other minorities. Reverse causality further complicates observed associations: poverty can cause inferior health status, but poor health can also affect the ability to earn income.

Health conditions, disabilities, and unhealthy behaviors can all have an effect on educational outcomes. Illness, poor nutrition, substance use and smoking, obesity, sleep disorders, mental health, asthma, poor vision, and inattention/hyperactivity have established links to school performance or attainment.[55,56] For example, compared to other students, children with attention-deficit/hyperactivity disorder are three times more likely to be held back (retained a grade) and almost three times more likely to drop out of school before graduation.[57] Children who are born with low birth weight also tend to have a lower IQ,[58] poorer educational outcomes,[59] and higher risk for special education placements.[60–62]

Perhaps the most difficult complexities involve intergenerational effects, such as the extent to which individuals' health reflects the conditions of their childhood and the social status of their parents and families.[63]

The clustering and interrelationships of these variables make it exceedingly difficult to discuss income, race, or any other individual social determinant of health in isolation,[64] and render impossible any attempt to quantify with certainty the degree to which that variable affects health outcomes. Research in this field makes regular use of statistical techniques, such as multiple logistic regression analysis, to adjust for confounding variables in an attempt to quantify individual effects. Such methods often yield inconsistent results across studies and are often inadequate to deal with the complex interrelationships between social factors.[65–67] The anatomy of these interrelationships is not well understood. This uncertainty poses questions about where responsibility for disparities lie and where policy interventions should be directed, but it also offers many potential targets for innovation and experimentation and is the focus of active research among social scientists and health services researchers. For example, complex systems modeling, which considers the dynamic and changing relationship of factors at multiple levels (e.g., biologic, behavioral, community) is a promising methodological approach to inform our knowledge of how specific policy interventions influence the health of populations.[68,69] There is also a growing interest in "big data," which refers to the very large datasets and new data streams (e.g., social media, crowdsourcing) that exist in the various domains that shape health—health care, health behaviors, social networks, socioeconomic conditions, the environment, policies and spending, etc.—and data platforms and supercomputers that allow for merging and management of these data at unprecedented speed.[70–73]

Analyzed by education, income, race, and ethnicity, individuals and families who face adverse social conditions have markedly inferior health outcomes on multiple measures, including lower life expectancies, higher prevalence rates for diseases, more severe complications, and higher morbidity and mortality rates. The magnitude of the disparities is profound.[74] Social factors are responsible for as many deaths as the number typically attributed to pathophysiological and behavioral causes.[75] In the United States, a black newborn is 2.2 times more likely than a white baby to die by age one.[31] Compared to white Americans, the black population loses an excess of two million years of life each year.[76] As a population, U.S. blacks would rank 69th in the world for male life expectancy and 59th in the world for female life expectancy; U.S. whites would rank 29th and 31st, respectively.[77]

These disparities are longstanding. Although mortality rates for the entire U.S. population—whites and blacks included—have declined steadily over recent decades, black mortality rates have remained consistently higher than those of whites.[11] The mechanisms by which socioeconomic status affects health outcomes have changed over time, but the strength of the relationship between poverty and health has not. In fact, as income disparities grow in the United States, the impact of poverty may increase since there is some evidence that relative poverty is predictive of poor health independent of absolute poverty.[78] Longitudinal studies in California from 1965 to 1994 also demonstrated a strong relationship between cumulative exposure to economic disadvantage (below 200 percent of poverty) and decreased life expectancy, physical disability, depression, pessimism, hostility, and cognitive problems.[79]

The remainder of this chapter gives closer scrutiny to the interface between social determinants and health, demonstrating in particular how social conditions influence the major modifiable health determinants—(1) personal choices, (2) the environment, and (3) health care.

THE INTERFACE BETWEEN SOCIAL DETERMINANTS AND HEALTH

Personal Choices

Social determinants affect health by influencing the choices people make in modifying health habits and other risk factors for disease, in seeking clinical attention, and in self-care of disease.

Health Habits and Modifiable Risk Factors

Many of the leading causes of death in the United States are more common among racial and ethnic minorities and persons with limited education or low incomes. Tobacco use, the leading preventable cause of death in the United States, is more common among persons with limited education. In 2012, the prevalence of current cigarette smoking among persons age 25 and older was 8 percent for persons with a bachelor's degree or higher, 20 percent for those with some college but no bachelor's degree, 26 percent for those with a high school diploma or General Educational Development (GED) high school equivalency diploma, and 26 percent for those with no high school diploma or GED.[31] Obesity is more common among women who are poor and less educated and for minorities of both sexes.[31,80] Between 2009 and 2012, the prevalence of overweight (including obesity) was 82 percent among black women, compared to 61 percent for non-Hispanic white women.[31] The disparity in overweight by poverty status may be stabilizing in general but has widened among adolescents.[81] The major causes of obesity—physical inactivity and unhealthy diets—differ by socioeconomic status. In 2012, failure to meet aerobic and muscle-strengthening guidelines during leisure time activities was more common among those with no high school diploma or GED (66 percent) and adults living in poverty (61 percent) compared to those with a college education (40 percent) and adults living at 400 percent of poverty or more (36 percent). Persons with higher education and income consume more fruits and vegetables.[82,83] Adolescents living in poverty also drink larger quantities of sweetened beverages.[84]

Other health behaviors also differ by social class. Use of child safety seats is less common among Hispanics and black Americans and among low-income populations.[85] In a 2006–2010 survey, the proportion of women who reported using a highly effective contraceptive method was 70 percent for whites, 58 percent for blacks, and 64 percent for Hispanics.[86] Studies have also reported an association between parental education and earlier age at initiation of sex[87] and increased sexual risk behaviors among black adolescents.[88] Low-income individuals and families face financial barriers to adopting healthy behaviors. Healthful food options tend to cost more than calorie-dense diets.[89–91] Individuals facing food insecurity are more likely to consume a calorie-dense diet and have a higher body mass index.[92]

The higher prevalence of unhealthy behaviors among disadvantaged populations has multiple explanations,[93] but social and environmental conditions exert a major influence. Educational attainment is associated with an increased knowledge of health-promoting behavior, but also generally leads to higher income, better access to resources and a healthier environment. Individuals with low educational attainment are more likely to have limited health literacy, and may know less about how to reduce risk. They also may know less about available resources and most effective strategies to help with behavior modification.[94] Limited literacy, language, and cultural barriers may limit the usefulness of information delivered by pamphlets, websites, public health announcements, or advice given by health professionals.

However, an equally important factor is that resources to promote healthy choices are often lacking in the communities in which disadvantaged persons reside. These environmental factors can limit the choices those individuals can make. For example, the built environment in many urban settings, such as the lack of sidewalks and pedestrian routes, is not conducive to physical activity.[95,96] High crime rates, few or unsafe parks, and other factors discourage children and adults from walking or engaging in more vigorous activities outdoors.[97] The consumption of fruits and vegetables is correlated with proximity to supermarkets,[98] but minority and poor communities have fewer supermarkets than do other neighborhoods and often live in what some describe as "food deserts."[99–103]

Minority communities are targets for advertising and marketing that promote unhealthy behaviors. The density of fast food restaurants and advertisements for their products are greater in low-income and minority neighborhoods.[104–108] Billboards and other media in minority communities promote tobacco products and alcoholic beverages with images and messages that cater to cultural and ethnic backgrounds.[109–113] Commercials aired on television programming targeted to black viewers include more food and beverage advertisements—for fast food, candy, soda, or meat products—than those aired on other television programs and these advertisements are more likely to feature African-American characters.[114–116]

Seeking Clinical Attention

The choice to seek health care is influenced by financial and logistical barriers (as described later in this section), such as lack of providers or health insurance coverage, but social conditions also exert a more subtle influence on the patterns of seeking and adhering to treatment.[117] Racially segregated neighborhoods with a high concentration of black residents tend to have lower access to primary care providers.[118] In health systems in which access and insurance coverage are equivalent for black and white patients, such as the Medicare program and the Veterans Administration, black patients often have higher cancer mortality rates, a disparity attributed in part to delays in detection.[119–121] Influenza vaccination is covered under Medicare, but black beneficiaries, who have lower immunization rates, express less positive attitudes about the vaccine.[122]

Patients with good access but limited education or literacy may be less likely to obtain screening tests (or to follow-up on abnormal results) because they do not know about the disease, that screening is recommended, or how to obtain the tests.[123–125] Patients with limited health knowledge may also not appreciate the clinical significance of worsening symptoms that require prompt attention, such as the warning signs of a stroke, and may be more likely to harbor misconceptions that cause delays in contacting clinicians. Working-class patients often cannot afford to take time off from their jobs or their family responsibilities.

The choice to seek health care is also influenced by cultural and ethnic factors, such as one's language.[126] Efforts to educate patients about the need for care or the logistics of obtaining services are usually unsuccessful when delivered in languages that patients cannot understand. The health beliefs and traditions of certain cultures and ethnic groups may dampen interest in medical care.[127–129] The logic behind preventive care, such as screening for diseases, can be countermanded by fatalism and beliefs that disease is spiritually ordained.

Culture, ethnicity, and race influence levels of trust in clinicians and may also contribute to delays in seeking care. Native Americans often prefer traditional healers, such as medicine men, over allopathic physicians.[130] In general, patients exhibit greater reluctance to seek care from individuals of a different ethnic or racial background.[131] Black patients experience well-documented problems with mistrust of white clinicians emanating from their long troubled history with whites, including research atrocities such as the Tuskegee syphilis experiments, circumstances surrounding the HeLa cell line research,[132] and subtle or overt racism in health care and daily life.[133] Although racial and ethnic concordance between patient and provider could help remove this impediment to care, there is a shortage of minority clinicians in disadvantaged areas,[134,135] largely because proportionally few minorities are trained in the health professions. However, a number of studies have demonstrated that patient trust and more effective communication are the key drivers of adherence regardless of the patient–physician racial/ethnic composition.[136–138]

Self-Care of Diseases

Among those who obtain care, the same tableau of social conditions influence the choice to follow through on recommendations: to undergo tests, obtain and use medication as instructed, follow treatment instructions, and return for follow-up appointments. Socioeconomic conditions may require patients to forego or delay these steps because they are too expensive or because patients or their caregivers give precedence to what they perceive as higher priorities, such as feeding the family, getting to work, and staying safe from violent crime.

Other factors noted previously—limited education, literacy and language barriers, cultural and ethnic values—also influence patients' choices and their motivation to follow the advice. The effectiveness of treatments for chronic diseases such as diabetes and heart failure depend on self-management by patients, which is a greater challenge for individuals with fewer resources to draw upon.[139] For patients of all backgrounds, the highly fragmented U.S. health care system makes it difficult to navigate the logistical complexities of obtaining clinical services, such as getting an appointment, obtaining referrals to specialists, tracking down test results, and negotiating with insurance companies.[140] Individuals with limited education and resources face a special disadvantage and are vulnerable to falling through the cracks of the health care system.

Policy and Environmental Exposures

Independent of the personal choices made by individuals, health status is also influenced by the social conditions in which people live. Individuals and families often have limited control over these environmental health risks and are often vulnerable to the choices made by communities, industries, and policymakers—and policy is often the primary channel for creating healthier environments.

The most obvious and proximal source of environmental exposures is the home itself. For example, aged housing stock and apartment buildings contaminated by lead-based paint or asbestos are more likely to be occupied by disadvantaged residents who cannot afford better housing.[141,142] More destitute conditions force individuals and families to become homeless, where they are exposed to health risks from outdoor threats (e.g., hypothermia, sexual assault) and from the crowded conditions at homeless shelters, such as increased susceptibility to infectious diseases (e.g., tuberculosis).

Building and land use are all aspects of the built environment that impact health. The way communities are designed and built affect travel patterns, transportation safety, physical activity, access to healthy food, and pollution, which are directly related to health issues such as asthma, motor-vehicle-related injuries, obesity and physical activity, and heart disease.[143–146] For example, the lack of sidewalks and pedestrian routes from home to shopping in many urban settings is not conducive to physical activity.[147–149] High crime rates, few or unsafe parks, and other factors discourage children and adults from walking or engaging in more vigorous activities outdoors.[150]

Factories, waste management facilities, and other sources of air, water, and soil pollution are generally located closer to impoverished residential areas and to minority communities than to more affluent suburbs. This issue, sometimes referred to as *environmental injustice*, has pernicious health consequences.[151] For example, black children in poverty have a three-fold excess risk of asthma relative to children residing in nonpoverty communities.[152]

Adults and children living in high-crime areas are at greater risk of violent personal injury from assault or homicide, but more subtle characteristics of communities under stress may also influence the health of their residents.[153–155] For example, the literature suggests that the health of the people in a community is influenced by *social capital* and *social cohesion*. These factors, according to Krieger,

> are proposed (and contested) as population-level psychosocial assets that potentially can improve population health by influencing norms and strengthening bonds of "civil society," with the caveat that membership in certain social formations can potentially harm either members of the group (for example, group norms encourage high-risk behaviors) or nongroup members (for example, harm caused to groups subjected to discrimination by groups supporting discrimination)."[27]

Most disadvantaged individuals and families lack the resources to escape such communities by moving to areas with greater social capital and healthier surroundings. Lacking the job opportunities and income to enable such a move, they remain mired in unhealthy communities where their best efforts at disease prevention can be undermined by frayed social infrastructure.[156] Health outcomes in such areas are often affected by languishing, underfunded school systems that compromise educational attainment, inadequate public transportation services that impede access to

supermarkets or medical appointments, local work settings that lack the resources for health promotion programs, and insufficient social service agencies, programs, personnel, and resources to help the disadvantaged. Lack of social cohesion has ripple effects, such as lowering participation in political activity (e.g., voting, serving on boards and committees) "which undermines the responsiveness of government institutions in addressing the needs of the worst off."[157]

Attempts have been made to create indices of multiple variables in order to assess risk of worse outcomes within specific geographies. The Townsend Index, one often used in the United Kingdom, is calculated using four variables: the proportion of people without an automobile, the proportion of households in overcrowded accommodations, the proportion of households that are not owner-occupied, and the proportion of people who are unemployed.[158] A positive Townsend score indicates material deprivation, whereas a negative score signifies comparative affluence. The association between the Townsend Index and unfavorable health outcomes has been widely validated and tends to be most predictive in urban areas. Figure 3–3 shows the distribution of the Townsend Index for New York City (note the high scores in the underprivileged western end of

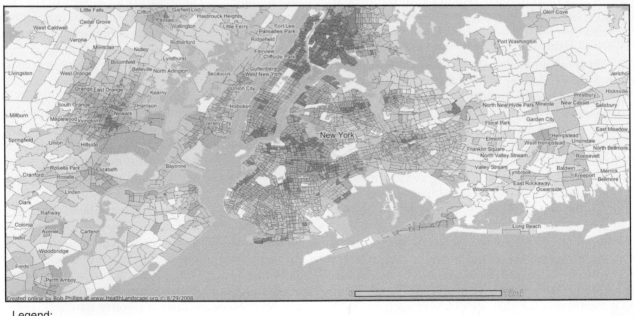

Legend:

Area-Based Socioeconomic Measures, 2000–Townsend Index	Area-Based Socioeconomic Measures, 2000–Townsend Index (Cont'd)
☐ −5— −2	▨ 5—10
▨ −2—0	▨ 10—20
▨ 0—5	▨ 20—30

FIGURE 3–3   Townsend Deprivation Index by Census Tract for New York City

Created online by Bob Phillips at www.healthlandscape.org © 8/29/2008

Long Island—the Bronx). Other recent measures used internationally include the Index of Multiple Deprivation, also used in the United Kingdom, which combines 38 indicators across seven distinct domains of deprivation[159] and the NZDep2013 Index of Deprivation used in New Zealand.[160] A similar research effort in the United States produced a parsimonious Social Deprivation Index of available social determinant data at the census tract level that demonstrates stable relationships with poor health and utilization outcomes, but which has not been applied to policy as yet.[161] The evolving use of "big data" is likely to improve the investigation of these relationships and to develop policy-relevant indices for use in the United States.

Economic inequality, a phenomenon that relates more to relative than to absolute income, is another potential environmental mediator of health. Some literature suggests that the adverse health of a population is associated with the steepness of its socioeconomic gradient.[162–165]After adjustment for confounding variables, Lynch *et al.* found that U.S. metropolitan areas with high income inequality had higher death rates than communities with more egalitarian distributions. Across 283 Metropolitan Statistical Areas, the combined impact of high levels of income inequality and low per capita income was associated with a burden of mortality equal to the combined total mortality from lung cancer, HIV/AIDS, unintentional injuries, diabetes, suicide, and homicide.[166] Intra-area differences (within regions) in income are more important than those between regions: just as income inequality within countries is more profound than cross-national comparisons, differences within states in the United States are more important than differences between states.[165] And differences within census tracts tend to be more striking than those between counties.

Several famous studies have validated the effects of social class or status on health outcomes. As defined by Krieger, "social class refers to social groups arising from interdependent economic relationships among people. These relationships are determined by a society's forms of property, ownership, and labor, and their connections through production, distribution, and consumption of goods, services, and information. Social class is thus premised upon people's structural location within the economy—as employers, employees, self-employed, and unemployed (in both the formal and informal sector), and as owners, or not, of capital, land, or other forms of economic investments."[27]

The seminal work on the relationship between social class and health was the Whitehall Study, a 25-year longitudinal study that observed that the position of government employees in the British civil service hierarchy was associated with a gradient of premature mortality.[167] The study heralded a body of research showing that health is influenced by social and geopolitical contexts. The effects occur in aggregate: although poverty or other single measures are helpful proxies for the collective influence, the *combination* of factors and their interrelationships contribute most to the relative gradient of social inequality.

The environmental conditions heretofore discussed—violent crime, frayed infrastructure, and social inequality—foster stress and emotional reactions, such as humiliation, resentment, and anger over the experience of deprivation and asymmetric power.[168] Stress and other emotions elicited by these conditions may have direct biological influences on health, physiological functions (e.g., nerve conduction, immunity, endocrine function), and disease progression,[3,169] and may precipitate depression, posttraumatic stress disorder, and other clinical disorders.[170] It may also foster unhealthy behaviors (e.g., alcohol and drug abuse, sexual promiscuity, domestic violence) as compensatory mechanisms. Living in a neighborhood with increased "psychological hazards" has been shown to have an independent association with cardiovascular disease.[171,172] In the United States, which has the highest reported incarceration rate in the world, 1 in 13 (12 percent) black men aged 30–34 is in jail or prison.[173] Even following release, a history of incarceration is associated with increased risk for a number of poor health outcomes,[174–176] as well as premature mortality.[177]

The influence of environmental conditions on health is perhaps most lasting for children, whose vulnerability to factors outside their control begins *in utero.* Maternal nutrition, behaviors (e.g., tobacco and substance abuse), and disease states that are brought about by social conditions have established influences on perinatal outcomes, such as infant mortality and low birth weight,[178] but a growing literature suggests that *in utero* exposures have a more prolonged influence on disease processes manifested later in life. For example, low birth weight appears to be a risk factor for the development of hypertension, diabetes, and stroke, heart attack, or heart disease in adulthood.[179–180]

Social conditions also shape the home surroundings and experience amid which children are raised. Children's growth and their physical and cognitive health and development are affected by the quality of meals they are served, the opportunities they are given for physical activity, the secondhand tobacco smoke they inhale, and other domestic conditions that, as noted previously, reflect the social conditions of the family. Stresses on parents and families fostered by austere living conditions can affect domestic stability, the quality of parenting, and the opportunity to encourage educational advancement and to promote healthy behaviors. Children in poverty face heightened exposure to emotional and physical trauma from marital discord, family dysfunction, and domestic violence.[181,182] Single-parent households are more common among the poor and minorities.[26] A turbulent community environment can affect children's sense of safety.[183]

Exposure to unfavorable living conditions in early childhood can have negative, lasting effects on health and well-being.[184] In the United States, 46 percent of children have been exposed to one or more "adverse childhood events," which include exposure to economic hardship; physical, emotional, or sexual abuse; parental divorce, incarceration or death; exposure to violence; and having parents with a mental illness or alcohol/drug problem.[185] A growing area of research is finding that children who are exposed to toxic stress from multiple adverse childhood events experience harmful changes in the architecture of the developing brain that affect cognition, behavioral regulation, and executive function[186-188] that can shape health outcomes decades later.[189-191] Children raised in poor families are also more likely to experience poverty as adults,[192,193] which not only affects their personal health status but also creates the conditions in which they, as parents, are at risk of repeating the same cycle with their own children.

Health Care

Social conditions affect the health care that patients receive, both in terms of access (including health insurance coverage) and the quality of care available to those with access.

Access to Health Care

Social conditions create well-known barriers to obtaining health care, which may be categorized as structural (e.g., lack of available health providers, transportation, time/hours, etc.), financial, and cognitive barriers (e.g., knowledge, literacy, communication).[194] In 2013, an estimated 26 percent of Americans confronted barriers to accessing health care; those with lower-income and racial/ethnic minorities reported the most barriers to care.[195] Access to care is more limited in rural areas, disadvantaged, and minority communities[196] where health care providers, hospitals, and other clinical facilities are either unavailable or inaccessible due to transportation difficulties.[197-199] Community Health Centers (CHCs) fill this role in some locales, providing a medical home to some 22 million people in 2013 who were mostly low-income and either uninsured or Medicaid/State Children's Health Insurance Program (SCHIP) beneficiaries, but CHCs are unavailable in some needy areas.[200,201] In 2012, CHCs that met the Community, Migrant, and Public Housing Health Center grant requirements and received federal funding from the Bureau of Primary Health Care served less than 10 percent of the nonelderly uninsured in 5 states and less than 20

percent in a total of 31 states.[202] CHCs also face staffing challenges that can limit service provision.[203,204] Growing evidence suggests that having a usual source of care in primary care can ameliorate some of the disparities in health care and outcomes wrought by social inequalities,[205-207] and that access to primary care is inversely related to hospitalization for conditions that should be preventable by receiving robust primary care ("ambulatory care–sensitive conditions").[208] In 2011, 77.3 percent of Americans had a usual source of primary care, but the likelihood of having a usual source of care was lowest for low-income/poor individuals and the uninsured.[195]

Throughout the latter decades of the twentieth century and the first decade of the twenty-first, the growing number of uninsured Americans became highly visible in headlines and in the hardships faced by the uninsured and the health systems and payers that provide and finance their care. The number of persons in the United States without health insurance coverage reached almost 50 million in 2010 (16.3 percent of the population) and remained at almost 48 million in 2012 (15.4 percent of the population). Disadvantaged persons and minorities are more likely to be uninsured or underinsured, a major health risk in the market-based health care system of the United States. By 2012, 24.9 percent of people in households with income under $25,000 were uninsured, compared to 21.4 percent with incomes $25,000 to $49,999, 15.0 percent with incomes $50,000 to $74,999, and 7.9 percent with income of $75,000 and over.[26] Rates of uninsuredness are highest among Hispanics, followed by non-Hispanic blacks (see Figure 3–4).[26]

Policy makers faced mounting pressure to adopt health reforms to improve coverage. After unsuccessful national health care reform efforts, including President Clinton's Health Security Act and the implementation of incremental efforts to expand coverage, such as the

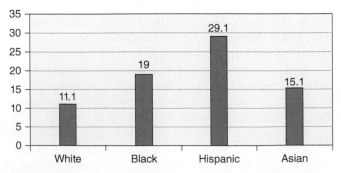

FIGURE 3–4   Percent of the U.S. population uninsured by race and Hispanic origin, 2012

DATA Source: DeNavas-Walt, Proctor, and Smith, 2013

1997 SCHIP,* the Patient Protection and Affordable Care Act (ACA) was passed in 2010 to expand and reform health insurance coverage. The ACA aimed to increase health insurance coverage by requiring most U.S. citizens and legal residents to have coverage (backed up by a tax penalty for those without coverage); imposing coverage requirements on businesses with 50 or more full-time employees; expanding Medicaid to all non-Medicare eligible individuals under age 65 with incomes up to 133 percent of the Federal Poverty Level based on modified adjusted gross income; providing premium credits and subsidies to income-eligible individuals and families; providing premium subsidies to small employers; and creating health insurance Exchanges for individuals and small businesses to purchase coverage (see Chapter 30 for more detail on the ACA). Extended coverage for young adults was implemented in 2010, and by December 2011 an estimated 3.1 million persons age 19 to 25 acquired insurance coverage.[209]

The first open enrollment on the insurance exchanges occurred October 2013 to March 2014. Rates of uninsuredness dropped in 2014 as people signed up for plans on the exchanges and as more people enrolled in Medicaid in those states offering the expansion. Considering all the health insurance expansions initiated by the ACA, an estimated 20 million Americans had gained coverage as of May 1, 2014.[210] These include one million young adults who gained coverage under parents' policies, eight million people who bought plans in the marketplaces, five million individuals who purchased coverage directly from insurers, and six million adults and children who enrolled in Medicaid or Children's Health Insurance Program (CHIP). It is not known exactly how many of these individuals were uninsured, but the Congressional Budget Office estimates that the law will decrease the number of uninsured by 12 million in 2014 and by 25 million by 2016.[211]

With the rapid growth in the costs of health care and prescription drugs, a growing population, including insured as well as uninsured persons, find it difficult to afford the steadily rising costs of copayments, deductibles, pharmacy bills, and medical supplies. In 2011, 17.5 percent of people under age 65 had expenses for health insurance premiums and out-of-pocket health expenditures that exceeded 10 percent of family income. Low-income individuals, those with activity limitations, and those with private, nongroup insurance were most likely to have premium and out-of-pocket costs exceeding 10 percent of family income.[195] Even for seniors with Medicare, out-of-pocket health expenses exceed total assets (including housing assets) in the last five years of life in an estimated 25 percent of cases.[212] Illness, and illness and health care spending may contribute to the majority of personal bankruptcy cases in the United States.[213–214]

Quality of Health Care

The quality of care for disadvantaged and minority patients can be compromised if clinicians who care for such patients have deficient training or if the quality of facilities and services to which they have access is limited. Specialists, surgical centers, and other ancillary services are less available to vulnerable populations.[215] Some patients with the same clinical presentation and health insurance coverage receive different care because of their race or ethnicity. Minority patients cared for by clinicians of a different race or ethnicity encounter difficulties with communication and trust and may be more likely to experience inferior outcomes.[216,217] Physicians less readily engage black patients in participatory decision making. A literature review by the Kaiser Family Foundation found 68 studies reporting racial or ethnic deficiencies in cardiac care.[218] In one widely cited study, physicians shown videotapes of simulated patients (actors) with identically scripted complaints were 40 percent less likely to recommend cardiac catheterization if the actor was black.[219]

THE CLIMATE FOR SOCIAL CHANGE

The existence of social conditions that compromise health status is as longstanding as civilization itself. Resources have always been concentrated among the aristocracy at the expense of the common man.[220] However, like individual determinants of health, social conditions are often modifiable. Modern countries and cultures differ in their tolerance of social injustice and the willingness of the public and the powerful to sacrifice self-interest to pursue aspirations for social equity.[221] In contrast to the United States, the public in many countries more willingly accepts high tax rates to finance social programs and rational distribution of medical services to ensure universal, equitable access to basic health care.[222]

The American public and its leaders have always found themselves caught in the crosswinds of two prevailing ethics: the utilitarian commitment to the

---

* SCHIP was designed to help states provide insurance coverage for children whose families did not qualify for Medicaid but could not afford private health insurance. Congress provided block grants to states over 10 years for SCHIP, which was reauthorized in 2009 and further extended under the Patient Protection and Affordable Care Act (Committee on Child Health Financing, 2014). As a result of CHIP, uninsurance rates for children dropped even while they were rising among adults.

common good and the spirit of individualism and entrepreneurialism on which the nation was founded. The latter fuels the popular sentiment that individuals hold personal responsibility for their success, that the disadvantaged should "pull themselves up by their bootstraps," and that limits exist on the duty of the state or of the affluent to lend assistance to the needy. Reflected in the dominant themes of conservative politics, many Americans are reluctant to expand government and entitlement programs or to pay higher taxes to address social problems.

> The inequality/health policy debate in the United States is caught in a fundamental conflict between the worship of individualism and varying impulses toward egalitarianism … Many Americans hold dear a national myth that effort always overcomes bad odds… [which] leads quite easily to the conclusion that individuals are responsible for themselves and that most get the resources they deserve most of the time. My larger point is that this cannot be the cultural myth of a generous society –Len Nichols[33]

Changes in public attitudes and the economic climate that are conspicuous at the time of this writing have produced more turbulent counterforces that could affect the social conditions discussed in this chapter. For example, poverty and income inequality resurfaced on the national agenda in the wake of the 2007 recession and the slow economic recovery that followed. The implications are best understood from the broad historical perspective. Following a period of intense interest in the 1960s—in which the War on Poverty was the domestic centerpiece of the Johnson administration and garnered visibility from the civil rights movement and outspoken leaders such as Robert F. Kennedy, Jr., Martin Luther King, Jr., and Marian Wright Edelman—the plight of the poor subsequently slipped out of the national consciousness for much of the remainder of the twentieth century. This period was punctuated by blunt reminders of the problem, most notably in 2005 when the nation was horrified by televised images of conditions in Ward 9 of New Orleans in the aftermath of Hurricane Katrina.

Attitudes about the poor were otherwise complacent. A period of relative economic prosperity in the 1990s created favorable conditions in which the vast majority of Americans felt comfortable enough to view the disadvantaged as an isolated sector of the population whose concerns were quite distinct from their own.[223] Circumstances changed in the new millennium as a recession in 2001, and a subsequent foreclosure crisis in which many Americans lost their homes, culminated in the Great Recession of 2007. This period witnessed the near collapse of global financial markets

and rescue efforts to save core U.S. industries, such as automobile manufacturing and large banks that were considered "too big to fail." Although Wall Street and major corporations eventually emerged from the crisis, American households suffered large losses in the net worth of their homes, savings, and other assets. Job insecurity pushed many upper-income workers into the middle class, and the incomes of many in the middle class fell below the poverty threshold, causing dramatic increases in poverty rates. By 2010 the U.S. poverty rate had reached 15.1 percent, its highest percentage since 1993.

Problems that had largely been considered the province of the poor—such as lack of health insurance and the inability to afford housing, medical bills, and other daily living expenses—increasingly became the problem of the middle class, a population that existing social safety net and entitlement programs were not designed to serve. An economic recovery ensued that mainly accrued to the benefit of large corporations. Salaries for most Americans did not rebound; median household income in the United States was lower in 2012 than at its peak in 1999. Financial burdens increased as stagnant wages faced rising household costs for health care, housing, child care, gasoline, and food, and government agencies struggling with fiscal shortfalls cut funding for the social safety net.

In the wake of these events, public discourse in recent years has turned increasingly to the widening income disparities in the United States. The ratio between the 90th and 10th percentiles of household income increased 14.5 percent between 1999 and 2012. News reports chronicle the enormous earnings of corporate executives and how the ratio between management and labor incomes has grown steeply in recent years. Economists warn that widening income inequality is threatening the nation's economic growth.[224,225] In 2011, resentment toward the advantages enjoyed by the 1 percent of wealthiest Americans spawned the Occupy movement, in which protestors occupied public spaces in more than 600 U.S. communities to draw attention to income inequality.

Opposing factions emerged in conservative politics in reaction to these conditions. Tea Party Republicans won landslide victories in the 2010 election by campaigning on the need for fiscal restraint and reducing the size of government, especially tax spending on social programs. More moderate Republicans began to take up concerns about poverty and income inequality, seeking to demonstrate sensitivity to the economic plight of American voters and to widen their base among minorities. By 2014, as the nation marked the 50th anniversary of Johnson's War on Poverty, leading moderate conservatives contemplating presidential campaigns in 2016 were introducing legislation and proposals to alleviate poverty. In general, however, the Tea Party movement forced many moderate conservatives out of office and pushed the policy compass to the right. Opportunities for compromise with progressive politicians diminished, creating gridlock on Capitol Hill and a polarized political environment for discussions of social justice issues. Proponents of new policies to strengthen the social safety net or to improve income, such as an increase in the minimum wage, enhanced job security, and job training programs, found greater opportunity in state and local government than in Washington, DC.

In recent years, the gaps in federal leadership to foster socioeconomic growth and opportunity have been filled by important movements in the private sector and local communities. For example, employers struggling with rising health care costs and decreased workforce productivity have embraced a business argument for investing in their communities with increasing attention to social determinants of health.[226] The financial industry—led by the initiatives of the Federal Reserve Bank of San Francisco—is exploring the role of new investment vehicles, such as social impact bonds, to invest in communities to improve socioeconomic conditions and public health.[227] Leaders of health care systems are making the case for investing in education, housing, and other social determinants as strategies to curb overutilization of health care.[228] Communities have begun to organize stakeholders to achieve collective impact in initiatives aimed at improving public health, economic growth, and other shared goals.[229]

In particular, the desire to improve educational attainment has increased with greater recognition of the primacy of the "knowledge economy"[16]—competitiveness in the global market depends on employers' and workers' mastery of science, technology, and other disciplines—and of the dismal performance of American students when compared to their counterparts in China, India, and other global competitors. Corporate leaders see a "business case" in investing in better education from pre-K through college, and many states have adopted policies to promote "STEM" (science, technology, engineering, and mathematics) education. State and local governments have sought to broaden access to early childhood education, and greater attention is being given to escalating college tuitions and loans that price low-income students out of higher education.

Along with heightened interest in addressing income and education, the subject of racial and ethnic disparities remains critically important. Following the seminal Institute of Medicine report on this topic in 2003,[217] the federal government, private foundations, and nonprofit organizations launched initiatives to document the ways and the severity with which race and ethnicity influence health status and health care and to explore and formally evaluate potential solutions. The tempo of these efforts is likely to increase as a result of demographic shifts in the U.S. population that will eventually make non-Hispanic whites a minority group (Table 3–1). The marked increase in the number of immigrants entering the United States is exerting profound influence on policy decisions about immigrant minorities.

A variety of initiatives seek to intervene at the interface in which social conditions affect health. Following are examples from each of the three nexuses discussed in this chapter: personal choices, environmental exposures, and health care.

Personal Choices

Various national and local initiatives seek to mitigate the conditions that heighten the exposure of disadvantaged adults and children to unhealthy behaviors. Examples include the work of some urban planners and developers to modify the built environment to encourage physical activity and to develop community gardens and farmers' markets to improve inner-city access to healthy food choices[230–232] and efforts to address lunch menus and vending machine offerings at low-income schools. Other examples include countermarketing activities in which ad messages are used to undermine the industry's promotion of tobacco products and alcoholic beverages to minorities.[233] The San Francisco Tobacco-Free Project (SFTFP) of the Community Health Promotion and Prevention section of the San Francisco Department of Public Health, addresses the tobacco epidemic by mobilizing community members and agencies to change environmental factors such as tobacco advertising and tobacco product access for minors that promote health inequity.[234]

Developers of health educational materials, websites, and public health campaigns are giving greater attention to targeted outreach by focusing on language barriers and the cultural concerns and health literacy of their audience.[235] Faith-based organizations and lay health workers are proving effective, especially in black and Hispanic communities, in disseminating health information and providing social support in seeking care.[236] The most innovative public schools organize classes for adults, offer parenting skills courses, screen children for abuse and neglect, involve parents in the classroom, and host community events.

To make the health care setting more inviting to minorities, and to thereby facilitate prompt clinical attention for screening or the evaluation of abnormal symptoms, health systems are devoting greater attention to cultural sensitivity and to expanding the size of the minority health care workforce. "Patient navigator" programs, the deployment of community health workers, and chronic disease management services are being developed and tested for disadvantaged patients.[237]

Employers, who increasingly recognize the connection between worksite health promotion and business productivity, offer programs and benefits such as exercise breaks, fitness facilities, heart-healthy cafeterias, occupational medicine clinics, and insurance coverage for preventive services.[238,239] Although the typical blue-collar worker is not employed by businesses that offer such benefits, that stereotype is beginning to change.

Environmental Exposures

Civil rights organizations have brought greater attention to environmental justice issues, and the public health community has continued its longstanding efforts to implement policies and regulations to reduce exposure to environmental and occupational toxins. For example, policies enacted in past years to eliminate lead from household paint and gasoline continue to yield benefits today, while current efforts focus on other initiatives, such as banning indoor use of tobacco.[240] The ability to move out of unsafe housing conditions and to avoid homelessness is facilitated by programs that offer rent support and foster home ownership.

A variety of public- and private-sector initiatives build infrastructure and social cohesion in disadvantaged communities. They range from the most practical—such as free or discounted bus services to enable residents to shop at supermarkets or visit a physician—to more elaborate programs to improve the home environment for children. Social cohesion can be strengthened by programs to reduce crime, arrange care for the homeless, build community social and health centers, and enhance job opportunities.

More imaginative efforts are envisioned for the future. For example, programs can actively intervene at key times in peoples' lives or when they are most vulnerable. The implementation in Britain of a universal program of home visits by community nurses after childbirth has enhanced childhood development scores and reduced child abuse. These programs are designed to support new parents during the first year of a child's life, offering parents a sense of control over their lives and tools for better parenting.[241,242] More recently, the ACA established the Maternal, Infant, and Early Childhood Visitation Program (MIECHV), which was the first nationwide expansion of home visiting services in the United States. The MIECHV program focuses on at-risk families and seeks to prevent child abuse and neglect, encourage positive parenting, and promote child development and school readiness. States are required to spend at least 75 percent of MIECHV funds on evidence-based program models such as the Nurse-Family Partnership[243] and Healthy Families America.[244]

The public health system in the United States is frequently overburdened by providing personal health care and ensuring preparedness for bioterrorism and other emergencies. Ideally, it should turn its attention to community-level interventions and programs to help resolve the effects of social disparities. Social determinants such as economic opportunity, vibrancy of neighborhoods, and access to education that so strongly influence health are set by society—not physicians, hospitals, or health plans.[245] Increasingly governments are being encouraged to consider the broader determinants of health as part of a more comprehensive approach to improving health and address health inequalities.[246,247] Under this "Health in All Policies" approach, policy makers are urged to consider the health implications and impact on health disparities of transportation, housing, education, tax, land use, and policies in nonhealth sectors. Collective impact is an effective approach to pulling together key people from different sectors to develop a shared vision for change and create a common agenda for solving a specific social problem that is being utilized by communities across the United States. An example of such an effort is the Live Well San Diego initiative of the County of San Diego, California (see Exhibit 3–1).[248] Other examples of effective community efforts are reviewed elsewhere.[249]

Health Care

In addition to expanding health insurance coverage, the ACA includes a range of provisions to reform private insurance, promote cost containment, improve health care quality/health system performance, and reduce health disparities.[250,251] The ACA would have doubled the capacity of CHCs with the goal of increasing access where the newly insured were most clustered; however, this expansion was slowed by Congress after passage of the ACA.[252,253] Safety net services are similarly hampered by failure to expand Medicaid, which restricts essential funding for CHCs and the capacity to care for those who are ineligible under state Medicaid rules and unable to afford private insurance.[254]

Despite gains in health insurance coverage and expansion of safety net services under the ACA, the federal government currently lacks the political will to follow through on this and other efforts to reduce social disparities. Disquiet about social injustice may not be sufficiently acute in the United States to motivate the public or its leaders to accept large sacrifices for equity, such as reordering the priorities of government or paying higher taxes. Most elected officials also lack the vision to understand that there may be offsets to higher taxes in greater productivity, lower crime rates, and improved intellectual advantage that come with a more robust middle class.

This leads to a second obstacle to dramatic social change: cost. Although, as discussed earlier, optimistic economic analyses forecast long-term net savings to society if it invests in improving education and other social determinants of health, the upfront costs remain problematic at this writing,[255] when the federal government is experiencing enormous budget deficits from financial crises and when many state and local governments are struggling to make ends meet. For example, most school districts rely on property taxes for revenue, and impoverished communities have few resources to draw upon to finance transformational changes in their school systems. Small businesses, the predominant employer for most of the middle class, cannot afford to offer health promotion benefits, such as membership in fitness clubs or weight-loss counseling. That said, major employers and business associations are reporting a return on investment from health promotion efforts.[256,257] And community-based interventions, such as programs to help parents and teachers of young children, are producing measurable results as early as age eight years.[258]

The third major challenge is the inherent complexity of the social tapestry itself, which renders unsuccessful many well-meaning attempts at social change, especially those that rely too much on simplistic expectations. Critics of antipoverty programs frequently cite their lack of success in alleviating poverty. Only a few strategies to improve educational attainment have been evaluated or proven effective in well-designed, controlled studies.[259] Successful efforts at social change are likely to require multipronged interventions across sectors. Apart from the sizable costs and the difficulties of "stove-piping" that such ambitious endeavors encounter, the ideal blueprint for such efforts remains speculative until social scientists acquire a better understanding of the interrelationships between social determinants of health.

Advocates for social justice find encouragement in the belief that all three of these major obstacles are surmountable with perseverance, and until then, progress in improving social conditions continues to occur at the local level and in a steady sequence of incremental national initiatives. Winston Churchill, Harry Truman, and Hubert Humphrey each quoted the maxim that nations are judged by how they treat the most vulnerable and disadvantaged segments of society. The alleviation of societal distress therefore stands not only as a means for improving public health but also as an expression of civilized society. The WHO Commission on Social Determinants of Health concluded in 2008 that we could close the gap in international health outcomes in a generation by working on three principles of action: improve the conditions of daily life (e.g., the circumstances in which people are born, grow, live, work, and age); tackle the inequitable distribution of power, money, and resources (the structural drivers of those conditions of daily life) globally, nationally, and locally; and measure the problem, evaluate action, expand the knowledge base, develop a workforce that is trained in the social determinants of health, and raise public awareness about these determinants.[260]

EXHIBIT 3-1   San Diego: A Case Study in Collective Impact

Led by the County of San Diego Health and Human Services Agency (HHSA), San Diego has committed itself to a transformational community-wide effort (Live Well San Diego) to improve health outcomes and to track measures for success. The initiative was launched in 2008, supported in part by federal Community Putting Prevention to Work and Community Transformation Grant funding from the Centers for Disease Control and Prevention. Live Well San Diego has transformed the theory of "Health in All Policies" into action, and has also fully embraced the principles of collective impact as described by Kania and Kramer[229]: a common agenda, shared measurements, mutually reinforcing activities, continuous communication, and a backbone organization. The stated goal of HHSA is for "cross-sector leaders within diverse organizations to focus on the same vision to address large-scale social problems." It has brought together local residents, schools, the health care community, businesses, military installations, nonprofit organizations, and the faith community—including more than 60 "recognized partners" in the community that have pledged a formal commitment to Live Well San Diego. These partners include the largest city in the County (City of San Diego) and four others (National City, Coronado, Chula Vista, Imperial Beach), California's largest elementary school district (Chula Vista Elementary School District), the state's largest health care district (Palomar), and the largest Chamber of Commerce on the West Coast. Championed by San Diego County's elected Board of Supervisors, this shared vision for healthy, safe, and thriving communities is supported by county government staff in every department. These recognized partners have agreed to a shared goal of optimizing health care, public health, and social services resources to improve health, safety, and thriving in San Diego. The initiative has a strong virtual presence on its website (http://www.LiveWellSD.org) as well as social and traditional media.

SUMMARY

The health of individuals and of populations is a product of multiple influences, including individual characteristics, environmental characteristics, and health care. Social determinants affect health in each of these three areas. At the individual level, social determinants influence the choices people make in modifying health habits and other risk factors for disease, in seeking clinical attention, and in self-care of disease. Independent of the personal choices made by individuals, health status is also influenced by the social conditions in which people live. Individuals and families often have limited control over these environmental health risks and are often vulnerable to the choices made by communities, industries, and policymakers. Social conditions also affect the health care that patients receive, both in terms of access and quality of care. The substantial prevalence of adverse social conditions, combined with their profound influence on health outcomes, creates the opportunity for social change to influence disease rates on a scale that rivals biomedical advances. A strategy to reduce disease in America should emphasize the alleviation of societal distress at least as much as medical advances.

REVIEW QUESTIONS

1. What is the causal relationship between social conditions and health status?

2. How do social determinants affect personal health-related choices, environmental exposures, and access to quality health care?

3. What is the prevalence of adverse social conditions in the United States?

4. What are the principal arguments for the contention that ameliorating social conditions can be more influential than advances in medical care?

5. What aspects of the current policy climate might foster interest in addressing social determinants of health, and what factors remain impediments?

REFERENCE

1. Centers for Disease Control and Prevention. *CDC Telebriefing: Potentially Preventable Deaths from the Five Leading Causes of Death* [Audio Recording]. May 1, 2014 at 12:00 ET. Available at: http://www.cdc.gov/media/releases/2014/t0501-preventable-deaths.html.

2. Danaie G, Ding EL, Mozaffarain D, *et al.* The preventable causes of death in the United States: Comparative risk assessment of dietary, lifestyle, and metabolic risk factors. *PLoS Med.* 2009;6(4):e1000058.

3. Tosevski DL, Milovancevic MP. Stressful life events and physical health. *Curr Opin Psychiatry.* 2006;19:184–189.

4. Taylor SE, Lerner JS, Sage RM, Lehman BJ, Seeman TE. Early environment, emotions, responses to stress, and health. *J Pers.* 2004;72:1365–1393.

5. National Research Council and Institute of Medicine. (2009). *Depression in Parents, Parenting, and Children: Opportunities to Improve Identification, Treatment, and Prevention. Committee on Depression, Parenting Practices, and the Healthy Development of Children. Board on Children, Youth, and Families. Division of Behavioral and Social Sciences and Education.* Washington, DC: The National Academies Press.

6. Burke T. Accountable care organizations. *Public Health Rep.* 2011;126(6):875–878.

7. Howard SW, Bernell SL, Yoon J, Luck J. Oregon's coordinated care organizations: A promising and practical reform model. *J Health Polit Policy Law.* 2014;pii: 2744450. [Epub ahead of print].

8. Davies GP, Perkins D, McDonald J, Williams A. Integrated primary health care in Australia. *Int J Integr Care.* 2009;9:e95.

9. Institute of Medicine. *Primary Care and Public Health: Exploring Integration to Improve Population Health.* Washington, DC: The National Academies Press; 2012.

10. U.S. Census Bureau. Educational Attainment in the United States: 2009. February 2012. Available at: http://www.census.gov/prod/2012pubs/p20-566.pdf. Accessed November 17, 2014.

11. National Center for Education Statistics. Performance of U.S. 15-Year-Old Students in Mathematics, Science, and Reading Literacy in an International Context-First Look at PISA 2012. December 2013. Available at: http://nces.ed.gov/pubs2014/2014024rev.pdf. Accessed July 24, 2014.

12. National Center for Education Statistics. Table PS1. Percentage distribution of 15-year-old students on PISA problem solving scale, by proficiency level and education system: 2012. April 2014. Available at: http://nces.ed.gov/surveys/pisa/pisa2012/xls/table_ps1.xls. Accessed July 24, 2014.

13. Nielsen-Bohlman L, Panzer AM, Kindig DA, eds. *Health Literacy: A Prescription to End Confusion.* Committee on Health Literacy, Institute of Medicine. Washington, DC: National Academy Press; 2004.

14. DeNavas-Walt C, Proctor BD, Smith JC. U.S. Census Bureau, Current Population Reports, P60-245, Income, Poverty, and Health Insurance Coverage in the United States: 2012, U.S. Government Printing Office, Washington, DC; 2013.

15. Krieger N. A glossary for social epidemiology. *Epidemiol Bull.* 2002;23:7–11.

16. Colby SL, Ortman JM. The Baby Boom Cohort in the United States: 2012 to 2060. *Current Population Reports*, P25-1141. U.S. Census Bureau, Washington, DC. 2014. Available at: http://www.census.gov/prod/2014pubs/p25-1141.pdf. Accessed on August 10, 2014.

17. Henry M, Cortes A, Morris S, Abt Associates. The 2013 Annual Homeless Assessment Report (AHAR) to Congress: Part 1 Point-in-Time Estimates of Homelessness. Available at: https://www.hudexchange.info/resources/documents/ahar-2013-part1.pdf. Accessed August 31, 2014.

18. Coleman-Jensen, Alisha, Mark Nord, and Anita Singh. *Household Food Security in the United States in 2012*, ERR-155, U.S. Department of Agriculture, Economic Research Service, September 2013. Available at: http://www.ers.usda.gov/media/1183208/err-155.pdf. Accessed September 17, 2014

19. Health, United States, 2013: With Special Feature on Prescription Drugs. Hyattsville, MD; 2014. Available at: http://www.cdc.gov/nchs/data/hus/hus13.pdf#summary. Accessed August 6, 2014.

20. Commonwealth Fund. *2012 Commonwealth Fund Biennial Health Insurance Survey.* April 2013. Available at: http://www.commonwealthfund.org/publications/surveys/2013/biennial-health-insurance-survey. Accessed July 28, 2014.

21. Hoyert DL. 75 years of mortality in the United States, 1935–2010 NCHS data brief, no 88. Hyattsville, MD: National Center for Health Statistics; 2012.

22. Satcher D, Fryer GE Jr, McCann J, Troutman A, Woolf SH, Rust G. What if we were equal? A comparison of the black-white mortality gap in 1960 and 2000. *Health Aff.* 2005;24:459–464.

23. National Center for Health Statistics. Detailed Tables for the National Vital Statistics Report (NVSR) "Deaths: Final Data for 2011." Available at: http://www.cdc.gov/nchs/data/nvsr/nvsr63/nvsr63_03.pdf . Accessed on September 16, 2014.

24. Woolf SH, Johnson RE, Fryer GE Jr, Rust G, Satcher D. The health impact of resolving racial disparities: An analysis of U.S. mortality data. *Am J Public Health.* 2004;94:2078–2081.

25. Woolf SH, Johnson RE, Phillips RL Jr, Philipsen M. Giving everyone the health of the educated: Would social change save more lives than medical advances? *Am J Public Health.* 2007;97(4):679–683.

26. Muennig P, Fahs M. The cost-effectiveness of public postsecondary education subsidies. *Prev Med.* 2001;32:156–162.

27. Muennig P. Health returns to education interventions. Available at: http://devweb.tc.columbia.edu/manager/symposium/Files/81_Muennig_paper.ed.pdf. Accessed November 4, 2006.

28. Graham PA, Stacey NG, eds. *The Knowledge Economy and Postsecondary Education: Report of a Workshop.* Committee on the Impact of the Changing Economy on the Education System, National Research Council. Washington, DC: National Academy Press; 2002. Available at: http://www.nap.edu/catalog/10239.html. Accessed November 4, 2006.

29. Lochner L, Moretti E. The effect of education on crime: Evidence from prison inmates, arrests, and self-reports. *American Econ Rev.* 2004;94:155–189.

30. Belfield C. The Promise of Early Childhood Education. Available at: http://devweb.tc.columbia.edu/manager/symposium/Files/72_Belfield_paper.ed.pdf. Accessed August 29, 2014.

31. Muennig PA, Woolf SH. Health and economic benefits of reducing the number of students per classroom in U.S. primary schools. *Am J Public Health.* 2007;97:2020–2027.

32. Rouse CE. The Labor Market Consequences of an Inadequate Education. Available at: http://devweb.tc.columbia.edu/manager/symposium/Files/77_Rouse_paper.pdf. Accessed July 12, 2014.

33. Nichols LM. The case for additional research on the relationship between socioeconomic status and health. In: Auerbach JA, Krimgold BK, eds. *Income, Socioeconomic Status, and Health: Exploring the Relationships.* Washington, DC: National Policy Association; 2001:132–136.

34. Bradley EH, Elkins BR, Herrin J, Elbel B. Health and social services expenditures: associations with health outcomes. *BMJ Qual Saf.* 2011;Oct;20(10):826–831.

35. Bradley EH, Taylor LA. *The American Health Care Paradox: Why Spending More is Getting Us Less.* New York: Public Affairs; 2013.

36. Woolf SH. Society's choice: The tradeoff between efficacy and equity and the lives at stake. *Am J Prev Med.* 2004;27:49–56.

37. National Head Start Association. *Special Report: Funding and Enrollment Cuts in Fiscal Year 2006.* Washington, DC: National Head Start Association Research and Evaluation Department; 2004. Available at: http://www.nhsa.org/download/research/FY2006_Budget_Cuts.pdf. Accessed October 21, 2005.

38. Report of the Committee on Commerce, United States Senate. *Investigation into Loss of* S.S. Titanic. Report No. 86, 62nd Congress. Washington, DC: Government Printing Office; 1912:5. Available at: http://www.senate.gov/artandhistory/history/resources/pdf/TitanicReport.pdf. Accessed August 1, 2014.

39. Henderson G. Introduction to Part II: The influences of social factors on health and illness. In: *The Social Medicine Reader.* Henderson GE, King NMP, Strauss RP, Estroff SE, Churchill LR, eds. 1997. Durham, NC: Duke University Press; 1997:103.

40. Link BG, Phelan J. Social conditions as fundamental causes of disease. *J Health Soc Behav.* 1995;Spec No:80–94.

41. Solar O, Irwin A. A conceptual framework for action on the social determinants of health: Social Determinants of Health Discussion Paper 2 (Policy and Practice). Geneva, Switzerland:World Health Organization; 2010. Available at: http://www.who.int/sdhconference/resources/ConceptualframeworkforactiononSDH_eng.pdf. Accessed July 12, 2014.

42. Doyal L, Gough I. *A Theory of Human Need.* London: Macmillan Press; 1991.

43. Carter-Pokras O, Baquet C. What is a "health disparity"? *Public Health Rep.* 2002 Sep–Oct; 117(5): 426–434.

44. Rawls J. *A Theory of Justice*, rev ed. Cambridge: Harvard University Press; 1999.

45. Sen A. *Inequality Reexamined.* Oxford: Clarendon Press, New York: Russell Sage Foundation, and Cambridge. MA: Harvard University Press; 1992.

46. United Nations. *The Millennium Development Goals Report.* 2013. Available at: http://www.un.org/millenniumgoals/pdf/report-2013/mdg-report-2013-english.pdf. Accessed on October 3, 2014.

47. Irwin A, Valentine N, Brown C, *et al.* The commission on social determinants of health: Tackling the social roots of health inequities. *PLoS Med.* 2006;3:e106.

48. National Research Center and Institute of Medicine. *U.S. Health in International Perspective: Shorter Lives, Poorer Health.* Washington DC: The National Academies Press; 2013.

49. Marmot M, Wilkinson RG, eds. *Social Determinants of Health.* Oxford: Oxford University Press; 1999.

50. Adler NE, Boyce WT, Chesney MA, Folkman S, Syme SL. Socioeconomic inequalities in health: No easy solution. *JAMA.* 1993;269:3140–3145.

51. Goldman N. Social inequalities in health disentangling the underlying mechanisms. *Ann NY Acad Sci.* 2001;954:118–139.

52. Marmot M, Bell R. Fair society, healthy lives. *The Marmot Review.* February 2010. Available at: http://www.instituteofhealthequity.org/projects/fair-society-healthy-lives-the-marmot-review. Accessed August 11, 2014.

53. Kilbourne AM, Switzer G, Hyman K, Crowley-Matoka M, Fine MJ. Advancing health disparities research within the health care system: A conceptual framework. *Am J Public Health.* 2006;96:2113–2121.

54. Lahelma E, Martikainen P, Laaksonen M, Aittomaki A. Pathways between socioeconomic determinants of health. *J Epidemiol Community Health.* 2004;58:327–332.

55. Case A, Fertig A, Paxson C. The lasting impact of childhood health and circumstance. *J Health Econ.* 2005;24:365–389.

56. Suhrcke M, de Paz Nieves C. *The Impact of Health and Health Behaviours on Educational Outcomes in High-Income Countries: A Review of the Evidence.* Copenhagen: WHO Regional Office for Europe; 2011.

57. Barbaresi WJ, Katusic SK, Colligan RC, Weaver AL, Jacobsen SJ. Long-term school outcomes for children with attention-deficit/hyperactivity disorder: A population-based perspective. *J Dev Behav Pediatr.* 2007;28:265–273.

58. Kormos CE, Wilkinson AJ, Davey CJ, Cunningham AJ. Low birth weight and intelligence in adolescence and early adulthood: A meta-analysis. *Am J Public Health.* 2014;36(2):213–224.

59. Quigley MA, Poulsen, Boyle E, Wolke D, Field D, Alfirevic Z, Kurinczuk JJ. Early term and late preterm birth are associated with poorer school performance at age 5 years: A cohort study. *Arch Dis Child Fetal Neonatal Ed.* 2012;97(3):167–173.

60. Avchen RN, Scott, KG, Mason CA. Birth weight and school-age disabilities: A population-based study. *Am J Epidemiol.* 2002;154:895–901.

61. Chapman DA, Scott KG, Stanton-Chapman TL. Public health approach to the study of mental retardation. *Am J Ment Retard.* 2008;113:102–116.

62. Litt JS, Taylor HG, Margevicius S, Schluchter M, Andreias L, Hack M. Academic achievement of adolescents born with extremely low birth weight. *Acta Paediatrica.* 2012;101(12):1240–1245.

63. Lawlor DA, Ebrahim S, Davey Smith G. Adverse socioeconomic position across the lifecourse increases coronary heart disease risk cumulatively: Findings from the British women's heart and health study. *J Epidemiol Community Health.* 2005;59:785–793.

64. Geyer S, Hemström O, Peter R, Vågerö D. Education, income, and occupational class cannot be used interchangeably in social epidemiology. Empirical evidence against a common practice. *J Epidemiol Community Health.* 2006;60:804–810.

65. Braveman PA, Cubbin C, Egerter S, Chideya S, Marchi KS, Metzler M, Posner S. Socioeconomic status in health research: One size does not fit all. *JAMA.* 2005;294(22):2879–2888.

66. Diez Roux AV. Complex systems thinking and current impasses in health disparities research. *Am J Public Health.* 2011;101(9):1627–1634.

67. Maglio PP, Sepulveda MJ, Mabry PL. Mainstreaming modeling and simulation to accelerate public health innovation. *Am J Public Health.* 2014;104(7):1181–1186.

68. Galea S, Riddle M, Kaplan GA. Causal thinking and complex system approaches in epidemiology. *Int J Epidemio.* 2010;39:97–106.

69. Livingwood WC, Allegrante JP, Airhihenbuwa CO, *et al.* Applied social and behavioral science to address complex health problems. *Am J Prev Med.* 2011;41(5):525–531.

70. Krumholz HM. Big data and new knowledge in medicine: The thinking, training, and tools needed for a learning health system. *Health Aff.* 2014;33(7):1163–1170.

71. Buxton B, Hayward V, Pearson I, Kärkkäinen L, Greiner H, Dyson E, *et al.* Big data: The next Google. *Nature.* 2008;455:8–9.

72. Roski J, Bo-Linn GW, Andrews TA. Creating value in health care through big data: Opportunities and policy implications. *Health Aff.* 2014;33:1115–1122.

73. Jain SH, Rosenblatt M, Duke J. Is big data the new frontier for academic-industry collaboration? *JAMA.* 2014;311:2171–2172.

74. Braveman PA, Egerter S. Overcoming Obstacles to Health in 2013 and Beyond. Princeton, NJ: Robert Wood Johnson Foundation; 2013. Available at: http://www.rwjf.org/content/dam/farm/reports/reports/2013/rwjf406474. Accessed August 26, 2014.

75. Galea S, Tracy M, Hoggart KJ, DiMaggio C, Karpati, A. Estimated deaths attributable to social factors in the United States. *Am J Public Health.* 2011;101(8):1456–1465.

76. Franks P, Muening P, Lubetkin E, Jia H. The burden of disease associated with being African-American in the United States and the contribution of socio-economic status. *Soc Sci Med.* 2006;62:2469–2478.

77. Data from the Statistical Annex of the World Health Report 2006 (http://www.who.int/whr/2006/annex/en/index.html) and Health, United States, 2006 (http://www.cdc.gov/nchs/data/hus/hus06.pdf#027) were used for ranking. Analysis by the Robert Graham Center.

78. Kondo N, van Dam RM, Sembajwe G, Subramanian SV, Kawachi I, Yamagata ZJ. Income inequality and health: The role of population size, inequality threshold, period effects and lag effects. *Epidemiol Community Health.* 2012;66:e11. doi:10.1136/jech-2011–200321.

79. Lynch JW, Kaplan GA, Shema SJ. Cumulative impact of sustained economic hardship on physical, cognitive, psychological, and social functioning. *N Engl J Med.* 1997;337:1889–1895.

80. Ogden CL, Lamb MM, Carroll MD, Flegal KM. Obesity and socioeconomic status in adults: United States 1988–1994 and 2005–2008. NCHS data brief no 50. Hyattsville, MD: National Center for Health Statistics; 2010.

81. Miech RA, Kumanyika SK, Stettler N, Link BG, Phelan JC, Chang VW. Trends in the association of poverty with overweight among U.S. adolescents, 1971–2004. *JAMA.* 2006;295:2385–2393.

82. Di Noia J, Byrd-Bredbenner. Determinants of fruit and vegetable intake in low-income children and adolescents. *Nutr Rev.* 2014;72(9):575–590.

83. Rasmussen M, Krølner R, Klepp KI, Lytle L, Brug J, Bere E, Due P. Determinants of fruit and vegetable consumption among children and adolescents: a review of the literature. Part I: Quantitative studies. *Int J Behav Nutr Phys Act.* 2006;3:22.

84. Han E, Powell LM. Consumption patterns of sugar-sweetened beverages in the United States. *J Acad Nutr Diet.* 2013;113:43–53.

85. Agran PF, Anderson CL, Winn DG. Violators of a child passenger safety law. *Pediatrics.* 2004;114:109–115.

86. Dehlendorf C, Park SY, Emeremni CA, Comer D, Vincett K, Borrero S. Racial/ethnic disparities in contraceptive use: Variation by age and women's reproductive experiences. *Am J Obstet Gynecol.* 2014;210:526.e1–9.

87. Santelli JS, Lowry R, Brener ND, Robin L. The association of sexual behaviors with socioeconomic status, family structure, and race/ethnicity among U.S. adolescents. *Am J Public Health.* 2000;90(10): 1582–1588.

88. Kann L, Kinchen S, Shanklin SL, *et al.* Youth risk behavior surveillance-United States, 2013. *MMWR* 2014;63(No. 4):1–168.

89. Drewnowski A. The cost of U.S. foods as related to their nutritive value. *Am J Clin Nutr.* 2010;92(5)1181–1188.

90. Monsivais P, Aggarwal A, Drewnowski A. Are socio-economic disparities in diet quality explained by diet cost? *J Epidemiol Community Health.* 2012;66(6):530–535.

91. Krukowski RA, West DS, Harvey-Berino J, Elaine Prewitt T. Neighborhood impact on healthy food availability and pricing in food stores. *J. Community Health.* 2010;35:315–320.

92. Widome R, Neumark-Sztainer D, Hannan PJ, Haines J, Story M. Eating when there is not enough to eat: Eating behaviors and perceptions of food among food-insecure youths. *Am J Public Health.* 2009;99(5):822–828.

93. Brownell KD, Kersh R, Ludwig DS, Post RC, Puhl RM, Schwartz MB, Willett WC. Personal responsibility and obesity: A constructive approach to a controversial issue. *Health Aff.* 2010;29(3):379–387.

94. Kakinami L, Gauvin L, Barnett TA, Paradis G. Trying to lose weight the association of income and age to weight-loss strategies in the U.S. *Am J Prev Med.* 2014;46(6):585–592.

95. Ferdinand AO, Sen B, Rahurkar S, Engler S, Menachemi N. The relationship between built environments and physical activity: A systematic review. *Am J Public Health.* 2012;102(10):e7–e13.

96. Ding D, Sallis JF, Kerr J, Lee S, Rosenberg DE. Neighborhood environment and physical activity among youth: A review. *Am J Prev Med.* 2011;41(4):442–455.

97. Schweitzer JH, Kim JW, Mackin JR. The impact of the built environment on crime and fear of crime in urban neighborhoods. *J Urban Technol.* 1999;6:59–73.

98. Morland K, Wing S, Diez Roux A. The contextual effect of the local food environment on residents' diets: The atherosclerosis risk in communities study. *Am J Public Health.* 2002;92:1761–1767.

99. Dutko P, Ploeg MV, Farrigan T. Characteristics and Influential Factors of Food Deserts. Economic Research Report ERR-140. U.S. Department of Agriculture; August 2012. Available at http://www.ers.usda.gov/publications/err-economic-research-report/err140.aspx#.U-zRZWP6TTo. Accessed August 17, 2014.

100. Powell LM, Slater S, Mirtcheva D, Bao Y, Chaloupka FJ. Food store availability and neighborhood characteristics in the U.S. *Prev Med.* 2007;44:189–195.

101. Moore LV, Diez Roux AV, Nettleton JA, Jacobs DR. Associations of the local food environment with diet quality—a comparison of assessments based on surveys and geographic information systems: the multi-ethnic study of atherosclerosis. *Am J Epidemiol.* 2008;167(8):917–924.

102. Larson NI, Story MT, Nelson MC. Neighborhood environments: Disparities in access to healthy foods in the U.S. *Am J Prev Med.* 2009;36(1):74–81.

103. Cannuscio CC, Tappe K, Hillier A, Buttenheim A, Karpyn A, Glanz K. Urban food environments and residents' shopping behaviors. *Am J Prev Med.* 2013;45(5):606–614.

104. Fleischhacker SE, Evenson KR, Rodriguez A, Ammerman S. A systematic review of fast food access studies. *Obes Rev.* 2011;12(5):e460–e471.

105. Bridging the gap. Exterior Marketing Practices of Fast-Food Restaurants. March 2010. Available at: http://www.rwjf.org/content/dam/farm/reports/issue_briefs/2012/rwjf72562. Accessed August 14, 2014.

106. Grier SA, Kumanyika SK. The context for choice: Health implications of targeted food and beverage marketing to African Americans. *Am J Public Health.* 2008:98(8):1616–1629.

107. Yancey AK, Cole BL, Brown R, *et al.* A cross-sectional prevalence study of ethnically targeted and general audience outdoor obesity-related advertising. *Milbank Q.* 2009;87(1)155–184.

108. Larson NI, Story MT, Nelson MC. Neighborhood environments: Disparities in access to healthy foods in the U.S. *Am J Prev Med.* 2009;36:74–81.

109. Primack BA, Bost JE, Land SR, Fine MJ. Volume of tobacco advertising in African American Markets: Systematic review and meta-analysis. *Public Health Reports.* 2007;122(5): 607–615.

110. John R, Cheney MK, Azad MR. Point-of-sale marketing of tobacco products: Taking advantage of the socially disadvantaged? *J Health Care Poor Underserved.* 2009;20(2):489–506.

111. Gentry E, Poirier K, Wilkinson T, Nhean S, Nyborn J, Siegel M. Alcohol advertising at Boston subway stations: An assessment of exposure by race and socioeconomic status. *Am J Public Health.* 2011;101(10):1936–1941.

112. Seidenberg AB, Caughey RW, Rees VW, Connolly GN. Storefront cigarette advertising differs by community demographic profile. *Am J Health Promot.* 2010;24(6):e26–e31.

113. Cohen EL, Caburnay CA, Rodgers S. Alcohol and tobacco advertising in black and general audience newspapers: Targeting with message cues? *Journal of Health Communication.* 2011; 6;566–582.

114. Grier SA, Kumanyika SK. The context for choice: Health implications of targeted food and beverage marketing to African Americans. *Am J Public Health.* 2008;98(9):1616–1629.

115. Williams JD, Crockett D, Harrison RL, Thomas KD. The role of food culture and marketing activity in health disparities. *Prev Med.* 2012;55(5):382–386.

116. Gilmore JS, Jordan A. Burgers and basketball: Race and stereotypes in food and beverage advertising aimed at children in the U.S. *J Children Media.* 2012;6(3)317–332.

117. Cuffee YL, Hargraves JL, Rosal M, *et al.* Reported racial discrimination, trust in physicians, and medication adherence among inner-city African Americans with hypertension. *Am J Public Health.* 2013;103(11):55–62.

118. Gaskin DJ, Dinwiddie GY, Chan KS, McCleary RR. Residential segregation and the availability of primary care physicians. *Health Serv Res.* 2012;47(6):2353–2376.

119. Ries LA, Wingo PA, Miller DS, *et al.* The annual report to the nation on the status of cancer, 1973–1997, with a special section on colorectal cancer. *Cancer.* 2000;88:2398–2424.

120. Etzioni DA, Yano EM, Rubenstein LV, *et al.* Measuring the quality of colorectal cancer screening: The importance of follow-up. *Dis Colon Rectum.* 2006;49:1002–1010.

121. Lantz PM, Mujahid M, Schwartz K, *et al.* The influence of race, ethnicity, and individual socioeconomic factors on breast cancer stage at diagnosis. *Am J Public Health.* 2006;96:2173–2178.

122. Groom HC, Zhang F, Fisher AK, Wortley PM. Differences in adult influenza vaccine-seeking behavior: The roles of race and attitudes. *J Public Health Manag Prac.* 2014;20(2):246–250.

123. Berkman ND, Sheridan SL, Donahue KE, Halpern DJ, Crotty K. Low health literacy and health outcomes: An updated systematic review. *Ann Intern Med* 2011;155:97–107.

124. Paasche-Orlow MK, Wolf MS. The causal pathways linking health literacy to health outcomes. *Am J Health Behav.* 2007; 31(Suppl 1):S19–S26.

125. von Wagner C, Steptoe A, Wolf MS, Wardle J. Health literacy and health actions: A review and a framework from health psychology. *Health Educ Behav.* 2009;36:860–877.

126. Helman CG. *Culture, Health and Illness, Fifth edition.* New York: Oxford University Press; 2007.

127. Simon CE. Breast cancer screening: Cultural beliefs and diverse populations. *Health Soc Work.* 2006;31:36–43.

128. Cykert S, Phifer N. Surgical decisions for early-stage, non-small cell lung cancer: Which racially sensitive perceptions of cancer are likely to explain racial variation in surgery? *Med Decis Making.* 2003;23:167–176.

129. Thornton Johnson RL, Powe NR, Roter D, Cooper LA. Patient–physician social concordance, medical visit communication and patients' perceptions of health care quality. *Patient Education and Counseling.* 2011;3: E201–E208.

130. Novins DK, Beals J, Moore LA, Spicer P, Manson SM, AI-SUPERPFP Team. Use of biomedical services and traditional healing options among American Indians: Sociodemographic correlates, spirituality, and ethnic identity. *Med Care.* 2004;42:670–679.

131. Chen FM, Fryer GE, Phillips RL, Wilson E, Pathman DE. Patients' beliefs about racism, preferences for physician race, and satisfaction with care. *Ann Fam Med.* 2005;3:138–143.

132. Skloot R. *The Immortal Life of Henrietta Lacks.* New York: Broadway Paperbacks;2011.

133. Smith DB. *Health Care Divided: Race and Healing a Nation.* Ann Arbor: University of Michigan Press;2002.

134. Gaskin DJ, Dinwiddie GY, Chan KS, McCleary RR. Residential segregation and the availability of primary care physicians. *Health Serv Res.* 2012;47(6):2353–2376.

135. Grumbach K, Mendoza R. Disparities in human resources: Addressing the lack of diversity in the health professions. *Health Aff.* 2008;27(2):413–422.

136. Jerant A, Bertakis K, Fenton JJ, Tancredi DJ, Franks P. Patient-provider sex and race/ethnicity concordance: A national study of healthcare and outcomes. *Med Care.* 2011;49(11):1012–1020.

137. Schoenthalera A, Allegrante JP, Chaplin W, Ogedegbe G. The effect of patient–provider communication on medication adherence in hypertensive Black patients: Does race concordance matter? *Ann Behav Med.* 2012;43(3):372–382.

138. Schoenthalera A, Montagueb E, Manwellc LB, Brownd R, Schwartza MD, Linzere M. Patient–physician racial/ethnic concordance and blood pressure control: The role of trust and medication adherence. *Ethn Health.*2014;19(5):565–578.

139. Bodenheimer T, Lorig K, Holman H, Grumbach K. Patient self-management of chronic disease in primary care. *JAMA.* 2002;288:2469–2475.

140. National Institutes of Health. *Voices of a Broken System: Real People, Real Problems.* 2001. Available at: http://deainfo.nci.nih.gov/advisory/pcp/archive/pcp00-01rpt/PCPvideo/voices_files/PDF-files/PCPbook.pdf. Accessed October 3, 2014.

141. Jacobs DE, Clickner RP, Zhou JY, *et al.* The prevalence of lead-based paint hazards in U.S. housing. *Environ Health Perspect.* 2002;110:A599–A606.

142. Hood E. Dwelling disparities: How poor housing leads to poor health. *Environ Health Perspect.* 2005;113:A310–A317.

143. Kent J, Thompson S. Health and the built environment: Exploring foundations for a new interdisciplinary profession. *J Environ Public Health.* 2012;2012:958175.

144. Marshall JD, Brauer M, Frank LD. Healthy neighborhoods: Walkability and air pollution. *Environ Health Perspect.* 2009;117(11):1752–1759.

145. Sallis JF, Saelens BE, Frank LD, *et al.* Neighborhood built environment and income: Examining multiple health outcomes. *Soc Sci Med.* 2009;68(7):1285–1293.

146. Dai D, Taquechel E, Steward J, Strasser S. The impact of built environment on pedestrian crashes and the identification of crash clusters on an urban university campus. *West J Emerg Med.* 2010;11(3):294–301.

147. Ferdinand AO, Sen B, Rahurkar S, Engler S, Menachemi N. The relationship between built environments and physical activity: A systematic review. *Am J Public Health.* 2012;102(10):e7–e13.

148. Ding D, Sallis JF, Kerr J, Lee S, Rosenberg DE. Neighborhood environment and physical activity among youth: A review. Am J Prev Med. 2011;41(4):442–455.

149. Humpel N, Owen N, Leslie E. Environmental factors associated with adults' participation in physical activity: A review. *Am J Prev Med.* 2002;22:188–199.

150. Schweitzer JH, Kim JW, Mackin JR. The impact of the built environment on crime and fear of crime in urban neighborhoods. *J Urban Technol.* 1999;6:59–73.

151. Morello-Frosch R, Lopez R. The riskscape and the color line: Examining the role of segregation in environmental health disparities. *Environ Res.* 2006;102:181–196.

152. Pearlman DN, Zierler S, Meersman S, Kim, HK, Viner-Brown SI, Caron, C. Race disparities in childhood asthma: Does where you live matter? *J Natl Med Assoc.* 2006;98(2):239–247.

153. Mackenbach JP, Kunst AE, Cavelaars AE, Groenhof F, Geurts JJ. Socioeconomic inequalities in morbidity and mortality in Western Europe. The EU Working Group on Socioeconomic Inequalities in Health. *Lancet.* 1997;349:1655–1659.

154. Diez Roux AV, Merkin SS, Arnett D, *et al.* Neighborhood of residence and incidence of coronary heart disease. *N Engl J Med.* 2001;345:99–106.

155. Kaplan GA. What is the role of the social environment in understanding inequalities in health? *Ann NY Acad Sci.* 1999;896:116–119.

156. Braveman P, Egerter S, Williams DR. The social determinants of health: Coming of age. *Annu Rev Public Health.* 2011;32:381–398.

157. Daniels N, Kennedy B, Kawachi I. Justice is good for our health. In: Daniels N, Kennedy B, Kawachi I. *Is Inequality Bad for Our Health?* Boston, MA: Beacon Press; 2000:14.

158. Townsend P, Phillimore P, Beattie A. *Health and Deprivation: Inequality and the North.* London: Croom Helm Ltd; 1988.

159. Department for Communities and Local Government.*The English Indicies of Deprivation 2010.* Available at: https://www.gov.uk/government/uploads/system/uploads/attachment_data/file/6871/1871208.pdf. Accessed on August 29, 2014.

160. Atkinson J, Salmond, C, Crampton P. *NZDep2013 Index of Deprivation.* Wellington: Department of Public Health, University of Otago. Available at: http://www.otago.ac.nz/wellington/otago069936.pdf. Accessed August 29, 2014.

161. Butler DC, Petterson S, Phillips RL, Bazemore AW. Measures of social deprivation that predict health care access and need within a rational area of primary care service delivery. *Health Serv Res.* 2013;48(2 Pt 1):539–559.

162. Olson ME, Diekema D, Elliott BA, Renier CM. Impact of income and income inequality on infant health outcomes in the United States. *Pediatrics.* 2010;126(6):1165–1173.

163. Wilkinson RG, Pickett KE. Income inequality and socioeconomic gradients in mortality. *Am J Public Health.* 2008;98(4):699–704.

164. Kondo N, Sembajwe G, Kawachi I, van Dam RM, Subramanian SV, Yamagata Z. Income inequality, mortality, and self rated health: Meta-analysis of multilevel studies. *BMJ.* 2009;339:b4471.

165. Wilkinson RG, Pickett KE. The spirit level: Why greater equality makes societies stronger. New York: Bloomsbury Press; 2009.

166. Lynch JW, Kaplan GA, Pamuk ER, *et al.* Income inequality and mortality in metropolitan areas of the United States. *Am J Public Health.* 1998;88:1074–1080.

167. Marmot MG, Smith GD, Stansfeld S, *et al.* Health inequalities among British civil servants: The Whitehall II study. *Lancet.* 1991:337:1387–1393.

168. Leventhal T, Brooks-Gunn J. Moving to opportunity: An experimental study of neighborhood effects on mental health. *Am J Public Health.* 2003;93:1576–1582.

169. Taylor SE, Repetti RL, Seeman T. What is an unhealthy environment and how does it get under the skin? *Annu Rev Psychol.* 1997;48:411–447.

170. Goldmann E, Aiello A, Uddin M, *et al.* Pervasive exposure to violence and posttraumatic stress disorder in a community: The Detroit neighborhood health study. *J Trauma Stress.* 2011;24(6):747–751.

171. Glass TA, Rasmussen MD, Schwartz BS. Neighborhoods and obesity in older adults: The Baltimore memory study. *Am J Prev Med.* 2006;31:455–463.

172. Augustin T, Glass TA, James BD, Schwartz BS. Neighborhood psychosocial hazards and cardiovascular disease: The Baltimore memory study. *Am J Public Health.* 2008;98(9):1664–1670.

173. The Sentencing Project. Facts about Prisons and People in Prisons. January 2014. Available at: http://sentencingproject.org/doc/publications/inc_Facts%20About%20Prisons.pdf. Accessed on August 8, 2014.

174. Wildeman C. Imprisonment and (Inequality in) Population Health. *Social Science Research.* 2012;41(1):74–91.

175. Massoglia M. Incarceration as exposure: The prison, infectious disease, and other stress-related illnesses. *J Health Soc Behav.* 2008;49(1):56–71.

176. Schnittker J, John A. Enduring stigma: The long-term effects of incarceration on health. *J Health Soc Behav.* 2007;48(2):115–130.

177. Pridemore WA. The mortality penalty of incarceration: Evidence from a population-based case-control study of working-age males. *J Health Soc Behav.* 2014;55:215–233.

178. Aizer A, Currie J. The intergenerational transmission of inequality: Maternal disadvantage and health at birth. *Science.* 2014;344(6186):856–861.

179. Barker DJ. The developmental origins of adult disease. *J Am Coll Nutr.* 2004;23(6 Suppl): 588S–595S.

180. Johnson RC, Schoeni RF. Early life origins of adult disease: National longitudinal population-based study of the United States. *Am J Public Health.* 2011;101(12):2317–2324.

181. Rutter M. Poverty and child mental health: Natural experiments and social causation. *JAMA.* 2003;290:2063–2064.

182. Freisthler B, Merritt DH, LaScala EA. Understanding the ecology of child maltreatment: A review of the literature and directions for future research. *Child Maltreat.* 2006;11:263–280.

183. Mijanovich T, Weitzman BC. Which "broken windows" matter? School, neighborhood, and family characteristics associated with youths' feelings of unsafety. *J Urban Health.* 2003;80:400–415.

184. Felitti VJ, Anda RF, Nordenberg D, Williamson DF, Spitz AM, Edwards V, Koss MP. Relationship of childhood abuse and household dysfunction to many of the leading causes of death in adults: The Adverse Childhood Experiences (ACE) Study. *Am J Prev Med.* 1998;14(4):245–258.

185. Sacks V, Murphey D, Moore K. Adverse childhood experiences: National and State-Level Prevalence. Available at http://www.childtrends.org/wp-content/uploads/2014/07/Brief-adverse-childhood-experiences_FINAL.pdf . Accessed on August 31, 2014.

186. Hackman DA, Farah MJ, Meaney MJ. Socioeconomic status and the brain: Mechanistic insights from human and animal research. *Nat Rev Neurosci.* 2010;11:651–659.

187. Hanson JL, Hair N, Shen DG, Shi F, Gilmore JH, Wolfe BL, Pollak SD. Family poverty affects the rate of human infant brain growth. *PLoS One.* 2013 Dec 11;8(12).

188. Hanson JL, Chung MK, Avants BB, Rudolph KD, Shirtcliff EA, Gee JC, Davidson RJ, Pollak SD. Structural variations in prefrontal cortex mediate the relationship between early childhood stress and spatial working memory. *J Neurosci.* 2012 Jun 6;32(23):7917–7925.

189. Shonkoff JP, Phillips DA, eds. *From Neurons to Neighborhoods: The Science of Early Child Development.* National Research Council and Institute of Medicine. Washington, DC: The National Academies Press; 2000.

190. Shonkoff JP. Building a new biodevelopmental framework to guide the future of early childhood policy. *Child Dev.* 2010;81(1):357–367.

191. Shonkoff JP, Garner AS; Committee on Psychosocial Aspects of Child and Family Health; Committee on Early Childhood, Adoption, and Dependent Care; Section on Developmental and Behavioral Pediatrics. The lifelong effects of early childhood adversity and toxic stress. *Pediatrics.* 2012 Jan;129(1):e232–e246.

192. Musick K, Mare RD. Recent trends in the inheritance of poverty and family structure. *Soc Sci Res.* 2006;35:471–499.

193. Long J, Ferie J. Intergenerational occupational mobility in Great Britain and the United States since 1850. *Am Econ Rev.* 2013;103(4): 1109–1137.

194. Carillo JE, Carrilo VA, Perez HR, Salas-Lopez D, Natale-Pereira A, Byron AT. Defining and targeting health care access barriers. *J Health Care Poor Underserved.* 2011;22(2): 562–575.

195. Agency for Healthcare Research and Quality. *2013 National Healthcare Disparities Report.* Publication No. 14-0006. Rockville, MD: U.S. Department of Health and Human Services; 2014. Available at: http://www.ahrq.gov/research/findings/nhqrdr/nhdr13/index.html. Accessed August 4, 2014.

196. Dower C, O'Neill E. Primary care health workforce in the United States. Research Synthesis Report No. 22. Princeton, NJ: Robert Wood Johnson Foundation; 2011.

197. Field K, Briggs D. Socio-economic and locational determinants of accessibility and utilization of primary health care. *Health and Social Care in the Community.* 2001;9:294–308.

198. Zuvekas SH, Weinick RM. Changes in access to care, 1977–1996: The role of health insurance. *Health Serv Res.* 1999;34:271–279.

199. Hendryx MS, Ahern MM, Lovrich NP, McCurdy AH. Access to health care and community social capital. *Health Serv Res.* 2002;37:87–103.

200. National Association of Community Health Centers, Robert Graham Center, The George Washington University School of Public Health and Health Services. Access transformed: Building a Primary Care Workforce for the 21st Century; 2008. Available at: http://www.nachc.com/client/documents/ACCESS%20Transformed%20full%20report.PDF. Accessed August 20, 2014.

201. Shin P, Ku L, Jones E, Finnegan B, Rosenbaum S. 2009. Financing Community Health Centers as Patient- and Community-Centered Medical Homes: A Primer. Available at: https://publichealth.gwu.edu/departments/healthpolicy/DHP_Publications/pub_uploads/dhpPublication_A186E838-5056-9D20-3D9EA92EB75DAC24.pdf. Accessed August 20, 2014.

202. National Association of Community Health Centers. A Sketch of Community Health Centers: Chart Book 2014. Available at: http://www.nachc.com/client//Chartbook_2014.pdf. Accessed August 1, 2014.

203. Forrest CB, Whelan EM. Primary care safety-net delivery sites in the United States: A comparison of community health centers, hospital outpatient departments, and physicians' offices. *JAMA.* 2000;284:2077–2083.

204. Rosenblatt RA, Andrilla CH, Curtin T, Hart LG. Shortages of medical personnel at community health centers: Implications for planned expansion. *JAMA.* 2006;295:1042–1049.

205. Starfield B, Shi L, Macinko J. Contribution of primary care to health systems and health. *Milbank Q.* 2005;83:457–502.

206. DeVoe JE, Tillotson CJ, Wallace LS, Lesko E, Angier H. The effects of health insurance and a usual source of care on a child's receipt of health care. *J Pediatr Health Care.* 2012;26(5)e25–e35.

207. Spatz ES, Sheth SD, Gosch KL, *et al.* Usual source of care and outcomes following acute myocardial infarction. *J Gen Intern Med.* 2014;29(6):862–869.

208. Rosano A, Loha CA, Falvo R, *et al.* The relationship between avoidable hospitalization and accessibility to primary care: A systematic review. *Eur J Public Health.* 2013;23(3):356–360.

209. Department of Health and Human Services. ASPE Issue Brief; July 9, 2012. Available at: http://aspe.hhs.gov/health/reports/2012/Young AdultsbyGroup/ib.pdf. Accessed on September 16, 2014.

210. Blumenthal D, Collins SR. Health care coverage under the Affordable Care Act--A progress report. *N Engl J Med.* 2014 Jul 17;371(3):275–281. doi: 10.1056/NEJMhpr1405667. Epub 2014 Jul 2.

211. Congressional Budget Office. Updated Estimates of the Effects of the Insurance Coverage Provisions of the Affordable Care Act. April 2014 Available at: http://www.cbo.gov/publication/45231. Accessed on August 31, 2014.

212. Kelley AS, McGarry K, Fahle S, Marshall SM, Du Q, Skinner JS. Out-of-pocket spending in the last five years of life. *J Gen Intern Med.* 2013; 8(2):304–309.

213. Himmelstein DU, Warren E, Thorne D, Woolhandler S. Illness and injury as contributors to bankruptcy. *Health Aff.* 2005 January–June;Suppl Web Exclusives:W5-63–W5-73.

214. Himmelstein DU, Thorne D, Warren E, Woolhandler S. Medical bankruptcy in the United States, 2007: Results of a national study. *Am J Med.* 2009;122(8):741–746.

215. Neuhausen K, Grumbach K, Bazemore A, Phillips RL. Integrating Community Health Centers into organized delivery systems can improve access to subspecialty care. *Health Aff.* 2012;31(8):1708–1716.

216. Cooper-Patrick L, Gallo JJ, Gonzales JJ, et al. Race, gender, and partnership in the patient-physician relationship. *JAMA.* 1999;282:583–589.

217. Smedley BD, Stith AY, Nelson AR, eds. *Unequal Treatment: Confronting Racial and Ethnic Disparities in Health Care.* Committee on Understanding and Eliminating Racial and Ethnic Disparities in Health Care, Board on Health Sciences Policy, Institute of Medicine. Washington, DC: National Academy Press; 2003.

218. Lillie-Blanton M, Rushing OE, Ruiz S, Mayberry R, Boone L. *Racial/Ethnic Differences in Cardiac Care: The Weight of the Evidence.* Publication No. 6041. Menlo Park, CA: The Henry J. Kaiser Family Foundation; 2002.

219. Schulman KA, Berlin JA, Harless W, et al. The effect of race and sex on physicians' recommendations for cardiac catheterization. *N Engl J Med.* 1999;340:618–626.

220. Tanner R. Governors wrestle with Medicaid changes. Associated Press. August 7, 2006. Available at: http://www.washingtonpost.com/wpdyn/content/article/2006/08/07/AR2006080700121_pf.html. Accessed December 12, 2014.

221. Muntaner C, Borrell C, Ng E, et al. Politics, welfare regimes, and population health: Controversies and evidence. *Soc Health Illn.* 2011;33(6):946–964.

222. Acemoglu D, Robinson JA. Why nations fail: The origins of power, prosperity and poverty. New York: Crown; 2012.

223. Phillips K. *Wealth and Democracy: A Political History of the American Rich.* New York: Broadway Books; 2002.

224. International Monetary Fund. Fiscal Policy and Income Inequality. January 2014. Available at: http://www.imf.org/external/np/pp/eng/2014/012314.pdf. Accessed on May 14, 2014.

225. Piketty T. *Capital in the Twenty-First Century.* Cambridge, MA: Harvard University Press; 2014.

226. National Business Group on Health. Health Determinants and Employees in Growth Countries. Washington, DC; 2011.

227. Federal Reserve Bank. *Investing in What Works for America's Communities: Essays on People Place & Purpose.* San Francisco: Federal Reserve Bank of San Francisco and Low Income Investment Fund; 2012.

228. Isham GJ, Zimmerman DJ, Kindig DA, Hornseth GW. HealthPartners adopts community business model to deepen focus on nonclinical factors of health outcomes. *Health Aff (Millwood).* 2013;32(8):1446–1452.

229. Kania J, Kramer M. Collective impact. *Stanford Social Innovation Review.* 2011; Winter:36–41. Available at: http://www.ssireview.org/images/articles/2011_WI_Feature_Kania.pdf. Accessed August 31, 2014.

230. Miller W, Simon P, Maleque S, eds. *Beyond Health Care: New Directions to a Healthier America.* Washington, DC: Robert Wood Johnson Foundation Commission to Build a Healthier America; 2009.

231. Miller WD, Pollack CE, Williams DR. Healthy homes and communities: Putting the pieces together. *Am J Prev Med.* 2011;40(1S1):S48–S57.

232. Brownell KD, Kersh R, Ludwig DS, et al. Personal responsibility and obesity: A constructive approach to a controversial issue. *Health Aff (Millwood).* 2010;29(3):379–387.

233. Siegel M, Biener L. The impact of an antismoking media campaign on progression to established smoking: Results of a longitudinal youth study. *Am J Public Health*. 2000;90:380–386.

234. Hofrichter R, ed. *Tackling Health Inequities Through Public Health Practice: A Handbook for Action*. Available at: http://www.naccho.org/topics/justice/upload/naccho_handbook_hyperlinks_000.pdf. Accessed December 1, 2014.

235. Niederdeppe J, Farrelly MC, Haviland ML. Confirming "truth": More evidence of a successful tobacco countermarketing campaign in Florida. *Am J Public Health*. 2004;94:255–257.

236. Brown SA, Garcia AA, Winchell M. Reaching underserved populations and cultural competence in diabetes education. *Curr Diab Rep*. 2002;2:166–176.

237. Alter JH. Social determinants of health: From bench to bedside. *JAMA Intern Med*. 2014;174(4):543–545.

238. Goetzel RZ, Ozminkowski RJ. The health and cost benefits of work site health-promotion programs. *Annu Rev Public Health*. 2008;29:303–323.

239. Baicker K, Cutler D, Song Z. Workplace wellness programs can generate savings. *Health Aff (Millwood)*. 2010;29(2):304–311.

240. CDC. State-specific prevalence of current cigarette smoking among adults and secondhand smoke rules and policies in homes and workplaces—United States, 2005. *MMWR*. 2006;55:1148–1151.

241. Kamerman SB, Kahn AJ. Home health visiting in Europe. *The Future of Children*. Available at: http://futureofchildren.org/futureofchildren/publications/docs/03_03_02.pdf. Accessed September 2, 2014.

242. Kendrick D, Elkan R, Hewitt M, *et al*. Does home visiting improve parenting and the quality of the home environment? A systematic review and meta analysis. *Arch Dis Child*. 2000;82:443–451.

243. Olds DL. The nurse–family partnership: An evidence-based preventive intervention. *Infant Ment Health J*. 2006; 27(1):5–25.

244. Galano J, Ed. *The Healthy Families America Initiative, Integrating Research, Theory and Practice*. New York: Routledge; 2007.

245. Woolf SH, Braveman P. Where health disparities begin: The role of social and economic determinants and why current policies may make matters worse. *Health Aff*. 2011;30(10):1852–1859.

246. Frieden TR. A framework for public health action: The health impact pyramid. *Am J Public Health*. 2010;100:590–595.

247. World Health Organization, Commission on Social Determinants of Health. Closing the gap in a generation: Health equity through action on the social determinants of health. Final report of the Commission on Social Determinants of Health. Geneva: WHO; 2008. Available at: http://whqlibdoc.who.int/publications/2008/9789241563703_eng.pdf. Accessed August 31, 2014.

248. County of San Diego. *Live Well San Diego!: Building Better Health*. Available at: http://www.sdcounty.ca.gov/dmpr/gfx/Live_Well_Annual_Report_2011-12/. Accessed August 22, 2014.

249. Hofrichter R, & Rajiv B, eds. *Tackling Health Inequities through Public Health Practice: Theory to Action*. Oxford University Press, 2010.

250. Kaiser Family Foundation. Summary of the Affordable Care Act. April 2013. Available at: http://kff.org/health-reform/fact-sheet/summary-of-the-affordable-care-act/. Accessed on August 1, 2014.

251. IOM (Institute of Medicine). How far have we come in reducing health disparities? Progress since 2000: Workshop summary. Washington, DC: The National Academies Press; 2012.

252. HRSA. The Affordable Care Act and health centers. Available at: http://bphc.hrsa.gov/about/healthcenterfactsheet.pdf. Accessed July 30, 2014.

253. Wood SF, Goldberg DG, Bruen BK, Johson K, Mead H. Community Health Centers in an Era of Health Reform: An Overview and Key Challenges to Health Center Growth. Available at: http://hsrc.himmelfarb.gwu.edu/cgi/viewcontent.cgi?article=1079&context=sphhs_policy_facpubs. Accessed July 30, 2014.

254. Ku L, Zur J, Jones E, Shin P, Rosenbaum S. How Medicaid expansions and future community health center funding will shape capacity to meet the nation's primary care needs. Washington, DC: George Washington University, School of Public Health and Health Services, Department of Health Policy. Available at: http://hsrc.himmelfarb.gwu.edu/cgi/viewcontent.cgi?article=1025&context=sphhs_policy_ggrchn . Accessed August 31, 2014.

255. Wadsworth M. Early life. In: *Social Determinants of Health*. Marmot M, Wilkinson RG, eds. Oxford: Oxford University Press; 1999: 44–63.

256. Berry LL, Mirabito AM, Baun WB. What's the hard return on employee wellness programs? *Harv Bus Rev*. 2010;88(12):104–112.

257. National Business Group on Health. The Business Case for Prevention: Why Investing in Prevention is Good for Business. Available at: http://www.businessgrouphealth.org/preventive/businesscase/index.cfm. Accessed September 4, 2014.

258. Brotman LM, Dawson-McClure S, Huang KY, *et al*. Early childhood family intervention and long-term obesity prevention among high-risk minority youth. *Pediatrics*. 2012;129:e621–e628.

259. Finn JD, Gerber SB, Boyd-Zaharias J. Small classes in the early grades, academic achievement, and graduating from high school. *J Educ Psychol*. 2005;97:214–223.

260. Marmot M, Friel S, Bell R, Houweling TAJ, Taylor S. Closing the gap in a generation: Health equity through action on the social determinants of health. *The Lancet*. 2008;372(9650):1661–1669.

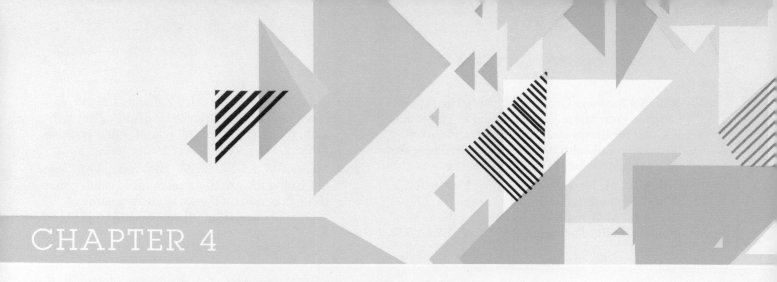

CHAPTER 4

Legal Basis of Public Health

Susan Allan, MD, JD, MPH

LEARNING OBJECTIVES

Upon completion of this chapter, the reader will be able to:

1. Identify the primary legal sources of public health authority.

2. Explain the distribution of public health authorities between the federal and state governments.

3. Define "police power" and explain how this relates to public health.

4. Describe the standard requirements of procedural due process.

5. Explain how the constitutional requirements of "equal protection" apply to public health actions.

6. Explain how the privacy requirements of the Health Insurance Portability and Accountability Act apply to public health agencies.

KEY TERMS

administrative law
equal protection
federalism
police powers
preemption
procedural due process
substantive due process

INTRODUCTION

The purpose of this chapter is to understand law as a major component of the practice of public health. This is important both in looking at the history of public health and as a re-emerging tool in improving opportunities for health in communities today. As noted elsewhere in this textbook, the history of public health to a great extent is a story of developing and enforcing laws and policies that improved sanitary conditions, required vaccinations, addressed hazards at work, reduced contamination of the food supply, and in many other ways reduced the environmental and infectious hazards of the conditions in which people lived and worked. In Chapter 1, Drs. Erwin and Brownson note that the public health successes described in "Ten Great Public Health Achievements of the 20th Century" identified by the Centers for Disease Control and Prevention (CDC) involved national, state, and local policies, laws, and ordinances.

Though there are many different definitions of "public health," all emphasize that a fundamental component is organized societal action to protect or promote health. One of the most fundamental and enduring forms of societal action is through the development and enforcement of laws.

> Law is foundational to U.S. public health practice. Laws establish and delineate the missions of public health agencies, authorize and delimit public health functions, and appropriate essential funds.[1] (p. 29)

The early history of the use of laws to improve health was for the most part the regulation and restriction of hazards—keeping sewage out of drinking water, isolating people with active smallpox from the general community until the period of infection had passed, limiting exposures of workers to toxic chemicals, and restricting sales of cigarettes to minors. In more recent years, there has been increased attention also to the potential for laws to be used not only to address emerging hazards, but also to promote opportunities for health—proposals such as using zoning rules to increase availability of sidewalks, requiring restaurant menus to list calorie counts, and using building codes to improve accessibility of stairs. While "health promotion" activities remain an important priority for public health, this is increasingly paired with efforts to use laws and regulations to change aspects of the environment to make health-promoting behaviors easier or more appealing.

This refreshed interest in law and policy within the public health community is discussed extensively in the 2011 Institute of Medicine report, *For the Public's Health: Revitalizing Law and Policy to Meet New Challenges*.[2] In noting the following list of activities as characteristic of public health law, the report makes the point that some of these directly affect primarily the public health department, while others affect other agencies or sectors.

Legal and public policy tools for the public's health include

▶ "taxation, incentives, and spending (e.g., cigarette and other "sin" taxes and allocation of the tax to combat the problem may include pricing policies and financial incentives);
▶ altering the informational environment (e.g., food or drug labeling and disclosure of health information);
▶ altering the built/physical environment (e.g., zoning, toxic waste);
▶ altering the natural environment (e.g., clean water, air, environmental justice);
▶ direct regulation (e.g., seat belts, helmets, drinking water fluoridation, folate fortification of grain-based products, iodized salt; licensure of medical care providers and facilities);
▶ indirect regulation (e.g., tort litigation in tobacco); and
▶ deregulation (e.g., distribution of sterile injection equipment or criminalization of HIV risk behaviors)." (p. 58)

An earlier Institute of Medicine report on public health education identified public health law as an important area of knowledge for all public health professionals (*Who Will Keep the Public Healthy?: Educating Public Health Professionals for the 21st Century*).[3] The Public Health Accreditation Board (PHAB) Standards include requirements for knowing, updating, and enforcing the public health laws for the jurisdiction.[4] One of the 10 Essential Public Health Services is to enforce laws and regulations, which is also an expectation of the National Public Health Performance Standards for assessing local and state public health system performance.[5]

This chapter addresses legal topics that are most often important in public health practice. Because laws are intrinsically governmental, most of the discussion pertains to governmental activities, while recognizing that many public health laws, such as requiring seatbelts in cars and removing lead from paint, have come about because of advocacy groups. It should be emphasized from the beginning that laws and their application vary from place to place and time to time. So when dealing with an actual or potential legal issue, it is highly advisable to obtain consultation from someone whose knowledge of the relevant law is current and specific.

SOURCES OF PUBLIC HEALTH LAW

Basic Sources of Law

Communities are subject to a complex network and interplay of laws from different levels of government—federal, state, local, tribal—and sometimes special jurisdictions (such as an airport authority, or health and hospital authority). In general, there are five basic sources of U.S. public health law:

▶ *Constitutions.* The U.S. Constitution is the source of all legal authority for the federal government. The U.S. Constitution and state constitutions are the source of all legal authority for states.

▶ *Statutes.* Congress passes laws giving power to agencies of the executive branch. Federal statutes establish federal public health agencies, programs, and services, and appropriate funds for federal and state public health work. State legislatures pass state statutes that establish analogous state functions.

▶ *Regulations.* Legislatures give agencies power to make regulations that have the same force as statutes. Regulations are usually the process for establishing standards and procedures to implement statutes, which typically are written with broader language. The authority to develop regulations (often called "rulemaking") allows agencies to quickly respond to new challenges or address technical issues, and allows the legislature to defer to that department's expertise on that particular subject matter. Procedures for "rulemaking" require opportunity for the public to participate.

▶ *Common law or case law.* This law is based on court decisions that create and reflect custom that provides judicial interpretation of statutes, regulations, etc. Court decisions establish "precedent" that is treated as authoritative. (This feature is unique to those governmental systems derived from the British legal system.)

▶ *Executive Orders.* This is a policy directive, typically by the top executive, that implements or interprets a federal or state statute. When legislatively authorized, an Executive Order has the force of law.

Distribution of Power Between Federal Government and States

The governmental power to make rules and decisions affecting the public's health is distributed between the federal and state governments. Federalism describes the division of power between the federal government and state governments. The basis of federalism is the Tenth Amendment to the U.S. Constitution, which states that any powers not "delegated to the United States by the Constitution, nor prohibited by it to the

States, are reserved to the States respectively, or to the people." Therefore the constitutional federal authority over public health matters is somewhat limited, and the majority of public health responsibilities and authorities are found at the state level. (Note that the public health authority of local governments is dependent upon delegation of state authority. This is discussed in more depth in Chapters 7 and 8 on the Federal and State contributions to Public Health.) The authority to take actions on behalf of the public's health is often spoken of as deriving from the broad governmental police powers that are established by the U.S. Constitution and further elaborated by state and local laws. "The police power is the right of the state to take coercive action against individuals for the benefit of society."[6]

Direct federal authority applies to a small number of public health circumstances, although these are often highly visible, such as at international borders and interstate/multistate threats. In addition, the federal authority to regulate interstate commerce has supported many actions affecting public health, such as the regulation of the safety of many products. In more recent years, the federal responsibility for homeland security has been invoked for the management of planning and response to certain high-risk infectious disease threats such as severe acute respiratory syndrome (SARS) and pandemic influenza that would have substantial national impact.

The federal government exerts substantial influence on public health activities beyond its direct authority through "the power of the purse"—that is, through making federal funds available with conditions and constraints for how the money may be used for public health activities. When states accept the funds, they must comply with the federal conditions. Because federal funding is a very large proportion of state and local public health resources, as a practical matter, through this "power of the purse," the federal government has a very significant influence on the state, local, and tribal public health activities. This has influenced not only direct public health activities such as disease surveillance, but also other state activities with public health impact, such as lowering speed limits as a condition of receiving federal highway funds.

Local Law

The distribution of power between local and state governments is defined by the state constitution, laws, and regulations. As described in more detail in Chapters 8 and 9 on the structure of public health systems at the state and local levels, the extent and degree of independence of local authority varies widely from state to state. Even in local jurisdictions that are defined as having Home Rule, the authority for relative independence is derived from the state, and there are usually specified situations, such as multicounty outbreaks, in which that state may assume primary responsibility. Many local health departments also have local programs that are authorized by laws or regulations by the local governing body (e.g., a county or city commission), local executive authority (e.g., a mayor or county executive), or a local board of health. In some jurisdictions, local boards of health have promulgated ordinances that have in effect become law, in the absence of higher state-level action, e.g., banning smoking in public places and requiring menu labeling.

Tribal Law

Federally-recognized tribes have legal status as sovereign nations, with the full rights of self-determination on tribal land. Because there is considerable variation in the legal structures and authorities for individual tribes, tribal law is a complex field, and each tribe should be approached as a unique instance. Federal, state, and local agencies only have jurisdiction on tribal lands or relation to tribal activities when authorized by the tribe through formal agreements. State and local health departments often engage in agreements with tribes to provide public health services such as epidemiology and control of infectious diseases or environmental services related to food safety and drinking water. Many tribes also have agreements with state and local health departments related to emergency preparedness and response. (See Chapter 10 for additional detail on tribal health.)

The Bill of Rights and Public Health Actions

The Bill of Rights of the U.S. Constitution (the first 10 Amendments) is the primary legal source for the protection of individual rights. Although originally written to apply to the actions of the federal government, because of the Fourteenth Amendment, many of these individual rights also apply to actions of state and local governments (see Exhibit 4-1). Of particular significance for public health actions, the Bill of Rights defines legal requirements for due process, equal protection, freedom of religion, and prohibition of unreasonable search and seizures. Table 4–1 includes public health-related protections in specific amendments.

Preemption

What happens when federal and state powers conflict? The Supremacy Clause of the U.S. Constitution provides that where a state and federal law conflict, the federal law preempts the state law. Generally, preemption assures national uniformity and sets a minimal standard of protection, allowing state and local governments to enact greater levels of protection of the public's health (see Exhibit 4-2). However, sometimes states are specifically prohibited by federal statute from enacting a standard that is either less or more strict than that set by federal law. For example, national health care reform legislation—the Patient Protection and Affordable Care Act (ACA) of 2010—established a new federal standard for menu labeling to be implemented by the states. The menu labeling provisions of the ACA provide that the federal law will preempt any state or local law on the same subject matter that are not "identical to" the provisions of the ACA. Although King County, Washington had passed one of the strictest menu labeling laws in the nation in 2008, it had to amend the regulation in 2010 to align with the national statute.

EXHIBIT 4-1 Amendment XIV. Section 1

No state shall make or enforce any law which shall abridge the privileges or immunities of citizens of the United States; nor shall any state deprive any person of life, liberty, or property, without due process of law; nor deny to any person within its jurisdiction the equal protection of the laws.

TABLE 4–1   Bill of Rights Protections Applicable to Public Health

Amendment	Protections	Example
1	Guarantees freedom of speech, religion, and assembly.	People can be exempted from vaccines for religious reasons.
4	Guards against unreasonable search and seizure.	There must be a reason for inspections of facilities.
5	Guarantees protection against deprivation of life, liberty, or property without "due process of law."	The government must fairly compensate landowners for property taken or restricted for public health benefit. People at risk of spreading disease cannot be confined nor have their movements restricted without appropriate notice and an opportunity for a hearing.

EXHIBIT 4-2

> The basis of "preemption" is the Supremacy Clause of the U.S. Constitution (Article VI, clause 2).

EXHIBIT 4-3

> In the century following the *Jacobson v. Massachusetts* decision, the case has been cited in 69 Supreme Court cases and numerous lower court cases to justify governmental action to protect the public's health.

PRINCIPLES OF PUBLIC HEALTH LAW

Governmental Authority to Protect the Public's Health

A key principle of public health law is the need to maintain constitutional balance—that is, the responsibility to promote the public good while protecting individual liberties. This concept—and the entire field of public health law—came into focus in the early 1900s. The state of Massachusetts had enacted a law empowering municipal boards of health to require vaccinations if necessary for the public's health or safety. A few years later, in response to a smallpox outbreak in the Boston area, the Cambridge Board of Health ordered all inhabitants of the city to be vaccinated against the disease. Reverend Henning Jacobson refused to get vaccinated, claiming that "a compulsory vaccination law is unreasonable, arbitrary and oppressive, and, therefore, hostile to the inherent right of every free-man to care for his own body and health in such way as to him seems best." (*Jacobson v. Massachusetts*, 197 U.S. 11 (1905))

A trial court convicted Jacobson and sentenced him to pay a fine of $5. This decision was upheld by the Massachusetts Supreme Judicial Court and subsequently by the U.S. Supreme Court (on February 20, 1905). Presiding Justice Harlan stated, "The safety and the health of the people of Massachusetts are for that Commonwealth to guard and protect. The legislature has the right to pass laws which... are adapted to prevent the spread of contagious diseases."[7]

Jacobson v. Massachusetts is widely regarded as the most important judicial decision in public health. The opinion written by Justice Harlan acknowledged the authority of state governments to set public health policy, while also setting standards to safeguard individual freedoms (see Exhibit 4-3).

While the principle of *Jacobson v. Massachusetts* is still relevant, for a comparable public health action today there is more critical attention to the demonstration of substantial risk to the public's health and more elaborated expectations regarding due process. A 1999 review of the use of governmental police power in public health described the increasing scrutiny by courts of the justifications for a coercive action and of the procedures followed. The authors concluded, "Reaching an acceptable balance between the rights of society and those of individuals is the central issue facing public health

in the next millennium, and the police power is at the center of this balance."[6] Examples of the police power authority in public health today include the power to compel persons to comply with treatment for tuberculosis (which may involve placing people under legal detention); requirements to complete vaccination for school attendance; requirements for providers to report cases of specified diseases to the health department; the authority to require licensing and inspections of food establishments; and, the authority to remove or restrict access to substances or premises that are hazardous to health. At the state level police powers are more often exercised for environmental issues such as drinking water, recreational waters (ponds, beaches, lakes), food sources and facilities, chemical and radiological sources, and sewage disposal. While the legacy of "Typhoid Mary" (and her subsequent incarceration and isolation) may be an extreme form of the police power in public health that is no longer practiced, governmental public health authorities still maintain a considerable legal mandate to act in order to protect the public's health.

Types of Authority

The actions of a public health department are authorized by one (or a combination) of three categories of powers:

▸ *"Broad powers.* These are usually general legislative statements granting agencies the authority to carry out their functions or missions. Also known as general grants of power or enabling legislation, broad powers allow a department to flexibly respond to problems.
▸ *Specified powers* grant specific and limited powers to agencies. Specified powers reflect the legislature's determination to direct a department to achieve specific goals and to limit changes in policy based on the circumstance.
▸ *Contingent powers* may be invoked only when triggered by a specific event. Many emergency powers are of this type, dependent upon the occurrence of certain types of events or declarations of public health emergency."

Administrative law is the body of law created by administrative agencies through rules, regulations, orders, and decisions. Through the development of rules and regulations, agencies provide details regarding standards, procedures, and penalties that enable statues to be translated into action. An administrative or a public health official may use various tools to enforce the department's authority. These administrative enforcement tools are specifically authorized by statutes or regulations. These enforcement tools may include administrative orders, court orders, or civil penalties such as fines or revoking the license of an establishment.

Due Process and Equal Protection

The constitutional requirements of due process and equal protection apply to any governmental action that affects liberty or property. Public health programs generally have established explicit and detailed rules and protocols that define the standards and the procedures for taking an action that limits someone's freedom in any way or that affects property. There are two components of due process:

▸ **Substantive Due Process:** Determination that governmental action is justified and appropriate, that the action serves a compelling public interest, such as public health and safety.
▸ **Procedural Due Process:** Defining required steps for how a government may proceed in an action.

Typically, a person is entitled to notice and an opportunity to present his case before the government may take any action that adversely affects a right. In most cases, an individual would also have a right to be represented by legal counsel and the right to a translator. There would usually also be provisions for an appeals process if the individual would like to challenge the action that is proposed or has been taken.

Although the general standard is that due process is implemented prior to taking an action, laws and regulations recognize some emergency situations in which immediate action may be justified. In such a case, the individual affected would still have rights of substantive and procedural due process that should be implemented as soon as reasonably possible after the event. In recent years, most states have updated their quarantine and isolation laws and procedures, providing explicit and multistep due process, while also defining standards for cases in which immediate action would be justified, with due process then provided typically no later than 72 hours after the action. As an example, if a health department learns that a person in an infectious state with a particularly serious form of tuberculosis is proposing to fly on a commercial airline, it may be necessary and appropriate to take immediate action such as notifying the airline that the person should not fly, or restricting him to his home. The patient should be provided an opportunity for an appropriate hearing no later than the time specified by that state's laws.

The concept of "least restrictive alternative" has developed from the requirement for substantive due process. This means that governmental action should be no broader or longer than what is needed to address a compelling public interest. In the example of the highly infectious tuberculosis patient, while he could not be permitted to get on a commercial airplane, he would not need to be forcibly confined to a hospital or medical unit if he agrees to stay in his house and his compliance could be monitored. Similarly, a restaurant with a nonfunctioning steam table may not need to be closed down if there are other foods they could continue to sell safely.

Another key concept to ensure that governmental action is reasonable and fair is that of equal protection. This requires that people in similar situations be treated similarly. If groups are treated differently, there must be a credible and substantive reason. There have been many cases in which the courts overturned a governmental action because it failed to provide equal protection. A 1900 San Francisco case is fairly typical: The board of health imposed quarantine during a bubonic plague outbreak on a 12-block district that was home to more than 15,000 residents. Because the quarantine restrictions were enforced almost exclusively against persons of Chinese origin, the court held that this was discriminatory.[8]

Property

Governmental public health agencies, including health departments, generally have powers to take, destroy, or restrict property use if necessary to protect the public's health. When facing pandemic influenza, a public health department might have to commandeer medical equipment, supplies, or facilities. In other situations, a department might have to close buildings; prohibit access to contaminated land; confiscate and destroy property, including food, animals, and crops; or regulate property use. As previously noted, a department must ensure due process before depriving individuals of their property interest.

Private property is also protected under the Takings Clause of the Fifth Amendment of the U.S. Constitution, which states: "nor shall private property be taken without just compensation." A governmental department may have to compensate the property owner for actions related to property, but that would not be required in most instances when this is in response to a threat to the public's health. As an example, the government does not need to pay the owner when restricting the use of dangerous property such as a taco cart whose operator knowingly sells contaminated food, a meth-contaminated vehicle or building, or an unvaccinated stray dog that has bitten people. A health department may close a facility as a public nuisance if it is unsafe after a fire, earthquake, or storm. However, the owner should be paid fair market value of the property when using private property for a governmental purpose, such as taking over a hotel to use as a quarantine or isolation facility during a pandemic. In all these instances, the requirements for substantive and procedural due process would apply, as well as those of equal protection.

Civil Versus Criminal Law in Public Health

Legal issues relevant to public health are typically civil law actions, such as issuing fines or taking an action related to property. However, occasionally public health may be involved in criminal cases, such as child abuse or otherwise willfully causing harm. Involvement in criminal cases may also arise when there has been forceful interference with public health officials in the conduct of their duties, such as threatening or attempting to bribe a restaurant inspector. While due process applies in both civil and criminal cases, an individual usually has more rights in a criminal case. For example, in civil cases individuals generally do not have the right to appointed counsel, and public health officials do not need probable cause to search property. By contrast, because in criminal cases, individuals are at risk of losing more constitutionally protected rights and liberties (e.g., freedom from confinement), people have the right to appointed counsel, and a search warrant based on probable cause may be needed to search property.

Other Legal Issues in Public Health Practice

Governmental agencies are complex enterprises that may encounter many other legal requirements and issues that relate to the basic rules of conducting business. Some of these are the execution and enforcement of a wide array of contracts, laws pertaining to the management of human resources, and property liability. While beyond the scope of the current discussion, these are important topics for public health officials and their legal counsel.

To some extent, the legal counsel for a public health department functions as part of the public health system. Some of the resources noted at the end of this chapter discuss the roles of legal counsel and how to work effectively with them. An important legal principle is that of Attorney-Client Privilege. An attorney cannot share a client's information with others unless it is necessary to prevent an imminent harm to one or more other people. (The most common example is that of a credible threat against another person that is voiced to legal counsel.) This is a traditional legal right that assures that information provided by an individual while talking with legal counsel will remain confidential and cannot be "discovered" during litigation.

PRIVACY LAWS

Overview

Federal, state, and local laws dictate how information can be collected and shared during public health surveillance and investigation activities, which are most frequently conducted by epidemiology, food safety, or other environmental health programs. Two key federal privacy laws are the Health Insurance Portability and Accountability Act (HIPAA)[9] and the Family Education Rights and Privacy Act (FERPA).[10] Public health departments also must be aware of other federal, state, or local laws that may be more restrictive or may apply in special circumstances, such as mental health or substance abuse treatment.

HIPAA

The Health Insurance Portability and Accountability Act (HIPAA) is a federal law that protects patient health data and plays a large role in how an organization must handle an individual's health information. Using its administrative authority, under HIPAA the Department of Health and Human Services (DHHS) created a set of national privacy standards for health information, known as the HIPAA Privacy Rule (see Exhibit 4-4). These standards provide patients with more control over how their personal health information (PHI) is used and disclosed, and create an obligation for health care organizations to protect this personal data. The HIPAA Privacy Rule may affect how a public health department can conduct, process, and collect information from other providers or institutions required to protect personal information. However, there are important exceptions to the HIPAA Privacy Rule that permit activities for public health purposes that would otherwise be restricted.

EXHIBIT 4-4 Disclosing Information

The Privacy Rule requires that a covered entity use, disclose, or request the minimum amount of personal health information necessary to meet the intended purpose.

EXHIBIT 4-5   Personal Identifiers include

1. Names
2. Geographic identifiers smaller than a state, with limited exceptions
3. Dates (except year) if directly related to an individual; and all ages over 89
4. Phone numbers, fax numbers
5. Email addresses
6. Social Security numbers
7. Medical record numbers
8. Health plan beneficiary numbers
9. Account numbers
10. Certificate/license numbers
11. Vehicle identifiers
12. Any other unique identifying number or characteristic

Protected Information

The Privacy Rule only protects the use and disclosure of certain types of information. This information is called protected health information (PHI). PHI includes all information that can be connected to a specific person (personal identifiers) and is related to

▸ Physical and mental health conditions
▸ Provision of health care
▸ Payment for health care

If any of the listed identifiers are associated with medical information, they will trigger protections required by HIPAA's Privacy Rule. Recognized identifiers include names, telephone numbers, email addresses, Social Security numbers, medical record numbers, and health plan beneficiary numbers (see Exhibit 4-5).

Covered Entities

HIPAA's Privacy Rule applies to "covered entities," as defined in the law. The following groups are generally considered covered entities:

▸ *Health plans.* Individual or group plans that provide or pay the cost of medical care (there are exceptions to this).
▸ *Health care providers.* Medical or health services (physicians, hospitals, clinics, dentists).
▸ *Health care clearinghouses.* Billing services, repricing companies, and community health information systems.

Whether a public health department or specific program is a covered entity can be a complicated question. Failure to comply with HIPAA's Privacy Rule can have severe civil, criminal, and monetary consequences. Breaches of privacy can also damage the credibility of a public health department or program. In addition, there may be state and local privacy laws that restrict the use of information gathered by a health department.

Privacy Requirements

Generally, covered entities cannot share protected health information. However, this rule is subject to specific exceptions. There are two cases when covered entities *must* disclose protected health information:

▸ When the person (to whom the information belongs) asks for their information
▸ When DHHS investigates a covered entity's compliance with the Privacy Rule

In addition, there may be state or local laws that require disclosing health information for reporting of notifiable conditions or for other public health purposes. There are also several instances when covered entities can disclose or use protected health information without the person's written consent. Permitted disclosures include:

▸ Exceptions for public health activities
▸ Judicial and administrative proceedings
▸ Victims of abuse, neglect, or domestic violence
▸ Law enforcement under certain circumstances
▸ Research data

There are strict guidelines to each of the permitted exceptions. One should always consult with counsel or a designated HIPAA expert when dealing with a disclosure.

Common Exceptions

The following two permitted exceptions are most relevant to public health programs:

▸ *Public health exception.* This is the provision that allows hospitals, laboratories, and doctors to share PHI related to reportable illnesses with public health agencies or officials. If a health care provider is unaware of privacy laws and exceptions, it may be necessary to provide a reference on the public health exception for HIPAA or refer them to the relevant state codes.
▸ *Judicial and administrative proceedings exception.* A public health department may be ordered to provide PHI gathered during an investigation. This might occur during a judicial hearing, or in response to a subpoena, request for discovery, or other legal process. In either of these situations, most agencies will consult with legal counsel. Only the information explicitly requested in the particular case should be disclosed. All other information remains protected health information.

FERPA—Investigation in Schools

The Family Education Rights and Privacy Act (FERPA) is a federal law that protects the privacy of student education records, which can lead to difficulties when investigating disease outbreaks or health hazards in a school setting or among students. FERPA applies to educational agencies and institutions that receive funds under any program administered by the U.S. Department of Education. This includes most public schools and school districts. Although records kept by the school could provide useful information in the investigation, the records kept by a nurse or other school employee are protected. The records can be accessed by obtaining written parental consent. The right to control access to the records transfers to the student when the student becomes 18 years of age or attends a school beyond the high school level.

There are also certain instances when educational records can be shared without written consent. Deidentified information is not protected under FERPA. Deidentification requires the educational institution or agency to remove all personally identifiable information (such as from records kept by the nurse). Then the agency must make a reasonable determination that the student's identity is safe, while taking into account previous information released by the agency or school and information available from other sources.

FERPA also allows limited disclosure without consent in connection with a health or safety emergency. The personally identifiable information may be disclosed to appropriate parties, during an emergency, when the information is necessary to protect the health and safety of the student or others. Though this exception has a narrow interpretation, there may be an argument that this exception applies during a disease outbreak, depending on the circumstances.

LEGAL COUNSEL FOR PUBLIC HEALTH DEPARTMENTS

For state and local public health departments, an important part of their work is addressing legal issues related to the health of their communities. The responsibility for public health department engagement with laws and regulations has been articulated in a number of descriptions of public health services. The widely referenced 10 Essential Public Health Services includes as Essential Service 6: "Enforce laws and regulations that protect health and ensure safety."[11] The accreditation standards developed by the Public Health Accreditation Board define the expectations for processes and capacities of public health departments for the enforcement of public health laws in the provisions of Domain 6.

As described in more detail elsewhere (particularly in Chapters 8–10), state public health departments typically are responsible for a large number and great diversity of programs. The routine work of many state public health programs may include legal activities such as administrative or judicial hearings, developing regulations, or updating laws and standards. This is typical of programs such as those that are regulatory or that involve licensing or certifying credentials. For many other state public health programs, engaging with the legal or legislative systems may occur less frequently, but it is seen by public health officials and by their communities as a key responsibility and opportunity.

As more fully discussed in Chapter 9, local health departments (LHDs) vary tremendously in size, resources, and types of programs. Although there are relatively few very large (serving more than one million people) local or regional public health departments, these may be similar to state public health departments in the number of programs and scope of responsibility, and also may be similar in frequency and types of engagement with legal issues. The majority of LHDs, with modest numbers of staff and programs, also need the capacity to identify and engage with legal issues, although this may be applied much less frequently.

To meet their responsibilities, state and local public health departments will often involve legal counsel, in addition to drawing on the knowledge and experience of program staff. In recent years, surveys were conducted for state public health departments and separately for LHDs to collect information about the roles and the types of arrangements for legal counsel.[12,13]

The survey results described similar roles for legal counsel for state and for local health departments. The main activities include:

- Provide formal opinions on laws, statutes, regulations, enforcement policies, and enforcement actions
- Assist in drafting laws, regulations, enforcement policies, and enforcement actions
- Provide informal advice on the legality or constitutionality of various laws, statutes, regulations, and policies
- Represent the department in legal matters
- Determine when to litigate or prosecute for violation of statutes and regulations.

States may draw their legal counsel from many different sources, and in practice they often draw from different sources for different kinds of legal actions. For example, it is common to use agency-based counsel for routine enforcements and for drafting regulations, but to use either different state legal counsel or outside contract attorneys for litigation, or for certain kinds of very technical actions. As shown in Table 4–2 below, almost two-thirds of state health departments have their own

TABLE 4–2   Legal Counsel Arrangements for Local and State Health Departments

Legal Counsel Arrangements	All LHDs*	SHDs**
Attorneys and legal staff assigned by local government	66%	4%
Attorneys and legal staff assigned by state health agency	23%	NA
Contracts with outside attorneys and legal staff	15%	9%
Employs own attorneys and legal staff	9%	62%
Attorneys and legal staff assigned by state Attorney General	9%	51%
Other arrangement	4%	9%
No legal counsel	1%	0%

* Local Health Departments. LHD data from the National Association of County and City Health Officials Profile of Local Health Departments, 2012. LHD percentages reflect weighting to produce national estimates.

** State Health Departments. SHD data from the Association of State and Territorial Health Officials Profile Survey, 2012. Agencies could select more than one option, thus totals are greater than 100%.

legal division that employs attorneys. Local health departments that serve large populations and those in decentralized states more frequently reported that they have their own legal division. Just over 50 percent of state health departments report that they use attorneys and legal staff assigned by the state attorney general.

As shown in Table 4–2, counsel for LHDs are derived from the same sources as those of state departments, but LHDs are much more likely to use attorneys assigned by the local jurisdiction, and are much less likely to have attorneys employed by the department who serve as legal counsel. A more detailed breakout of the local data shows some variation with the size of the health department. For example, 19 percent of the largest LHDs (those serving a population of more than half a million) employ legal counsel within the department, while 11 percent of moderately sized LHDs (serving populations of 50,000–499,000) employ legal counsel. It is also common for LHDs to obtain legal counsel from the state, either from the state public health department (23 percent) or assigned by the state attorney general (9 percent). Moderately sized LHDs are somewhat more likely (14 percent) to obtain legal counsel by assignment by the state attorney general.

The effective use of law on behalf of the public's health can be a powerful tool to protect and promote health. However, many legal counsel and many public health officials may not come to their roles fully prepared to understand and use public health law or to work together effectively. As Kaufman and colleagues note:

Typically, legal counsel for health departments are not formally trained in public health.

Schools of law offer limited or no teaching of public health law, and faculty lack the specific training to do so. Most law schools offer courses in health law, but few offer public health law courses that examine the role law plays in keeping our communities healthy….The same can be said of most M.P.H. students who are not required to take a public health law course as part of their training.[14]

Fortunately, the increasing attention in recent years to the field of public health law has resulted in the development of training and other resources that are available to strengthen the knowledge and skills of public health professionals and their legal counsel.

RESOURCES ABOUT PUBLIC HEALTH LAW

In recent years, there has been an increase in academic and practitioner interest in the field of public health law. In response to the terrorism events of 2001, the focus was particularly on public health laws related to emergencies, but attention has since expanded to consideration of the broad range of ways that law can protect and promote the public's health. As previously noted, in 2011 the Institute of Medicine produced a full study entitled *"For the Public's Health: Revitalizing Law and Policy to Meet New Challenges,"* describing the importance and urging renewed attention of the role of law for public health. There are now a number of centers that teach, conduct research, or provide training regarding public health law and that serve as resources for public health or legal practitioners seeking information about current, emerging, or potential public health laws and policies. Three of these valuable resources are the Public Health Law Program at the Centers for Disease Control and Prevention (CDC), the Network for Public Health Law, and the national program for Public Health Law Research. Some additional sources for training and teaching are also briefly noted below.

The Public Health Law Program at the CDC "works to improve the health of the public by developing law-related tools and providing legal technical assistance to public health practitioners and policy makers in state, tribal, local, and territorial (STLT) jurisdictions."[15] The program's offerings include a newsletter (*Public Health Law News*), articles and reports, bench books (guidance used by judges), draft memoranda of understanding, issue briefs, toolkits, and trainings. The program also provides consultation that may include identification of laws that impact the public's health and comparative analysis of laws across jurisdictions.

The Network for Public Health Law, supported by the Robert Wood Johnson Foundation, consists of public health attorneys and practitioners located at a National Coordinating Center and five Regional Centers. The Network "provides insightful legal assistance, helpful resources and opportunities to build connections for local, tribal, state and federal officials; public health practitioners; attorneys; policy makers; and advocates."[16] Each of the centers has specialized expertise in some key areas of public health law, but the network is structured so that each center serves as a single entry point to access the experts affiliated with any part of the Network. The Network has an extensive collection of information that is readily available, including fact sheets, issues briefs, and a newsletter. It also provides technical assistance in response to requests from public health practitioners or attorneys. A particular emphasis of the Network is to provide prompt and practical information and analysis about urgent or emerging legal issues through publications and webinars.

The national program for Public Health Law Research (PHLR), based at Temple University in Philadelphia and also supported by the Robert Wood Johnson Foundation, "is dedicated to building the evidence base for laws that improve public health. PHLR funds research, improves research methods, and makes evidence more accessible to policy makers, the media, and the public."[17] The overall goal of the program's activities is to support and develop research to identify effective regulatory, legal and policy solutions that improve public health, and to promote the awareness and increased use of evidence-based legal approaches. The program's resources include a research library organized by topics, and the LawAtlas, which is "an online platform developed by PHLR as a model resource for the systematic collection, measurement and display of statutes, regulations, court decisions and other legal policies that matter to health."[18] The program, along with partner organizations, is also involved in tracking the trends and characteristics of laws, or "policy surveillance."

Additional public health law resources for public health practitioners and their counsel include:

General Resources

▷ Change Lab Solutions, http://changelabsolutions.org/

▷ O'Neill Institute for National and Global Health Law, http://www.law.georgetown.edu/oneillinstitute/

▷ Association of State and Territorial Health Officials, Emergency Law toolkits, http://www.astho.org/ (Go to the site and search under "toolkits")

▷ National Association of County and City Health Officials, Public Health Law, http://www.naccho.org (Access the site and follow the links from *Programs* to *Public Health Infrastructure and Systems*)

▷ Northwest Center for Public Health Practice, University of Washington School of Public Health, https://www.nwcphp.org
  - Public Health Law Training Database - Access the site and search under "Public health law training database".
  - Public Health Law Training Project - Access the site and search under "Public health law training project"; includes several training modules, resources, and toolkits
  - Practical Law for Public Health Officials (online training module) – Access the site and search under "Practical law for public health officials"

▷ L. O. Gostin, Public Health Law: Power, Duty, Restraint, 2nd ed. (Berkeley: University of California Press, New York: Milbank Memorial Fund, 2008).

▷ RA Goodman, *et al.* Law in Public Health Practice, 2nd ed. (Oxford University Press, New York, 2007).

SUMMARY

Public health law has been an important component of achieving major advances in public health in the past, and continues to be an important responsibility of public health departments and community organizations for advancing the public's health. Federal, state, and local laws and regulations form an interconnected system, with distinctive roles but also some overlap of jurisdiction. Several provisions of the U.S. Constitution are important as the source of state and local public health authority, and also define principles that limit governmental actions against individuals and property. Key constitutional principles for public health action include substantive and procedural due process, equal protection, and protection of property rights by the Takings Clause.

Public health departments have an obligation to protect information about individuals under federal privacy laws, particularly HIPAA and FERPA. However, the public health exception in HIPAA allows public health departments to obtain or use certain types of individual information that would otherwise be protected.

Legal counsel are important partners for effective use of the law by public health departments. State and local departments have many different types of arrangements for obtaining legal counsel, with most state public health departments having internal legal staff or divisions, and most LHDs using counsel assigned by the local government. Few attorneys and few public health officials have had specific training in public health law; however, the field of public health law has been receiving more attention in recent years, and there are opportunities for training and technical assistance that can strengthen the knowledge and skills of public health and legal practitioners. Effective public health practitioners use the law not only for reacting to risks and hazards to the public's health, but also to shape new laws that can further promote the public's health.

REVIEW QUESTIONS

1. Considering two of the 10 Great Public Health Achievements presented in Chapter 1, what were the contributions of laws or regulations to the control of infectious diseases and motor-vehicle safety? (A useful exercise would be to consider the role of laws in the remaining eight Great Achievements.)

2. How would procedural and substantive due process apply when proposing to isolate a seriously ill tuberculosis patient who refused to take medications or to stay away from public places?

3. You are investigating what appears to be a serious foodborne disease outbreak at a well-known local restaurant. What information about the sick people and the restaurant could reasonably be released to news reporters?

4. Your legal counsel tells you that he would prefer that the health department maternity clinic be closed, because it creates too much legal liability for the local government. How could you respond?

5. A new form of a very contagious and severe respiratory disease has hit communities in several U.S. states. It appears that this disease originated in another country, and several other countries are taking extreme measures to control the disease. Describe the federal, state, and local public health roles in responding to the situation.

REFERENCES

1. Goodman R, Moulton A, Matthews G, *et al.* Law and Public Health at CDC. *MMWR. Morbidity and Mortality Weekly Report.* 2006;55:29–33.

2. Institute of Medicine Committee on Public Health Strategies to Improve Health. *For the Public's Health: Revitalizing Law and Policy to Meet New Challenges.* National Academies Press; Washington DC; 2011.

3. Hernandez LM, Rosenstock L, Gebbie K. *Who will Keep the Public Healthy?: Educating Public Health Professionals for the 21st Century.* National Academies Press: Washington, DC; 2003.

4. Public Health Accreditation Board. Public Health Accreditation Board Standards and Measures, version 1.5. 2013; http://www.phaboard.org/wp-content/uploads/SM-Version-1.5-Board-adopted-FINAL-01-24-2014.docx.pdf. Accessed December/02, 2014.

5. Centers for Disease Control and Prevention. The National Public Health Performance Standards Program. 2008; http://www.cdc.gov/od/ocphp/nphpsp/. Accessed August/25, 2010.

6. Richards III EP, Rathbun KC. The role of the police power in 21st century public health. *Sexually Transmitted Diseases.* 1999;26(6):350–357.

7. *Jacobson v. Massachusetts,* 197 U.S. 11 (1905).

8. *Jew Ho v Williamson.* 103 F 101900.

9. Health Insurance Portability and Accountability Act of 1996 (HIPAA) Pub. L. No. 104-191, 110 Stat. 1936 (1996).

10. Family Education Rights and Privacy Act 34 CFR Part 99 (1974).

11. U.S. Public Health Service, Public Health Functions Steering Committee. *Public Health in America.* Washington, DC; 1994.

12. National Association of County and City Health Officials. 2013 National Profile of Local Health Departments 2013; http://www.naccho.org/topics/infrastructure/profile/upload/2013-National-Profile-of-Local-Health-Departments-report.pdf. Accessed January 27, 2015.

13. Association of State and Territorial Health Officials. Profile of State Public Health 2010; http://www.astho.org/profiles/. Accessed June/18, 2013. Personal communication of data from the 2012 ASTHO Profile Survey, for Association of State and Territorial Health Officials. ASTHO Profile of State Public Health, Volume Three. Washington, DC: Association of State and Territorial Health Officials. 2014. Personal communication of data from the 2010 Profile questionnaire, for NACCHO (National Association of County and City Health

Officials), 2010 National Profile of Local Health Departments, Washington, DC; 2011.

14. Kaufman N, Allan S, Ibrahim J. Using public health legal counsel effectively: Beliefs, barriers and opportunities for training. *J Law Med Ethics.* Mar 2013;41 (Suppl 1):61–64.

15. Public Health Law Program, Centers for Disease Control and Prevention, http://www.cdc.gov/phlp/about.html. Accessed December 20, 2014.

16. Network for Public Health Law, https://www.networkforphl.org/about_the_network. Accessed December 21, 2014.

17. Public Health Law Research, http://publichealth-lawresearch.org. Accessed January 22, 2015.

18. The Policy Surveillance Portal, LawAtlas, http://LawAtlas.org. Accessed January 24, 2014.

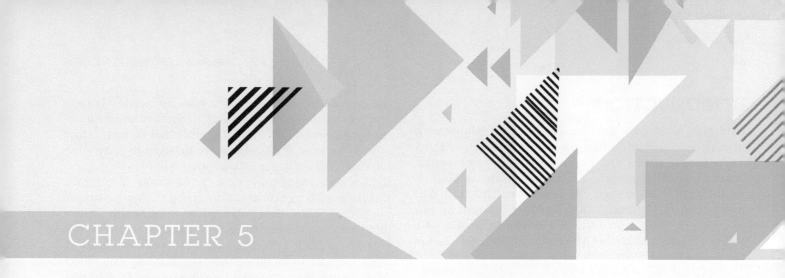

CHAPTER 5

Public Health Ethics

James C. Thomas, MPH, PhD

LEARNING OBJECTIVES

Upon completion of this chapter, the reader will be able to:

1. Distinguish public health ethics from medical ethics.
2. Provide an orientation to ethical foundations in public health research.
3. Describe the contributions of utilitarianism and human rights to the ethics of public health practice.
4. Identify core values underlying public health ethics.
5. Describe the steps in ethical decision making.
6. Identify resources for encouraging the ethical practice of public health.
7. Contextualize public health ethics in contemporary public health.

KEY TERMS

45 CFR 46
applied ethics
Belmont Report
bioethics
common rule
human rights
informed consent
institutional review boards (IRBs)
medical ethics
morally defensible decision
public health ethics
public health practice
research
Siracusa principles
tyranny of the majority
Universal Declaration of Human Rights
utilitarianism
vulnerable individuals

INTRODUCTION

In 2012, New York City mayor Michael Bloomberg proposed a city-wide ban on soft drinks larger than 16 ounces, citing the negative role of sweetened drinks in public health. The city's Board of Health unanimously approved the limit, but the state Supreme Court declared it illegal before it could be implemented.[1,2] Critics of the law invoked the idea of a "Nanny State" restricting the rights of individuals for their own good.

This debate embodies the key questions in public health ethics. How do we balance the rights of individuals against the good of the community? What are the respective rights and obligations of the government and private industry? This chapter describes how public health ethics fits in the broader ethics landscape, the principles of public health ethics that guide discussions, and issues that remain to be addressed.

THE ETHICS LANDSCAPE

A basic question to start with is whether ethics is another word for morality. Are they the same thing? The short answer is, basically, yes. The longer answer is that some people think of morality as being more practical and based in action, and ethics as being more theoretical. More narrowly, the term morality has been used frequently in religious contexts, often around issues of sex and sexuality. To philosophers, however, the term moral philosophy is virtually synonymous with ethics. In this chapter, the term ethics will refer to both theory and practice.

At a university, the philosophy department will primarily teach ethical theory while professional schools, such as medicine, engineering, business, law, journalism, and public health, will teach applied ethics. Ethical theory includes concepts such as deontology (ethics based on a sense of duty) and consequentialism (ethics based on fairness of outcomes), and schools of thought such as utilitarianism, virtue ethics, and human rights. Applied ethics is concerned with prescribed actions or policies in ethical situations commonly encountered in a particular profession. Of course, applied ethics is rooted in ethical theory and ethical theories arise from practical situations. So, the differences are in terms of emphasis and what people spend most of their time thinking about.

Research versus Practice

Applied ethics can be further divided into research and practice. In the case of public health, research is defined as the intent to obtain knowledge that can be generalized to settings and populations other than the ones from which the data were collected.[3] For example, an epidemiologic study of factors affecting the transmission of HIV may be published in a scientific journal because the findings are thought to clarify the infection and epidemic in ways that will benefit populations around the country or even the world. In contrast, public health practice is concerned with a particular population. Thus, data collected by a city health department on the occurrence of HIV infections is not considered research as long as the disease surveillance is intended only to facilitate the planning and evaluation of programs to control the transmission of HIV in that city. If the surveillance data are later used to understand transmission in a way that is applicable to other cities, the use of the data becomes research and additional ethical guidelines, discussed below, are brought to bear.

Distinctions between Medical and Public Health Ethics

Among the health-related professions, the articulation of ethics in public health is a very recent development.[4] While the American Medical Association adopted a code of ethics in 1847, a code of ethics for public health wasn't adopted until 2002. A reason for this 150-year lag may be that for centuries physicians were considered the experts to turn to for all things related to health. Moreover, public health leadership positions were often filled by physicians. They would naturally refer to the ethical guidelines either received in their training or adopted by the professional (medical) societies to which they belonged. In the last few decades, however, nonmedical professionals, such as health administrators and epidemiologists, have assumed more leadership in public health and have not reflexively turned to the medical community for guidance in ethics (see Exhibit 5-1).

A key reason that nonmedical ethical guidance is needed for public health is that the field of public health presents ethical dilemmas different from those in medicine. The professional situation most commonly giving rise to ethical dilemmas in medicine is the patient-provider interaction. In the clinic room, the physician is in his or her own setting with symbols of status and power such as diplomas on the wall, a white coat and stethoscope, and knowledge of things that can heal the patient. In contrast, the patient is often undressed or scantily covered, in need of healing, and mystified by the pharmaceuticals and tools used by the physician. This setting in which the patient is dependent upon and vulnerable to the physician gives rise to most of the ethical dilemmas faced by physicians. Thus, medical ethics concerns itself with preserving the autonomy of the patient and forbidding the physician from knowingly causing any harm.

The principal setting giving rise to the most common ethical dilemmas in public health is not a one-on-one interaction, but one that is many-on-many; it is the interaction between a health department and the population it serves. Therefore, interactions entail group discussion and democratic processes. Also, public health is often concerned with prevention rather than cure of disease. Thus, it has an extra burden of proof to justify intervening in the life of a person who is already healthy (see Exhibit 5-1).

A fundamental reality of populations is that one person's actions affect others. This is particularly evident with some infectious diseases. For example, a person with influenza can transmit the infection to others and make them sick. Conversely, by staying isolated, the infected person can prevent transmission to others. Out of concern for those who are well, a health department may infringe on the autonomy of individuals, at times through imposed isolation, but also through required vaccination or regulation of industries. The tension between preserving the health of the community and respecting the rights of individuals is the most common ethical dilemma arising in public health (see Figure 5-1).

Bioethics and Public Health Ethics

Although medical and public health ethics arise from different situations, one might think that these two categories of applied ethics would reside together under the big tent of bioethics. Along with them would be nursing ethics, environmental ethics, and any other ethics pertaining to living things. In practice, however, centers, books, and courses on bioethics most often address applications of technology affecting the beginning and end of human life. Common concerns are contraception, abortion, gene therapy, termination of life-support, and the right to health care. All of these topics also dominate medical ethics. Thus, although medical ethics is logically a subcategory of bioethics, in reality the two are nearly synonymous. Some centers for bioethics are branching out to include public health ethics (e.g., the University of Toronto Center for Bioethics), but many view ethics through a medical lens and thus overlook public health.

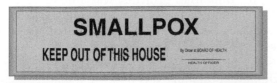

FIGURE 5-1   **Signs Used in Quarantine against Smallpox**

EXHIBIT 5-1 Distinguishing Between Medical Ethics and Public Health Ethics

Key Principles in Medical Ethics
- *Autonomy:* The right of a person to govern himself or herself; the right not to be coerced
- *Nonmaleficence:* The absence of an intent to do harm
- *Beneficence:* To act with the best interests or benefit of the patient
- *Justice:* An equitable distribution of resources and opportunities.

Key Principles in Public Health Ethics
- *Interdependence:* People rely on each other for companionship, safety, and survival. Each person's actions are felt by others.
- *Participation:* Input on public health decision-making processes and policy development from people who will be affected by them.
- *Scientific evidence:* The use of the scientific method to provide a relatively objective means of identifying the factors necessary for health in a population, and for evaluating policies and programs to protect and promote health.

ETHICS IN PUBLIC HEALTH RESEARCH

Research ethics is the component of public health ethics that bears the closest relationship to medical ethics, in part because many public health studies include interactions between a researcher and a respondent, resembling the interactions between a clinician and a patient. The current guidelines for research ethics have their origins in response to medical experiments conducted on German concentration camp internees during the World War II. Following the war, the Nuremberg War Crime Trials led to the creation of the Nuremberg Code in 1947, articulating basic principles for ethical research involving human subjects. The key underlying principle was ensuring that research participation is truly voluntary. Ensuring voluntary participation requires that potential participants be fully aware of what the research entails, including all the likely risks and benefits. The process by which voluntary participation is ensured came to be known as informed consent.

While the principle of informed consent was being articulated in Nuremburg, a study in the United States that did not adhere to this principle was more than 10 years under way. Although conducted by the U.S. Public Health Service, it came to be known as the Tuskegee Study because the Tuskegee Institute, located near the site of the study, was a collaborator. The study aimed to assess the health outcomes of untreated syphilis. The participants were not informed of the true purpose of the study. Instead, they were told they would receive treatments for the infection. However, the "treatments" they received were actually procedures for monitoring the progress of the infection. This deception was possible, in part, because the study subjects were low income, uneducated men from rural Alabama. Much of the medical world was a mystery to them; they simply trusted the word of the highly educated physicians conducting the study.[5]

The deception became even more egregious with the discovery of penicillin in the early 1940s. This cure for syphilis was withheld from the men in the study so the researchers could learn what would happen if syphilis were allowed to follow its natural course. The ethical lapses of the Tuskegee study were compounded by race relations. The researchers were white while the study subjects were black. One might argue that racial attitudes blinded the researchers to the ethical lapses of the study; that is, they held a lower standard for the treatment of poor and uneducated black men. An extension of this argument would be that the Western world recoiled from the medical experiments of the Holocaust in part because the study subjects were white Westerners themselves.

The Tuskegee study of untreated syphilis ended in scandal in 1974. Initially, research ethics were articulated by international bodies. The U.S. government had not fully owned the need for research ethics by developing its own guidelines. This situation was remedied a few years after the end of the Tuskegee Study. The first U.S.-based report on research ethics was published in 1979 by the National Commission for the Protection of Human Subjects of Biomedical and Behavioral Research. Known as the **Belmont Report**, it reinforced and elaborated on the principles of the Nuremberg Code.[6] Three key ethical principles were identified: respect for persons, beneficence, and justice. These principles were then manifested in the practices of informed consent, weighing the risks and benefits to study subjects, and protecting **vulnerable individuals** such as minors, pregnant women, and prisoners.

The practices were codified into federal regulations in 1981. A publication (or "Title") of the Code of Federal Regulations (CFR) addressing human welfare concerns of the Department of Health and Human Services included a section on protection of human subjects. Because it was the 46th section of Title 45, the regulations are referred to as **45 CFR 46**.[7] Also referred to as "The **Common Rule**," they establish the role of **institutional review boards (IRBs)** for research on human subjects. Institutions that receive government funds for research are required to have their research approved by an IRB. Large institutions, such as universities where much research is conducted, typically have several IRBs. Moreover, researchers receiving government funds are now required to receive training in research ethics. This is often done online through a site such as the CITI Program (http://www.citiprogram.org). The training modules teach the viewer about the origins of IRBs, the values that guide them and the processes they follow. Viewers are taught the elements of informed consent and the concerns for vulnerable populations.

The regulated policies of research ethics have helped establish an ethical work environment in research settings. They have brought ethics to the front and center of the minds of researchers. Unfortunately, the required processes are viewed by some researchers as burdensome, consuming time and creating delays in the research. In some instances, the policies are followed mechanically and resentfully. In this way they can deaden one's ethical sensitivity rather than sharpen it. As ethics in public health practice (i.e., apart from research) becomes more institutionalized, one challenge will be to avoid mechanical routinization of tasks and to stimulate ethical sensitivity and skills.

ETHICS IN PUBLIC HEALTH PRACTICE

Ethical principles in public health practice have not been developed along such a well-defined path. And rather than having their origins in the deliberations of international bodies, practice ethics have been country-specific. The following sections include descriptions of the ethical schools of thought relevant to public health practice and the values and beliefs inherent to a public health perspective.

Schools of Ethical Thought Relevant to Public Health Practice

The ethical principles in public health, as well as the values and beliefs, do not come from one particular philosophy or ethical school of thought. Rather, several philosophies are prominent in public health ethics.[8] The two most dominant are **utilitarianism** and **human rights**.

Writing in England at the turn of the nineteenth century, Jeremy Bentham articulated the principle of "the greatest happiness of the greatest number,"[9] typically understood today as "the greatest good for the greatest number." With public health's orientation to populations, the utilitarian principle was a natural fit for its ethical deliberations, and is manifested today in such policy-making tools as the ranking of diseases by incidence and the prioritization of programs by cost-benefit analyses.

Utilitarian thinking was influential among the Philosophic Radicals in Great Britain in the early nineteenth century.[10] This group included early epidemiologists, biostatisticians, and one of the most prominent of the public health reformers, Edwin Chadwick. An intellectual and great admirer of Bentham, Chadwick was appointed as secretary of the Royal Commission to inquire into the Poor Laws of England. Through work on this commission, Chadwick and others brought attention to the dire health conditions of the new majority in the population, the urban working class, with the publication in 1842 of the pivotal public health document, the "Report . . . on an inquiry into the Sanitary Condition of the Labouring Population of Great Britain."[10] Using the emerging sciences of epidemiology and statistics, this report identified conditions such as polluted water supplies and filthy living conditions that were associated with epidemic diseases observed in Great Britain at the time.[11] Thus, a public health approach that identified the conditions associated with the most prevalent diseases found a natural ally in a utilitarian perspective that also argued for those actions that would benefit the majority of the population.

One of the limitations of utilitarianism is the need for data to enable decisions. In a cost-benefit analysis, for example, one is often missing important information on either the costs or the benefits. Conversely, in some situations, the amount of data available can overwhelm the ability to consider it all. In either situation, too little or too much information, the result can be inaction.

Another limitation is that, although its egalitarianism and principle of maximization place the majority in the spotlight, bringing attention to the problems of the "masses," a simple utilitarian outlook risks pushing out of the spotlight those not in the majority. In a utilitarian calculus, each individual becomes a unit and his or her concerns are folded in with those of others, yielding a sum or average that lacks a human face. In this way, the experience of one individual can get swept aside by the momentum of larger numbers. When state laws sanction this "tyranny of the majority," it can have devastating consequences: examples include slavery and eugenics.

It was in reaction to the eugenic atrocities of the Third Reich's Holocaust that the **Universal Declaration of Human Rights** was drafted in 1948 as a statement of the minimum protection and benefits due to each human being (see Exhibit 5-2). Half a decade after the Holocaust, the inadequacy of a utilitarian perspective is evident again in the AIDS pandemic. The overwhelming suffering caused by AIDS has disproportionately affected those in resource-poor areas of the world[12] and groups that have been traditionally marginalized and disenfranchised in resource-rich countries.[13] In neither situation are those with AIDS the people who control the distribution of goods in resource-rich countries. Nor are people living with AIDS around the world likely to figure prominently in a utilitarian

EXHIBIT 5-2 Article 25 of the Universal Declaration of Human Rights

> Everyone has the right to a standard of living adequate for the health and well-being of himself and of his family, including food, clothing, housing and medical care and necessary social services, and the right to security in the event of unemployment, sickness, disability, widowhood, old age or other lack of livelihood in circumstances beyond his control.

SOURCE: UN General Assembly, *Universal Declaration of Human Rights*, 10 December 1948, 217 A (III)

calculation of maximizing happiness among the populations in resource-rich nations. It was in this context that Dr. Jonathan Mann of the United Nations Global Program on AIDS invoked human rights as an ethical guiding force in public health.[14]

A human rights perspective is important in public health because of the equal dignity and worth it places in each human being.[15] Equal dignity demands a minimum standard of treatment and respect for each person, providing a needed correction to utilitarianism, in which the dignity and worth of a minority can get lost in the desires of the majority. Modern human rights also bring global attention to the determinants of an individual's health and well-being; including liberty, security, self-determination, access to basic health care, education, nutrition, and a clean environment. Their general acceptance around the world also makes human rights a functionally powerful ethical paradigm.

The social, political, and legal natures of human rights, however, are arguably more important than their ability to stand alone as the only ethical paradigm in public health. In some respects a narrow human rights interpretation is at odds with some public health values. Notably modern human rights are principally individualistic, whereas public health is community oriented. Moreover, human rights have traditionally been invoked to redress abuses by a state against its citizens. These appeals to rights represent only one of several conceptions of the relationship between individuals and their state, tending to focus on negative rather than positive interactions.

Although humans are individualistic to some extent, they are also inherently social. Some of the most rewarding and meaningful moments in life are when we care for or nurture another person, and when we receive that care. The word *community*, itself, is rooted in the idea of communing, or sharing things in common. Interdependence and community, rather than independence and individualism, are more central to the values of public health.

Human rights have traditionally been invoked following political and civil abuses by a state against its citizens. Even though one purpose of a government is to enable healthy human interaction, there remains the possibility that it will fail in this function to the point of harming its citizens. There is no doubt that protections and recourse for individuals are needed in this event. However, governments also serve functions that enable, or perhaps even ennoble, people to care for one another. This is seen in part through the redistribution of income and services in the form of taxes, and the creation of public spaces that encourage human interaction. It is this latter role of government that is more akin to public health values.

In addition to interpretations of modern human rights that are not consonant with a public health perspective, a human rights ethic is a tool that is inadequately refined for charting an ethical course for public health. Rights have a binary quality; either they exist or they don't, there are no gradations of a right. Even among those rights that people agree upon, there is no agreement on the relative weight of one right against another when two rights come into conflict. When two rights are not in conflict, there is no guidance as to which should be pursued first or most aggressively. It is in these situations that a utilitarian or data-based approach can be helpful.

Other ethical schools of thought that have been applied in public health are virtue ethics, focusing on the character of the public health professional,[16] and care ethics, with its principal attention to the interdependence of people and our obligations to care for one another.[8] Religiously motivated ethics have also had their influence on public health. For example, the Civil Rights movement, based largely in African American churches, addressed the inequities of segregation, many of which were manifested in racial health disparities.

Values and Beliefs Underlying a Public Health Perspective

In practical ethics, principles are born from common situations in which the practitioners find themselves. They are also rooted in the core beliefs and values of the profession. A belief is something held to be true and a value is something given priority in decision making. Public health is a diverse field, composed of professionals with a wide range of skills, so unanimity in values and beliefs is seldom realized. Nonetheless, there are discernible, dominant shared beliefs and values. They are enumerated in the supporting documents for the Public Health Code of Ethics developed by the Public Health Leadership Society and endorsed by national public health organizations. The values and beliefs are grouped in three topics: health, community, and the bases for action below, extracted from the Code documents (http://www.phls.org/home/section/3-26/).

Health

Humans have a right to the resources necessary for health. The public health code of ethics affirms Article 25 of the Universal Declaration of Human Rights, which states in part, "Everyone has the right to a standard of living adequate for the health and well-being of himself and his family. . . ."

Community

Humans are inherently social and interdependent. Humans look to each other for companionship in friendships, families, and community; and rely upon one another for safety and survival. Positive relationships among individuals and positive collaborations among institutions are signs of a healthy community. The rightful concern for the physical individuality of humans and one's right to make decisions for oneself must be balanced against the fact that each person's actions affects other people.

The effectiveness of institutions depends heavily on the public's trust. Factors that contribute to trust in an institution include the following actions on the part of the institution: communication; truth telling; transparency (i.e., not concealing information); accountability; reliability; and reciprocity. One critical form of reciprocity and communication is listening to as well as speaking with the community.

Collaboration is a key element to public health. The public health infrastructure of a society is composed of a wide variety of agencies and professional disciplines. To be effective, they must work together well. Moreover, new collaborations will be needed to rise to new public health challenges.

People and their physical environment are interdependent. People depend upon the resources of their natural and constructed environments for life itself. A damaged or unbalanced natural environment, and a constructed environment of poor design or in poor condition, will have an adverse effect on the health of people. Conversely, people can have a profound effect on their natural environment through consumption of resources and generation of waste.

Each person in a community should have an opportunity to contribute to public discourse. Contributions to discourse may occur through a direct or a representative system of government. In the process of developing and evaluating policy, it is important to discern whether all who would like to contribute to the discussion have an opportunity to do so, even though expressing a concern does not mean that it will necessarily be addressed in the final policy.

Identifying and promoting the fundamental requirements for health in a community are a primary concern to public health. The way in which a society is structured is reflected in the health of a community. The primary concern of public health is with these underlying structural aspects. While some important public health programs are curative in nature, the field as a whole must never lose sight of underlying causes and prevention. Because fundamental social structures affect many aspects of health, addressing the fundamental causes rather than more proximal causes, is more truly preventive.

Bases for Action

Knowledge is important and powerful. We are to seek to improve our understanding of health and the means of protecting it through research and the accumulation of knowledge. Once obtained, there is a moral obligation in some instances to share what is known. For example, active and informed participation in policy-making processes requires access to relevant information. In other instances, such as information provided in confidence, there is an obligation to protect information.

Science is the basis for much of our public health knowledge. The scientific method provides a relatively objective means of identifying the factors necessary for health in a population, and for evaluating policies and programs to protect and promote health. The full range of scientific tools, including both quantitative and qualitative methods, and collaboration among the sciences is needed.

People are responsible to act on the basis of what they know. Knowledge is not morally neutral and often demands action. Moreover, information is not to be gathered for idle interest. Public health should seek to translate available information into timely action. Often, the action required is research to fill in the gaps of what we *don't* know.

Action is not based on information alone. In many instances, action is required in the absence of all the information one would like. In other instances, policies are demanded by the fundamental value and dignity of each human being, even if implementing them is not calculated to be optimally efficient or cost-beneficial. In both of these situations, values inform the application of information or the action in the absence of information.

Principles in the Ethical Practice of Public Health

The values and beliefs inherent to a public health perspective underlie the 12 principles of the public health code of ethics presented in Exhibit 5-3. Each principle also relates to one or more of the 10 Essential Public Health Services articulated by Public Health Functions Steering Committee. You can view the correspondence between the principles and the services by downloading the code of ethics materials from the Public Health Leadership Society website, http://www.phls.org. The code is a working document. As the world changes, public health professionals will become sensitized to new ethical issues.[17] When gaps in the code arise, it will need to be updated accordingly.

EXHIBIT 5-3 The Public Health Code of Ethics

1) Public health should address principally the fundamental causes of disease and requirements for health, aiming to prevent adverse health outcomes.
2) Public health should achieve community health in a way that respects the rights of individuals in the community.
3) Public health policies, programs, and priorities should be developed and evaluated through processes that ensure an opportunity for input from community members.
4) Public health should advocate and work for the empowerment of disenfranchised community members, aiming to ensure that the basic resources and conditions necessary for health are accessible to all.
5) Public health should seek the information needed to implement effective policies and programs that protect and promote health.
6) Public health institutions should provide communities with the information they have that is needed for decisions on policies or programs and should obtain the community's consent for their implementation.
7) Public health institutions should act in a timely manner on the information they have within the resources and the mandate given to them by the public.
8) Public health programs and policies should incorporate a variety of approaches that anticipate and respect diverse values, beliefs, and cultures in the community.
9) Public health programs and policies should be implemented in a manner that most enhances the physical and social environment.
10) Public health institutions should protect the confidentiality of information that can bring harm to an individual or community if made public. Exceptions must be justified on the basis of the high likelihood of significant harm to the individual or others.
11) Public health institutions should ensure the professional competence of their employees.
12) Public health institutions and their employees should engage in collaborations and affiliations in ways that build the public's trust and the institution's effectiveness.

SOURCE: Thomas JC, Sage M, Dillenberg J, Guillory VJ. A code of ethics for public health. *Am J Public Health.* 2002;92(7):1057–1059

The code of ethics is not the only place that ethical principles in public health have been articulated. Following the international epidemic of sudden acute respiratory syndrome (SARS) in 2002, and in anticipation of a pandemic of influenza, a number of groups have identified ethical principles for the distribution of scarce resources, social distancing to limit transmission, keeping the public informed, the obligations and rights of health care staff who care for the ill, and more. The World Health Organization Project on Addressing Ethical Issues in Pandemic Influenza Planning identified four principles for public health measures:[18]

1. *Public health necessity.* A government should exercise its public health police powers on an individual or group only if the person or group poses a threat to the community, such as the likelihood of spreading an infection.

2. *Reasonable and effective means.* The methods by which a threat is addressed should have a reasonable chance of being effective.

3. *Proportionality.* The human burden imposed by a public health regulation should be proportionate to the expected public health benefit.

4. *Distributive justice.* The risks, benefits, and burdens of public health action should be fairly distributed, thereby precluding the unjustified targeting of an already socially vulnerable population.

Speaking about the tension in public health between the rights of individuals and the good of the community, this group noted The *Siracusa Principles*, a set of principles regarding internationally recognized limitations on human rights, established at a meeting in Siracusa, Italy.[19] The four principles for restricting rights for the benefit of the community are as follows: (1) the restriction is provided for and carried out in accordance with the law, (2) the restriction is in the interest of a legitimate objective of general interest, (3) the restriction is strictly necessary in a democratic society to achieve the objective, and (4) there are no less intrusive and restrictive means available to reach the same objective.

The Relation between Ethics and Law

The first of the Siracusa Principles says that individual rights should only be restricted in accordance with the law. This begs the question of the ethical nature of the law. Utilitarianism tells us that, in a democratic society, the majority can enact legislation that systematically oppresses or neglects the minority. Intuitively, we might think that laws are the way a society codifies its ethics. While that is the case with murder, for example, in other situations a law may have little to do with ethics; and

in many instances, ethics are not encoded in the law. An example of a law that is largely unrelated to ethics is the requirement that the President of the United States be at least 35 years old. The rationale behind setting the age at 35 was, in all likelihood, an approximation of an age at which one would be mature enough to fulfill the obligations of the office (this was perhaps a reaction to child kings and queens in history). Experience tells us, however, that there are some people over 35 who do not have the maturity needed for the presidency, and we might well imagine a 34 year old who is wise and experienced beyond his or her years who would do well in the office. In this and other instances, the law is more about politics and pragmatic issues than about right and wrong.

In some cases, pragmatism works in conjunction with ideology to achieve the greatest public health benefit, as is the case for school vaccination requirements. Although public health research demonstrates a clear public health benefit to requiring children to be vaccinated prior to entering the school system and a clear danger to allowing abstentions, 48 states offer exemptions from school vaccination requirements for religious or philosophical reasons.[20] Setting aside the clear tension between individual freedoms and protecting the health of the community that occurs when families choose not to vaccinate their children for religious or philosophical reasons, historical evidence demonstrates that providing an exemption option together with quality health education decreases social resistance to school vaccinations, increasing the public health achievements of programs.[21] In other words, optimizing vaccination rates in many communities requires a dose of pragmatism alongside considerations of public health ethics.

The "right to a standard of living adequate for health and well-being" mentioned in the Universal Declaration of Human Rights is an example of an ethical tenet not encoded in law. It is not illegal in the United States to be homeless.

From these examples, we see that the door into ethics is not necessarily law (Figure 5-2). In fact, making our public health systems more ethical may entail changing existing laws or enacting laws that don't exist.

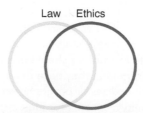

FIGURE 5-2   **The Overlap between Law and Ethics**

ETHICAL DECISION MAKING

If the law does not necessarily tell us what is ethical in public health, how do we make decisions and enact policies that are ethical? There are procedures and steps to aid us in this process, but before describing them it is worth clarifying what we can reasonably expect from them. We cannot expect to identify a particular answer that is indisputably ethical or, in other words, *the* right answer. One can seldom, if ever, be sure that all relevant considerations have been taken into account for a particular decision. And not everyone gives the same weight or importance to each consideration. One person or group will favor civil liberties for individuals and another will favor restriction of some liberties to benefit the health of the whole community.

What we *can* expect is to arrive at a **morally defensible decision**, one that was determined by a fair process and that took into consideration factors that are commonly regarded as important. With different groups of people, a variety of decisions may be made with a similar process and information, but in each case the group can account for an ethical process of decision making.

Because public health policy is carried out by an agency, usually part of the government, and it effects a population, decision making is a group process. Not only does it entail several people within an agency or at various levels of government, but the Public Health Code of Ethics would dictate that representatives from the public be included in the process. Thus, the foundation of ethical decision making in public health is a fair process of deliberation, which is generally considered to have five characteristics.

▸ *Transparency.* The process by which decisions are made should be evident to all who are interested (otherwise known as stakeholders) and the decisions made should be publicized.

▸ *Inclusiveness.* The interests of all stakeholders should be considered and stakeholders or their representatives should have an opportunity to contribute to the decision-making process.

▸ *Reasonableness.* Decisions should be made on the basis of the best evidence available, and to the degree possible should reflect values shared among the stakeholders.

▸ *Responsiveness.* Deliberations should address the concerns that led to the deliberations and there should be opportunities to evaluate decisions and outcomes as new information becomes available.

▸ *Accountability.* There should be a means to hold the decision-makers accountable for their decisions.

A group that is deliberating in this manner should then follow a multistep process. Although the following steps are listed in a particular order, often in reality the order gets jumbled or a group may return to an earlier step after more information is obtained.

1. *Clarify the facts of the situation.* If the ethical question involves a health outcome, what is the occurrence of the disease? What are the risk factors? How do rates compare between males and females, or between different ethnicities? What is the history of the situation? What led to the ethical question arising? What are the financial costs involved?

   The list of relevant facts can be quite extensive and seldom are all the desired facts available. Discussion of the remaining steps will sometimes refine the question and allow a group to zero in on particular concerns or to reorient entirely the facts considered relevant. Inevitably, however, the group will have to make a decision with incomplete information.

2. *Identify the ethical questions.* The process of ethical decision making often begins with an individual or a group identifying an ethical dilemma. The group that deliberates over a response to the dilemma may identify additional ethical questions that were previously unrecognized. They may even conclude that the original question brought to them is not the most important one. Keeping in mind that responsiveness to the original concern is a component of a fair process, the deliberators should confer with the ones who brought the initial concern to either persuade them that their question needs to be reframed or to inform them of the priority of their question among the others identified. In any case, the group should continue the process for only one well-defined ethical question at a time.

3. *Identify the stakeholders and what each stands to lose or gain.* The principal intent of this step is to look at the ethical question through the eyes of each group that will be most affected by the decision. The more narrowly stakeholders can be described, the more helpful this step will be. For example, if a question concerns Hispanic immigrants, the deliberating group may wish to consider separately single men, mothers, and dependent children; or those who can speak English and those who cannot. This step will be greatly aided if the fair process principle of inclusion is followed and representatives of the various stakeholder groups are among the deliberators.

4. *What do the various schools of ethical thought highlight?* In the previous step, the deliberating group looked at the ethical question through the eyes of various stakeholders. In this step the group

considers the question through the lens of various ethical schools of thought. What does a human rights perspective bring to light? Is it different from what one would concentrate on with a utilitarian perspective? One or more of the stakeholder groups may adhere to a particular religion. What would be the principal concerns, prescriptions, and proscriptions of those faith perspectives?

5. *What do professional ethical principles, standards of practice, and law suggest?* Here the process turns to resources such as the codes of ethics in public health and other relevant professions. Perhaps there are established "best practices" or even laws to consider. Hopefully, these professional guidelines and laws will move the group towards ethical courses of action. However, it is also possible that flaws in the guidelines or laws may be identified in this process. Then the group of deliberators will have to decide whether to let their recommended actions be constrained by existing policies and law or to override them with what they consider to be a truly ethical course of action. In the latter case, they must be willing to deal with a legal challenge or punishment.

6. *Identify possible alternative courses of action.* The options available to a group are seldom as narrow or constrained as they initially appear. In many instances, there is room for nuanced actions in which the pain of the most offensive implications of a decision is blunted with exceptions or modifications for certain stakeholders or in certain situations.

7. *Choose the alternative best supported by the preceding analysis.* At this point, the time has come for the group to make a decision. As stated earlier, decisions are inevitably made with inadequate information. But by the time the group has reached this step, they have followed a process that has been fair and they have systematically considered the most important facets. They should make their decision by a process agreed upon in the beginning, whether by a simple majority vote, consensus (in which some of the group may not agree

with the others, but not so strongly that they prevent a decision), or unanimity.

8. *Evaluate the actions taken and their eventual outcomes.* This step is perhaps the hardest, principally because once a decision has been made, people generally want to move on to other concerns. It takes a high level of commitment to track the effects of a decision and then, in spite of other pressing issues, to consider the quality of a decision made in the past. Yet, in a fully ethical process, those who make a decision truly care about the outcome, not only for those affected by the decision, but to inform future ethical decisions.

RESOURCES FOR ENCOURAGING ETHICS IN PUBLIC HEALTH

The process just described is rarely implemented. Not many in public health are trained to recognize ethical dilemmas and address them. But ethics is increasingly regarded as an important component of public health and resources for imparting ethical skills are becoming available. The Public Health Code of Ethics is one such resource. In addition, a list of competencies and skills in public health ethics has been made available online (http://www.phls.org) to inform the development of courses and training materials. Many of those competencies were incorporated into the competencies for certification in public health, as devised by the Association of Schools and Programs of Public Health (http://www.aspph.org).

Ready-made materials for teaching or learning ethics are also available free of charge online, including a series of modules presented through slides and voice-over (http://nciph.sph.unc.edu/tws/training_list). A number of textbooks and electronic readers on public health ethics are good sources for information on ethical theory and ethics in public health history.[22-34] There remains a need, however, for materials that impart skills in ethical decision making. A number of websites with helpful information on public health ethics are listed in Exhibit 5-4.

EXHIBIT 5-4 International and National Institutions Addressing Public Health Ethics

World Health Organization
   http://www.who.int/ethics/en/
Centers for Disease Control and Prevention (United States)
   http://www.cdc.gov/od/science/integrity/phethics/

The Provincial Health Ethics Network (Canada)
   http://www.phen.ab.ca/
National Ethics Advisory Committee (New Zealand)
   http://www.neac.health.govt.nz/

CURRENT, COMPELLING QUESTIONS IN PUBLIC HEALTH ETHICS

The obesity epidemic and the serious health consequences of climate change increasingly dominate contemporary discussions in public health. According to the Centers for Disease Control and Prevention, in the United States approximately one-third of adults and one-fifth of children and adolescents are obese.[35,36] Obesity is a major risk factor for potentially life-threatening noncommunicable diseases, such as cardiovascular problems, diabetes mellitus Type 2, and certain types of cancers, in addition to associated quality-of-life and psychosocial problems.[37] Climate change is adversely impacting health, for example by increasing the spread of disease-carrying vectors, damaging air quality, and straining water supplies, consequences that effect poor and vulnerable populations disproportionately.[38–42]

For obesity and climate change, the causes are largely structural—industrialized agriculture, the absence of healthy food in communities, and built environments that do not support healthy and green lifestyle choices. Perhaps not surprisingly, both the obesity epidemic and climate change are increasing health disparities, with poor populations most affected by structural causes of obesity and vulnerable to the serious health ramifications and unpredictable nature of climate change.[38–40,43–46] The similarly complex roots of these two major public health issues lend themselves to cohesive and integrated government policy strategies to transform our environment to promote healthy and eco-friendly living. Lawrence Gostin (University Professor, Georgetown University Law Center) defines the "new public health" as a focus on such solutions that address up-stream risk factors in everyday life and the human habitat.[43] In essence, he reaffirms the first principle of the Public Health Code of Ethics whereby "public health should address principally the fundamental causes of disease and requirements for health." While he focuses on obesity, "the new public health" could easily be extended to tackling climate change; indeed climate and obesity solutions are often complementary.[39]

What Gostin adds to this principle is a call for government accountability to the obesity epidemic, whereas the government's role in the Public Health Code of Ethics is conspicuously absent. In light of these contemporary health challenges we are faced with a series of ethical questions about the role of the government in public health. If these major public health issues necessitate government action to mitigate major population level health consequences, does the government have an ethical responsibility to act? What level of government intervention is appropriate in order to promote community health without violating the rights of individuals? What role does the government and other arms of public health have to address disparities, key factors associated with poor health outcomes? Does the Public Health Code of Ethics provide guidance to inform answers to these questions or should its content be revisited?

These compelling public health issues present a new frontier in the battle between individual rights and utilitarianism. Critics of government intervention are rightly concerned about infringing on individual liberties to promote the health of the community. In addition, as society and practitioners probe the limits of infringing on individual liberties to improve health, scientists across disciplines question how autonomous we really are in our decision making. For example, New York City's ban on soft drinks larger than 16 ounces mentioned in the beginning of the chapter may cause us to question whether freedom to purchase large sodas is a question of individual liberty since the soft drink industry has been gradually increasing the volume of soda available to consumers since sodas were first introduced in the market.[43] In this case, the choices are based on the evolution of marketing practices, whether or not we agree with them.

Private companies also have an important role to play in climate change, for example, by lowering carbon emissions from coal plants. What is the private sector's duty to public health? Are there other means of encouraging positive contributions to public health beyond regulation? There are no obviously right answers; rather, we are being pushed to address new ethical questions rooted in enduring tensions in public health practice towards the pursuit of a healthier society.

Alongside debates over critical issues in domestic public health, are debates over ethical issues arising from the proliferation of global public health research and practice activities financed by American institutions both governmental and nongovernmental. Advances in international travel have heightened the international potential of epidemics and the relevance of the health of one country to the well-being of another. The globalization of trade, communication, migration, information, and lifestyles has blurred the lines traditionally dividing domestic and global health.[47] As previously mentioned, the global HIV pandemic (see Figure 5-3) has squarely focused international attention on the moral imperative for rich countries to provide essential medicines and health services to poorer countries. Indeed the moral obligation of rich countries to limit carbon production and mitigate the effects of climate change in poor countries is an increasingly urgent need as the effects of climate change become more severe.

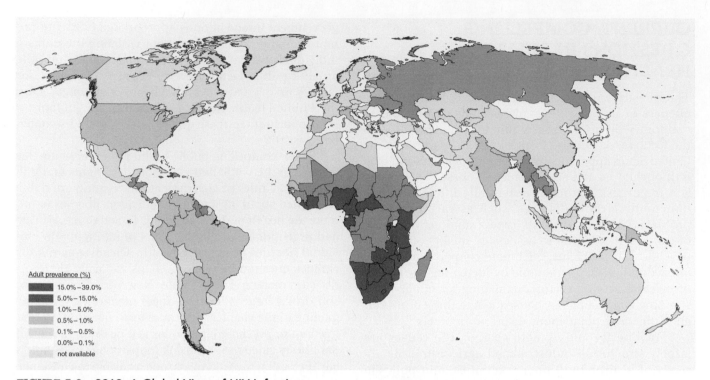

FIGURE 5-3   2010: A Global View of HIV Infection

Reprinted from http://www.who.int/hiv/facts/hiv2003/en/, World Health Organization. Reprinted by permission.

The expansion of domestic public health into global health domains has brought with it a very different set of ethical questions. Human rights frameworks are central in global health. But who has the duty to "respect, protect, and fulfill" a population's right to health?[48] Initially, the obvious answer would be the country government where the population resides. But what happens when the country is financially unable or politically unwilling to fulfill those rights? Whose duty is it to step in and under what circumstance? What happens when the rights of the rights-holders and duty bearers conflict? For example, a big challenge for the AIDS epidemic is the issue of providing antiretroviral treatment for millions of people throughout the world. Here we see the tension between the property rights of pharmaceutical companies in rich countries where they conflict with the right to health in poorer countries.[49] While the World Trade Organization has taken the stance that health rights should be prioritized over property rights of companies in the case of health emergencies, and many NGOs argue for prioritizing health rights over property rights, this remains a difficult ethical leap for some as populations are challenged to expand their moral considerations to include people in remote parts of the world.[49–51]

We encounter a whole new set of issues when we probe the ethical perspectives of the foreign countries, NGOs, and private foundations providing health services or conducting health research versus those receiving the assistance. Values underlying community health and health priorities differ markedly from country to country. To further obscure clear courses of action, few countries have articulated an ethic related to public health.[52] There is a very real risk that foreign institutions will dominate the priority-setting process due to their financial power, raising difficult ethical questions about development work. These pressing questions have no easy answers. However, it is important to have an understanding of the ethical perspectives of different countries and cultures, to anticipate differences, and to establish means of working together while also demonstrating mutual respect.

ACHIEVING ETHICAL PRACTICES IN PUBLIC HEALTH

Ethical frameworks that don't result in action are something less than ethics. What are the factors that result in an ethical framework having real traction, that is, that make a difference in the actions taken? Guidelines, such as the Siracusa Principles and the Public Health Code of Ethics are helpful. They are usually borne out of experience and reflect more than just theory. However, they are largely aspirational and not binding unless they are woven into law, regulations, or systems for professional sanctions. In contrast, research ethics are tied to review boards and mechanisms for stopping the flow of research funds if necessary. In medicine, a physician can be sued or have his or her license taken away in the case of a severe ethical breach. But there is no such system for public health. This is in part because, as noted above, public health administration is seldom tied to an individual and is usually carried out by an office or a board.

Some public health obligations are indeed woven into law and regulations. They address disposal of human waste, vaccination for students in public schools, carbon emissions of industrial plants, and more. But there are no regulations pertaining to several of the principles of the public health code of ethics, such as addressing fundamental causes of poor health outcomes, or ensuring opportunity for input from community members. The absence of a mechanism to enforce these principles may be one reason that public health ethics is most often addressed by people with legal training and perspectives. Laws provide them traction to achieve ethical practice.

Although not as forceful, there is also traction in altruism. In a study of the follow-through of state governments' stated intentions to create systems that support public health ethics in the event of an influenza pandemic, we found that those that had made progress were health departments in which the director had a strong commitment to ethics.[53] Strong leadership, then, can make a difference. But by the same token, turnover in leadership can result in the lapse of ethical progress. This can be mitigated somewhat by educating the public health work force in public health ethics.[54] Thus, rising leaders can be familiar with the standards of the profession, increasing the chances that the standards will remain salient. Even so, this falls short of enforcement and thus points to two other factors that can lead to achieving ethical practices in public health. The first of these is shame. Too often, we recognize a breach in ethics only when confronted by the reality of oversights or how a situation appears in the public light. For example, the Tuskegee study of syphilis ended only after it was exposed in the *Washington Star* and the *New York Times.* Since progress towards preparation for ethical challenges in the context of public health emergencies has occurred in only a few states, the need for ethical guidelines may be appreciated only when the response to an actual emergency goes badly.[51]

The other factor that can facilitate ethical practices in public health is the institutionalization of professional standards for individuals and agencies, along with sanctions for not meeting the standards. The establishment of standards and sanctions are often an element of professionalization of a field. Progress on this question will likely occur through discussions within and between public health organizations, such as the American Public Health Association (APHA), the Association of State and Territorial Health Officials (ASTHO), and the National Association of County and City Health Officials (NACCHO). Such a discussion could also be informed by a review of standards and sanctions in professions other than public health and in public health in other countries.

Because public health addresses health and the distribution of resources for whole populations, it is a fundamentally ethical endeavor. There are principles and laws that form the outline of an ethical foundation. But in the view of this author, that foundation is under-formed relative to the ethical implications of the profession. To ensure the ethical practice of public health, there remains much work to complete that foundation and to build upon it.

SUMMARY

This chapter provides a framework for how fundamental questions of rights and obligations are addressed in public health practice, particularly in how we balance the rights of individuals against the good of the community. While medical ethics have guided medical practice for over 150 years, public health ethics have only recently been articulated, and there are important differences between the two. Most importantly, medical ethics focus on the individual, while public health ethics reflect a communitarian perspective. Key principles of public health ethics include interdependence, participation, and scientific evidence. The values and beliefs that underlie public health ethics include having the right to the resources necessary for health; recognizing that humans are inherently social and interdependent; and understanding that the effectiveness of institutions depends heavily on the public's trust. Research ethics is the component of public health ethics that bears the closest relationship to medical ethics, in part because many public health studies include interactions between a researcher and a respondent. Ethical violations in research have resulted in the promulgation of federal guidelines (e.g., The Common Rule) to protect research participants.

A public health code of ethics, developed by the Public Health Leadership Society, is based on 12 principles which relate to the essential public health services, providing guidance to the public health practitioner for how she or he engages with communities. Ethical decision making in public health is a fair process of deliberation, involving transparency, inclusiveness, reasonableness, responsiveness, and accountability. While ethical frameworks are important for guiding ethical decision making, and the interplay of ethics, laws, and regulations provide legal justification for action, the application of public health ethics is ultimately dependent on the experience and leadership of the practitioner as well as the practitioner's sense of altruism. The institutionalization of professional standards for individuals and agencies, along with sanctions for not meeting the standards, can further ensure the application of public health ethics in the practice setting.

REVIEW QUESTIONS

1. The autonomy of the patient is a prominent ethical principle in medical ethics. In contrast, interdependence between people in a population, and thus the need to sometimes restrict individuals' rights, is more prominent in public health ethics. Why is this?

2. Name one strength and one weakness of utilitarian ethics.

3. Name one strength and one weakness of human rights ethics.

4. What are the Siracusa Principles, and how do they relate to human rights?

5. What are the elements of a fair process of decision making?

6. Describe a contemporary issue in public health that evidences a tension between individual rights and utilitarianism, and explain why.

ACKNOWLEDGMENTS

The author would like to thank Reid Elizabeth Miller for contributing the section on "Current, compelling questions in public health ethics" and her thoughtful input on the chapter.

REFERENCES

1. Colvin J. New York Soda Ban Approved: Board of Health OKs Limiting Sale of Large-Sized, Sugary Drinks. *Huffington Post* September 13, 2012; http://www.huffingtonpost.com/2012/09/13/new-york-approves-soda-ban-big-sugary-drinks_n_1880868.html. Accessed June 15, 2014.

2. *NY Statewide Coalition of Hispanic Chambers of Commerce v. NYC Board of Health, Supreme Court of New York, New York County, WL 1343607,* (N.Y. Sup. March 11, 2013).

3. MacQueen KM BJ. Ethics, practice, and research in public health. *Am J Public Health.* June 2004;96(6):928–931.

4. Kass NE. An ethics framework for public health. *Am J Public Health.* 2001;91(11):1776–1782.

5. Jones JH. *Bad Blood: The Tuskegee Syphilis Experiment.* New York: Free Press; 1993.

6. The Belmont Report: Ethical Principles and Guidelines for the Protection of Human Subjects of Research. Washington, DC: US Government Printing Office; 1979.

7. Code of Federal Regulations. Title 45, Part 46, Protection of Human Subjects. Revised June 23, 2005; http://www.hhs.gov/ohrp/humansubjects/guidance/45cfr46.html. Accessed August 29, 2014.

8. Roberts MJ, Reich MR. Ethical analysis in public health. *The Lancet.* 2002;359(9311):1055–1059.

9. Bentham J. *A Fragment on Government and an Introduction to the Principles of Morals and Legislation.* Oxford: Blackwell Publishers; 1948.

10. Rosen G. *A History of Public Health (expanded ed).* Baltimore, MD: The Johns Hopkins University Press; 1993.

11. Lewis RA. *Edwin Chadwick and the Public Health Movement 1832-1854.* London: Longmans & Green; 1952.

12. Joint United Nations Program on HIV/AIDS (UNAIDS). Report on the Global HIV/AIDS Epidemic. 2000; http://data.unaids.org/pub/Report/2000/2000_gr_en.pdf. Accessed August 29, 2014.

13. Centers for Disease Control and Prevention. HIV/AIDS Surveillance Report. Vol 1, No. 2. Atlanta, GA: Center for Disease Control and Prevention. 1999; http://www.cdc.gov/hiv/pdf/statistics_hasr1102.pdf. Accessed August 29, 2014.

14. Mann JM. Human rights and AIDS: the future of the pandemic. In: Mann JM GS, Grodin MA, Anna GJ, ed. *Health and Human Rights: A Reader.* New York: Springer; 1999:223.

15. Mann JM GL, Gruskin S, Brennan T, Lazzarini Z, Fineberg H. Health and human rights. In: Mann JM GS, Grodin MA, Annas GJ ed. *Health and Human Rights: A Reader.* New York: Routledge; 1999:7–20.

16. Columbia University Mailman School of Public Health. About us: Public Health Code. 2014; http://www.mailman.columbia.edu/about-us/mission-and-history/public-health-oath. Accessed August 29, 2014.

17. Thomas JC, Sage M, Dillenberg J, Guillory VJ. A code of ethics for public health. *Am J Public Health.* 2002;92(7):1057–1059.

18. World Health Organization. Project on Addressing Ethical Issues in Pandemic Influenza Planning. Draft paper for Working Group Two: Ethics of Public Health Measures in Response to Pandemic Influenza. October 2006; http://apps.who.int/eth/ethics/PI_Ethics_draft_paper_WG2_6_Oct_06.pdf. Accessed August 29, 2014.

19. United Nations, Economic and Social Council. Siracusa Principles on the Limitation and Derogation Provisions in the International Covenant on Civil and Political Rights. Vol E/CN.4/1985/4, Annex (1985). 1985.

20. Diekema DS. Personal belief exemptions from school vaccination requirements. *Annual Review of Public Health*. 2014;35(1):275–292.

21. Leavitt JW. Public resistance or cooperation? A tale of smallpox in two cities. *Biosecurity and Bioterrorism: Biodefense Strategy, Practice, and Science*. 2003;1(3):185–192.

22. Bayer R, Gostin LO, Jennings B, Steinbock B, eds. *Public Health Ethics: Theory, Policy, and Practice*. New York: Oxford University Press; 2007.

23. Coughlin SS. *Case studies in public health ethics*. Washington, DC: American Public Health Association; 2009.

24. Dawson A, Verweij M, eds. *Ethics, Prevention, and Public Health*. New York: Oxford University Press; 2009.

25. Faden R, Shebaya S. Public Health Ethics. Stanford Encyclopedia of Philosophy (Summer 2010 Edition). April 12, 2010; http://plato.stanford.edu/entries/publichealth-ethics/. Accessed August 28, 2014.

26. Gostin LOE. *Public Health Law and Ethics: A Reader*. 2nd ed. Oakland, CA: University of California Press; 2010.

27. Holland S. *Public Health Ethics*. Cambridge, UK: Polity Press; 2007.

28. Beauchamp DE, Steinbock B, eds. *New Ethics for the Public's Health*. New York: Oxford University Press; 1999.

29. Powers M, Faden RR. *Social Justice: The Moral Foundations of Public Health and Health Policy*. New York: Oxford University Press; 2006.

30. Anand S, Peter F, Sen A, eds. *Public Health, Ethics, and Equity*. New York: Oxford University Press; 2006.

31. Boylan ME. *International Public Health Policy and Ethics*. Vol 42. Dordrecht, NY: Springer; 2008.

32. Peckham S, Hann, A. ed *Public Health Ethics and Practice*. Bristol, UK: The Policy Press; 2010.

33. Dawson AE. *Public Health Ethics: Key Concepts and Issues in Policy and Practice*. Cambridge, UK: Cambridge University Press; 2011.

34. Hirschberg I, Marckmann G, Strech DE. *Ethics in public health and health policy [electronic resource] : concepts, methods, case studies*. Vol 1. Dordrecht, NY: Springer; 2013.

35. Centers for Disease Control and Prevention. Adult Overweight and Obesity. 2012; http://www.cdc.gov/obesity/adult/index.html. Accessed June 26, 2014.

36. Centers for Disease Control and Prevention. Adult Overweight and Obesity. 2013; http://www.cdc.gov/obesity/childhood/index.html. Accessed June 26, 2014.

37. Ogden CL, Carroll MD, Curtin LR, Lamb MM, Flegal KM. Prevalence of high body mass index in US children and adolescents, 2007-2008. *JAMA*. 2010;303(3):242–249.

38. Friel S, Marmot M, McMichael AJ, Kjellstrom T, Vågerö D. Global health equity and climate stabilisation: a common agenda. *The Lancet*. 2008;372(9650):1677–1683.

39. Frumkin H, Hess J, Luber G, Malilay J, McGeehin M. Climate change: the public health response. *Am J Public Health*. 2008;98(3):435–445.

40. Wiley LF, Gostin LO. The international response to climate change: an agenda for global health. *JAMA*. 2009;302(11):1218–1220.

41. Confalonieri U, Menne B, Akhtar R, et al. Climate Change 2007: Impacts, Adaptation and Vulnerability: Contribution of Working Group II to the Fourth Assessment Report of the Intergovernmental Panel on Climate Change. In: Parry ML CO, Palutikof JP, van der Linden PH, Hanson CE ed. *Human Health*. Cambridge, UK: Cambridge University Press; 2007:291–431.

42. Bates B, Kundzewicz ZW, Wu S, Palutikof J. Climate change and water. Intergovernmental Panel on Climate Change (IPCC). 2008; https://www.ipcc.ch/pdf/technical-papers/ccw/frontmatter.pdf. Accessed August 29, 2014.

43. Gostin LO. Bloomberg's Health Legacy: Urban Innovator or Meddling Nanny? *Hastings Center Report*. 2013;43(5):19–25.

44. Pomeranz JL, Gostin LO. Improving laws and legal authorities for obesity prevention and control. *The Journal of Law, Medicine & Ethics*. 2009;37(s1):62–75.

45. ten Have M. Ethical aspects of obesity prevention. *Best Practice & Research Clinical Gastroenterology*. 2014;28(2):303–314.

46. Gostin LO. Trans Fat Bans and the Human Free-
    dom: A Refutation. *The American Journal of Bioeth-
    ics.* 2010;10(3):33–34.

47. Gostin LO, Taylor AL. Global health law: a defi-
    nition and grand challenges. *Public Health Ethics.*
    2008;1(1):53–63.

48. United Nations Committee on Economic, Social
    and Cultural Rights. The right to the highest attain-
    able standard of health (general comments). Vol
    E/C.12/2000/4: United Nations; 2008.

49. World Trade Organization. Declaration on the
    TRIPS agreement and public health. Adopted
    November 14, 2001; http://www.wto.org/english/
    thewto_e/minist_e/min01_e/mindecl_trips_e.htm.
    Accessed August 29, 2014.

50. Commission on Intellectual Property Rights.
    Integrating Intellectual Property Rights and

Development Policy. September 2002; http://
www.iprcommission.org/papers/pdfs/final_report/
ciprfullfinal.pdf. Accessed August 6, 2014.

51. DanChurchAid. *'You Reap What You Sow' A Call
    for a Declaration on the TRIPs Agreement and Food
    Security.* Copenhagen: DanChurchAID;2005.

52. Thomas JC. Ethical Concerns in Pandemic Influ-
    enza Preparation and Responses. SERCEB Policy,
    Ethics and Law Core. 2007; http://www.unc
    .edu/~thomasjc/documents/pandemic_flu_white_
    paper_Thomas.pdf. Accessed August 29, 2014.

53. Thomas JC, Young S. Wake Me Up When There's
    a Crisis: Progress on State Pandemic Influenza
    Ethics Preparedness. *Am J Public Health.*
    2011;101(11):2080.

54. Thomas JC. Teaching ethics in schools of public
    health. *Public Health Reports.* 2003;118(3):279.

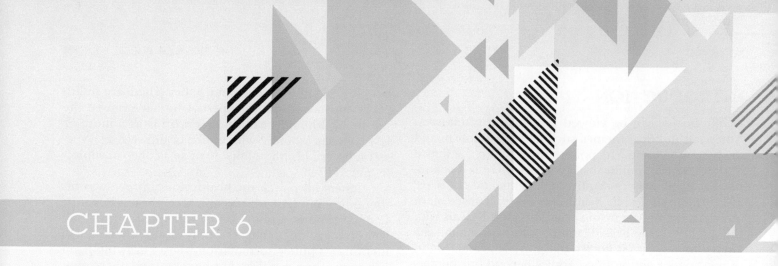

CHAPTER 6

The Policy Basis of Public Health

Thomas C. Ricketts, PhD, MPH

LEARNING OBJECTIVES

Upon completion of this chapter the reader will be able to:

1. Understand the major theories that drive policy making and politics in public health in the United States.

2. Describe the policy-making process in public health in the United States as a form of storytelling.

3. Understand the basic structure of overall public policy making and be able to recognize the institutions where this takes place.

4. Understand the major frameworks for understanding policy making in the United States and to act within them.

5. Recognize and be able to use key terms in public health policy making including the role of numerical data, facts and evidence, symbols, and timing in the process as it relates to public health.

KEY TERMS

advocacy
agendas
policy
policy making
politics
professionals
stakeholders

INTRODUCTION

Public health can be viewed as a fusion of classical American political themes such as individualism and the "common good." Its politics fit well into the thread of the American political story where there is a continuous struggle between individual rights and collective responsibilities. Public health touches practically all of the elements of American society because it deals with the quality of the lives of the people who inhabit the United States, thus it finds a place in the general world of governance and politics. Forces beyond our borders also affect the public's health, and while policy making in public health easily stretches into international affairs, our focus here is on the United States. There are extensions of public health policy making into other, perhaps unexpected domains. The physical structure of the land and the buildings we inhabit has an effect on our health, allowing the policies for public health to intersect with the politics and policy making of engineering, infrastructure, and the environment. Given its breadth, it might appear to the casual observer that the politics of public health may be either too broad to be usefully characterized or made up of a shifting set of special political rules and structures impossible to coherently describe or intervene upon. Public health is just one of many political and policy streams in the American context that can be interpreted and "explained" using general political theory and policy frameworks. In this chapter "storytelling" will be used to help the practitioner follow the politics and policy making in public health.

In this chapter the description of public health politics will unfold as a story much like one would describe an event in a newspaper. A good journalist is often reminded that a story must answer the following questions: who, what, when, where, how, and why something happened. This storytelling approach does not deviate very much from the guidance given by a well-accepted definition of politics. Harold Lasswell described **politics** as "who gets what, when (and) how" and titled his influential analysis of American politics with those words.[1] That definition is repeated to this day because it explains so well what politics is all about. But to complete the description, the additional questions of where and why are justifiably added.

John Kingdon uses much the same taxonomy in describing how **policy** is generated.[2] He describes a wide range of elements important to policy creation that fall into the journalist's categorical questions but he places more or less emphasis on some elements than others. His book, *Agendas, Alternatives and Public Policies*, is one of the most widely used texts in courses that focus on health and public health policy although it is intended for a general audience of people seeking to understand policy. There are political scientists and policy experts who have viewed the public health and health policy worlds as a more or less coherent whole[3,4] with public health seen as a special subset of health politics [5,6] or as a coherent subject in and of itself.[7]

Others have seen the health policy process as fitting into a model with recognizable phases. Beaufort Longest promotes this form of structured conceptualization to guide managers in the health system.[8] He identifies a policy formulation phase, drawing from Kingdon, then a policy implementation phase that feeds back to the formulation process via a policy modification stage. His emphasis is on formal legislation; he suggests that that form of policy direction fits better with the management of formal institutions. Others see the policy process as something that can be better understood through the lessons of case studies and the specific history of individual issues. Harrington and Estes continue a series of volumes that cover a range of issues in the 4th edition of their book,[9] and McLaughlin and McLaughlin make use of many specific policy examples within a general structure of policy analysis to give a sense of how health policy works.[10] The use of anecdotes and histories of how past policy has emerged followed by the application of a generalized model has been the standard way to describe health policy making and elaborate the processes of health policy.

The state or local public health practitioner may find that understanding the story of policy making that affects their own work may be useful if they are to shape those policies or react as constructively as possible. The framework described in this chapter is intended to allow the practitioner to describe the policy and political contexts that affect them to allow them to succeed in their mission and profession.

WHO CONTROLS POLITICS, *WHO* MAKES POLICY?

It is fitting to start with a description of the people who take the lead in politics and policy because politics is a "people" activity. While we can speak easily about a decision being subject to "politics" and played out in "institutions" we know that it is the politicians who drive this process. The same can be said for **policy making**, it is a people process. This is true at the local as well as national levels. To be successful, a public health official must understand the people for and with whom she works, be they legislators, state cabinet members or agency chiefs. They, in turn, react to others who "run the show"—those "elites" who dominate politics and policy. "Elites" is a negative term in current political discussions and these "influentials" are often called by other names, such as: business leaders, political operatives, professional spokespeople, prominent fundraisers, even as "great" people, a term used in political science. Understanding the people who lead political discussions goes a long way toward understanding politics and policy.

Elites

It should come as no surprise to most Americans that there is a relatively small group of elites who make most political decisions. It is widely recognized that there are identifiable people whose economic or social position give them more "weight" in politics than their role as a single voter or individual claimant on government. It is also easy for most Americans to accept that some "types" of people are more politically influential. Theories that describe the political dominance of elites go beyond that simple observation and posit that practically all decisions are made by the same small set of elite actors, and the elites can be identified by their social, economic, or occupational characteristics.

Even in local public health systems, boards and commissions are often controlled by the more powerful sectors of society and the economy. These people, who are charged with representing the community as a whole, often are chosen from the well-educated and financially successful elements of their communities. The decision-making process in local public health has been described as a process whereby "The result is that elites discuss the problem and work through solutions with other elites, not citizens."[11]

While we may feel that public health is an activity that is antithetical to elite dominance, we find many instances of elites either leading reform in public health or exerting great influence on the direction of public health policy through foundations and corporate boards. The Robert Wood Johnson Foundation, the Commonwealth Fund, the Milbank Memorial Fund, the W.K. Kellogg Foundation and the Kaiser Family Foundation are but a few of the many philanthropic organizations who take an active role in influencing the direction of public health policy, either through direct funding of experimental and model programs or the training and socialization of leaders. The W.K. Kellogg and Robert Wood Johnson Foundations have programs whose goals are to develop individuals who will make up the elite of public health. These programs orient emerging experts and practitioners to the world of power and government with a goal of bettering the nation's health by creating leadership capital. To be effective leaders, they will either become part of the elite or they will have to work closely with elites.

Professionals

In the sphere of health care and public health, there is a tradition of interpreting the emergence of policies from a viewpoint that considers professionals and professional roles as dominating the process. Where professionals are given strong social and legal powers, they may take a position as independent arbiters of behavior—determining who is and is not ill or capable of exercising their roles as citizens. This might be "great people" theory of control and change in a restricted sense, and, indeed health care and public health professionals have special social and economic leadership and decision-making roles that they play that are not replicated in other policy domains.

The states have retained the power to license and regulate the healing professions through their police power to protect the health, safety, and welfare of the public. This provides a complementary legal justification for the professional role of public health professionals that is tied to the protective power of the state governments expressed through state departments of public health. Paul Starr in his excellent review of the history of medicine in America, *The Social Transformation of American Medicine*, pointed out the special role that professionals play in our society. Starr's work traces this parallel process where the "sovereign" profession of medicine acts as a stimulating force in the emergence of professional public health with most health departments being organized, then led, by physicians.[12]

Health professionals are expected to behave "benevolently" and this may extend to a sense of public responsibility that often translates into a "public" health role. Recently health professionals have discovered that "the benevolence of their work world is eroding in the face of growing concern over their responsiveness to public needs."[13] This clash of the professional tendency to benevolent (often considered paternalistic) activity and of market responsiveness is not a new one but it is creating problems for medical professionals once comfortable with their dominant role in society.

Bureaucrats and Bureaucracies

This is an example of the "who's" getting mixed with the "what" of government. The bureaucracy is a necessary part of the system, but bureaucrats behave in ways that transcend and, in many ways, defy organizations and their missions. Some might say that studying bureaucracy has more of a place in administration than politics, but the nature and structure of bureaucracy makes many policy options either infeasible or can facilitate their implementation. Understanding how bureaucrats work and how much power they can wield in the implementation of policies is a necessary political skill. Any policy analysis that is considering options and alternatives for future action must include an assessment of the capacity of the bureaucracy to achieve the stated goals for policy.

California issued a report in 2004 that called for a general restructuring of the public health authority and a formal reorganization of the public health system in that state. (You can review the report by accessing http://www.lhc.ca.gov and searching under "Report 170.") The major recommendations from that report were for bureaucratic restructuring and a focus on establishing the right overall scale and developing mechanisms for accountability. Any enterprise whose constituency is the entire population will require careful and close attention to the demands and needs of bureaucracy if it is to make any meaningful change in individual or collective behavior beyond what occurs as a result of natural competition for money and power.

Scientists/Academics

The role of scientists and academics in policy making and politics differs to some degree from that of professionals in public health and is reflected in a delineation between the academic, or "ivory tower" world of research and teaching, and the practical day-to-day work of delivering services. Academics have influence in policy making where there is a high degree of complexity and technical language is the norm. This is somewhat parallel to the power derived from mastery of knowledge on the part of medical professionals, but, in the case of public health, the knowledge base is much wider, encompassing issues of pollution, water quality management, disease propagation, risk factors, and the relative effectiveness of prevention versus control measures.

Academics have been criticized for holding themselves aloof from the worlds of practical policy making and politics[14] and often see themselves as clearly separate and untainted by the quotidian. In fact, the research and academic worlds have long been enmeshed in political battles and their influence and participation remains substantial. This is particularly so in public health where the academic homes of the field grew from practical needs to understand the nature of vectors and diseases and how to organize and manage a relatively uniform public service structure. A contemporary program such as the Community-Campus Partnerships for Health highlights the practical involvement of the academy in local policy making and governance (http://depts.washington.edu/ccph).

Media

The media serve a unique function in modern democracies. Some have called it a separate branch of government that provides another check to power in the tradition of the "fourth estate."[15] Others see it as a political player on its own, functioning as a form of special interest group.[16] In public health policy, the media are important in the dissemination of information from central and professional sources and are often seen as functioning more like messengers rather than shapers of policy. However, the media may not recognize important "news" that the public needs until it fits into their expectations of what is newsworthy or interesting to the public. For example, in the coverage of AIDS, the disease and its threat were an isolated and technical issue until a major film star and other personalities were revealed to be infected or died from the disease. The media could then focus the issue with the drama of the struggle of recognizable "personalities."[17]

One use of the media to promote public health has seen the rise of "social marketing."[18] This is the use of the media to foster social change and promote behaviors and beliefs that either experts or elites consider beneficial for society as a whole. The process of social marketing has the potential for influence in policy making as well because the messages flow "down" to the public as well as "up" to policy makers. Social marketing may be somewhat akin to a political "campaign" intended to generate policy change, or to elect someone to office. The same principles apply of clarity and simplicity of message, repetition, and the use of persuasive symbols. The antitobacco advertising program was intended not only to change individual behavior but also to foster political changes.[19]

The People, the Public

Alan Wolfe argues that Americans have adequate access to democratic mechanisms but that the quality of democracy has degraded because participation is both uninformed as well as heavily influenced by "special interests."[20] Public health is a beneficiary of all of the avenues of participation in the democratic process with a range of national interest groups and coalitions engaged at all levels of government. These include groups such as the American Public Health Association and the American Cancer Society. Local interests are reflected by organizations such as the "Healthy Ansonians" (in Anson County, NC) that are grassroots groups whose organizations are concerned with health in a broad sense but focus their work on a local system or government structure.

The media and interest groups often offer more direct connections between the public and policy makers. This is especially true in the case of elections and in recalls or referenda. Whether the public is more or less engaged in public health policy making is open to debate. Policy making does ebb and flow with the public mood and the public has been, at times, able to express preferences for complex problems in health care and public health.[21,22] The American public is aware of public health issues and there is formal participation at the local level through membership on boards and commissions but more often the public's involvement is viewed through the lens of "community."[23] Much of the democratic engagement of Americans in public health is through groups who are concerned with the general health of their fellow citizens or of a specific group of people at risk or suffering from a disease. These groups represent single, usually local, issues and involve constituencies that cross traditional political lines. Threats to health are often seen as being "above politics." This may, ironically, weaken the formal political power of the public's involvement in policy making for public health because groups focused on a specific disease may destabilize the normal political process in the name of a single suffering victim—causing legislation to pass that favors that class of individuals at the expense of larger, less visible groups. This can be said to be true of "named" legislation, such as the Ryan White Act, that may focus attention and funds on a specific problem, one that "has a face."

Policy Entrepreneurs

Policy making in the United States has become an industry in itself. The emergence of multiple "think-tanks" and advocacy groups has created a well-developed "market of policy ideas." Many of these entities have been created around single ideas that were promoted by individuals. Tom Oliver pointed out the significant role that policy entrepreneurs played in the politics of health reform as well as in broader public health policy making.[24] Most of the important leaders in public health can be viewed as policy entrepreneurs of some form as they seek to promote their vision of change through formal policy making or in the political arena.

In public health there are individuals who are closely identified with specific policy solutions. For those policies that are successfully implemented, the recognition of those individuals places them more in the "great people" category. While they are struggling to attract policy attention to their ideas, they are viewed more as entrepreneurs trying to build support for a policy or an approach. *Moments in Leadership: Case Studies in Public Health Policy* (Pfizer, 2008) highlights the struggle of some of these policy entrepreneurs who were eventually successful in bringing public health policies into being. The policy innovations they promoted did not necessarily have a unique and inevitable pathway toward implementation. The development of the *Guide to Clinical Preventive Services*[25] promoted by Michael McGinnis, for example, led to adoption by both public agencies and private groups. The policy innovation in this instance was a more general policy solution to a broad scale problem. The downstream policies are yet to be realized, but the promotion of evidence-based guidance for clinical prevention is now a well-established idea.

Great People

In the nineteenth and early twentieth century, the driving forces of history and social progress were often embodied in the lives of "great men." One way to look at the history of the American polity and its economy is that it grew and prospered because of efforts of the "founding fathers," such as Washington, Franklin, Jefferson, then later Lincoln, and the Roosevelts. Our industry thrived given the vision and energy of Carnegie, Rockefeller, and Edison. Public health had its own great men and women: Lemuel Shattuck, William Gorgas, William Sedgewick, Dorothea Dix, and Clara Barton are often invoked to explain why certain decisions were made and the course of events changed to bring "progress." The role of great people in making policy and influencing politics is an important consideration in understanding politics, but it is also a way by which subsequent political positions and policy platforms are promoted by invoking an important historical figure as being somehow connected to the decisions of the present. Great people do make important differences in their time, but they may have even greater influence when they are used as symbols by their successors.

Luther Terry and C. Everett Koop are often regarded as influential individuals in the history of public health for their contributions to the political dialog and the policies that emerged while they served as Surgeon General.[26] They gave voice to positions that were unpopular in government because the policy decisions that had to flow from their words would impose heavy costs on entrenched interests. They used their position to "speak truth to power." The post they held survives, but in name only; reorganization in the U.S. Department of Health and Human Services has left the Surgeon General as a largely ceremonial office with only a role as titular head of the U.S. Public Health Service Commissioned Corps. The "Bully Pulpit" of the Surgeon General has been largely torn down by recent administrations who see the role of the Surgeon General more as a symbol than as an actor.[27]

Interest Groups

The power of interest groups in American politics and policy making is perhaps the dominant interpretive lens for understanding how policy emerges. Interest groups are embedded deeply in our political systems since they were given explicit support by the founding fathers (e.g. Madison's "factions") and their implicit recognition in the Constitution (the right to petition government) combined with the ease with which we allow groups to coalesce and receive formal recognition. The U.S. tax code recognizes several types of voluntary organizations that can influence the political process. Nonprofit organizations (i.e. 501(c)(3) organizations) are "absolutely prohibited from directly or indirectly participating in, or intervening in, and political campaigning on behalf of (or in opposition to) any candidate for elective public office." (See http://www.irs.gov/charities.) However, these organizations can participate in "voter education" activities, which is a very gray area. Those not-for-profit, tax-exempt associations can also participate in lobbying activity attempting to influence legislation so long as it is not the majority of their activity. Other more political organizations can be recognized as 501(c)(4) corporations but donations to those organizations are not tax-exempt and their open participation in politics is permitted. These include the American Association of Retired Persons, the National Rifle Association, MoveOn.org, and the Christian Coalition.

So-called "527" organizations have recently emerged as another vehicle for financing political activities. They are formed to influence issues, not candidates, and are not regulated by the Federal Elections Commission. They are influential in conservative and liberal movements and include groups such as Emily's List, Swift Boat Veterans for Truth, and the Sierra Club. The role of these organizations in politics has only expanded in the recent past after the "Citizens United" decision by the U.S. Supreme Court.[28] While much of the recent expanded activity of pressure groups has focused on national elections, they have also turned their attention to the states. One example of this new use of interest group money is the efforts by the American Legislative Exchange Council (ALEC) to support repeal or modification of state laws that regulate pharmaceuticals, air quality, food safety, and in support of efforts to privatize some traditional state public health activities including inspections and certifications. ALEC's support is not public but the organization acknowledges large donations from corporate givers including Exxon and Koch Industries. So-called "progressive" interest groups also push legislative agendas at the state level and make use of the same funding opportunities and the ability to conceal their donors.[29]

The current role of interest groups in health policy is found to be most effective when they function as advocacy coalitions.[30] Interest groups are not always successful in achieving their goals. For example, there has long been a recognition that rural economic interests have not been powerful players in national policy[31] but the interest group coalition surrounding rural health care, especially rural hospitals, has been especially effective in getting attention and favorable policies in Congress.[32]

In public health, there is a very fluid structure to interest group activity. There are many factions and **stakeholders** in the public health field who see their claim to policy attention as paramount. The American Public Health Association (APHA) itself can be viewed as more of a federation of groups working under a "big tent" of related interests. APHA includes many Sections, Caucuses, and Special Primary Interest Groups (SPIGs) that have titles as varied as podiatric health, disability, homelessness, laboratory, food and nutrition, and chiropractic. These groupings allow individuals who may identify professionally more with a specific discipline (e.g. epidemiology) or profession (e.g. chiropractic) to combine for common advocacy and support of programs. APHA has attracted criticism by conservatives as being too much concerned with a "social justice agenda" and not focused on practical public health policy issues.[33] This "drift" in focus and message can impair an advocacy group in their ability to provide a clear and cogent message. However, when there is a need for a broad-based coalition to motivate a large number of supporters in a coherent campaign, these larger associations can provide the breadth of support necessary to motivate politicians. These broad scale movements are often confused with "grassroots," citizen-generated movements that arise spontaneously.

Public health leaders and practitioners are often involved in their professional associations and these organizations often promote political activity by their members. The effectiveness of an organization is a function both of its size (members as potential voters) and the funding it can bring to elections and issues campaigns, but also by the quality of its message and the reputation of its advocates and membership. As a public health practitioner, one can engage in policy making activity directly at the local level through membership on boards and commissions. These entities are often put in the middle of political disputes and issues and an individual's professional activity can be transformed into political tasks very easily.

WHAT IS PUBLIC HEALTH POLITICS AND POLICY MAKING ALL ABOUT?

The "whats" of policy making in public health are the topics and issues that are being considered and for which "**policy**" is being made. These are intangible things in a system that is largely devoted to the distribution of resources, favors, or restraint on actions. What we are debating or considering on any given day will certainly change but there are issues that tend to always be under discussion and which rise and fall in the degree of attention they receive in the policy-making process. Describing an "agenda" for policy making has been one of several useful interpretive structures that help outside observers as well as policy makers themselves understand what is going on.

Agendas and Plans

At any time in the political life of the nation, there are some issues that seem to dominate the news and the attention of the public. This is true for public health, whether it be smoking cessation or preparedness for bioterrorism; however, there are only a few topics that tend to rise to the top of the political agenda in any given year. There is only so much time available to legislators and administrators to make policy changes. The most important issues that these individuals and institutions confront at any given time are generally termed the *policy agenda*. The idea of an "agenda" with a limited set of issues is an established idea in political analysis. Anthony Downs described an "issue-attention cycle" that tracked how the attention of politicians and policy makers was dominated at times by specific issues which then faded away over time.[34] John Kingdon emphasizes the importance of the somewhat restricted policy agenda and described how specific topics came onto or dropped off of the national policy agenda.[2] Baumgardner and Jones argued that the narrow focus that the agenda-setting process brings to a few issues tends to hide the overall continuity that underlies the system where there is a relatively constant process of policy building more or less behind the scenes.[35] Their public health-oriented example of tobacco and pesticide legislation traced a pattern of relatively constant and incremental policy formation that allowed more distributed benefits of regulation to trump the concentrated costs to specific industries. This notion of the balance of benefits and costs was posited originally by James Q. Wilson, who suggested that there were paradoxical situations where the concentration of costs on a particular industry or social sector would negate the ability of policy advocates to pass legislation that had diffuse benefits. An example of such situations is emissions abatement in electrical production to clean the air of pollutants.[36] However, there are multiple examples of how these "imbalanced" policies have been enacted to benefit the public's health (Figure 6-1).[24]

Client politics can be considered the "normal" politics of redistribution of resources that benefit well-organized interest groups; in health care the use of Medicare funds for graduate medical education is an example. The *Entrepreneurial* politics quadrant is where public health politics are most often played out, for example, with pollution abatement, seat belt laws, vaccine requirements and other policies that burden individuals or small groups but distribute the benefits widely across populations, and were viewed by Wilson as entrepreneurial in nature.[37] They require aggressive, creative arguments for policy makers to grasp the benefits of their passage, and widespread acceptance on the part of the political community and the public.

Laws, Rules, Regulations

The "laws of the land" are distributed across the Constitution of the United States and the separate constitutions of the several states as well as the enacted codes of the nation, states, and local government. These form only a part of the formal legal structure for the nation as there are many other sets of rules, codes, regulations,

		BENEFITS	
		Concentrated	Diffuse
COSTS	Diffuse	Client politics *Politically attractive*	Majoritarian politics
	Concentrated	Interest Group politics	Entrepreneurial politics *Politically Unattractive*

Concentrated Effects	Diffuse Effects
• Large magnitude • Occur immediately • Direct traceable impact • Identifiable group or geography	• Small in magnitude • Occur over time • Indirect less traceable impacts • Broad, less identifiable population

FIGURE 6-1 Wilson's Framework for Policy Analysis

ADAPTED from: Oliver TR. The politics of public health policy. *Annu Rev Public Health*. 2006;27:195–233 24 and Wilson JQ. American Government: Institutions and Policies. Lexington, MA: D.C. Health and Company; 1992.

statutes, and policies that either guarantee certain rights, set obligations, or guide or restrict action in some way. Public health law is often described as having its primary basis in the common law "police powers" reserved to the states. In reality, in the twenty-first century there is a robust mix of statutes and legal structures that affect the public's health or the public health structure and which draw on a broad range of legal sources. The stability of this mixed set of legal authorities was jolted by the terrorist attacks of 2001 where the jumbled overlap of multiple jurisdictions and conflicting authorities were revealed to be, in themselves, threats to the protection of the public.[38]

The process of "modernizing" public health law was underway before the attacks but they served as focusing events that opened a window of opportunity for sweeping change in public health law. Following the attacks of 9/11, efforts were set in motion to modernize state public health and emergency powers acts, and model statutes were disseminated and distributed. This was met with some resistance as debates erupted over how much additional "coercive" power should be given to government. The politics of this debate brought left-wing civil libertarians together with right-wing traditional libertarians, both concerned with erosion to individual rights and freedoms. This resistance blunted some of the most aggressive efforts to centralize command and control of threats to the public and the changes that were made in the following years tended toward incremental and clarifying rather than broadly reforming.

Political struggles sometimes emerge as one or more of the 50 states or other jurisdictions contend with the federal government over the applicability or the intensity of some specific law or regulation. This federal-state-local tension is apparent in public health law as localities often react to strong concentrated pressure from groups to restrain behavior (antismoking ordinances) or to regulate industry (abatement rules) that may exceed their statutory powers or conflict with interests whose abilities to sway legislatures is much greater than their ability to move local councils.

Symbols

Politics is often described symbolically as a "game" or even a "war" (. . . against cancer, against poverty). Politics plays out with many symbols being invoked to promote policies or to rally support for programs.[1,39] Public health, itself, can be used in a symbolic sense by politicians when they call for "more funding for public health" or for programs that "protect the public's health" when they are actually reducing programs but promoting behavior change. Those two uses convey very different meanings depending on the context. The rhetoric of politics requires the use of symbols to both define

concepts as well as align supporters and policies.[40] The ability to manipulate symbols is now considered to be a key attribute of the successful politician or political movement. The careful crafting of political messages brought Newt Gingrich to power, and his method of "capturing the rhetorical high ground" is a lesson learned by both the left and right.[41]

Public health has been viewed as the expression of "social justice" by some (a moral symbol) and as a pragmatic mechanism to ensure national productivity by others (an economic symbol).[42,43] The use of metaphors is important to the conduct of debate as it is to the development of policy. Structuring a public health debate around a notion of a healthy "ecology" would generate substantially different outcomes than a debate where the dominant theme was the creation of healthy individuals or a healthy economy. In recent years, public health improvement has focused on the role of "place" and neighborhood in creating the opportunities and conditions in which people can live healthier lives.[44] This use of place-based metaphors and identifiers has shifted policy discussions away from "personal behavior" toward more general mechanisms to intervene to improve health. When we speak of a person's health status being affected by their ZIP code we are shifting both responsibility and the pathway to solutions toward their context and away from the individual.

Rights and Freedoms

The basis for government, it is argued by some, is the protection of individual rights. John Locke argued that "civil government is the proper remedy for the inconveniences of the state of nature."[45] To Locke, that "state of nature" is freedom, and government's proper role is to preserve that freedom mainly by preserving our fundamental rights of property and autonomy. In public health the essential rights we often speak of are those that protect us from interferences and harm. These are often called negative rights in contrast to positive rights that entitle us to some benefit, such as health care, even to privacy. However, the complex relationship between liberty and rights creates a tension that is very apparent in public health. Mill's principle that our liberties, meaning rights to freedom of action, end where we begin to harm others is not sufficient to justify a robust public health approach.[46] Prevention and protection provides a form of extension of our positive rights that allow us freedom to enjoy cleaner air, safe water, and longer lives.

Arguments over rights in public health can pit the collective and the individual in stark terms. The "right to smoke" cigarettes may be invoked by some who are more concerned with their right not to be interfered with rather than their lack of concern for health. Likewise, the rights of others to "clean air" is expressed more effectively when it is cast as a protection rather than a guarantee of noninterference. Mary Ann Glendon sees these conflicts over contending rights as misplaced and reflective of a society "obsessed with laws."[47] Public health is often more comfortable set in the context of a contractual world where the balance between fungible interests can be resolved. Absolute rights create irresolvable conflicts. Dan Beauchamp sees public health as a social and governmental process that is essentially pragmatic in nature, an expression of democracy itself, not a "thing" guaranteed in a structure of law-based rights.[48] That pragmatic approach to resolving conflicts between contending rights is the essence of politics but few like to admit to giving ground on the rights they believe in.

The relationship between universal human rights and public health was made forcefully by Jonathan Mann who argued that people could not function with dignity without their health and that public health systems were the best means of producing and protecting health.[49] This connection is now recognized as a movement of its own with the journal *Health and Human Rights*, founded by Mann, expressing the central arguments that promoting the public's health promotes justice and prosperity and is a moral obligation of governments and individuals.[50] Mann's belief was that "in the modern world, public health officials have, for the first time, two fundamental responsibilities to the public: to protect and promote public health and to protect and promote human rights."[51]

WHEN DOES PUBLIC HEALTH POLICY MAKING HAPPEN?

"Timing is everything in politics" is an oft-repeated nostrum likely to be heard or written in relationship to any specific issue. In public health, the reliance on protections in the infrastructures of water quality, workplace safety, air quality, as well as the responsiveness to immediate and overwhelming threats such as AIDS, severe acute respiratory syndrome (SARS), and bioterrorism present political challenges to public health. The field must maintain and regenerate its infrastructure as a continuing process that relies on annual budgets and long-term commitments, as well as being able to react swiftly and effectively in uncertain political terrain when new issues arise, often overnight. The combination of long-term predictability (there will always be disasters) and short-term unpredictability (where the next disaster will strike) creates pressure for public health leaders to assume Janus-like capabilities which can challenge even experienced political operatives.

Windows of Opportunity

Policy windows are those periods in the policy-making process when things can and do change, when ideas emerge "whose time has come" or when a series of coincident events create conditions that are favorable to the implementation of a policy that was formerly "premature" or "unacceptable." The brute force of big events, such as a terrorist attack, can create conditions where there is broad scale reform in the public health structure, or the force of such an event can be dissipated in endless discussions of changes that need to be made while the real political power, in the form of funding or leadership, is lacking.

There are temporal factors in the politics of public health that reflect broader political trends and cycles. These "windows of opportunity" occur in specific cycles tied to elections and budgets. However, the force of history looms large in political consideration in many fields, but especially in public health where we are often given only the lesson of history to help anticipate what may happen in the future or cope with unexpected events. The contemporary terrain includes a potential massive outbreak of avian influenza or Ebola, and, although we have plans to cope with them, they thrust policy making onto new ground. For an emerging Ebola crisis we may have only the 1918 influenza outbreak to serve as a template for action as well as a mechanism for stimulating attention.

Recent "concentrating" events in public health that opened windows of opportunity include the rise of HIV/AIDS that stimulated changes in research funding, treatment access, laws and rules of privacy, and the perception of the public toward various high-risk groups. The practical political impact is reflected in the rise in influence of pressure groups interested in fast-track research.

Election Cycles

In government, windows of opportunity open often when the people in charge change, and this cycle is somewhat regular due to the American tradition of fixed date elections and term limits. The power of elections to change the political landscape has recently been demonstrated. In the words of William Roper, former CDC and Health Care Financing Administration (HCFA), chief, writing in November of 2006 after the Democrats gained control of the House and Senate "There will be a window of opportunity in 2007 to legislate on some key health and health care issues, but by early 2008 that window will have closed, as the presidential campaign will then be in full swing."[52] This speaks to the powers of elections past as well as anticipated. The national policy process is punctuated by regular congressional and presidential elections that open up windows of opportunity for policy change especially if there is a sharp change in the power structure. The new leadership in Congress or the White House will sometimes see a "mandate for change."

Funding Cycles

The politics of public health are, in a sense, dominated by our annual budgeting process. Although we do create long-term authorizations and, in general, recurring budgets are relatively stable, we also pass state and local budgets every year or biennium. This puts almost every aspect of governmental public health "at risk" for legislative involvement. The annual crisis-driven budget cycle in the Congress known as "reconciliation" has become well known as the source of ill-considered and often extensive policy making. The Congress has set itself certain rules for its budget process, but divided government, with Democrats in the majority or in office in the Presidency and Republicans holding the other branch, created budget stalemates that required extraordinary processes to pass appropriations. These so-called Omnibus bills (OBRA, SOBRA, COBRA, TEFRA, BBA, and BBRA) included many enabling and directive laws that changed public health policy. Some were considered in hearings and the "normal" legislative process and included in final passage, others were the result of rushed compromises as part of huge and often contradictory enactments. The Patient Protection and Affordable Care Act (ACA) resembles this sort of "omnibus" approach where many disparate pieces of legislation were combined in the name of "comprehensive" reform.

Selected public health issues have become leverage points in the legislative process. Stem cell research and late-term abortions, for example, have been "hot-button" items which are inserted in larger bills with the goal of forcing a vote that will in effect stall passage of appropriations for "normal" government activities. Because these are germane to health they are often inserted in the appropriations bills for Labor, Health and Human Services, and Education—the cluster of appropriations that covers much of federal health activities. This often slows or even completely stalls final action on the funding bills. The solution necessary to keep government running, is to pass continuing resolutions which essentially set in place funding levels of the previous year's appropriations. In February of 2007, the Congress essentially agreed to give up on passing appropriations for many parts of government including Health and Human Services by extending the relevant continuing resolution through Fiscal Year 2007. This is an unusual approach even in a process that has apparently no set rules and is an outgrowth of the divided government that has become common early in the twenty-first century.

Agendas as Schedules

The budget cycle is one temporal element of the agenda-setting process. Election cycles and the natural history of policy proposals, the "issue-attention cycle" mentioned earlier, are also important to the timing of policy events. There are also contrived **agenda** that presidents, agency heads or congressional leaders or caucuses set and which control the ascent of issues into the policy-making process. Presidents are now fond of declaring a 100-day agenda; Newt Gingrich created a "Contract with America" that was essentially an agenda for a large voting bloc in Congress; and in the 109th Congress, Speaker Nancy Pelosi declared a 100-hour schedule in the House of Representatives with specific legislative goals. These structured agendas can be derailed—Gingrich's plans were interrupted by a breakdown in Medicare reform when rural hospital interests balked at budget cuts—but they also can be very powerful in keeping issues out of the process as much as they are to promoting policies. Secretary of Health and Human Services Michael Leavitt entered office with a 500-day plan (http://www.hhs.gov/500DayPlan) that essentially signaled to his agency that no substantive work would be done on anything except what was included in the list.

WHERE DOES PUBLIC HEALTH POLITICS AND POLICY MAKING HAPPEN

The notion of place in policy making is a subtle concept but often the geographical context of a policy decision is the most important factor shaping how it evolves and is applied. The United States is a large and largely self-sufficient nation and its politics reflect a particularism and tradition of independence that often rejects other national models. These conditions hold in public health; the nation was built on a tradition of self-reliance and invention that followed necessity and its social and political structures as well as its public health system emerged from pragmatic local as well as national accommodations to the realities of a rapidly growing, industrializing nation that had immense natural resources to exploit.

Geography

The geography of the United States reflects historical, geological, and meteorological realities. The nation was settled or conquered from east to west (by the Anglophones); the indigenous peoples were pushed into the sparsely settled and arid Western lands, then largely ignored as those places had little economic value. The South embraced slavery and created a disenfranchised population that, when freed, sought to migrate to places where there was more tolerance and opportunity. These realities of place and people created the basis for persisting inequities and disparities in health.[53] The geography of race and ethnicity once saw concentrations of groups in certain places: Hispanics in the Western border states and poor blacks in the rural South and central Northern cities. Those patterns are quickly breaking down as populations continue to be very mobile and new immigrants move to places where jobs are available far away from the "traditional" settling places. There remain significant geographic and regional clusters of poverty and lack of development that create regional political pressures. Those areas are also marked by their very poor public health indicators.[54]

The region that includes and immediately borders the Appalachian Mountains were long synonymous with persistent rural poverty. To address poverty in those towns and counties, regional, quasi-political structures were created to build infrastructure and support development. The Tennessee Valley Authority and later the Appalachian Regional Commission were created to focus efforts in places that were common in their economic and social characteristics but crossed many state boundaries. These regional solutions to common geographic problems are not well accepted in the federal structure; the power base to support them is diffuse and unorganized and often conflicts with claimants and stakeholders in the states and localities who are included in the region.

Other regional "authorities" have been developed with the intent of closing persistent economic gaps. These also include substantial attention to health and public health issues. The Delta Regional Authority and Denali Regional Commissions promote direct support for health care delivery and prevention and public health.

Federalism

The federal structure of American government is a unique characteristic of the American polity that is very important to public health policy.[55] When we speak of federalism, we are referring to the system of government where the original, sovereign powers of government rested within the several states, and those states ceded specific powers to the federal or central government by ratifying the Constitution. The states retained the common law "police powers" which reserved to the states the responsibility and the power to protect the public's health, safety, and welfare. In order to exercise this power, the states, themselves, were free to create other levels of government as they saw fit: counties, towns,

municipalities, authorities. This left the nation with a very complex structure of state, local, and national government, but the principal responsibility for public health was held by the states.

This complexity, as it relates to public health, is viewed as both a weakness and a strength.[56] Federalism, to Oliver, allows us to experiment to some degree with policy formation where the states operate as the "laboratories of democracy" but that can create bewildering variation in policies in some sectors.[24]

While the legal basis for public health laws may rest in the states and common law, the federal government assumed a leadership role in protecting the public using other clauses in the Constitution, most notably the Commerce Clause, to justify the Food and Drug Act, then protections for workers and subsequently for clean air and water. For much of the twentieth century, it could be said that the notable advances in public health were the result of federal legislation that was built *via* federal political structures and processes. Toward the end of the twentieth century, the federal government, the Congress and the executive branch, backed away from active promotion of public health issues and the states were left to either act or to remain passive as the "new federalism" devolved the initiative for further public activity to the states.[55] There remain substantial forces alive for further public health regulation and policy making in Congress and the national executive branch, but individual states have been more active in recent years as they recognize the opportunity to regulate behavior to protect lives (e.g. smoking restrictions) or the need to restructure and modernize bureaucracies (e.g. pandemic flu or a bioterrorism attack).

WHY PUBLIC HEALTH POLICY; WHY PUBLIC HEALTH POLITICS?

Politics and policy making in the United States can be seen to be driven by our collective desires to achieve the goals set out in the Preamble to the Constitution. Public health as promoting the general welfare may seem most relevant to some while others may see the establishment of justice as the primary principle that guides our collective decision making. However, as the debates in the 13 original state assemblies that led to the adoption of the Constitution revealed, there was as much concern about the maintenance of trade and the economy as there was concern with fundamental, philosophical liberties and rights. The practical evolution of public health agencies emerged from practical collective decisions made by local authorities under their interpretation of the reserved police powers. This dependence on pragmatics and local authority complicates any attempt to identify a central answer to the question of "why?" in public health policy making. Over time, we have developed some main themes that can be used to categorize the justifications for public health policy.

Liberal Traditions

The heart of our legal as well as philosophical traditions has been the idea that all persons enjoy individual and inviolable rights which the government is bound to protect. The liberal traditions of American politics are at the core of the public health policy paradox: how collective action can occur in a nation that values individual liberty. The United States has a long history of balancing the powers of government and the prerogatives and freedoms of the individuals. Many of the central conflicts of the republic have come over issues surrounding public health that saw individual rights in conflict with the collective powers and needs of the nation or state.

Liberal justice emphasizes individual responsibility, restricted collective action, and freedom from collective obligations except to respect the fundamental rights of others. John Stuart Mill's essay "On Liberty" remains a much-read guide to the limits of government and the responsibilities of individuals.[57] Liberal justice historically has sought to limit the range of interests people can claim in conditions conducive to well-being, but in recent years a more libertarian model of justice has surfaced that stresses traditional values. F.A. Hayek, a libertarian much admired by the new conservatives, sees the social structures, uniformities, and regularities by which public health advances the common health as merely "spontaneous orders" produced by individuals and organizations, and the dream of social justice as a "mirage."[58]

The alternative to the libertarian theme is one of social justice where the underlying problems of inequality and injustice are taken as a problem and not a condition. This recognition of inequality, or in modern public health parlance, disparity and inequities, are problems subject to policy interventions, and this fits well into Kingdon's description of how issues move on to an agenda and eventually find a match with policy solutions.

Economics

From the founding of the republic there has been a tension between the demands of commerce and the health of the people; Nancy Milio posed the contrast starkly by asking "Is a healthy profit compatible with a healthy population?"[59] Conflicts between economic interests and public health are often very public and dramatic. The pressures for profits drive corporations to pollute water and air, which in turn creates measurable health consequences, the Love Canal example being just one of many.[60] The role of business is often seen as naturally oppositional to public health interests. Political scientist and economist Charles Lindblom described the "market prison" that forces elected officials and bureaucrats to favor market expansion over health or public protection.[61] However there have been significant constraints placed on the freedom of business to ignore the health of the public and equally significant restraints on personal behavior, such as smoking, that have important effects on the viability of business.

The ability of the United States to control the negative health effects of market activity is seen as somewhat surprising by some who see the regulatory advances of the 1970s, including the Clean Air and Clean Water Acts and the Occupational Safety and Health Act as somewhat out of step with American traditions.[62] However, aggressive agencies that confront business often "have their wings clipped" as did the Environmental Protection Agency (EPA) and the Occupational Safety and Health Administration (OSHA) when their enthusiastic enforcement of the laws in the 1980s was met with subsequent administrative and congressional opposition.[63] However, the important thing is that those agencies persisted beyond the 1980s into the twenty-first century and their mechanisms to control pollution or occupational hazards remain in place and their effects have created an overall better environment and workplace than would have occurred without their work.[48,64]

Values in Public Health: Justice and Utility

Amartya Sen, a Nobel Laureate in economics, speaks of democracy's values as *intrinsic* (one vote, one person, etc.), *instrumental* (giving voice to the hitherto powerless), and *constructive* (forging new interests and needs in the conditions for social justice through conflict and democratic discussion); these may be seen as values more aligned with notions of justice than with the general welfare.[65] In a more philosophical vein, Dan Beauchamp wrote an important essay that equated public health with social justice.[43] That juxtaposition has helped structure arguments for expanded government activity in public health as well as greater personal responsibility for health. The notion of public health as social justice ties together the separate components of Sen's democratic values, giving us an example of how democracy should work, balancing the needs of individuals with the pressures and compulsions of the commons. Indeed, Beauchamp points to the resurgence of democracy as the stimulus for public health progress:

> Surely that 10-year increase in life expectancy since 1950 is mostly due to societal sea changes like the sharp decline in smoking from public health campaigns, causing a big drop in heart disease and lung cancer, or to safer highways, less poverty, less discrimination, and cleaner air. For all that, and for Medicare and Medicaid, we can thank resurgent democracy during the Great Society era and the coming to the fore of public health agencies and activism.[66]

The contrast of utilitarian ideals with those of justice does not present an either-or choice. Each presents a schema that can help guide practical policy choices. The elaboration of the utilitarian idea into careful cost-benefit studies that consider the widest possible set of externalities can be matched with a careful assessment of the degree to which principles of justice can be applied. This is accomplished through democratic structures and processes that give voice to both sides. Those structures are forums for honest and open debate as well as the electoral process; however, the latter seldom considers public health.

HOW DOES PUBLIC HEALTH POLICY AND POLITICS GET DONE?

Policy making is the creation of laws, rules, regulations as well as the structured codes and laws of the states and the federal government. It is the "stuff" that politics does. But, how is it done? Most of the guidance a student gets in introductory politics and policy classes focuses on the formal structure of law making, and this is covered extensively in texts and guides. "How a Bill Becomes Law" is a classic title of a description of the steps legislation takes before final passage (see, for example, http://thomas.loc.gov/home/holam.txt for a description). Unfortunately that process is more the exception than the rule in the U.S. Congress and most state assemblies. Public health law making is like any other legislative process and it enjoys no special stature, as for example, budgeting might. The entire policy-making process in public health extends well beyond the passage of laws as there are public health policy decisions that control the lives and actions of people and institutions that are made by even the lowliest sanitation inspector in the application of local ordinances. The inspector may have a degree of flexibility, a pattern that amounts to a policy decision. Policy can be made at the street level and often is.[67]

Law Making

Public Health law expert Michelle Mello wrote: "The law is firmly established as a powerful instrument of public health."[68] That close relationship has created a sense that we can, with the wise use of legal means, improve the health and well-being of Americans by tackling the recognizable threats to health. However, this creates in some minds an overreliance on legal mechanisms. The current controversies over how to deal with rising rates of obesity exemplifies the attraction of legal remedies for public health problems as we try to make certain products and practices "illegal." This dependence on formal regulation and law making puts public health in a position of a constant participant in the formal governmental process, where legal language and adherence to procedures becomes paramount.

Public health policy to protect the population is characterized by Turshen as falling into three major realms: cleansing the environment, eradicating disease, and containing disease.[69] These options are contrasted with the preferred option of prevention, which, in Turshen's view, is less often available to public health policy makers. Public health law and policy is more often reactive and structured to clean up after hazards are produced (as in Super Fund legislation), to eradicate vectors after they have spread (as in polio vaccines), or to contain threats when that is the only option (as in pandemic influenza preparedness). Cleansing the environment can be more progressive and effective if it anticipates the impact of emerging threats. However, the process of cleansing often entails transporting and storing hazardous materials that no one wants. The resistance to siting of landfills and hazardous waste containment facilities can be intense and generates a "NIMBY—Not In My Backyard" response as communities are targeted for these uses.

The lawmaking process is a function of the institutions of Congress, the Administration, and bureaucracy, and that process is replicated across the 50 states. The staggering of terms, the varieties of rules and customs, and the natural tensions of one branch against the other multiplied by the federal structure makes law making a complex and inherently conservative process. In public health, this is especially so due to the relative place of the states in terms of their public health responsibilities.

Intergovernmental Processes

The federal system is an important defining element of the public health structure in the United States. The state governments are often said to have the original jurisdiction in public health matters by virtue of their police powers, but the proximity of interest groups and stakeholders often makes it difficult for the states to enact restrictive policies and laws that affect producers and communities. Where an industry is an important local contributor to the economy, state legislators are loathe to require controls and set standards that would affect profits.[70] By the same token states and localities have been able to pass laws that set stringent air quality levels, restrict smoking, and change the fat content of cooking oils. This is due to their responsiveness to public pressure that outweighs their sensitivity to organized economic pressures.

The federal government does not have a constitutional power to protect the public's health, but does have the power and ability to control interstate commerce as well as to set national standards for air and water quality or passenger vehicle safety. These powers come with the deep pockets of tax revenues and a borrowing capacity that allows immense federal support to flow to programs to advance health-promoting regulations, support prevention and surveillance programs, and directly provide services such as vaccinations for the general population. However, many programs and initiatives that form the core of public health are actually state-based with significant but minority federal input. Vital statistics and monitoring, for example, are collaborative efforts where state agencies adopt shared standards, and grant-in-aid funds are provided by the federal government to supplement state funds. Maternal and child health programs in the states function with substantial federal block grants, with some states far exceeding the federal commitment, while others barely supplement it.

Political scientist Tom Oliver argues that, in public health, federalism has produced an unhealthy variation in policies to address common problems;[24] this was recognized in public health by its leaders and a "public health statute modernization collaborative" was created with the support of the Robert Wood Johnson and W. K. Kellogg Foundations to align the laws and procedures of the states to allow them to better meet the challenges of public health need and external threats (http://www.turningpointprogram.org). This process has generated initiatives to compare and assess the performance of state public health agencies.[71] That development threatens to weaken the traditional independence and autonomy of the states as they become subject to the politics of comparisons—where they must keep up with other states and not "go it alone."

It is often local governments that bear the greatest burden of enforcing public health laws and making policy that restricts individual and business behaviors. The National Association of County and City Health Officials (NACCHO) estimates that there are 2,864 local health departments in the United States.[72] These are often overseen by elected or appointed boards with executive powers and authority and they contend with state laws set by statewide agencies as well as federal standards and rules and occasionally direct responsibility to report to federal officials. This very complex system can be seen as chaotic in one sense, but it is drawn together by a common notion of the unique profession of public health as well as a broad agreement on the core functions and responsibilities of public health.

Markets for Policy

The economist Paul Feldstein sees policy making and politics subject to market rules, where policy makers are merely balancing their demands with those of other stakeholders and exchanges of values are accomplished in legislative or administrative "markets."[73] This notion of "trading" in policy is described by Feldstein as an "economic version of interest group theory of legislation" where it is the special interests who are the primary demanders of legislation rather than the people whom legislators represent. The suppliers of legislation are the legislators themselves who redistribute resources, taxes, and power, and the administrative branch that enforces those decisions. The applicability of this framework to public health is more difficult than for other health policy domains. Feldstein noted that legislation to combat AIDS was not forthcoming until established and recognizable interest groups demanded support for drug research. The evolution of environmental policies that cleaned the air and water are even harder to fit into this theory. Feldstein found that the policies were enacted largely due to a stalemate between contending industrial interests. In the end, he says that the solutions that were put in place were economically inefficient largely because the Congress did not want to cede its power to the market, thus supporting his notion of legislators as suppliers of policy and suppliers who could dominate the market if they chose to.

Politics of People and "Stories"

There is a school of thought that sees policy making as structured and subject to scientific rules and patterns if not fundamental laws. The study of policy analysis has moved itself away from politics, something seen as emotional and chaotic which can be manipulated by the unscrupulous or the single issue advocate. However, it is the chaos and the struggle that creates the effective "stories" of politics, and these stories that create the real themes that support policy making, even in a professionally dominated, complex world such as public health.

"Organizations, government or private, when they reach a certain size, become 'organized anarchies.'"[74] The anarchic nature of large government is recognizable in the United States in public health policy making. The system is very complex, structurally and conceptually, the stakeholders varied and, at any given time, any group can dominate. This makes it difficult to apply a "formula" to any description of the process and tends to make it possible to just "tell the story" as it happens. This is where the idea of pure politics comes into play, the point where it is the combination of the personalities, the place, and the time that conspires to make a thing happen or not. In the United States, the tendency is toward less, rather than more change, given the consciously designed and unconscious complexity of the system; however, the dominance of people and ideas is evident in the politics. In their book describing the failure of President Clinton's health reform plan, David Broder and Haynes Johnson emphasize how it is flesh-and-blood people with their personal stories that make politics run.[75] They emphasize how the people involved in policy making could stand up to institutions and waves of popular sentiment to bring an "idea whose time had come" to a halt. They also made the point that it is people's stories that change people's minds in the process and they gave us examples of real stories from the emergency rooms of Los Angeles to the manufactured story of Harry and Louise; the former may have moved the reform forward, but the latter served to thwart it. The power of storytelling is the power behind policy making. In public health, the stories are a bit different but almost always personal, whether coming from Love Canal or the family of Ryan White; these stories are the heart of the politics (see Table 6–1).

TABLE 6–1   The Journalistic Approach to Policy Assessment: A Review

Q's The Questions)	Sub Q's (The Sub-Questions)	Brief Description
Who	Elites	The people who run things. They sometimes get elected but more often are found running the primary institutions.
	Professionals	Doctors, dentists, lawyers. In public health there is an emerging trend toward more professionalization.
	Bureaucrats	In and out of government, they have enormous negative, less often recognized positive, power including the ability to manage and complete very complex tasks.
	Scientists/Academics	People with a "code" of science who are respected by the public. Their sustenance comes from a mix of public and private sources and their values underpin some aspects of public health: the primacy of data and inquiry.
	Media	Once this was restricted to journalists but the role of media is now becoming much more diffuse.
	"The People," the public	They are voters. They appear in public opinion polls and they function as communities with specific demands.
	Policy Entrepreneurs	They push solutions, generate ideas, and try to make them policy.
	Great People	Public health has strong historical figures, but the field is not seen as a place where individual power can be exercised. Great people emerge as role models.
What	Agendas and Plans	The political agenda for parties and groups form the starting framework for political debates and controversies.
	Laws, Rules, Regulations	They guide human behavior.
	Customs	These are not written down but they also guide behavior.
	Institutions	Banks, hospitals, the Congress, the Administration, interest group systems.
	Symbols	The flag, equality, efficiency, "15% of the GNP," access, health.
	Rights	The few guaranteed versus the many claimed.

TABLE 6–1 (Continued)

Q's The Questions)	Sub Q's (The Sub-Questions)	Brief Description
	Governments	The 7,000 jurisdictions, boards, commissions, and authorities that tax and distribute benefits.
	Communities	The innumerable ways people get together and relate to each other. Politics is often practiced most intensively at this level.
When	Windows of Opportunity	Kingdon's classic "idea whose time has come." Usually either by the confluence of forces or an unexpected event (death, war, election).
	Election Cycles	They influence behavior and what can be done.
	Funding Cycles	The creation of budgets in the United States is a regular cycle in legislation and opens opportunities to change substantive laws at the same time as appropriations are set.
	Agendas and Schedules	The legislative and policy-making process has limits to the volume of issues. Timing and priority are very important.
	History	It looms large in policy, as we look to past decisions to guide.
Where	American Values	We have a manifest destiny, we lead the world, we are a melting pot, we are dominated by Judeo-Christian ideas.
	Border Realities	In reality we are a continental nation that has two very different borders, Canada (like us) and Mexico (unlike us).
	Regional Concerns	"We don't care how you did it up North" is seen on license plates in the South and there's no denying that there are regional values and health realities for the Appalachians or the upper Midwest.
	Federalism	The states do have power in health; policies can change dramatically as one crosses a state border.
Why	Liberal Traditions	We are individuals, with individual freedoms, and science and knowledge lead the way (with a dose of Judeo-Christian authority).
	Economics	Adam Smith said we all seek our own satisfaction and that benefits the masses. Likewise, the complexity of the system reflects the efficiencies gained by the division of labor. However, people often do not seek to optimize nor is health a compartmentalized process.
	Values	Judeo-Christian, humanistic. Either take care of the next person directly or let the market do it while maintaining autonomy. Americans embody a paradox where strong individuals conform to common patters of consumption and belief.
	Justice	A super-value in that all systems and theories claim to create or promote justice.
How	Law Making	The "classic" process of passing legislation, but it has rules and almost all laws take their own special and unique routes to passage.
	Intergovernmental Processes	America is a federal republic with a unique balance of powers between the central government and the states. Power and politics are often devolved to localities—counties, cities . . . all have influence over public health.
	Market for Policy	Policies compete for attention and acceptance, like ideas. Some are "superior" and accepted, other rejected.
	Politics	The exercise of power, for its own sake, is a real factor in what policies are adopted.
	Making Deals	"How things really get done," the interaction of people and policies, within the constraints of institutions and time

Policy making and politics in public health follow the "normal" pathways to law making and the implementation of regulations, but there are important differences. These can best be understood if we follow the "story" of public health and understand: who is making the laws, what they are all about, where the laws and rules are applied so that they match the American context, when they fit into the cycles of the legislative process, budgeting, or if they react to "focusing" events, why they try to balance the tension between individual freedom and collective needs, and how the process works in the real world.

SUMMARY

The conduct of politics and the policy-making process in public health can be better understood when viewed through a journalistic lens. By asking **who** is involved in the process, **what** the options and mechanisms are, **where** the specific programs are intended to work while considering the American context, **when** the procedures and institutions will allow for change, **how** the process works and how politics function, and lastly, **why** policy changes are needed, the student of the health policy system can capture almost all of what they need to function effectively and change public health policy and politics.

REVIEW QUESTIONS

1. Describe a "journalistic" approach to policy analysis and identify the key individual elements that fall within the core questions a policy analyst should ask.

2. What are the differences between politics and policy making? Describe how values may influence both.

3. Provide arguments for why "windows of opportunity" can trump carefully crafted policy agendas and give examples of how each interpretation of policy making can be applied to recent policy changes.

REFERENCES

1. Lasswell HD. *Politics: Who Gets What, When, How.* 11th printing ed. New York: The World Publishing Company; 1971.

2. Kingdon JW. *Agendas, Alternatives and Public Policies.* Second ed. New York: HarperCollins; 1995.

3. Heaney MT. Brokering health policy: coalitions, parties and interest group influence. *Journal of Health Politics, Policy and Law.* October 2006;31(5):887–944.

4. Oliver TK, Jr., Tunnessen WW, Jr., Butzin D, Guerin R, Stockman JA, 3rd. Pediatric work force: data from the American Board of Pediatrics. *Pediatrics.* 1997;99(2):241–244.

5. Litman TJ, Robins LS, eds. *Health Politics and Policy.* Third ed. Albany, NY: Delmar Publishers; 1997.

6. Morone JA, Litman TJ, Robins LS, eds. *Health Politics and Policy.* 4th ed. Clifton Park, NY: Delmar Cengage Learning; 2008.

7. Patel K, Rushevsky ME. *The Politics of Public Health in the United States.* New York: M.E. Sharpe; 2005.

8. Longest BB. *Health Policymaking in the United States.* 4th ed. Chicago: Health Administration Press; 2004.

9. Harrington C, Estes CL, eds. *Health Policy.* 4th ed. Boston: Jones and Bartlett; 2004.

10. McLaughlin CP, McLaughlin CD. *Health Policy Analysis an Interdisciplinary Approach.* Boston: Jones and Bartlett; 2008.

11. Scutchfield FD, Ireson C, Hall L. The voice of the public in public health policy and planning: the role of public judgment. *Journal of Public Health Policy.* 2004;25(2).

12. Starr P. *The Social Transformation of American Medicine.* New York: Basic Books; 1982.

13. Begun JW, Lippencott RC. *Strategic Adaptation in the Health Professions.* San Francisco: Jossey-Bass; 1993.

14. Jacobson N, Butterill D, Goering P. Consulting as a strategy for knowledge transfer. *Milbank Quarterly.* 2005;82(2):299–321.

15. Schultz J. *Reviving the Fourth Estate: Democracy, Accountability & the Media.* Cambridge: Cambridge University Press; 1998.

16. Fallows J. *Breaking the News: How the Media Undermine American Democracy.* New York: Pantheon Books; 1996.

17. Singhal A, Rogers EM. *Combating AIDS: Communication Strategies in Action.* Thousand Oaks, CA: Sage; 2003.

18. Grier S, Bryant CA. Social marketing in public health. *Annu Rev Public Health.* 2005;26: 319–339.

19. Siegel M. Mass media antismoking campaigns: a powerful tool for health promotion. *Ann Intern Med.* Jul 15 1998;129(2):128–132.

20. Wolfe A. *Does American Democracy Still Work?* New Haven, CT: Yale University Press; 2006.

21. Soroka SN, Lim ET. Issue definition and the opinion-policy link: public preferences and health care spending in the US and UK. *British Journal of Politics and International Relations.* November 2003(5):4.

22. Blendon RJ, Altman DE. Voters and health care in the 2006 election. *N Engl J Med.* Nov 2 2006;355(18):1928–1933.

23. Institute of Medicine. *The Future of the Public's Health in the 21st Century.* Washington, DC: National Academy Press; 2003.

24. Oliver TR. The politics of public health policy. *Annu Rev Public Health.* 2006;27:195–233.

25. *The Guide to Clinical Preventive Services 2014: Recommendations of the U.S. Preventive Services Task Force.* Rockville (MD)2014.

26. Stobbe M. *Surgeon General's Warning: How Politics Crippled the Nation's Doctor.* Oakland, CA: University of California Press; 2014.

27. Harris G. Surgeon General Sees 4-Year Term as Compromised. *New York Times.* July 11, 2007, 2007.

28. Wilst WH. Citizens United, Public Health, and Democracy: The Supreme Court Ruling, Its implications, and Proposed Action. *American Journal of Public Health.* July, 2011;101(7):1172–1179.

29. Garrett KN, Jansa JM, Carsey TM. Networks and Interest Group Influence in the Diffusion of Regulation 2014.

30. Sabatier PA, Jenkins-Smith HC. The advocacy coalition framework, an assessment. In: Sabatier PA, ed. *Theories of the Policy Process.* Boulder, CO: Westview Press; 1999.

31. Browne WP. Rural failure: the linkage between policy and lobbies. *Policy Studies Journal.* 2001;29(1):108–117.

32. Lambrew JM. The heartland's heartstrings: the power, challenges and opportunities of rural health advocacy in Washington. *North Carolina Medical Journal.* 2006;67(1):55–57.

33. Satel S. Public Health? Forget It; Cosmic Issues Beckon. *The Wall Street Journal.* December 13, 2001.

34. Downs A. Up and down with ecology: the issue attention cycle. *Public Interest.* 1972;28(1):38–50.

35. Baumgadner FR, Jones BD. *Agendas and Instability in American Politics.* Chicago: University of Chicago Press; 1993.

36. Wilson JQ, Dilulio JJ. *American Government: Institutions and Policies.* 9th ed. New York: Houghton Mifflin; 2004.

37. Wilson JQ. *American Government: Institutions and Policies.* Lexington, MA: D.C. Health and Company; 1992.

38. Gostin LO. Public health and civil liberties in an era of bioterrorism. *Crim Justice Ethics.* Summer 2002;21(2):2, 74–76.

39. Stone D. *Policy Paradox: The Art of Political Decision Making.* Second ed. New York: W. W. Norton & Company; 1997.

40. Stone D. Symbols. *Policy Paradox: The Art of Political Decision Making.* Second ed. New York: W. W. Norton & Company; 1997a:137–162.

41. Lemann N. Conservative opportunity society. *The Atlantic.* May 1985:22–36.

42. Beauchamp D. Public health, privatization, and market populism: a time for reflection. *Qual Manag Health Care.* 1997;5(2):73–79.

43. Beauchamp DE. Public health as social justice. *Inquiry.* 1976;13(1):3–14.

44. Kawachi I, Berkman LF. *Neighborhoods and Health.* New York: Oxford University Press; 2003.

45. Locke J. *Second Tretise of Civil Government.* New York: Liberal Arts; 1951.

46. Beauchamp DE. *The Health of the Republic. Epidemics, Medicine, and Moralism as Challenges to Democracy.* Philadelphia: Temple University Press; 1988.

47. Glendon MA. *Rights Talk: The Impoverishment of Political Discourse.* New York: Free Press; 1991.

48. Beauchamp D. Health, Social Justice and the Other Great Society. University of North Carolina at Chapel Hill; 2007.

49. Gostin LO. Public health, ethics and human rights: a tribute to the late Jonathan Mann. *Journal of Law Medicine & Ethics.* 2001;29:121–130.

50. Tarantola D, Gruskin S, Brown TM, Fee E. Jonathan Mann: founder of the health and human rights movement. *Am J Public Health.* Nov 2006;96(11):1942–1943.

51. Mann JM. Medicine and public health, ethics and human rights. In: Beauchamp DE, Steinbock B, eds. *New Ethics for the Public's Health.* New York: Oxford; 1999:83–93.

52. Roper B. A Republican perspective on the impact of the 2006 elections on U.S. health policy. *Health Affairs Blog* 2006; http://healthaffairs.org/blog/2006/11/09/politics-a-republican-perspective-on-the-impact-of-the-2006-elections-on-us-health-policy/. Accessed June 5, 2008.

53. Swift EK, ed *Guidance for the National Healthcare Disprites Report.* Washington, DC: Institute of Medicine; 2002.

54. Pickle LW, Mungiole M, Jones GK, White AA. *Atlas of United States Mortality.* Hyattsville, MD: U.S. Department of Health and Human Services; 1996.

55. Turnock BJ, Atchison C. Governmental public health in the United States: the implications of federalism. *Health Affairs.* 2002;21(6):68–78.

56. Institute of Medicine. Committee for the Study of the Future of Public Health. *The Future of Public Health.* Washington, DC: National Academy Press; 1988.

57. Mill JS. On Liberty. Bartleby.com; 1999: www .bartleby.com/130/.

58. Hayek FAV. *The Mirage of Social Justice.* London: Routledge and Kegan Paul; 1976.

59. Milio N. *Public Health in the Market.* Ann Arbor, MI: University of Michigan Press; 2000.

60. Wolff S. Love Canal revisited. *Jama.* Mar 16 1984;251(11):1464.

61. Lindblom C. The Market as Prison. *The Journal of Politics.* 1982;44:324–336.

62. Beauchamp D. The law, the market, and the health of the body politic. *Hastings Cent Rep.* Jul–Aug 2002;32(4):44–46.

63. Dryzek JS. The good society versus the state: Freedom and necessity in political innovation. *The Journal of Politics.* 1992;54(2):518–540.

64. Milikis SM, Mileur JM, eds. *The Great Society and the High Tide of Liberalism.* Amherst, MA: The University of Massachusetts Press; 2005.

65. Sen A. Democracy as a universal value. *Journal of Democracy.* 1999;10(3):3–17.

66. Beauchamp DE. Health care spending: the democracy connection. *talesofcoppercity.com* 2006; www.talesofcoppercity.com/talesofcoppercity/ public_health/index.html. Accessed March 23, 2007.

67. Lipsky M. *Street Level Bureaucracy.* 30th Anniversary Expanded Edition ed. New York: Russell Sage Foundation; 2010.

68. Mello MM, Studdert DM, Brennan TA. Obesity—the new frontier of public health law. *N Engl J Med.* Jun 15 2006;354(24):2601–2610.

69. Turshen M. *The Politics of Public Health.* New Brunscwick, NJ: Rutgers University Press; 1989.

70. Freudenberg N, Galea S. The impact of corporate practices on health: implications for health policy. *Journal of Public Health Policy.* 2008;29(1):86–104.

71. Mays GP, Halverson PK. Conceptual and methodological issues in public health performance measurement: results from a computer-assisted expert panel process. *Journal of Public Health Management and Practice.* 2000;6(5):59–65.

72. Leep CJ. *National Profile of Local Health Departments.* Washington, DC: National Association of County & City Health Officials; 2006.

73. Feldstein PJ. *The Politics of Health Legislation an Economic Perspective.* 2nd ed. Chicago: Health Administration Press; 1996.

74. Cohen MD, March JG, Olsen JP. A garbage can model of organizational choice. *Administrative Science Quarterly.* 1972;17(1):1–25.

75. Johnson H, Broder D. *The System, the American Way of Politics at the Breaking Point.* Boston: Little, Brown and Company; 1995.

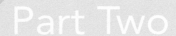

Part Two

THE SETTINGS OF PUBLIC HEALTH PRACTICE

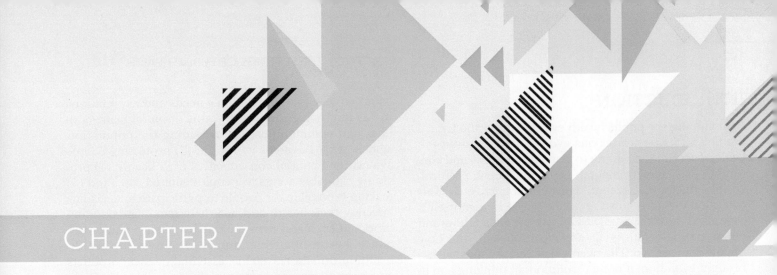

CHAPTER 7

The Federal Contribution to Public Health

Georgia A. Moore, MS • Craig W. Thomas, PhD • Judith A. Monroe, MD

LEARNING OBJECTIVES

Upon completion of this chapter, the reader will be able to:

1. Describe the various components of the federal government as they relate to public health.

2. Analyze the authorities, roles, and responsibilities of federal agencies in public health.

3. Examine examples of federal influence on and contributions to the public health system.

4. Assess emerging trends and possible future directions for public health from a federal perspective.

KEY TERMS

federal regulation
role of the federal government
health system transformation
National Center for Health Statistics (NCHS)
public health infrastructure
Surgeon General

INTRODUCTION

As it should, the public health system within the United States and its territories has evolved and continues to evolve over time according to population needs and conditions (e.g., environmental, economic, legal, political, social, educational, technological, biological, etc.). This evolution includes how the public health system itself is organized, how the parts fit and work together, how and where public health goals are accomplished, and how impact is measured. The twenty-first century thus far has brought evolution, if not a revolution, in thinking and in approach to these issues. This chapter provides an overview of the current roles, responsibilities, and contributions of the federal government to public health ("federal public health"), and of developments that are shaping the future of federal public health.

FEDERAL ROLES AND RESPONSIBILITIES IN PUBLIC HEALTH

The U.S. public health system is not centralized. Public health activities in the United States and its territories are carried out through the collective actions of governmental agencies and private-sector organizations working at national, state, local (includes cities, counties, regions), tribal, and territorial levels. These stakeholders have diverse interests, values, areas of focus, authorities, roles, resources, tools, and influence in the overall system. As previously discussed, most public health legal authorities reside with state, tribal, local, and territorial governments, and most public health services are delivered by and within those jurisdictions.

General Roles and Responsibilities

In a decentralized and continuously changing system, the overarching role of the federal government is to ensure the health system functions as well as possible. A well-functioning public health system responds in a balanced way to a population's needs and expectations by (1) improving the health status of individuals, families, and communities; (2) defending the population against what threatens its health; (3) protecting people against the financial consequences of ill health; (4) providing equitable access to people-centered care; and (5) making it possible for people to participate in decisions affecting their health and health system.[1] The building blocks of such a system include leadership and governance, health financing, human resources for health, health information systems, essential medical products and technologies, and service delivery.

The federal government plays an important role in facilitating communication, coordination, and collaboration across the decentralized system. It facilitates a shared vision (e.g., "Healthy people in healthy communities"),[2] a shared mission (e.g., "Promote physical and mental health and prevent disease, injury, and disability"),[2] and a shared functional framework (e.g., the 10 Essential Public Health Services).[3] Some of the general roles and responsibilities of the federal government are listed in Exhibit 7-1. In addition, as will be discussed in more detail later in this chapter, an important new role of the federal government is supporting changes related to connecting investments in the health of an individual with investments in the health of the entire community, with the goal of maximizing use of resources and better protecting and improving health.

All three branches of the federal government play a role in the health of the public according to their separate functions as follows (see Chapter 6):

- Legislative Branch – Creates statutes that establish and empower executive agencies; regulates various activities; provides agencies authority to promulgate regulations and oversee regulated activities; appropriates money; and makes certain activities crimes.
- Executive Branch – Implements authority provided by legislature; promulgates regulations, if authorized; prescribes the standards that people and companies must follow in order to be lawful while engaging in

EXHIBIT 7-1 Federal Public Health – General Roles and Responsibilities

- Ensure all levels of government have the capabilities to provide essential public health services.
- Act when health threats may span more than one state, a region, or the entire nation.
- Act where the solutions may be beyond the jurisdiction of individual states.
- Act to assist the states when they lack the expertise or resources to effectively respond in a public health emergency (e.g., a disaster, bioterrorism, or an emerging disease).
- Facilitate the formulation of public health goals (in collaboration with state and local governments and other relevant stakeholders).

SOURCE: Trust for America's Health. Public Health Leadership Initiative: An Action Plan for Healthy People in Healthy Communities in the 21st Century. Washington, DC. 2006

a certain activity; and enforces standards established in statutes and regulations. The President is the head of the executive branch of the government, which includes many departments and agencies.[4] These agencies are responsible for day-to-day enforcement and administration of federal laws.

▶ Judicial Branch – Resolves disputes between parties; makes "case law," interpreting the Constitution, statutes, and regulations while ruling on disputes between parties; and creates rulings that "attach" to statutes and regulations that are interpreted and ruled upon.

Figure 7-1 illustrates how the U.S. government is organized, and Figure 7-2 illustrates how the Department of Health and Human Services (DHHS) is organized. Figure 7-3 provides fiscal year 2014 budget information for select DHHS operating divisions. In fiscal year 2014, more than 90 percent of the budget for DHHS was appropriated for mandatory programs such as Medicare ($513.1 billion), Medicaid ($308.6 billion), and the Children's Health Insurance Program ($12.3 billion) administered by the Centers for Medicare and Medicaid Services (CMS), and mandatory programs of the Administration for Children and Families. The operating division that received the largest discretionary

appropriation ($30.1 billion) was the National Institutes of Health (NIH). Because of the intricacy of agency budgets and differences in what is included or excluded from totals in various snapshots, readers are encouraged to visit the budget section of each agency's website to view its "operating plan" for the year and to obtain more in-depth and comprehensive budget information.

Roles of Select Federal Agencies in Public Health

Through authorizing legislation, Congress establishes and defines the roles and scope of federal agencies and, often, individual programs within those agencies. Congress can modify, add to, or take away any of these authorities at any time; therefore, the roles, focus, and activities of federal agencies are fluid. In addition, multiple federal agencies may be authorized to address some of the same issues, but in specific and complementary ways. The most visible example of these complementary roles/functions in action is when federal agencies collectively address the various health, safety, and human services needs of citizens after a natural disaster. A list of each agency's authorities can be found in the U.S.

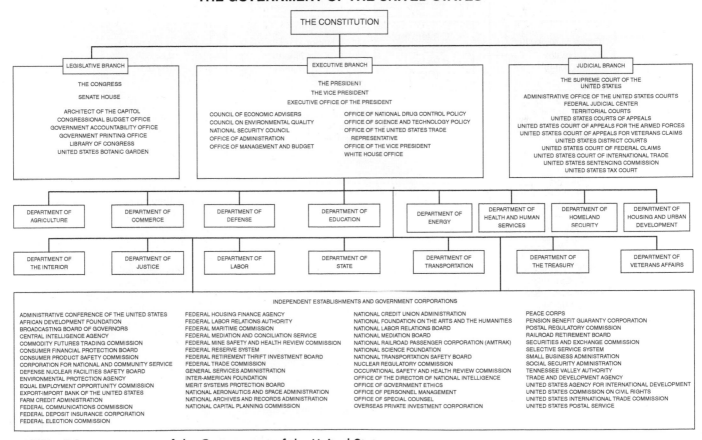

FIGURE 7-1   Organization of the Government of the United States

Courtesy of the U.S. Government Publishing Office

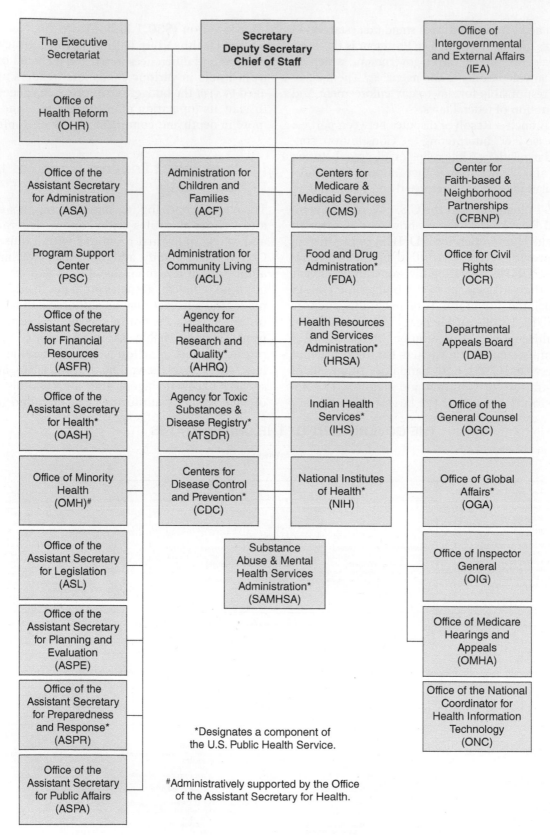

FIGURE 7-2   Department of Health and Human Services Organizational Chart
Courtesy of the Department of Health and Human Services

Operating Division	Mandatory and Discretionary Budget Authority (Dollars in Millions)
Food and Drug Administration[1]	$2,642
Health Resources and Services Administration	$9,142
Indian Health Service	$4,590
Centers for Disease Control and Prevention (includes funding for the Agency for Toxic Substances & Disease Registry)	$7,170
National Institutes of Health	$30,142
Substance Abuse and Mental Health Services Administration	$3,497
Agency for Healthcare Research and Quality (Program Level)	$464
Centers for Medicaid & Medicare Services[2]	$850,810
Administration for Children and Families	$51,158
Administration for Community Living	$1,647
Public Health and Social Services Emergency Fund	$1,243

SOURCE: Fiscal Year 2015 DHHS Budget in Brief; http://www.dhhs.gov/budget/fy2015/fy-2015-budget-in-brief.pdf. This is a useful rough budgetary snapshot; however, because of the intricacy of agency budgets and differences in what is included or excluded from totals in various snapshots, readers are encouraged to visit the Budget section of each agency's website to view each agency's "operating plan" for the year and to obtain more in-depth and comprehensive budget information.

[1] The Budget Authority levels for FDA are based on factors described in the Appendix of the "Fiscal Year 2015 DHHS Budget in Brief" and will differ from levels displayed in the FDA section of that same document. In FY 2013, the difference was due to the timing and availability of user fee collections, and in FY 2014, the inclusion of sequestered user fees made available in FY 2014.

[2] Budget Authority includes Non-CMS Budget Authority for Hospital Insurance and Supplementary Medical Insurance for the Social Security Administration and MedPac.

FIGURE 7-3   Fiscal Year 2014 Budgets for Select Department of Health and Human Services' Operating Divisions
Courtesy of the Department of Health and Human Services

Code,[5] and usually in each agency's annual budget request and on their websites. This section provides an overview of the roles and relationships of key federal agencies in terms of public health.

Table 7-1 (Federal Agencies and Their Relationship to Public Health) provides a snapshot of select federal agencies (1) that are dedicated exclusively to public health and public health practice across the system, (2) have an exclusive or significant focus on *specific areas* of public health or population health, (3) have a focus complementary to public health (e.g., health care or human services), and (4) that conduct some activities, usually situational, related to public health, or conduct activities that help address the social determinants of health. Table 7-1 illustrates the following:

▸ The majority of health-related federal activities are housed in DHHS. DHHS is the U.S. government's principal agency for protecting the health of all Americans and providing essential human services, especially for those who are least able to help themselves.[6]

▸ The Centers for Disease Control and Prevention (CDC) is the federal agency dedicated exclusively to supporting public health and public health practice across the system. Many other federal agencies play a significant direct role in addressing specific areas of public health, either by conducting discrete activities related or complementary to public health or by addressing the social determinants of health.

▸ The roles and relationships of these federal agencies point to the reality and importance of "Health in All Policies," which is defined as "a collaborative approach to improving the health of all people by incorporating health considerations into decision-making across sectors and policy areas."[7]

Federal agencies collaborate and contribute to each other's work in two major ways. First, they provide each other with information and data to inform decisions, programs and practice, and impact evaluation. For example, the Food and Drug Administration (FDA), Occupational Safety and Health Administration (OSHA), and Environmental Protection Agency (EPA) use the CDC's health statistics and investigatory data to inform and evaluate the impact of health-related regulations. Second, they actively collaborate on issues of joint interest. For example, multiple federal agencies such as the

TABLE 7-1   Federal Agencies and Their Relationship to Public Health

Relationship to Public Health and Public Health Practice	Agency	Department	Mission	Website
Focused exclusively on public health and public health practice across the system	Centers for Disease Control and Prevention (CDC)	Health and Human Services (DHHS)	Protect America from health, safety and security threats, both foreign and in the U.S. CDC's role is to (1) detect and respond to new and emerging health threats, (2) tackle the biggest health problems causing death and disability for Americans, (3) put science and advanced technology into action to prevent disease, (4) promote healthy and safe behaviors, communities and environment, (5) develop leaders and train the public health workforce, including disease detectives, and (6) take the health pulse of the nation.	www.cdc.gov
Exclusive or significant focus on specific areas of public health or population health	Agency for Toxic Substances and Disease Registry (ATSDR)	DHHS	Prevent exposure to toxic substances and the adverse health effects and diminished quality of life associated with exposure to hazardous substances from waste sites, unplanned releases, and other sources of pollution present in the environment.	www.cdc.atsdr.gov
	Environmental Protection Agency (EPA)	N/A	Protect human health and the environment, including developing and enforcing regulations to prevent or reduce environmental risks to health.	www.epa.gov
	Food and Drug Administration (FDA)	DHHS	Protect the public's health • Assure that foods (except for meat from livestock, poultry and some egg products which are regulated by USDA) are safe, wholesome, sanitary and properly labeled • Ensure human and veterinary drugs, and vaccines and other biological products and medical devices intended for human use are safe and effective • Prevent hazardous or unnecessary radiation exposure from radiation-emitting electronic products • Assure cosmetics and dietary supplements are safe and properly labeled • Regulate tobacco products • Help speed product innovations.	www.fda.gov
	Health Resources and Services Administration (HRSA)	DHHS	Improve access to health care by strengthening the health care workforce, building healthy communities and achieving health equity. Includes providing health care to people who are geographically isolated or economically or medically vulnerable. Also has five priority areas specific to public health: (1) achieving health equity and improving health outcomes, (2) linking and integrating public health and primary care, (3) strengthening research and evaluation, assuring availability of data, and supporting health information exchange, (4) assuring a strong public health and primary care workforce, and (5) increasing collaboration and alignment of programs within HRSA and among its partners.	www.hrsa.gov

	Homeland Security (DHS)	Ensure a homeland that is safe, secure, and resilient against terrorism and other hazards. These missions are enterprise-wide, and not limited to DHS; people from across the federal government, state, local, tribal, and territorial governments, the private sector, and other nongovernmental organizations are responsible for executing these missions, including public health agencies.	www.dhs.gov
	Labor	Occupational Safety and Health Administration (OSHA) — Assure safe and healthful working conditions for working men and women by setting and enforcing standards and by providing training, outreach, education and assistance.	www.osha.gov
	DHHS	Substance Abuse and Mental Health Services Administration (SAMHSA) — Lead public health efforts to advance the behavioral health of the nation. SAMHSA's mission is to reduce the impact of substance abuse and mental illness on America's communities.	www.samhsa.gov
	Agriculture (USDA)	Provide leadership on food, agriculture, natural resources, rural development, nutrition, and related issues based on sound public policy, the best available science, and efficient management. Public health-related activities and programs include (1) activities related to food safety and security, (2) the Supplemental Nutrition Assistance Program (SNAP), (3) the Special Supplemental Nutrition Program for Women, Infants, and Children (WIC), and (4) various nutrition education activities.	www.usda.gov
Complementary – primary focus on human care/services	DHHS	Agency for Healthcare Research and Quality (AHRQ) — Produce evidence to make health care safer, higher quality, more accessible, equitable, and affordable, and to work within DHHS and with other partners to make sure that the evidence is understood and used.	www.ahrq.gov
	DHHS	Centers for Medicare & Medicaid Services (CMS) — Administer the Medicare program, the Federal portion of the Medicaid program and State Children's Health Insurance Program, the Health Insurance Marketplace, and related quality assurance activities.	www.cms.gov
	DHHS	Indian Health Service (IHS) — Provide a comprehensive health service delivery system for American Indians and Alaska Natives who are members of federally recognized Tribes (currently 566) across the United States.	www.ihs.gov
	DHHS	National Institutes of Health (NIH) — Support biomedical and behavioral research domestically and abroad, conducts research in its own laboratories and clinics, trains promising young researchers, and promotes acquisition and distribution of medical knowledge.	www.nih.gov

TABLE 7-1 (Continued)

Relationship to Public Health and Public Health Practice	Department	Agency	Mission	Website
Complementary – primary focus on human services	DHHS	Administration for Children and Families (ACF)	Promote the economic and social well-being of families, children, individuals, and communities through a range of educational and supportive programs in partnership with states, tribes, and community organizations.	www.acf.gov
	DHHS	Administration for Community Living (ACL)	Increase access to community support and resources for the unique needs of older Americans and people with disabilities across the lifespan.	
	Veterans Affairs (VA)		Administer benefit programs for veterans, their families, and their survivors. These benefits include pension, education, disability compensation, home loans, life insurance, vocational rehabilitation, survivor support, medical care, and burial benefits.	www.va.gov
Complementary – conduct some activities, usually situational, related to public health OR conduct activities that help address the social determinants of health	Education		Promote student achievement and preparation for global competitiveness by fostering educational excellence and ensuring equal access.	www.ed.gov
	Housing and Urban Development (HUD)		Create strong, sustainable, inclusive communities and quality affordable homes for all. HUD is working to strengthen the housing market to bolster the economy and protect consumers; meet the need for quality affordable rental homes; utilize housing as a platform for improving quality of life; build inclusive and sustainable communities free from discrimination, and transform the way HUD does business.	www.hud.gov
	Transportation (DOT)		Ensure a fast, safe, efficient, accessible, and convenient transportation system that meets vital national interests and enhances the quality of life of the American people, today and into the future.	www.dot.gov

Substance Abuse and Mental Health Services Administration (SAMHSA), the CDC, the FDA, the National Institute on Drug Abuse, the Department of Justice, and others are working together to address the issue of prescription drug misuse and abuse. Two high-impact historical examples include health and environmental agencies working together to remove harmful lead from gasoline and paint, and health and transportation agencies working together to lower speed limits and increase use of seat belts to prevent injury and death.

In addition to the leaders of federal health agencies, the Surgeon General of the United States holds a position with significant influence on the public health system. The Surgeon General is dedicated to focusing the nation's attention on important public health issues and providing the best scientific information available to improve the nation's health.[8] The Surgeon General's reports[9] and calls to action[10] highlight essential prevention messages about tobacco, obesity, and other important topics. Perhaps the most well-known of these reports is the landmark 1964 report on smoking and health;[11] in 2014, the Surgeon General released "The Health Consequences of Smoking—50 Years of Progress: A Report of the Surgeon General."[12] The Surgeon General is nominated by the President with advice and consent of the Senate for a four-year term.[13] The Office of the Surgeon General is part of the Office of the Assistant Secretary for Health in DHHS. The Surgeon General also (1) oversees the U.S. Public Health Service Commissioned Corps (USPHS), an elite group of more than 6,800 uniformed officer public health professionals working throughout the federal government whose mission is to protect, promote, and advance the health of the Nation;[14] (2) oversees the Civilian Volunteer Medical Reserve Corps, a national network of more than 200,000 volunteers committed to improving the public health, emergency response, and resiliency of their communities;[15] and (3) chairs the National Prevention Council, which provides coordination and leadership among 20 executive departments with respect to prevention, wellness, and health promotion activities.[16]

Centers for Disease Control and Prevention (CDC)

Because the CDC is the federal agency with a mission dedicated solely to supporting public health and public health practice across the system, this section will explore the CDC's roles and activities, specifically: (1) the CDC connects state and local health departments across the United States, recognizing disease patterns and making state responses to health problems more effective; (2) the CDC and its state and local partners are key to homeland security, by maintaining the ability to detect and respond to outbreaks and natural and man-made disasters; (3) the CDC is a key source of evidence for health action — monitoring health, informing clinical and policy decision-making, and providing individuals the information they need to take responsibility for their own health; and (4) the CDC supports state and local public health partners with training and guidance to ensure nationwide lab capacity for detecting and responding to health threats, and the capacity to save lives by addressing key risk factors for premature death, injury, and disease.[17] Some of the CDC's priorities for the twenty-first century are listed in Exhibit 7-2.

The importance of public health infrastructure in the United States, and the CDC's role in it, is worth noting in particular. According to *Healthy People*, a federal initiative that provides science-based, 10-year national objectives for improving the health of all Americans, key to ensuring an effective and efficient public health system is the continuous development and maintenance of a strong public health infrastructure.[18] Public health infrastructure—which includes but is not limited to workforce, data and information systems, communications, partnerships, policy, and organizational competencies (e.g., leadership/governance)—is fundamental to the provision and execution of public health services at all levels; it provides the capacity to prepare for and respond to both acute (emergency) and chronic (ongoing) threats to the nation's health. It is the foundation for planning,

EXHIBIT 7-2 The Centers for Disease Control and Prevention in the Twenty-First Century

- **On the cutting edge of health security** – confronting global disease threats through advanced computing and lab analysis of huge amounts of data to quickly find solutions.
- **Putting science into action** – tracking disease and finding out what is making people sick and the most effective ways to prevent it.
- **Helping medical care** – bringing new knowledge to individual health care and community health to save more lives and reduce waste.

- **Fighting diseases before they reach our borders** – detecting and confronting new germs and diseases around the globe to increase our national security.
- **Nurturing public health** – building on our significant contribution to have strong, well-resourced public health leaders and capabilities at national, state, and local levels to protect Americans from health threats.

SOURCE: CDC Mission, Role and Pledge; http://www.cdc.gov/about/organization/mission.htm; accessed 8/1/14

delivering, and evaluating public health services. As with other forms of infrastructure in the United States, public health infrastructure is often at risk due to economic, social, and political factors (e.g., cuts in public health budgets that result in loss of workforce, programs, or services). In addition, the return on investment/impact of basic public health infrastructure is difficult to measure due to the fragmented nature of the system, and a "base level" of investment is yet to be determined.

Since its inception, the CDC has supported public health infrastructure at all levels—federal, state, tribal, local, and territorial—and great strides have been made in the United States, as evidenced by the list of great public health achievements to date (see Chapter 1). However, much of the funding for public health infrastructure is scattered across health issue-specific budget lines (e.g., chronic disease, infectious disease, environmental health), making it more difficult to plan and invest in infrastructure in a coordinated, effective, and efficient manner at all levels. In response to this and other needs, in 2010 the CDC created the Office for State, Tribal, Local and Territorial Support (OSTLTS) to advance U.S. public health agency and system performance, capacity, agility, and resilience. OSTLTS supports health departments specifically in building, maintaining, and improving infrastructure capacities and capabilities for effectively and efficiently providing essential public health services.[19] OSTLTS recognizes health departments as the front line of prevention and promotes a systems approach working across sectors, partners, and programs to tackle the complex community and economic challenges that have an impact on the public health system and the public's health.

FEDERAL SUPPORT TO THE PUBLIC HEALTH SYSTEM

The following are common activities and contributions of federal agencies whose primary mission is, or which have significant programs focused on, public health (i.e., on delivery of essential public health services).

Provide Funding

Federal agencies provide essential funding to state, tribal, local, and territorial grantees to build and sustain public health infrastructure, capacities, and capabilities to deliver public health services, and to develop, implement, and evaluate public health activities in their jurisdictions. The most common sources of funding for the governmental public health system are (1) federal funds, which are a mixture of population-based formula grant programs, incidence-based or prevalence-based formulas, and a series of competitive grants; (2) state and local funds, which also vary dramatically based on

state governance and health department structure and activities and (3) county and city revenues, which are also quite variable.[20] The reach of federal funding is wide. The federal government makes awards directly to health departments at all levels, nonprofits, academia, businesses, community organizations, etc. Awards made to state-level entities may be shared with local entities and/or benefit the whole state. In addition, awards to national associations are used to carry out national public health programs and may include sub-awards to other entities. Major sources of information on federal funding for public health include the following: (1) USASpending.gov, a searchable website that includes some information on each federal award made by every federal agency;[21] (2) CDC Grant Funding Profiles tool, which provides summaries and searchable data sets for CDC funding to grantees within states and U.S. territories, starting with fiscal year 2010;[22] and (3) the DHHS.gov/OPEN Prevention and Public Health Fund site, which provides information on the planned use of funds, funding opportunities, and the recipients of awards.[23]

Provide Data for Decision Making

Health statistics can be used to create fundamental knowledge and to guide health policy and programs. The CDC's National Center for Health Statistics (NCHS)[24] is the primary Federal government resource for collecting, analyzing, and distributing data on health and health care.[25] NCHS provides free downloadable public-use data files to researchers, teachers, students, and others through its Public-Use Data Files and Documentation site.[26] NCHS also houses the Health Indicators Warehouse (HIW), which serves as a federal data hub for DHHS's health data initiative. It provides a single, user-friendly source for national, state, and community health indicators, including population health (such as life expectancy, mortality, disease incidence or prevalence, or other health states); determinants of health (such as health behaviors, health risk factors, physical environments, and socioeconomic environments); and health care access, quality, and use. In addition, every federal agency houses some data specific to their programs and missions. The document "Shaping a Health Statistics Vision for the 21st Century"[27] describes a strategic vision for health statistics and the health statistics enterprise in the United States going forward.

In addition to health statistics, some CDC programs provide snapshots on progress on specific health issues in states or other jurisdictions, including disease trends, policy/guideline adoption and implementation, and success stories. For example, the CDC provides maps detailing the prevalence of obesity for all U.S. states based on the Behavioral Risk Factor Surveillance System (BRFSS)[28] each year. Another example is the

Prevention Status Report (PSR), which highlights—for all 50 states and the District of Columbia—the status of public health policies and practices designed to prevent or reduce select, important public health problems such as HIV, tobacco use, and health-care-acquired infections. The PSRs provide information in a simple, easy-to-use format that decision makers and other stakeholders can use to examine their state's status and identify areas for improvement. Other examples are the CDC's "2013–2014 National Snapshot of Public Health Preparedness"[29] and "The State Indicator Report on Fruits & Vegetables, 2013."[30]

Conduct, Support, and Translate Research Results into Public Health Practice

Federal agencies conduct and/or support clinical and other types of scientific and public health practice research that inform public health programs and practice. For example, the NIH is the largest source of funding for medical research in the world;[31] NIH scientists also conduct intramural research. The NIH increased its investment in translation of basic clinical research into practice in 2011 by establishing its National Center for Advancing Translational Sciences (NCATS).[32] Translation is the process of turning observations in the laboratory and clinic into interventions that improve the health of individuals and the public — from diagnostics and therapeutics to medical procedures and behavioral changes. The NIH and other agencies are supporting "community-based participatory research" (CBPR).[33] CBPR is an applied collaborative approach that enables community residents to more actively participate in the full spectrum of research (from conception, design, conduct, analysis, interpretation, conclusions, and communication of results) with a goal of influencing change in community health, systems, programs, or policies. Another body of research growing in urgency and importance is public health services and systems research (PHSSR), which federal agencies such as the NIH and the CDC are supporting through funding and other activities. In 1999, the AcademyHealth's Public Health Systems Research Interest Group provided a consensus definition of PHSSR as "a field of study that examines the organization, financing, and delivery of public health services within communities and the impact of these services on public health." It is a multidisciplinary field of study that recognizes and investigates system-level properties and outcomes that result from the dynamic interactions among various components of the public health system and how those interactions affect organizations, communities, environments, and population health status.[34] Results of PHSSR and other public health research are available in scientific journals and other publications, and agency websites. (See Chapter 17 for more detail on PHSSR.) In addition, some federal agencies publish journals themselves, such the CDC's *Emerging Infectious Diseases*,[35] *Preventing Chronic Disease*,[36] and the *Morbidity and Mortality Weekly Report (MMWR)* series.[37]

Develop, Implement, Enforce, and Evaluate the Impact of Health-Related Regulations

Federal regulation is one of the basic tools government uses to carry out public policy.[38] Agencies create regulations (also known as "rules") when Congress provides the authority to do so. The public plays an extremely important role in the rulemaking process by commenting on proposed rules. Regulations.gov is the site through which the federal government solicits and obtains public input to draft regulations, and houses copies of federal regulations and associated documents.[39] DHHS provides a site specific to its agencies' areas of regulatory authority.[38] Major federal regulatory agencies that have a role in health are the following: the Consumer Product Safety Commission (CPSC), which enforces federal safety standards; EPA, which establishes and enforces pollution standards; FDA, which administers federal food purity laws, drug testing and safety, and cosmetics; and OSHA, which develops and enforces federal standards and regulations ensuring safe working conditions. In addition, the CDC has been given regulatory authority in a limited number of cases, such as minimum standards for birth certificates, and some aspects of select agents and toxins, occupational safety and health, and quarantine.[40]

Build Capacity to Use Law as a Public Health Tool

Law has been critical in attaining public health goals, serving as a foundation for governmental public health activities.[41] Many of public health's greatest successes, including high childhood immunization rates, improved motor vehicle safety, safer workplaces, and reduced tooth decay, have relied heavily on law, and law is playing an increasingly important role in addressing emerging public health threats. Federal agencies also assist others in using law as a public health tool. One example is the CDC's Public Health Law Program, which, in collaboration with other CDC programs and external partners, develops law-related tools and provides legal technical assistance to public health practitioners and policy makers in state, tribal, local, and territorial jurisdictions.[42] In addition, the CDC provides funding and other resources to grantees to identify, implement, and evaluate public health policy options.

Conduct and Support Health Education Efforts

In addition to providing public health workforce educational resources, federal agencies educate and empower the public to make healthier decisions, such as through health education campaigns (e.g., the CDC's "Tips from Former Smokers" campaign).[43] They also make educational materials available free of charge through their websites, ordering features, or online syndication. Provision of these resources saves practitioners in the field time and resources. For example, CDC's Stacks[44] and CDC-INFO on Demand[45] sites provide access to books, fact sheets, pamphlets, CDC research articles, toolkits, and other health education materials. CDC's Content Syndication[46] site allows users to import content from CDC websites directly into their own websites or applications.

Support Advisory Bodies That Make Public Health Policy and Practice Recommendations to the Federal Government

Some of these advisory bodies are formal Federal Advisory Committee Act (FACA) committees;[47] as of May 2014, an average of 1,000 advisory committees with more than 60,000 members were advising the President and the Executive Branch on issues, according to the U.S. General Services Administration.[48] The CDC alone is advised by 24 public health-related advisory committees, ranging from those focused on disease-specific issues to those focused on cross-cutting public health system issues, such as CDC support to health departments[49] and emergency preparedness and response. Others are independent advisory bodies such as the Institute of Medicine (IOM), which works outside of government to provide unbiased and authoritative advice to decision makers and the public.[50] Prominent advisory bodies related to public health include the Advisory Committee on Immunization Practices,[51] the Community Preventive Services Task Force,[52] and the U.S. Preventive Services Task Force.[53]

Develop and Use Evidence-Based Guidelines and Recommendations

The CDC provides an online one-stop shop for guidelines or recommendations developed by the CDC, by the CDC working in collaboration with other organizations or agencies, and by CDC federal advisory committees.[54] These documents contain statements that include recommendations, strategies, and/or information that assists decision makers (such as health care providers, federal, state or private agencies, employers, public health officials, or the public) in choosing between alternative courses of action in specific situations. Ultimately, these documents are focused on providing actionable steps to address a specific issue of importance to public health.

Lead or Support the Development of National Health Initiatives, Strategies, and Action Plans

These efforts inform, enhance, and guide public health efforts across the United States by providing a shared understanding of the issues; roles and responsibilities of stakeholders; and goals, strategies, activities, measures, and targets. One of the most well-known of these plans is *Healthy People*, which provides science-based, 10-year national objectives for improving the health of all Americans.[55] For three decades, *Healthy People* has established benchmarks and monitored progress over time. Examples of other plans from across the public health system are listed on the CDC's "National Health Initiatives, Strategies, and Action Plans" webpage.[56]

Increase Consistency and Quality Across the Public Health System

Over the past several decades, the public health sector has shown increased interest in describing, standardizing, measuring, and improving public health practice. There are many efforts underway to standardize and otherwise improve the quality, effectiveness, and efficiency of individual parts of the system (e.g., public health laboratories, and surveillance systems). There are also efforts that target cross-cutting and foundational aspects of public health infrastructure and practice. The National Public Health Performance Standards (NPHPS) and public health department accreditation are two notable examples. Initiated in 1998, the NPHPS is a collaborative effort of the CDC and national public health organizations dedicated to improving public health practice and the performance of state and local public health systems, as well as governance (e.g., local boards of health). Public health practitioners can use the NPHPS framework to help identify areas for system improvement, strengthen state and local partnerships, and ensure that a strong system is in place for addressing public health issues.[57] Another example is CDC support for national voluntary public health accreditation for public health departments.[58] The nonprofit Public Health Accreditation Board (PHAB), which serves as the accrediting body and which the CDC has supported since its inception, seeks to advance the quality and performance of public health departments through nationally established consensus standards.[59] Based on the 10 Essential Public Health Services, PHAB accreditation offers a means to ensure comprehensive and quality programs across a range of public health areas for approximately 3,000 state, local, tribal, and territorial health agencies. As of September 2015, 80 public health departments (local and state) have achieved national accreditation, with approximately 300 more health departments in process.[60,61] The CDC also plays a role in supporting health department readiness for and obtaining accreditation through funding, incentives, technical assistance, training, and other resources. For example, from 2010 through 2013, CDC/OSTLTS' National Public Health Improvement Initiative (NPHII) provided 73 state, local, territorial, and tribal health agencies with funding and assistance to prepare for accreditation and to strengthen agencies' performance management and quality improvement capacity.[62] NPHII was the first noncategorical cooperative agreement at CDC that supported assessment against the PHAB standards to address critical gaps in service delivery and the implementation of quality improvement methods and practices for greater program efficiency and effectiveness.

Support Development and Sustainability of a Well-Trained, Diverse Public Health Workforce

Federal agencies provide workforce training resources, on-the-job training opportunities (e.g., internships, fellowships), and funding for workforce development activities in the field, and some embed federal staff in state, tribal, local, and territorial health-related agencies or organizations to provide hands-on technical assistance and subject matter expertise. Examples include the public health workforce programs and activities of the CDC (e.g., CDC Learning Connection,[63] Division of Scientific Education and Professional Development,[64] and Professional Development Opportunities site[65]) and the Human Resources and Services Administration (Public Health Training Centers program).[66] Examples of well-known CDC workforce development programs are the Epidemic Intelligence Service (EIS) and Public Health Associate Program (PHAP). EIS is a unique two-year postgraduate training program of service and on-the-job learning for health professionals interested in the practice of applied epidemiology. EIS officers are on the public health frontlines, conducting epidemiologic investigations, research, and public health surveillance both nationally and internationally.[67] PHAP is a two-year training program for entry-level public health professionals (recent graduates with at least a bachelor's degree) to gain hands-on, frontline experience in the day-to-day operation of public health programs. Associates are assigned to a state, tribal, local, or territorial public health agency and work on prevention alongside other professionals across a variety of public health settings.[68]

Provide Short-Term Technical Assistance

Some federal agencies, such as the CDC, provide short-term technical assistance upon request to state, local, tribal, and territorial agencies. For example, at the request of the public health authority of a jurisdiction, the CDC provides short-term assistance for an urgent public health problem requiring predominantly epidemiologic methodologies (known as an "Epi-Aid").[69]

Support Preparation for and Response to Emergencies

The Stafford Disaster Relief and Emergency Assistance Act constitutes the statutory authority for most federal disaster response activities.[70] The Act states that "it is the intent of the Congress, by this Act, to provide an orderly and continuing means of assistance by the Federal Government to State and local governments in carrying out their responsibilities to alleviate the suffering and damage which result from such disasters."[71] It also required preparation of a Federal Response Plan and individual state Emergency Operations Plans. The latest federal plan, the National Response Frameworks,[72,73] describes the coordinating structures and alignment of key roles and responsibilities for the whole community. These frameworks are integrated to ensure interoperability across all mission areas. Under the national frameworks, the DHHS Secretary can declare a public health emergency. Federal support to public health agencies ranges from helping states and localities build capacity to identify and respond to emergencies (preparation, including Crisis and Emergency Risk Communication); to providing scientific and logistic expertise, and deploying personnel and critical medical assets to the site of an emergency (response); and to recovering and restoring public health (recovery).

Provide and Support Laboratory Services and Systems

Federal agencies such as the CDC, FDA, NIH, and EPA have laboratories that develop knowledge, assessments, and scientific methods and tools that benefit the nation. Some of these federally owned laboratories have capabilities not present in any other U.S. laboratory, and some serve as the last-resort reference laboratory, able to confirm or rule out certain organisms or substances. They also support state, tribal, local, and territorial entities in building their laboratory capacity and capabilities, and improve the quality of laboratory testing and related practices in the United States and globally through the development and evaluation of standards and innovative training. One example of a federal assurance activity is implementation of the Clinical

Laboratory Improvement Amendments of 1988 (CLIA) regulations.[74] CLIA regulations include federal standards applicable to all U.S. facilities or sites that test human specimens for health assessment or to diagnose, prevent, or treat disease. The CDC, CMS, and FDA support the CLIA program and clinical laboratory quality.

FUTURE DIRECTIONS

As previously noted, federal public health agencies work to ensure all levels of government have the capabilities to provide essential public health services. They also will act when health threats span more than one state, region, or the entire nation, and where the solutions may be beyond the jurisdiction of individual states. Two of the most significant factors affecting the future of public health fall into those cross-cutting categories of federal action: (1) current and emerging global health threats, and (2) the need to improve and sustain the U.S. health system itself. Global public health threats such as infectious agents, antibiotic resistance, and climate change are urgent issues to be addressed. No less urgent is making the U.S. health system economically sustainable and more effective and efficient.

Federal agencies are applying, and will continue to apply, their public health resources and tools (i.e., funding, data, technical assistance, standards, regulations, policies, and guidelines) to these current and future challenges. The following are examples of current and continuing federal actions related to global health threats and health system change in particular.

Global Health Security

There is increasing awareness that global health security is a crucial component of national security, and many nations are taking action. Today's health security threats come from at least three sources: the emergence and spread of new microbes, the rise of drug-resistant pathogens, and the intentional creation and spread of infectious agents.[75] All of these threats are now amplified by the globalization of travel and food supply. The United States is partnering with other countries to build global health security capacity, with the goals of finding threats faster, stopping them closer to the source, and preventing them wherever possible.[76] The partners have created and are implementing a Global Health Security Agenda.[77] As of 2014, the following federal agencies are playing a role in the agenda: the Departments of Health and Human Services, State, Defense, and Agriculture, and the U.S. Agency for International Development.[78] These U.S. agencies are working with national and international partners to conduct activities such as the following: establishing emergency operations

centers, building information systems, and strengthening laboratory security; providing technical and operational support for preventing, detecting and responding to new emerging zoonotic disease threats; implementing emergency communication protocols for information sharing among the health, agriculture, security, and foreign affairs sectors; working with partners to rapidly detect, diagnose, and manage especially dangerous animal diseases in affected and high-risk countries; and developing formal processes for the rapid assessment and notification of potential public health emergencies of international concern.

Antibiotic Resistance

Antibiotic Resistance (AR) is a rapidly growing threat to the nation and the world.[79] Some antibiotic resistant infections are already untreatable. In response, the Interagency Task Force on Antimicrobial Resistance (ITFAR) is coordinating the activities of federal agencies in addressing AR.[80] The latest ITFAR "Public Health Action Plan to Combat Antimicrobial Resistance" (2012) addresses the three areas of federal action: surveillance, prevention, and control; research; and regulatory pathways for new products.[81] The Action Plan outlines goals and actions that the participating federal agencies and departments are pursuing or planning to pursue in an effort to respond to the complex public health risk posed by AR.

Climate Change

Federal agencies and other organizations are increasing their efforts to address the current and growing threat of climate change. "The President's Climate Action Plan" is a broad-based plan to cut the carbon pollution that causes climate change and affects public health.[82] The federal government will act with its partners in three key areas: (1) cut carbon pollution through tough new rules that protect the health and move the U.S. economy toward American-made clean energy sources that will create good jobs and lower home energy bills; (2) prepare the United States for the impacts of climate change (e.g., help state and local governments strengthen roads, bridges, and shorelines to better protect people's homes, businesses, and way of life from severe weather); and (3) lead international efforts to do the same, particularly among the major carbon pollution emitting countries. Examples of two resources specific to public health departments in addressing climate change are "Building Resilience against Climate Effects—A Novel Framework to Facilitate Climate Readiness in Public Health Agencies,"[83] and "Assessing Health Vulnerability to Climate Change: A Guide for Health Departments."[84]

Health System Transformation

Economic and other pressures are currently driving all parts of the health system, including public health and clinical care, to become more effective and efficient. This health system transformation process requires evaluating (and re-evaluating) how the system is and should be organized, how the parts fit and work together, who pays and how, how and where health goals are accomplished, and how impact and value are measured. The following are just a few of the many examples in which federal health agencies are supporting state, tribal, local, and territorial jurisdictions in regards to system change:

- Using federal data systems to monitor performance of the health system, identify issues that need to be addressed and possible solutions, and measure the impact of system changes.
- Providing funding and other types of support for development and testing of innovative public health and clinical service financing and delivery models. For example, the CMS/Center for Medicare and Medicaid Innovation (CMMI) was established in 2010 to test "innovative payment and service delivery models to reduce program expenditures ... while preserving or enhancing the quality of care" for those individuals who receive Medicare, Medicaid, or the Children's Health Insurance Program (CHIP) benefits.[85] CMMI aims to achieve better health care for the individual, improved population health, and lower costs, which will ultimately lead to better value for the nation's investment in health. The CDC is working with CMMI to help health departments, hospitals, and community leaders align their aims and resources and develop more comprehensive state health improvement plans.
- Bridging medicine and public health into one health system for the United States. To effectively build a seamless system will require both medicine and public health to make significant changes in how they conduct business, and strong leadership to overcome the barriers to successful transformation. In March 2012, the IOM released the report *Primary Care and Public Health: Exploring Integration to Improve Population Health*[86] in response to a request from HRSA and CDC for recommendations on this topic. HRSA and CDC developed a closer working relationship to take action on the recommendations, and primary care and public health partners were spurred to form collaborations at the national level. In addition, the de Beaumont Foundation, Duke Community and Family Medicine, and the CDC launched a new initiative – *A Practical Playbook:*

Public Health & Primary Care Together – in March 2014.[87] The initiative has three objectives: to improve population health, to better manage illness (especially chronic disease), and to mitigate health care costs. With the input of many stakeholders, the three partners developed and released the *Practical Playbook for Integrating Public Health and Primary Care*,[88] a web-based tool designed to promote and facilitate collaborative health projects between public health officers and primary care providers.

- Supporting creation and implementation of a sustainable governmental public health funding model. This includes encouraging cross-jurisdictional sharing of public health services[89] through initiatives, tools, education, and funding opportunity announcement provisions (e.g., see the CDC's Cross-Jurisdictional Sharing of Public Health Services website).[90] These activities also include supporting the identification of a "minimum package of public health services" (which includes foundational capabilities and basic programs that all public health departments should have) and the creation of a "chart of accounts" for use by all public health agencies to enable better tracking of revenue and expenditures, and how both relate to health outcomes.[91] Federal agencies are participating on national advisory bodies, such as the IOM committees on population health and public health financing and other bodies to advise on these issues and to feed this information into federal agency program and funding decision making.

In current and future conditions, federal public health agencies will continue to ensure that the health system functions as well as possible, especially in terms of providing leadership, expertise, and resources, and facilitating communication, coordination, and collaboration across the decentralized system.

SUMMARY

The public health system within the United States and its territories has evolved and continues to evolve over time according to population needs and conditions. It is a decentralized system; therefore, the overarching role of the federal government is to ensure the system functions as well as possible. The CDC is the federal agency dedicated exclusively to supporting public health and public health practice across the system. Many other federal agencies (e.g., CMS, FDA, HRSA, NIH, and SAMHSA) play a significant direct role in addressing specific areas of public health, either by conducting discrete activities related or complementary to public health or by addressing the social determinants of health.

Federal support to the public health system includes but is not limited to providing funding, technical assistance, data for decision making, evidence-based guidelines and recommendations, policy options and tools, regulations, health education and communication materials, and national health initiatives, strategies, and action plans. Federal agencies also support development and maintenance of essential public health infrastructure, such as emergency preparedness and response capabilities and capacities; public health laboratory services and systems; public health surveillance systems; workforce development; and consistency and quality across the public health system.

The future contributions of federal agencies to public health will be shaped by health threats and system changes. This includes evolution in how the public health system itself is organized, how the parts fit and work together, how and where public health goals are accomplished, and how impact is measured. Global threats include the emergence and spread of new microbes, the rise of drug-resistant pathogens, the intentional creation and spread of infectious agents, and global climate change. In terms of improving and sustaining the public health system, the following issues are being explored: creating and implementing a sustainable governmental public health funding model; more efficient and cost effective models for delivering public health services; new models for financing community health and prevention; and primary care and public health coordination and integration. This new emphasis on population health improvement in transforming the health system provides great opportunities as well as challenges for public health.

REVIEW QUESTIONS

1. What are the *general* roles and responsibilities of federal public health?

2. What branch of government is responsible for day-to-day enforcement and administration of federal laws; what department within that branch contains the majority of federal health-related activities; and what operating division within that department is *exclusively* dedicated to supporting public health and public health practice?

3. List three common contributions of the federal government to public health and public health practice.

4. What is the role and importance of having a strong national public health infrastructure?

5. What are three current and emerging threats to the public's health?

REFERENCES

1. World Health Organization. Key Components of a Well Functioning Health System. 2010; http://www.who.int/healthsystems/EN_HSSkeycomponents.pdf?ua=1. Accessed November 18, 2014.

2. U.S. Department of Health and Human Services. Public Health in America. 2008; http://www.health.gov/phfunctions/public.htm. Accessed November 18, 2014.

3. Harrell JA, Baker EL. The essential services of public health. *Leadership Public Health*. 1994;3(3):4.

4. U.S. Government. Federal Executive Branch. 2014; http://www.usa.gov/Agencies/Federal/Executive.shtml#Executive_Departments. Accessed November 18, 2014.

5. U.S. Government Printing Office. United States Code. http://www.gpo.gov/fdsys/browse/collectionUScode.action?collectionCode=USCODE. Accessed November 18, 2014.

6. U.S. Department of Health and Human Services. About DHHS. 2014; http://www.DHHS.gov/about/. Accessed August 11, 2014.

7. Rudolph L, Caplan J, Ben-Moshe K, Dillon L. *Health in All Policies: A Guide for State and Local Governments*. Washington, DC and Oakland, CA 2013. https://www.apha.org/~/media/files/pdf/fact%20sheets/healthinallpoliciesguide169pages.ashx. Accessed November 24, 2014

8. U.S. Department of Health and Human Services. The Surgeon General's Initiatives. http://www.surgeongeneral.gov/initiatives/index.html. Accessed November 18, 2014.

9. U.S. Department of Health and Human Services. Reports of the Surgeon General, U.S. Public Health Service. http://www.surgeongeneral.gov/library/reports/index.html. Accessed November 18, 2014.

10. U.S. Department of Health and Human Services. Surgeon General's Call to Action. http://www.surgeongeneral.gov/library/calls/index.html. Accessed November 18, 2014.

11. Surgeon General's Advisory Committee on Smoking and Health. *Smoking and Health: Report of the Advisory Committee to the Surgeon General of The Public Health Service*. 1964. 1103. http://profiles.nlm.nih.gov/ps/access/NNBBMQ.pdf

12. U.S. Department of Health and Human Services. *The Health Consequences of Smoking - 50 Years of Progress. A Report of the Surgeon General*. Atlanta, GA 2014. http://www.surgeongeneral.gov/library/reports/50-years-of-progress/full-report.pdf

13. U.S. Department of Health and Human Services. About the Office of the Surgeon General. http://www.surgeongeneral.gov/about/index.html. Accessed November 18, 2014.

14. U.S. Department of Health and Human Services. Commissioned Corp of the U.S. Public Health Service. http://www.usphs.gov/. Accessed November 18, 2014.

15. Medical Reserve Corps. Division of the Civilian Volunteer Medical Reserve Corps. https://www.medicalreservecorps.gov/HomePage. Accessed November 18, 2014.

16. U.S. Department of Health and Human Services. National Prevention Council. http://www.surgeon-general.gov/initiatives/prevention/about/. Accessed November 18, 2014.

17. Centers for Disease Control and Prevention. CDC Facts. 2014; http://www.cdc.gov/24-7/cdcfast-facts/cdcfacts.html. Accessed November 18, 2014.

18. U.S. Department of Health and Human Services. Healthy People 2020: Public Health Infrastructure. 2014; http://www.healthypeople.gov/2020/topics-objectives/topic/public-health-infrastructure?topicid=35. Accessed November 18, 2014.

19. Centers for Disease Control and Prevention. State, Tribal, Local, and Territorial Public Health Professionals Gateway. 2014; http://www.cdc.gov/stltpublichealth/aboutostlts/. Accessed November 18, 2014.

20. Trust for America's Health. Investing in America's Health: A State-By-State Look at Public Health Funding and Key Health Facts. 2012; http://healthyamericans.org/report/94/. Accessed November 18, 2014.

21. U.S. Government. USASpending.gov. http://usaspending.gov/. Accessed November 18, 2014.

22. Centers for Disease Control and Prevention. FY 2013 Grant Funding Profiles. http://wwwn.cdc.gov/FundingProfiles/FundingProfilesRIA/. Accessed November 18, 2014.

23. U.S. Department of Health and Human Services. Prevention and Public Health Fund. http://www.DHHS.gov/open/recordsandreports/prevention/index.html. Accessed November 18, 2014.

24. Centers for Disease Control and Prevention. National Center for Health Statistics…Monitoring the Nation's Health. 2014; http://www.cdc.gov/nchs/. Accessed November 18, 2014.

25. National Center for Health Statistics. *Data Access and Resources: A Guide for Obtaining NCHS Reports and Accessing Data.* http://www.cdc.gov/nchs/data/data_access_and_resources_booklet_web.pdf. Accessed November 24, 2014.

26. Centers for Disease Control and Prevention. Public-Use Data Files and Documentation. 2012; http://www.cdc.gov/nchs/data_access/ftp_data.htm. Accessed November 18, 2014.

27. U.S. Department of Health and Human Services. *Shaping a Health Statistics Vision for the 21st Century.* 2002. http://www.ncvhs.DHHS.gov/21st%20final%20report.pdf. Accessed November 24, 2014.

28. Centers for Disease Control and Prevention. Obesity Prevalence Maps. 2014; http://www.cdc.gov/obesity/data/prevalence-maps.html. Accessed November 18, 2014.

29. Centers for Disease Control and Prevention. Download 2013-2014 National Snapshot of Public Health Preparedness. 2014; http://www.cdc.gov/phpr/pubs-links/2013/download.html. Accessed November 18, 2014.

30. Centers for Disease Control and Prevention. *State Indicator Report on Fruits and Vegetables* 2013. http://www.cdc.gov/nutrition/downloads/State-Indicator-Report-Fruits-Vegetables-2013.pdf

31. U.S. Department of Health and Human Services. About NIH. 2014; http://www.nih.gov/about/. Accessed November 18, 2014.

32. U.S. Department of Health and Human Services. About NCATS. http://www.ncats.nih.gov/about/about.html. Accessed November 18, 2014.

33. National Institutes of Health. Community-Based Participatory Research. http://search.nih.gov/search?utf8=%E2%9C%93&affiliate=nih&query=community-based+participatory+research&commit.x=0&commit.y=0. Accessed November 18, 2014.

34. Health Services Research. Public Health Services and Systems Research: A Special Issue of HSR. *Health Services Research.* 2009;44(5).

35. Centers for Disease Control and Prevention. Emerging Infectious Diseases. 2014; http://wwwnc.cdc.gov/eid/. Accessed November 18, 2014.

36. Centers for Disease Control and Prevention. Preventing Chronic Disease. 2014; http://www.cdc.gov/pcd/index.htm. Accessed November 18, 2014.

37. Centers for Disease Control and Prevention. Morbidity and Mortality Weekly Report. 2014; http://www.cdc.gov/mmwr/. Accessed November 18, 2014.

38. U.S. Department of Health and Human Services. Regulations. http://www.DHHS.gov/regulations/. Accessed November 18, 2014.

39. U.S. Government. Regulations.gov: Your Voice in Federal Decision-Making. http://www.regulations.gov/#!home. Accessed November 18, 2014.

40. Centers for Disease Control and Prevention. Regulations at CDC. http://intranet.cdc.gov/od/ocs/cdcreg/regulations.html. Accessed November 18, 2014.

41. Centers for Disease Control and Prevention. Public Health Law Program: About Us. 2013; http://www.cdc.gov/phlp/about.html. Accessed November 18, 2014.

42. Centers for Disease Control and Prevention. Public Health Law Program. 2014; http://www.cdc.gov/phlp/. Accessed November 18, 2014.

43. Centers for Disease Control and Prevention. Tips From Former Smokers Campaign. 2014. http://www.cdc.gov/tobacco/campaign/tips/. Accessed November 18, 2014.

44. Centers for Disease Control and Prevention. CDC Stacks. http://stacks.cdc.gov/. Accessed November 18, 2014.

45. Centers for Disease Control and Prevention. CDC-INFO on Demand - Publications. 2014; http://wwwn.cdc.gov/pubs/cdcinfoondemand.aspx. Accessed November 18, 2014.

46. Centers for Disease Control and Prevention. Content Syndication. 2014; https://tools.cdc.gov/syndication/. Accessed November 18, 2014.

47. U.S. General Services Administration. Federal Advisory Committee Act (FACA) Management Overview. 2014; http://www.gsa.gov/portal/category/21242. Accessed November 18, 2014.

48. U.S. General Services Administration. The Federal Advisory Committee Act (FACA) Brochure. 2014; http://www.gsa.gov/portal/content/101010. Accessed November 18, 2014.

49. Centers for Disease Control and Prevention. CDC Federal Advisory Committees. http://www.cdc.gov/maso/FACM/facmCommittees.htm. Accessed November 18, 2014.

50. Institute of Medicine. About the IOM. http://www.iom.edu/About-IOM.aspx. Accessed November 18, 2014.

51. Centers for Disease Control and Prevention. Advisory Committee on Immunization Practices (ACIP). 2014; http://www.cdc.gov/vaccines/acip/. Accessed November 18, 2014.

52. Community Preventive Services Task Force. Community Preventive Services Task Force Members. 2014; http://www.thecommunityguide.org/about/task-force-members.html. Accessed November 18, 2014.

53. U.S. Preventive Services Task Force. Home. U.S. Preventive Services Task Force. 2014; http://www.uspreventiveservicestaskforce.org/Page/BasicOne-Column/28. Accessed November 18, 2014.

54. Centers for Disease Control and Prevention. CDC Stacks: Guidelines and Recommendations. http://stacks.cdc.gov/cbrowse?pid=cdc%3A100&parentId=cdc%3A100. Accessed November 18, 2014.

55. U.S. Department of Health and Human Services. Healthy People 2020: About Healthy People. 2014; http://www.healthypeople.gov/2020/About-Healthy-People. Accessed November 18, 2014.

56. Centers for Disease Control and Prevention. National Health Initiatives, Strategies, and Action Plans. 2013; http://www.cdc.gov/stltpublichealth/Strategy/index.html. Accessed November 18, 2014.

57. Centers for Disease Control and Prevention. National Public Health Performance Standards (NPHPS). 2014; http://www.cdc.gov/nphpsp/. Accessed November 18, 2014.

58. Centers for Disease Control and Prevention. National Voluntary Accreditation for Public Health Departments. 2014; http://www.cdc.gov/stltpublichealth/Accreditation/index.html. Accessed November 18, 2014.

59. Public Health Accreditation Board. Welcome to the Public Health Accreditation Board. http://www.phaboard.org/. Accessed November 18, 2014.

60. Public Health Accreditation Board. Accredited Health Departments. http://www.phaboard.org/news-room/accredited-health-departments/. Accessed November 18, 2014.

61. Public Health Accreditation Board. 301 Health Departments in e-PHAB. 2014; http://www.phaboard.org/wp-content/uploads/Applicant-Map_September-2-2014.pdf

62. Centers for Disease Control and Prevention. National Public Health Improvement Initiative. 2013; http://www.cdc.gov/stltpublichealth/nphii/about.html. Accessed November 18, 2014.

63. Centers for Disease Control and Prevention. CDC Learning Connection. 2014; http://www.cdc.gov/learning/. Accessed November 18, 2014.

64. Centers for Disease Control and Prevention. Division of Scientific Education and Professional Development. 2014; http://www.cdc.gov/OPHSS/CSELS/DSEPD/. Accessed November 18, 2014.

65. Centers for Disease Control and Prevention. Professional Development. 2014; http://www.cdc.gov/stltpublichealth/professional/index.html. Accessed November 18, 2014.

66. Health Resources and Services Administration. Public Health Training Centers (PHTC). http://

bhpr.hrsa.gov/grants/publichealth/phtc.html. Accessed November 18, 2014.

67. Centers for Disease Control and Prevention. Epidemic Intelligence Service. 2009; http://www.cdc.gov/eis/. Accessed November 18, 2014.

68. Centers for Disease Control and Prevention. Public Health Associate Program (PHAP). 2014; http://www.cdc.gov/phap/. Accessed November 18, 2014.

69. Centers for Disease Control and Prevention. *Epi-Aid–Epidemiologic Assistance.* http://intranet.cdc.gov/ophss/csels/dsepd/documents/eis-epiaid-overview.pdf

70. Federal Emergency Management Agency. Robert T. Stafford Disaster Relief and Emergency Assistance Act (Public Law 93-288) as amended, 42 U.S.C. §5121 et seq. 2014; http://www.fema.gov/robert-t-stafford-disaster-relief-and-emergency-assistance-act-public-law-93-288-amended. Accessed November 18, 2014.

71. Robert T. Stafford Disaster Relief and Emergency Assistance Act, as amended, 42 U.S.C. §5121 et seq. 2013; http://www.fema.gov/media-library-data/1383153669955-21f970b19e8eaa67087b7da-9f4af706e/stafford_act_booklet_042213_508e.pdf

72. U.S. Department of Homeland Security. *Overview of the National Planning Frameworks.* 2014; https://s3-us-gov-west-1.amazonaws.com/dam-production/uploads/1406718145199-838ef5be-d6355171a1f2d934c25f8ad0 FINAL_Overview_of_National_Planning_Frameworks_20140729.pdf

73. Federal Emergency Management Agency. National Response Framework. 2014; http://www.fema.gov/national-response-framework. Accessed November 18, 2014.

74. Centers for Disease Control and Prevention. Clinical Laboratory Improvement Amendments (CLIA): Overview. 2014; http://wwwn.cdc.gov/clia/default.aspx. Accessed November 18, 2014.

75. Centers for Disease Control and Prevention. *CDC-Global Health Security Program.* http://www.cdc.gov/fmo/topic/Budget%20Information/FY-2015-Fact-Sheets/Global-Health-Security.pdf. Accessed November 24, 2014.

76. U.S. Department of Health and Human Services. Global Health Security. http://www.globalhealth.gov/global-health-topics/global-health-security/index.html. Accessed November 18, 2014.

77. U.S. Department of Health and Human Services. The Global Health Security Agenda. http://www.globalhealth.gov/global-health-topics/global-health-security/ghsagenda.html. Accessed November 18, 2014.

78. U.S. Department of Health and Human Services. What the U.S. Government is Doing. http://www.globalhealth.gov/global-health-topics/global-health-security/usgovernmentrole.html. Accessed November 18, 2014.

79. Centers for Disease Control and Prevention. *CDC-Detect and Protect Against Antibiotic Resistance.* http://www.cdc.gov/fmo/topic/Budget%20Information/FY-2015-Fact-Sheets/Detect-and-Protect-Against-Antibiotic-Resistance.pdf. Accessed November 24, 2014.

80. Centers for Disease Control and Prevention. Interagency Task Force on Antimicrobial Resistance (ITFAR): U.S. Government Agencies unite to combat Antimicrobial Resistance. 2014; http://www.cdc.gov/drugresistance/itfar/. Accessed November 18, 2014.

81. Centers for Disease Control and Prevention. Public Health Action Plan to Combat Antimicrobial Resistance. 2014; http://www.cdc.gov/drugresistance/itfar/introduction_overview.html. Accessed November 18, 2014.

82. The White House Executive Office of the President. *The President's Climate Action Plan.* June, 2013 2013. http://www.whitehouse.gov/sites/default/files/image/president27sclimateactionplan.pdf

83. Marinucci GD, Luber G, Uejio CK, Saha S, Hess JJ. Building Resistance against Climate Effects - A Novel Framework to Facilitate Climate Readiness in Public Health. *International Journal of Environmental Research and Public Health.* 2014;11(6):26.

84. Manangan AP, Uejio CK, Saha S, et al. *Assessing Health Vulnerability to Climate Change: A Guide for Health Departments.* Centers for Disease Control and Prevention; 2014. http://www.cdc.gov/climate-andhealth/pubs/AssessingHealthVulnerabilityto ClimateChange.pdf. Accessed November 24, 2014.

85. Centers for Medicare & Medicaid Services. About the CMS Innovation Center. http://innovation.cms.gov/about/index.html. Accessed November 18, 2014.

86. Institute of Medicine. *Primary Care and Public Health: Exploring Integration to Improve Population Health.* Institute of Medicine; March 28, 2012. http://www.iom.edu/Reports/2012/Primary-Care-and-Public-Health.aspx. Accessed November 24, 2014.

87. Practical Playbook for Public Health and Primary Care Aims to Improve Population Health; Cut Health Care Costs [press release]. de Beaumont Foundation 2014. http://www.debeaumont.org/2014/03/05/practical-playbook-for

-public-health-and-primary-care-aims-to-improve-population-health-cut-health-care-costs/. Accessed November 24, 2014.

88. de Beaumont Foundation, Duke Department of Community and Family Medicine, Centers for Disease Control and Prevention. A Practical Playbook: Public Health. Primary Care. Together. 2014; https://practicalplaybook.org/. Accessed November 18, 2014.

89. Center for Sharing Public Health Services. A Roadmap to Develop Cross-Jurisdictional Sharing Initiatives. In: Center for Sharing Public Health Services, ed: Center for Sharing Public Health Services; 2013:1-4. http://www.phsharing.org/wp-content/uploads/2013/12/RoadmapBrochureV2.pdf

90. Centers for Disease Control and Prevention. Cross-Jurisdictional Sharing of Public Health Services. 2014; http://www.cdc.gov/stltpublichealth/cjs/index.html. Accessed November 18, 2014.

91. Institute of Medicine. *For the Public's Health: Investing in a Healthier Future.* Institute of Medicine; April 10, 2012. http://iom.edu/Reports/2012/For-the-Publics-Health-Investing-in-a-Healthier-Future.aspx?utm_medium=etmail&utm_source=Institute%20of%20Medicine&utm_campaign=04.10.12%2BReport%2B-%2BFor%2Bthe%2BPublic%27s%2BHealth&utm_content=New%20Reports&utm_term=Government. Accessed November 24, 2014.

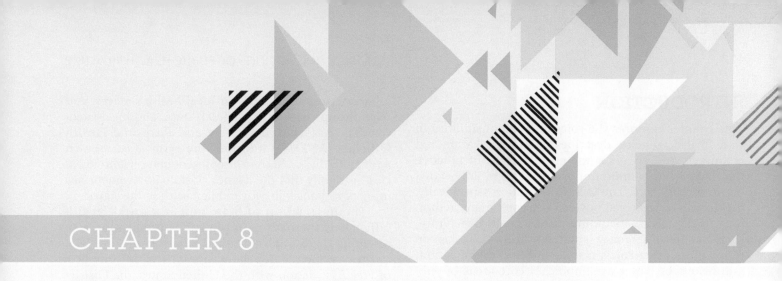

CHAPTER 8

The State Public Health Agencies

Paul E. Jarris, MD, MBA • Katie Sellers, DrPH, CPH

LEARNING OBJECTIVES

Upon completion of this chapter, the reader will be able to:

1. Understand the history and roles of state public health agencies (also called "state health agencies")

2. Give examples of state health agency activities in the following key areas: communicable disease control; chronic disease and injury prevention; environmental health; maternal, child, and family health; access to and linkages with clinical care; and emergency preparedness and response.

3. Recognize the leadership role of state health agencies in helping to create health information exchange networks, promote health equity, and facilitate coordination between clinical and public health services.

4. Understand the relationship between federal, state, and local health agencies.

5. Describe the roles and qualifications of state health officials.

6. Recognize the challenges associated with funding state and local public health programs with federal, state, local, and private funds.

7. Apply the information and resources provided in this chapter to foster further learning about state health agencies and track changes in state health agency roles, programs, and health concerns.

KEY TERMS

health equity
Health in All Policies
meaningful use
public health informatics
state health agency
surveillance
umbrella agency

INTRODUCTION

This chapter explores the roles and responsibilities of state health agencies, describes their organization and resources, and covers some critical areas of practice that have been gaining importance and rapidly evolving in recent years. The U.S. Constitution (specifically, the doctrine of reserved powers) delegates many authorities to the states, including public health; therefore, each state health agency is different from the others in terms of its exact roles, responsibilities, organization, and resources. There are important core areas of public health practice that all state health agencies cover in some way, and there are some recurring types of organizational structures that are described in this chapter. All state health agencies receive both federal and state funds, but the mix is different in each state.

This chapter will not provide a comparison between state health agencies and local health departments, nor will it attempt to delineate the many differences and/or overlapping characteristics between state and local health departments. Chapter 9 will focus exclusively on local health departments. The student is thus encouraged to take the full measure of Chapters 8 and 9 together in being able to draw distinctions in the roles and responsibilities of these two levels of governmental public health.

HISTORY

In 1869, Massachusetts became the first state to take responsibility for the health of its people by creating a state board of health. By 1909, all states had health departments and focused primarily on recording births and deaths (vital records) and controlling communicable diseases. Today, state health agencies have expanded their activities to include improving the health of children and pregnant women, controlling chronic diseases, preventing injuries, regulating health care facilities, performing epidemiological functions (such as disease surveillance and laboratory testing), developing emergency medical services and other health care resources, preparing and responding to emergencies, and protecting the environment.

The 1988 Institute of Medicine (IOM) report on *The Future of Public Health* noted that states are close enough to their inhabitants to understand population needs and preferences, and large enough, in most cases, to command the resources necessary to get important jobs done.[1] State health agencies were created to meet the differing needs and preferences of the people in each state, therefore each of these may vary widely in agency functions and activities, organizational structure, per capita expenditures, staffing patterns, political influence, responsibilities for local health services, and relationships with other federal, state, and local agencies. The Association of State and Territorial Health Officials (ASTHO) adopted the term state health agency (SHA, or SHAs to represent state health agencies) to signify that the agency of state government has primary responsibility for public health in the state.[2]

The Association of State and Territorial Health Officials is the national nonprofit organization representing the 50 SHAs in the United States, five U.S. territories, three independent nations with Compacts of Free Association with the United States, the District of Columbia, and over 100,000 public health professionals that these agencies employ. ASTHO's history began in 1879, when the idea of forming a national association of health officials was first discussed during a meeting of the Sanitary Council of the Mississippi Valley regarding measures to control the spread of cholera. By the turn of the twentieth century, the U.S. Surgeon General and state and territorial health officials began meeting annually to discuss medical and scientific aspects of controlling yellow fever and other diseases prevalent at the time. ASTHO was officially incorporated in 1942.[3] Today, ASTHO's primary function is to track, evaluate, and advise its members on the impact and formation of public or private health policy that may affect them and to provide them with guidance and technical assistance for improving the nation's health.[4]

ORGANIZATION OF STATE HEALTH AGENCIES

Agency Structure

The structure of a SHA varies depending on its placement within the state's larger departmental or organizational structure. A state public health agency can be either a freestanding agency or a unit of a larger agency, often referred to as an umbrella agency or a superagency.

In 1952, only Maine and Missouri had state public health functions in an umbrella agency. By 1969 there were eight states with such arrangements, by 1972 there were 16 states, and by 1980, 22 states were configured this way.[4,5] Results remained similar in 2012, with 20 states reporting being a unit of a larger umbrella agency.[6]

Bringing together several separate departments under one roof is meant to increase coordination between programs serving the same population groups and provide more political control over policy decisions. State public health agencies located within a larger agency often reside together with other programs such as Medicaid (the government-run health insurance program for those with low incomes) and Medicare (the government-run health insurance program for those over 65 years of age and with certain disabilities), social services, and substance abuse and mental health services.

State and Local Governance

The governance relationship between a SHA and a local health department (LHD) differs across states, and in some cases, within states. These governance differences have important implications for the coordination and delivery of essential public health services. Identifying these differences is integral to understanding roles, responsibilities, and authorities across levels of government. The following decision tree (Figure 8-1) outlines criteria to determine how states and the District of Columbia are classified according to their governance structure.

Nearly 30 percent of states (n=14) have a centralized or largely centralized governance structure, where local health units are primarily led by state employees and the state retains authority over most decisions related to finances, public health orders, and the selection of local health officials. Approximately 10 percent (n=4) have a shared governance system, where local health units may be led by state or local government employees. If they are led by state employees, the local government has the authority to make key decisions. In states with a shared governance system where LHDs are led by local employees, the SHA retains the authority to make certain key decisions. Over half of states (n=27) have a decentralized or largely decentralized system, in which local health units are primarily led by local government employees and the local governments retain authority over most key decisions. Twelve percent of states (n=6) have a mixed governance structure, in

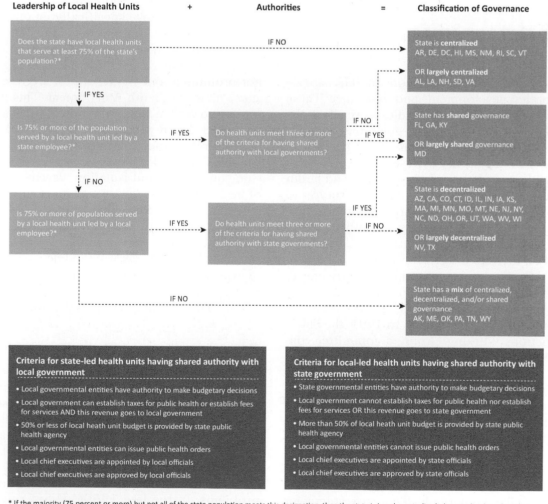

FIGURE 8-1   **State and Local Health Department Governance Classification System**

which some local health units are led by state employees and some are led by local government employees. In states with a mixed governance structure, no one arrangement predominates in the state.[7]

State Boards of Health

In the late 1800s, state governments created boards of health before SHAs made rules to prevent the spread of diseases and improve general sanitary conditions in the states. As these boards hired employees to enforce the rules, they created health departments. In 1972, all but four states had a state board of health in some form. In the 2012 ASTHO Profile survey, 26 of the 49 responding states reported having a board of health.[6] Nine of the 26 boards of health operate only in an advisory capacity, while the others have governing or policy-making authorities. Specific responsibilities among the 26 boards include advising the state health officer (85 percent), advising the governor (42 percent), and adopting and enforcing statutes (38 percent).[8]

ROLES OF STATE HEALTH AGENCIES

The three core public health functions of SHAs are assessment, policy development, and assurance. These functions imply an agenda-setting role, especially at the state level. Each SHA must identify goals and strategies to improve the health of its citizens. To set and implement this agenda, the agency assesses the health status and needs of the population, plans strategies and health programs to address unmet needs, obtains resources to support these plans, sets and enforces standards, provides technical assistance to LHDs and other governmental and nongovernmental agencies, and, in limited circumstances, delivers direct health services. In most states, LHDs are the primary government entity providing public health services to local communities.

Expert guidance for defining SHA roles and responsibilities comes from many sources. In 1994, the Public Health Functions Working Group, a committee convened by the U.S. Department of Health and Human Services (HHS) with representatives from all major public health constituencies, agreed on a list of the essential services of public health.[9] This list of services translates the three core functions into a more concrete set of activities known as the 10 Essential Public Health Services.

More recently, the Public Health Accreditation Board (PHAB), in defining standards and measures required for accreditation, has added concrete criteria for each of the 10 essential services, as well as two additional domains: administration and management, and

governance. The IOM's 2012 report on public health finance, *For the Public's Health: Investing in a Healthier Future*,[10] called for public health to define a minimum package of services, to include "an array of basic services that no health department can be without," and "foundational capabilities" — the underlying skills and infrastructure needed to perform basic public health functions such as assessment and communication. In 2013, the Robert Wood Johnson Foundation convened the Public Health Leadership Forum to define these concepts set forth by the IOM report. This work will allow public health to better define and describe the core services everyone should have access to, regardless of where they live, allow researchers to estimate the cost of providing these services, and assist advocates in their efforts to secure funding for public health departments to provide the minimum package of services.

Federal, State, and Local Authorities

The U.S. Constitution allocates power between state and federal levels of government. Federal governmental powers include those specifically enumerated in the Constitution, such as the power to tax and spend and the power to regulate interstate commerce. Those powers not expressly reserved for the federal government, nor prohibited to it by the states, are reserved to the states under the Tenth Amendment. This includes the "police power," meaning the power to enact measures to "preserve and protect the safety, health, welfare, and morals of the community." Examples of public health-related police powers exercised by the states include quarantine and isolation, vaccination, licensure of health care providers, water fluoridation, and standards for food and drinking water. While broad, state police powers have been upheld by the courts; they must be balanced against fundamental constitutional rights, including the First Amendment right to freedom of expression and the right to privacy.[11] Local governments are subsidiaries of the states and therefore their powers must be delegated from the state.[12]

Core Functions of State Health Agencies

Until the 1940s, SHAs focused almost solely on six basic public health services: vital records and statistics collection, control of communicable diseases, environmental sanitation, laboratory services, public health education, and maternal and child health. As antibiotics and vaccines became available to control the spread of communicable diseases, citizens voiced their desire for state government to give attention to other health problems. In the late 1950s, U.S. Congress began offering states federal funds to support new categories of services for certain groups of people and for specific diseases. These categorical programs addressed issues including heart disease, diabetes, developmental disabilities, migrant labor, ethnic and racial minorities, and the construction of new health facilities, such as hospitals and clinics.

This expansion of SHA activities has continued, stimulated by the increasing recognition of chronic diseases as the most prominent drivers of morbidity and mortality and the need to address the health impacts of natural and manmade disasters.

Assessment (Surveillance)

Two major functions of SHAs are collecting and preserving population health data and analyzing and using the information. According to the World Health Organization (WHO), "public health surveillance is the continuous, systematic collection, analysis and interpretation of health-related data needed for the planning, implementation, and evaluation of public health practice."[13] Syndromic surveillance involves using health data from sources such as clinics and hospitals, sent to SHAs in real time, to provide information that could help mitigate disease outbreaks.[14] SHAs collect information for vital records electronically in 46 states;[12] additionally, they may also keep records of marriages, divorces, and fetal deaths. Several examples of surveillance systems are provided in more detail in Chapters 12 and 20.

Epidemiology is "the study of the distribution and determinants of health-related states or events (including disease), and the application of this study to the control of diseases and other health problems," according to the WHO.[15] Epidemiologists use data from vital records, disease registries, populations, health providers, facility surveys, disease case reports, screening programs, syndromic surveillance systems, and laboratory results to study disease patterns, identify racial, ethnic, and other health disparities (e.g., sex, sexual identity, age, disability, socioeconomic status, and geographic location), and identify factors associated with the disease. Epidemiologists at the state level play a critical role in using data to inform decisions throughout the SHA; the results of their analyses influence the creation, continuation, or modification of policies and programs, identify disease patterns and outbreaks, determine priorities for resource allocation, and plan health care delivery sites and facilities.

Policy Development and Support

Policy, whether developed through the legislative process, formally enacted through rules or regulations, or handled internally (such as in the case of health agency worksite wellness policies), is a powerful tool to protect and promote health. State health agencies communicate regularly with their state legislators, the governor's office, and other stakeholders to shape health policy. State health agencies develop and support policies related to all of the public health topics in Table 8-1, as well as topics that may not be primarily health-focused, but may have an impact on health.

A key way SHAs participate in policy development is through encouraging a Health in All Policies (HiAP) approach to policy making throughout federal, state, or local government. Health in All Policies is a collaborative approach that integrates and articulates health considerations into policy making and programming across sectors, and at all levels, to improve the health of all communities and people. Health in All Policies requires public health practitioners to collaborate with individuals in other sectors, including transportation, education, agriculture, land use, housing, and public safety to define and achieve mutually beneficial goals.[16] Since the policies of other sectors outside of public health and health care have such a large impact on the health and equity of all people, making improvements requires genuine collaboration among sectors to define and achieve mutually beneficial goals. Good health and well-being are universally shared values, and addressing the determinants of health equity and environmental justice are a shared responsibility. Health equity is the attainment of the highest level of health for all people. Achieving health equity requires valuing everyone equally with focused and ongoing societal efforts to address avoidable inequalities, historical and contemporary injustices, and the elimination of health and health care disparities.[17] Health in All Policies serves to strengthen accountability of policy makers in all sectors and at all levels.[18]

Health impact assessment (HIA) is a primary tool for a Health in All Policies approach to decision making. The National Research Council defines an HIA as "a systematic process that uses an array of data sources and analytic methods, and considers input from stakeholders to determine the potential effects of a proposed policy, plan, program, or project on the health of a population and the distribution of those effects within the population. Health impact assessments provide recommendations on monitoring and managing those effects."[19] Health impact assessments also help evaluate the potential health effects of a plan, project, or policy before it is built or implemented, and can provide recommendations to increase positive health outcomes and minimize adverse health outcomes. In this way, it is also a tool to help achieve environmental justice. Major steps in conducting an HIA include the following: identifying projects for which an HIA would be helpful, identifying the appropriate health effects to consider, assessing the risks and benefits of the program, developing recommendations, presenting results to decision makers, and monitoring and evaluating the effect of the HIA on the decision.[20]

Traditional Programmatic Responsibilities

Efforts are currently underway to identify both foundational areas and capabilities for public health agencies.[21] The foundational areas are core components of public health work that all public health agencies have the responsibility to carry out: communicable disease control; chronic disease and injury prevention; environmental health, maternal, child, and family health; and access to and linkage with clinical care. The foundational capabilities are the underlying infrastructure and skills that a public health agency must have access to in order to carry out the critical work outlined in the foundational areas. The foundational capabilities include assessment (surveillance, epidemiology, and laboratory capacity), all-hazards preparedness and response, policy development and support, communications, community partnership development, and organizational competencies (including leadership and governance; health equity; accountability, performance management, and quality improvement; information technology; human resources; financial management; and public health law). The foundational capabilities must underlie the agency's ability to provide services in the foundational areas. Individual health agencies will engage in important public health work that is well beyond the foundational areas and capabilities, and different health departments will need to emphasize different components of the foundational areas. All residents should have access to all of the foundational services, regardless of where they live. It is worth noting that the core functions of assessment and policy development are considered foundational capabilities, while the third core function, assurance, is considered a foundational area (access to and linkage with clinical care).

Moving from a conceptual framework to empirical data, the list in Table 8-1 shows the responsibilities most commonly taken on by a SHA. The extent of state-level activities for each of the responsibilities listed in Table 8-1 will differ from state to state. In addition, there is considerable variation among the states in the levels of activities at the state versus the local health department level, and no one description of how these responsibilities are assigned or carried out at the state and local levels will suffice for all situations. The reader is again encouraged to take into account the more detailed description of local health department activities in Chapter 9 to get a better sense of the distinctions between state and local health department responsibilities. In many instances, but by no means all, the state provides overall programmatic guidance, sets policy, and channels resources, while the local health departments provide direct service delivery. So, for example, for immunizations, the state health agency might be responsible for interpreting and ensuring federal immunization policies as well as providing federal and state resources for vaccine purchase. The local health department might then be primarily responsible for actually providing immunizations in a clinic setting.

Communicable Disease Control

The prevention, detection, and control of communicable disease is an important function of public health.

TABLE 8-1   Typical Responsibilities of a State Health Agency

Communicable Disease Control
- Immunization programs
- Sexually transmitted disease counseling and partner notification
- Laboratory testing for infectious diseases
- Tuberculosis control
- HIV/AIDS screening

Chronic Disease and Injury Prevention
- Tobacco prevention services
- Data collection on behavioral risk factors
- Cholesterol, diabetes, and cardiovascular disease screening
- Injury prevention and control

Environmental Health
- Environmental epidemiology
- Food safety training/education
- Radiation control
- Toxicology
- Indoor air quality testing
- Lead inspection
- Inspecting laboratories

Maternal, Child, and Family Health
- Nutritional support for pregnant women, infants, and children (WIC)
- Services for children with special health care needs
- Maternal and child health home visits
- Early intervention programs
- Family planning services
- Well-child services

Access to and Linkage with Clinical Care
- Health disparities and minority health initiatives
- Rural health services
- Emergency medical services
- Outreach and enrollment for medical insurance
- Designation of health professional shortage areas
- Prevention of health-care-associated infections

Emergency Preparedness and Response
- Bioterrorism agent testing
- Syndromic surveillance
- Emergency medical services regulation, inspection, and licensing
- Hazmat response

Examples of morbidity and mortality caused by infectious diseases can be found throughout history (polio, pandemic influenza) and today (Ebola virus disease, West Nile virus). The public health system successfully addressed many infectious diseases through immunization, water quality improvements, waste removal, and blood screening, among other interventions, but threats remain with new and re-emerging diseases. The key components of an infection control program at a SHA include surveillance, epidemiologic investigation, laboratory capacity, risk communications, and public education. Effective public health systems require strong partnerships with health care providers and facilities for timely disease reporting, strong infection control practices, and ongoing communications.

Chronic Disease and Injury Prevention

As the leading causes of death have shifted from communicable to chronic diseases, SHAs have increased their attention to preventing chronic disease and injury. Moving beyond educating the population on public health issues, SHAs' health promotion efforts often use policy approaches to improve health. Public health practitioners are seeking to change the social and physical environments in which people live, in order to make the healthy choice the easy choice. Many current public health promotion efforts are focused on obesity as the United States is facing an unprecedented public health epidemic of overweight adults and children, which may in turn lead to the first generation in our nation's history to have shorter lives than their parents. The projected long-term health care costs of this epidemic are staggering. All ages, races, and genders are affected directly or indirectly by this epidemic. State health agencies are working with all public health sectors to develop a focused, consistent, and coordinated approach to create a culture and environment that promotes health. In the context of obesity, public health practitioners try to make it easy for communities to make healthy choices by advocating for bike lanes and public transportation, encouraging stores to offer fresh fruits and vegetables in low-income neighborhoods, and working with communities and law enforcement to increase neighborhood safety to make physical activity convenient.

In June 2011, the U.S. Surgeon General's Office released the National Prevention Strategy (NPS), which identified strategies and priorities to guide the nation in the most effective and achievable means for improving health and well-being. The NPS prioritizes prevention across multiple settings to improve health and save lives. The strategy provides the core recommendations necessary to build a prevention-oriented society and provide evidence-based recommendations to reduce the burden of the leading causes of preventable death and illness.[22] Overall, approximately 5 percent of SHA expenditures are targeted to chronic diseases prevention and control.

According to the National Center for Injury Prevention and Control, in 2011 over 50 percent of all deaths among people 1-44 years of age were due to injuries, whether unintentional or violence-related.[23] Given that many injuries are preventable, state public health agencies play a central role in implementing evidence-based policies and programs to improve outcomes for their jurisdictions. The tremendous variety of injury and violence prevention action areas present opportunities and challenges for SHAs, as these areas range from unintentional poisoning, suicide, traumatic brain injury, motor-vehicle safety, to the prevention of falls in older adults. State public health agencies regard injury prevention as a high priority, yet many agencies face budgetary constraints to fund services, with injury representing only about 1 percent of SHA expenditures.[6] Partnerships and collaboration are essential mechanisms for SHAs to provide leadership and extend their resources to prevent injury and violence. For example, collaborations with state substance abuse agencies, law enforcement, community-based agencies, and other partners can work together to address the current epidemic of prescription opioid drug abuse, misuse, and overdose.

Environmental Health

Historically, traditional environmental health programs have been implemented and overseen by state and local health agencies. However, with the creation of the Environmental Protection Agency (EPA) in 1970, state environmental health programs and activities began to move out of health agencies and become independent organizations or separate state agencies, mirroring federal changes. The result of these changes was the splintering of environmental health programs across multiple agencies and programs. State departments of environmental quality, environmental protection, and environmental services began administering traditional environmental health programs along with environmental protection programs. Environmental health programs today reflect the impact of the restructuring in the 1970s. Many health agencies have robust environmental health programs that provide a host of environmental health services; however, there are other agencies that only have responsibility for a few programs, or they are shared with other state agencies. In addition to sharing responsibility for environmental health programs and activities with other state agencies, SHAs also share responsibility with LHDs.

Examples of core environmental health activities carried out by SHAs include environmental monitoring, surveillance, and epidemiology; food safety and sanitation inspections, oversight, and training; water safety protection for groundwater, drinking water, and recreational sites; radiation control; hazardous waste and chemical safety activities; vector control and surveillance; indoor environments and housing hazard surveillance and mitigation; and the identification of other public health hazards related to environmental factors in accordance with federal, state, and local laws and regulations. Again, in many instances, the SHA provides programmatic oversight, while actual delivery of services may be through the local health department; for example, states may develop restaurant inspection programs, policies, and guidelines, while the actual inspection of restaurants may be by staff at the local health department.

Maternal, Child, and Family Health

Improving the health and wellness of mothers, infants, and children helps ensure that the next generation of children is born healthy and continues to enjoy good health throughout the lifespan. Programs and policies that effectively improve the health of these populations must continue to improve quality in existing services and functions, such as the newborn screening program, which includes monitoring specimens, improving short and long-term follow-up with affected newborns, and convening stakeholders and advocates. Maternal and child health services must also target emerging issues, such as lowering primary cesarean section rates, improving access to highly effective contraception, preventing and monitoring uptake of new forms of tobacco for children, adolescents, and pregnant women, and increasing access to care for these populations during the transformation of the health system.

Federal agencies, such as the Health Resources and Services Administration's (HRSA) Maternal and Child Health Bureau (MCHB), enhance state capacity to build data infrastructure and provide expertise to support programs and quality improvement (see Chapter 19). Within the state, health agency-based maternal and child health programs serve as the backbone for infrastructure-building services, population-based services, enabling services, and direct services aimed at women, infants, children, and their families.[24] The Maternal and Child Health Block Grant, the core funding for these services, is the only federal program that provides services within all four of these areas. Infrastructure-building services include needs assessments that determine the essential health services needed and gaps within the state's maternal and child populations, and the monitoring, training, quality assurance, and standards development for the systems of care and programs that meet those needs. Population-based services are provided to the entire maternal and child health population and include lead screening, immunizations, and newborn screening. Enabling services help families access other services, including transportation, translation services, and case management coordination with Medicaid, WIC, and other educational or health programs. Direct services are intended to cover gaps within the care system for maternal and child populations. These include health services for children and youth with special health care needs and obstetric care in areas with low access to providers.

EXPANDED AND EMERGING RESPONSIBILITIES

Emergency Preparedness and Response

From major disease outbreaks to extreme weather, events related to public health preparedness are often major news stories. Not often covered, however, is the behind-the-scenes work that public health preparedness professionals and volunteers do to prepare for and respond to these events. Public health preparedness involves building, maintaining, activating, and implementing the systems required to anticipate, respond to, and recover from all hazards, such as natural disasters, bioterrorism, or disease outbreaks. Recent examples of state and territorial public health preparedness activities include performing surveillance and laboratory services to determine the scope and patterns of chikungunya, a mosquito-borne virus causing flu-like symptoms and severe joint pain; responding to the West African Ebola outbreak; disseminating early warnings and alerts for the public to protect themselves from adverse effects of an oil spill; and coordinating the distribution of medical supplies and personnel following a fertilizer plant explosion. Emergency preparedness and response capacities, capabilities, activities, and accountabilities are covered in more detail in Chapter 26.

State health agencies also play an important role in coordinating federal, state, tribal, and local partners. While federal agencies, such as the CDC's Office of Public Health Preparedness and Response and the U.S. Department of Health and Human Services' Office of the Assistance Secretary for Preparedness and Response, provide much of the funding for public health preparedness, the states and territories are responsible for programmatic and fiscal management of federal public health preparedness programs. States seek to ensure that assets are allocated appropriately within their jurisdictions, build statewide capacity such as sophisticated epidemiological capacity, public health labs and health alert systems, and supplement and provide backup to local health jurisdictions.

Access to and Linkage with Clinical Care

State health agencies have been charged with protecting not only the health status of communities, but also the public's access to quality health care. Health departments recruit physicians for medically underserved areas and provide scholarships and loans for medical and nursing students.[25] Most SHAs serve a regulatory function with respect to hospitals (81 percent), the state's trauma system (81 percent), and the emergency medical system in the state (79 percent).[6] These regulatory roles are critical because medical error is a major cause of death and disability.[26] Health-care-associated infections are also a critical challenge to patient safety. At any given time, about one in 25 patients has a health-care-associated infection while receiving care in a U.S. hospital.[27] These infections result in up to $33 billion in excess medical costs every year. State health agencies are leading efforts to assure patient safety in hospital settings, including encouraging adoption of best practices and system modifications to reduce the probability of errors during medical procedures and in prescribing practices.

Health Care Delivery

Involvement of SHAs in direct delivery of care began with clinics for pregnant women and children. As federal and state funds have become available, direct services have expanded to include family planning, cancer screening, dental health, treatment for tuberculosis, HIV, sexually transmitted diseases, and most recently, primary medical care. In each of these undertakings, the state's role is centered on planning programs, setting and enforcing standards, developing procedures, and providing technical assistance and funding. Some public health agencies provide clinical services, including access to care for rural populations and other areas with clinical workforce shortages. Public health agencies are a vital part of the safety net and work with other components, such as retail clinics and health centers, to improve access to services. State health agencies carefully coordinate with these safety net providers to ensure high-quality services are provided to vulnerable populations. State health agencies also provide specialized clinics that offer services to treat tuberculosis and sexually transmitted infections, and provide immunization and family planning services, among others.

Financing Medical Care

A state's participation in financing medical care usually resides outside the state health agency. When the Medicaid program started in 1965, states had to select a single state agency to manage the program. Initially, some states assigned this role to the SHA. As Medicaid grew both in finances and number of participants, responsibility for operating the program shifted to either a separate state agency, social services, or a welfare agency.

Coordination and Control of Medicaid Services   When a SHA retains responsibility for the Medicaid program, the agency can use the same delivery system to better

integrate Medicaid-financed services with other public health services. Thus, both federal Medicaid and state public health funds can be coordinated to provide services to eligible patients. State health officials have a range of responsibilities and relationships with the state Medicaid agency. In seven states, the state health official has statutory oversight of Medicaid (Alabama, Kansas, Maryland, Montana, New York, Oklahoma, and Utah) and in 15 additional states the SHA and Medicaid are part of an umbrella agency. In 28 states the SHA and Medicaid report separately to the governor, and in the District of Columbia the agency reports to the mayor.

In the SHAs where the state health official does not have direct oversight of Medicaid, the flow of information and opportunities are largely dependent on the working relationships between the state health official and Medicaid leadership. Additionally, the public health workforce, from leadership to program experts, often have limited understanding of Medicaid processes and policies. Equally, Medicaid leadership can be limited by their lack of understanding of the unique expertise of public health. Therefore, when working with colleagues in Medicaid, this knowledge divide on both sides can prevent the development of strategic opportunities to improve population health and address escalating costs.

Importantly, there are new opportunities to identify the innovations occurring across states based on State Innovation Model (SIM) awards which are given to states by the Center for Medicare and Medicaid Innovation (CMMI) (see Chapter 30). In the first year of SIM (2013), 25 states received testing, pretesting, and design awards, and the second round SIM grantees were announced at the end of 2014. CMMI's ongoing use of demonstration projects in states and other jurisdictions presents opportunities that will require ongoing coordination and support at a national level to assure adequate understanding of rapidly emerging innovations. Importantly, the CMMI leadership has set as its goal the "three part aim": better care for individuals, better health for populations, and reduced expenditures. This critical partnership between public health agencies and Medicare and Medicaid at federal and state levels demonstrates the role that public health has in improving population health outcomes, articulating public health's contributions to new innovations, and developing payment mechanisms that support governmental public health.

Public Health Integration with Health Care

Since the IOM issued its report in 2012, *Primary Care and Public Health: Exploring Integration to Improve Population Health*,[28] there has been an increase in attention to the opportunities for public health and health care to work together to improve population health. This integration is a high priority for SHAs[29] and is covered in detail in Chapter 24.

Assessment (Informatics)

Another key role related to assessment involves internal and community-wide public health and health services informatics activities. **Public health informatics** can be defined as "the systematic application of information and computer science and technology to public health practice, research and learning."[30] Data collection and analysis are critical functions for SHAs. These activities help identify changing needs for health programs and emerging threats to the public's health. As information systems have evolved, new methods and tools are being developed for using technology to enhance SHAs' ability to identify and assess current and future priorities for policies, funding, and program activities. Nearly all activities of public health are now supported by some form of information technology.

Meaningful Use and Public Health

The Centers for Medicare and Medicaid Services' Electronic Health Care Record (EHR) Incentive Programs (commonly referred to as **meaningful use**) incentivize eligible hospitals, critical access hospitals, and eligible professionals to adopt, implement, and upgrade certified EHR systems to demonstrate meaningful use of these technologies. Meaningful use was enacted as a section of the American Recovery and Reinvestment Act of 2009 known as HITECH (Health Information Technology for Economic and Clinical Health). Meaningful use is comprised of three iterative stages of EHR functionality and reporting requirements. Stages 1 and 2 are underway, and Stage 3 requirements are expected to be released for public comment in spring 2015. The Stage 3 reporting period is scheduled to begin in 2017.

Meaningful use provided an unprecedented opportunity for SHAs to engage in electronic data exchange with clinical providers. In Stages 1 and 2, meaningful use participants are required to engage in public health data reporting with the public health agency (local or state) in their jurisdiction. Public health objectives for Stages 1 and 2 are detailed in Table 8-2. In Stage 1, participants are required to choose only one of the menu public health objectives and to conduct a data submission test. Although it is not required as part of Stage 1, providers are encouraged to establish ongoing data submission to their public health agency. In Stage 2, participants are subject to a mix of core, required, and menu public health objectives. Stage 2 also includes a requirement for participants to register their intent to submit data to their public health agency within 60 days of the start of their reporting period, and a requirement to establish ongoing data submission following a successful test.

TABLE 8-2   Summary of Meaningful Use Public Health Objectives[31]

	Stage 1		Stage 2	
	Eligible Professionals	**Eligible Hospitals**	**Eligible Professionals**	**Eligible Hospitals**
Capability to submit electronic data to immunization registries or Immunization Information Systems and actual submission	Menu*	Menu*	Core‡	Core‡
Capability to submit electronic data on reportable (as required by state or local law) lab results to public health agencies and actual submission	N/A	Menu*	N/A	Core‡
Capability to submit electronic syndromic surveillance data to public health agencies and actual submission	Menu*	Menu*	Menu*	Core‡
Capability to identify and report cancer cases to a state cancer registry	N/A	N/A	Menu*	N/A
Capability to identify and report specific cases to a specialized registry (other than a cancer registry)	N/A	N/A	Menu*	N/A

Note: Objectives do not supersede local, state, or federal requirements or each public health registry's requirements. "N/A" indicates that this objective was not a part of Stage 1.

* Menu objectives provide choice for Eligible Professionals and Hospitals to select one public health objective to qualify for meaningful use payment.

‡ Core objectives must be met to qualify for meaningful use payment.

State Health Information Exchanges

With increasing health information technology adoption both in SHAs and in the clinical health sector, SHAs collect, receive, and exchange increasing amounts of program-specific information electronically. Over half of SHAs collect information electronically for all areas except water wells, electronic health records, and onsite waste water treatment systems.[6] For all topic areas, data are collected primarily with the state system for more than 80 percent of SHAs. It is much less common for data to be collected primarily with local systems. Bidirectional data reporting and exchange is greatest for electronic health records (71 percent), Medicaid billing (56 percent), and lab results (53 percent). Much of this data exchange still occurs through direct connections between SHAs' information systems and clinical information systems.[6]

Public Health Community Platform

The CDC-funded Public Health Community Platform (PHCP) is being developed to provide an accessible, flexible, and secure public health information technology platform of interoperable shared solutions for the public health community. The PHCP is intended to be governed by the public health community and enable user-driven development, implementation, and collaboration to efficiently address public health priorities.

Clinical and laboratory providers are often unsure of how, to whom, and which notifiable conditions should be reported to public health authorities. Illustrating the usefulness of a centralized platform, a common decision support tool could be maintained with the appropriate notifiable condition triggers for EHRs and laboratories, and route common data elements necessary to instigate public health follow-up. This approach provides one point of reference (the PHCP) for the health care community and decreases the need for public health to maintain jurisdiction-specific triggers and routing. Public health agencies will receive a more complete picture of notifiable conditions within their jurisdictions and will be able to share their methods and findings with others, while minimizing the cost of hosting and maintaining a complex technology solution.

Syndromic Surveillance

Nearly all SHAs perform some syndromic surveillance activities, defined as population-level surveillance of clinical syndromes that have a significant impact on public health. In 2012, 94 percent of SHAs reported conducting syndromic surveillance, up from 79 percent in 2010.[6] To facilitate sharing of data and information among these jurisdictions and with federal partners, the CDC launched its BioSense program in 2003. BioSense now allows a shared environment for data among participating jurisdictions, support of shared analytical capabilities, a shared governing body, and the use of cloud computing technology. The goal of BioSense is to provide nationwide and regional situational awareness for hazardous health threats and to support national, state, and local responses to those various threats. Advances in public health informatics and the evolution of the BioSense program have helped syndromic surveillance become an increasingly important component of the biosurveillance enterprise.

Communications

Effective communication is an important tool in public health practice. State health agencies must deliver key messages to the public in times of emergency, such as whether or not to drink tap water, or how to avoid catching a deadly virus. Agencies also play a key role in communicating information from the federal government to local governments, such as how to comply with federal grant regulations, or how to interpret other federal guidance in the context of state law. Cross-sectoral collaboration, "Health in All Policies" approaches, and integration of public health and health care all require public health practitioners to speak the language of other disciplines, challenging the effectiveness of public health's traditional ways of communicating. Technology's rapid evolution also requires public health practitioners to embrace new methods of communication to reach members of the public less likely to access older methods. Current examples of this include social media and other forms of digital communication as alternatives to telephones and print media.

Community Partnership Development

State health agency partnerships with community leaders and organizations are critical to effective agency functioning in many ways. First, community partnerships allow agencies to gain insight into community health concerns and seek community buy-in for agency priorities. While evidence may suggest that a certain intervention is effective in preventing disease, agencies must engage communities with at-risk populations to determine if the intervention is culturally acceptable. Agencies can also work with community partners to ensure that key health messages are heard by community members who are unlikely to be reached by traditional channels such as local news or messages provided by health care providers. Finally, solid community partnerships can support agency efforts to develop effective health policy. If the community understands the need for what might otherwise be an unpopular policy, community members can vote for legislators who support that policy. State health agencies work directly with community partners, and work closely with local health departments in collaboration with community partnerships as well.

Organizational Competencies

In order for a SHA to successfully provide needed public health services, the agency itself must function effectively. The organizational competencies required for an effective and efficient agency include strong leadership or governance, a focus on health equity, attention to accountability, performance management, and quality improvement, and strong information technology, human resources, financial management, and legal capabilities. Many of these organizational competencies are necessary for most any organization or business, whether in the health field or not. We highlight key competencies specific to public health below.

Accountability, Performance Management, and Quality Improvement

As the national trend continues toward accountability and quality in SHAs, the public health system is working to reinforce and increase awareness and implementation of performance management and quality improvement (QI) activities and practices. Ongoing engagement in performance management and QI activities can help health agencies demonstrate sound financial, infrastructure, and program deployment decisions, as well as inform the implementation of effective cost-savings advancements that are appropriately linked to improved population health outcomes.

Health Equity

One of the central priorities driving the public health agenda is to achieve health equity. The World Health Organization suggests that "the objective of good health is twofold: the best attainable average level – goodness – and the smallest feasible differences among individuals and groups – fairness."[32] State and territorial health officials and health agency leadership staff can play a critical role in setting and progressing a health equity agenda across programs and departments.

Current data show significant inequities and disparities in key health indicators such as: infant mortality rates, life expectancy, and rates of disease; key risk factors such as smoking and access to care, nutrition, and physical activity; and in social determinants of health, which include poverty, inadequate housing, and unsafe working conditions. Health disparities that have their roots in social determinants of health are referred to as health inequities, which are a reflection of the persistent barriers to health that exist in American society. For example, infant mortality among African Americans

in 2011 occurred at a rate of 11.5 deaths per 1,000 live births, more than twice the national non-Hispanic white rate of 5.1 deaths per 1,000 live births.[33] The combined direct and indirect costs of health inequities in the United States between 2003 and 2006 were $1.24 trillion.[34]

Environmental and social exposures, education and economic opportunities, health behaviors, access to and quality of health care, and genetics are all major determinants of health status. Contributors to health inequities are interconnected and must be addressed through multifaceted and multisectoral approaches. In addition, structural and individual racism and other forms of discrimination affect health outcomes.[35]

AREAS OF SIGNIFICANT VARIATION IN STATE HEALTH AGENCY ROLES

Before 1960, almost all state public health programs were under the umbrella of SHAs. As programs became more complex and demands for new types of services increased, many public health activities were assigned to other state agencies. Table 8-3 shows the wide variation in responsibilities performed directly by health agencies in 2010 and 2012, and Table 8-4 shows other agencies that share responsibility for some public health activities.[6]

THE STATE PUBLIC HEALTH WORKFORCE

State Health Officials

The title of the chief executive of a SHA is usually Secretary, Director, or Commissioner, but more important than the title is who makes the appointment. Whether the state health official (SHO) is appointed by the governor, a board, or the head of an umbrella agency or superagency is a critical factor in determining the SHO's level of authority, access to state policy makers, and participation in health policy decisions.

State health officials are appointed by the governor in 37 states, by the secretary of state health and human services in three states, by the state board of health or commission in three states, and by other entities in three states.[6] If the SHO reports directly to the governor, there may be greater opportunity to influence health policy in both the executive and legislative branches. When emergencies arise, SHOs typically have extensive interaction directly with the governor.

Traditionally, medical requirements were part of state law, and only physicians could hold the position

TABLE 8-3 Diversity in State Health Agency Programs and Functions

Public Health Function or Program	Performed by State Health Agency Directly, 2010	Performed by State Health Agency Directly, 2012
Public water supply safety	52%	48%
Lead inspection	66%	77%
Food safety training and education	90%	83%
Hospital regulation, inspection, and licensing	83%	81%
Professional licensure of physicians	26%	24%
Rural health services	42%	25%
Trauma system coordination	81%	88%
Medical Examiner	23%	25%
Mental health treatment services	21%	17%
Newborn screenings	69%	63%
WIC	54%	56%

SOURCE: Association of State and Territorial Public Health Officials, ASTHO Profile of State Public Health, Volume Three (2014).

TABLE 8-4 Health Responsibilities Often in State Agencies Other Than the State Health Agency

State Agency/Department	Health-related Responsibilities
Department of Agriculture	Inspects grocery stores Inspects food-processing plants
Department of Education	Supervises development of wellness policies Supervises implementation of school nutrition programs
Department of Environmental Quality	Monitors air quality and pollution Monitors water quality and pollution Oversees radiation programs
Department of Labor and Industry	Regulates occupational health and safety
Department of Medical Assistance Services (Medicaid)	Finances medical care for low-income and categorically needy Funds a health status screening program for children
Department of Mental Health, Behavioral Health, and Substance Abuse Services	Operates psychiatric hospitals Directs community mental health and substance abuse services

of SHO. At first, most of these physicians had no formal training in public health. As public health schools were created, however, physicians who were trained specifically for positions in public health administration directed most SHAs. In 1977, all but six states had SHOs who were physicians.[36] Twenty-three of these 44 physicians were specialists in public health and preventive medicine, and 30 had public health degrees.

As of 2012, 26 states require the SHO to be a physician, while eight require a Master of Public Health and seven require experience in public health practice or teaching. Three other states require either a medical degree or another doctoral degree, while 14 states have no statutory requirements for the qualifications of the SHO. Eight states require executive management experience.[6] Figure 8-2 demonstrates the variation in SHO qualifications at the time of the survey.[6]

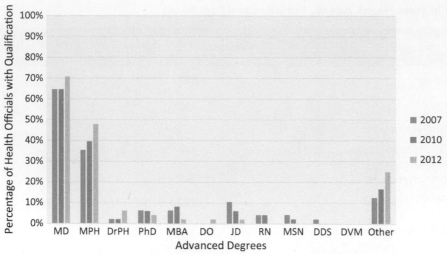

FIGURE 8-2   Advanced Degree Qualifications of State Health Officials, 2007–2012 (n=48)

DATA SOURCE: ASTHO Profile of State Public Health, Volume Three. Washington, DC: Association of State and Territorial Health Officials, 2014.

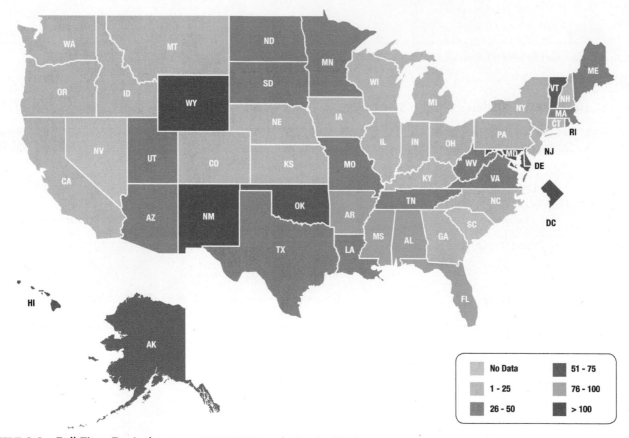

FIGURE 8-3   Full-Time Equivalents per 100,000 Population in 2012

DATA SOURCE: ASTHO Profile of State Public Health, Volume Three. Washington, DC: Association of State and Territorial Health Officials, 2014.

Public Health Workforce

Many factors influence the number and types of staff that a SHA employs. These include the agency's specific roles and responsibilities, distances between population centers, types and numbers of regulated health care facilities, density and economic status of populations served, degree of responsibility for direct delivery of services, and the number, size, autonomy, and sophistication of LHDs. Community values and goals can also affect SHA programs and staffing needs. There are approximately 101,000 full-time equivalents in the state public health workforce.[6] The number of full-time equivalents per 100,000 for each state is displayed in Figure 8-3.

The following are other key findings on the state public health agency workforce from the 2012 ASTHO Profile Survey:

▸ On average, 71 percent of SHA employees are female.
▸ On average, nearly three-quarters of all SHA employees are white, with the next largest percentage being black or African American (14.9 percent) and another 5 percent being Hispanic or Latino. On the whole, the racial composition of a SHA is relatively similar to that of the racial composition of the United States in 2012.
▸ Public health faces a rapidly aging workforce whose average age is 47.3 years.
▸ The average age of new employees is 40.6 years.
▸ SHAs report that the percentage of employees eligible for retirement over the next five years is as high as 70 percent in some SHAs, and the average percent of employees eligible for retirement across all SHAs in the next five years is 25 percent.
▸ Current vacancy rates are as high as 41 percent in some states; the average vacancy rate among the responding SHAs is 12 percent.[12]

Clearly there are challenges ahead if we hope to maintain an adequate workforce to staff our nation's SHAs.

FUNDING

Expenditures

As with staffing patterns, SHA expenditures are difficult to compare across the nation because agency responsibilities vary so widely. In fiscal year (FY) 2010, agency expenditures totaled approximately $26.5 billion, while in FY2011 they were just over $28 billion. Average per capita expenditures were $99 for FY2010 and $98 for FY2011. Median per capita expenditures were somewhat lower at $80 for FY2010 and $78 for FY2011. In FY2011, the largest percentage of funds was spent on improving consumer health (which includes clinical services) and the Special Supplemental Nutrition Program for Women, Infants, and Children (WIC), each accounting for approximately one-quarter of all SHA expenditures. Vital statistics, injury prevention, and health data accounted for the lowest amount of expenditures, with only 1 percent of total expenditures spent on each of the three categories (see Figure 8-4).[6]

Sources of Funds

In FY2011, SHAs received 53 percent of their revenue from federal funds, 24 percent from state general funds, 4 percent from fees and fines, 10 percent from other state funds, and 9 percent from other sources. The single largest source of federal funds (55 percent)

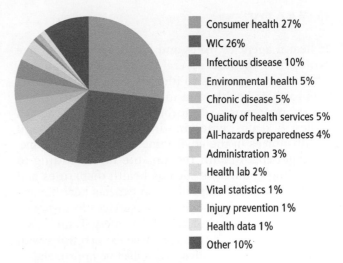

■ Consumer health 27%
■ WIC 26%
■ Infectious disease 10%
■ Environmental health 5%
■ Chronic disease 5%
■ Quality of health services 5%
■ All-hazards preparedness 4%
■ Administration 3%
■ Health lab 2%
■ Vital statistics 1%
■ Injury prevention 1%
■ Health data 1%
■ Other 10%

Note: Not all states reported values for all expenditure categories or sources of revenue. Ns ranged from 40 to 49.

FIGURE 8-4   Percentage of State Health Agency Expenditures by Expense Category for FY 2011 (n=49*)

DATA SOURCE: ASTHO Profile of State Public Health, Volume Three. Washington, DC: Association of State and Territorial Health Officials, 2014.

was the U.S. Department of Agriculture, which oversees WIC. CDC and HRSA were the next highest sources of health agencies' federal funds, accounting for 16 percent and 10 percent of federal revenue among SHAs, respectively.[6]

Categorical and Block Grants

Federal funds come to states both as categorical grants, which focus on a particular health problem or population group, and as block grants, which have a broader public health focus. In general, categorical grant programs are controlled by extensive federal regulations and lengthy reporting requirements and may lack the flexibility to address variations in state needs.

Block grants were created in the early 1980s to achieve greater financial flexibility, including more efficient use of tax dollars and more cost-effective services to recipients. Twenty-one previously separate programs were consolidated into block grant areas. States and members of Congress favor block grants because they provide opportunities to meet unique state priorities and fill gaps in federal and state funding. However, if states are able to use the funds in different ways, it can be a challenge to demonstrate the collective impact of the funding. Initiatives are underway to improve collection of block grant impacts while maintaining necessary state flexibility. The Title V Maternal and Child Health block grant and the Preventive Health and Health Services block grant continue to be important sources of financial support for all SHAs.

SUMMARY

State health agencies' roles and functions will continue to evolve over the next several decades. The public depends on state agencies to identify new and emerging threats to their health, and increasingly, needs protection from new causes of morbidity and mortality, such as violence, drugs, emerging infectious diseases, and toxic substances in the environment. At the same time, health agencies remain responsible for attending to longstanding challenges such as health disparities and infectious diseases. The public also expects health agencies to regulate health facilities and services to assure effective treatment and protect patient safety. Tomorrow's SHAs will be required to meet these expectations with new policies and innovative, cost-effective approaches.

REVIEW QUESTIONS

1. What is the difference between a freestanding state health agency and an umbrella agency?

2. Describe the following governance relationships between state and local health agencies: centralized, shared, decentralized, and mixed.

3. How do SHAs carry out the core public health function of assessment? How is public health informatics related to assessment?

4. Give an example of SHA responsibilities in each of the following key areas: communicable disease control; chronic disease and injury prevention; environmental health; maternal, child, and family health; access to and linkages with clinical care; and emergency preparedness and response.

5. List three organizational competencies important for SHAs.

6. Describe the process of appointing a state health official. What should his or her qualifications be?

7. From where do SHAs receive funding? Describe the difference between categorical and block grants.

REFERENCES

1. Institute of Medicine, Committee for the Study of the Future of Public Health. *The Future of Public Health*. Washington, DC: National Academy Press; 1988.

2. Association of State and Territorial Health Officials. By-laws. Washington, DC.

3. Association of State and Territorial Health Officials. History of ASTHO. Arlington, VA. http://www.astho.org/About/History/. Accessed December 23, 2014.

4. Public Health Foundation. SHAs-freestanding agencies v. super-agencies. *Public Health Macroview*. Washington, DC; 1995;7(1):1.

5. Public Health Foundation. Public Health Agencies 1980. A Report on Their Expenditures and Activities. Washington, DC; 1981.

6. ASTHO Profile of State Public Health, Volume Three. Washington, DC: Association of State and Territorial Health Officials, 2014.

7. Meit M1, Sellers K, Kronstadt J, Lawhorn N, Brown A, Liss-Levinson R, Pearsol J, Jarris PE. Governance typology: a consensus classification of state-local health department relationships. *J Public Health Manag Pract*. 2012 Nov;18(6):520–528.

8. Fenton GD. The status of state boards of health in 2010. *J. Public Health Manag. Pract*. 17(6):554–559. http://www.ncbi.nlm.nih.gov/pubmed/21964368. Accessed September 26, 2012.

9. Public Health Functions Steering Committee Report, *Public Health In America*. Washington, DC; 1994. Available at: http://www.health.gov/phfunctions/public.htm. Accessed June 1, 2007.

10. Institute of Medicine. *For the Public's Health; Investing in a Healthier Future*. Washington, DC: The National Academies Press; 2012.

11. Gostin LO. *Public Health Law: Power, Duty, Restraint*. 2nd ed. Berkeley, CA: University of California Press; 2008: 78–82; 141.

12. Gostin LO. *Public Health Law: Power, Duty, Restraint*. 2d ed. Berkeley, CA: University of California Press; 2008: 78–82.

13. Health Topics: Public Health Surveillance, World Health Organization, 2014. http://www.who.int/topics/public_health_surveillance/en/. Accessed December 23, 2014.

14. Henning KJ. Overview of syndromic surveillance, *Morbidity and Mortality Weekly Report (MMWR)* Supplement, September 24, 2004 / 53(Suppl);5–11. http://www.cdc.gov/mmwr/preview/mmwrhtml/su5301a3.htm. Accessed December 23, 2014.

15. Epidemiology, World Health Organization, 2014; http://www.who.int/topics/epidemiology/en/. Accessed December 23, 2014.

16. ASTHO. Health in All Policies. http://www.astho.org/Programs/HiAP/

17. Recommendations For Health Equity Language In ASTHO Written Publications, Association of State and Territorial Health Officials, 2013.

18. World Health Organization. Health in all Policies: Helsinki statement. Framework for country action. Finland: World Health Organization and Ministry of Social Affairs and Health. 2013.

19. Committee on Health Impact Assessment; National Research Council. *Improving Health in the United States: The Role of Health Impact Assessment.* Washington, DC: National Academies Press; 2011.

20. Centers for Disease Control and Prevention. Health Impact Assessment. http://www.cdc.gov/healthyplaces/hia.htm. Accessed October 22, 2014.

21. This work is being developed in an iterative process that is still underway at the time of writing.

22. U.S. Department of Health and Human Services, Office of the Surgeon General. National Prevention Strategy. http://www.surgeongeneral.gov/initiatives/prevention/strategy/index.html. January 28, 2015.

23. Centers for Disease Control and Prevention, National Center for Injury Prevention and Control: Web-based Injury Statistics Query and Reporting System (WISQARS). http://www.cdc.gov/injury/wisqars/index.html.

24. Health Resources Services Administration (HRSA)/ Maternal and Child Health Bureau (MCHB). MCH Programs Overview: Program Categories. http://mchb.hrsa.gov/programs/. Accessed November 21, 2014.

25. For example, see California's Health Profession Education Foundation website. http://www.healthprofessions.ca.gov/progfacts.htm. Accessed June 6, 2007. Information on the national Health Resources and Services Administration (HRSA) program can be seen at http:// nhsc.bhpr.hrsa.gov/jobs/. Accessed June 6, 2007.

26. For example, see the Institute of Medicine's reports, *To Err is Human: Building A Safer Health System* and *Crossing the Quality Chasm: A New Health System for the 21st Century.* http://www.iom.edu/?id=12735 and http://www.iom.edu/?id=12736. Also see Aspden, P, Wolcott, J, Bootman, JL, Cronenwett, LR. (Eds.) *Preventing Medication Errors: Quality Chasm Series.*

27. Magill SS, Edwards JR, Bamberg W, et al. Multistate Point-Prevalence Survey of Health Care–Associated Infections. *N Engl J Med* 2014;370:1198–208.

28. Institute of Medicine. *Primary Care and Public Health; Exploring Integration to Improve Population Health.* Washington, DC: National Academies Press; 2012.

29. Montero JT and Terrillion A. Reintegrating Health Care and Public Health: A population health imperative. *J. Public Health Manag. Pract.* 2013: 19(5):493–496.

30. What is public health informatics? Johns Hopkins University. http://www.jhsph.edu/departments/health-policy-and-management/certificates/public-health-informatics/what-is-health-informatics.html. Accessed December 23, 2014.

31. CMS "Public Health Registry Tipsheet." http://www.cms.gov/Regulations-and-Guidance/Legislation/EHRIncentivePrograms/Downloads/PublicHealthRegistry_Tipsheet-.pdf. Accessed November 10, 2014.

32. World Health Organization. *The World Health Report 2000.* Geneva: WHO, 2000.

33. Kids Count Datacenter. Infant Mortality by Race. http://datacenter.kidscount.org/data/tables/21-infant-mortality-by-race#detailed/1/any/false/867,133,38,35,18/10, 11,9,12,1,13/285,284

34. LaVeist, TA, Gaskin, DJ, Richard, P. "The Economic Burden of Health Inequities in the United States." Joint Center of Political and Economic Studies. September 2009. https://www.ndhealth.gov/heo/publications/The%20Economic%20Burden%20of%20Health%20Inequalities%20in%20the%20United%20States.pdf. Accessed October 20, 2014.

35. Healthy People 2020. http://www.healthypeople.gov/2020/about/DisparitiesAbout.aspx. Accessed October 17, 2014.

36. Terris M. Letter to all state health officials on results of questionnaire on training and experience. New York Medical College; December 2, 1977.

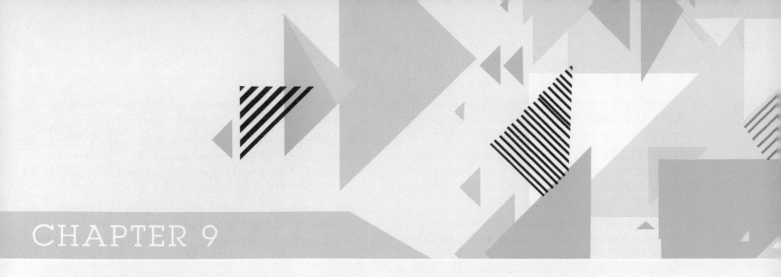

CHAPTER 9

The Local Health Department

Carolyn J. Leep, MS, MPH • Sarah J. Newman, MPH • Robert M. Pestronk, MPH • Ivey Wohlfeld, BA

LEARNING OBJECTIVES

Upon completion of this chapter, the reader will be able to:

1. Describe the factors that affect local governmental public health practice.

2. Distinguish the different types of local health department governance models.

3. Recognize the large differences in size among local health departments, in terms of population served, budget, and staffing.

4. Describe how local health department operations are financed.

5. Describe the roles of the local health department in carrying out each of the 10 Essential Public Health Services.

6. List activities and services frequently provided by local health departments.

7. Identify the occupations typically employed by local health departments of various sizes.

KEY TERMS

accreditation
governance
local health department
workforce

INTRODUCTION

The **local health department** (LHD) is "an administrative or service unit of local or state government, concerned with health, and carrying some responsibility for the health of a jurisdiction smaller than the state."[1] Where they are a unit of local government, they typically are part of county, city, or town government. Regardless of whether they rest within state or local government, partisan, political, social, and economic interests along with the availability of technology and a well-trained workforce affect the work of LHDs.

This chapter provides an overview of, and historical perspectives about, LHDs, their organizational form, the work they perform, and the workforce, tools, and technologies employed by them. It discusses issues that LHDs currently face and are likely to face in the future.

At the LHD and in the LHD's jurisdiction, the themes and components of the public health enterprise described in this book's chapters all intersect and play out in daily practice. To a great extent, the goals of LHDs have remained, and will remain, constant: prevent poor health, enable equity and quality of life, and protect people from threats to life and health. LHDs will continue to accomplish this through leadership, knowledge, partnership, and the strategic use of their own resources and those administered by others.

OVERVIEW OF LOCAL HEALTH DEPARTMENTS

In contrast to a panel of patients served in a clinical practice, the major focus for the LHD is the entire population of their jurisdiction. Simply put, the job of the LHD, working with other people and organizations, is to make health easier and more likely for everyone and to stimulate the design of environments which encourage healthy decision making by default. It is easier, for example, for residents of a community served by a community drinking water system not to be infected or intoxicated by waterborne agents if the municipal system is designed to deliver clean and safe drinking water. Safe water can be assumed by default. Each resident need not make an individual decision about whether to treat the water emerging from the tap.

This mission of the LHD is accomplished through core functions which have been characterized as assessment, policy development, and assurance.[2] Through assessment, the LHD collects, analyzes, and shares information about the health of people in its jurisdiction. For example, LHDs (increasingly together with others in the jurisdiction) use data from local, state, and federal sources to contrast the health status of people in their jurisdiction with that of other jurisdictions. Likely causes for poor health are elucidated. With leadership, processes to identify high-priority problems and which commit the LHD and others to improving performance and outcomes can result from the assessment. Metrics, whereby progress over time can be measured, may also be established.

All organizations adopt policy to orient their own internal operations. LHDs typically possess the additional authority to adopt policy (law, regulation, ordinance), or to inform the adoption of policy by their governing boards, which creates an expectation, rule, or requirement for those living in the LHD's jurisdiction. This local authority is akin to the lawmaking authority of a state legislature or Congress. LHD authority applies to the jurisdiction for which the LHD has responsibility. If public spaces and worksites are free of tobacco smoke, this probably reflects the policy-making activity of an LHD or of another governmental body which has been informed by the work of LHDs. In rural areas, policy adopted by an LHD may determine where wells for drinking water may be drilled or where and whether septic systems can be installed. A Health in All Policies approach[3] is increasingly promoted by LHDs in recognition of the extent to which the decisions of other organizations influence or shape the health of a jurisdiction's residents. Some LHDs may produce health impact assessments as a means to explore the impact of policy before a final decision is reached.[4]

As might be imagined, the use of this unusual power engages the department in several ways: in the use of data from its assessment; in the discovery of evidence of what remedy might best improve health; and with the political process needed to gain support from elected or appointed officials and, of course, from the residents of the jurisdiction. In a democratic society, the ballot enables residents of a jurisdiction to collectively express their aspirations for their elected officials and government. The direction for those aims and their intensity change over time and influence the orientation and work of LHDs.

The trust and support of local residents is important. Their voices can facilitate or impede the adoption of policy. Their votes often elect the people responsible for choosing the director of the LHD and for the budget with which the LHD operates. Elected officials want to be responsive to their constituents or at a minimum not irritate them to the point of convincing them of the need to cast their vote for an opponent. When asked by a new local health official what the most important aspect of his job was, one chairman of a county board of commissioners (the governing body for the LHD) replied, "The ability to count to five" (Personal Communication, Sylvester Broome, 1986). There were nine commissioners on the county board. Five were needed to adopt or oppose any measure or to replace the local health official.

While an understanding of local health status and the use of law to express intent, to reward, and/or to punish for noncompliance are necessary foundations, they are insufficient for continuous improvement in health. Assurance includes activities such as community education campaigns to help residents understand the causes for better or poor health and to increase the likelihood of compliance with law. Where adoption will limit personal freedoms, support can be enhanced for the tradeoff between freedom and health. Through assurance, LHDs monitor activities within the jurisdiction to determine compliance with licensing or operating requirements for businesses. LHDs may inspect restaurants, daycare centers, and recreation facilities. They may assess fines or require change in process or practice. The process for exercising and challenging LHD authority may be outlined in administrative law. Challenges questioning the limits of authority may be resolved by the judicial system.

Assurance also involves the delivery of services to people for whom access would otherwise be limited or of poor quality or because it is more efficient to provide a service *en masse*, such as screening programs, mass vaccination, or pharmaceutical delivery campaigns. LHDs may deliver primary care or certain categorical services such as vaccination, family planning, and programs to increase access to healthy food. They may screen for or treat disease or provide home health care. Unlike the assessment and policy development functions, which require LHDs to examine or address the population as a whole, some assurance activities involve the delivery of services to one person at a time.

While many people associate LHD work with the clinical service which members of their family receive from it, the broader scope of LHD work is revealed during outbreaks of disease or emergencies, when media are used to heighten visibility to prevalent or incipient health problems, or when businesses are required to close until hygienic practices are routine. Real estate developers platting new subdivisions interact with LHDs in the design of water and sewer systems. Businesses required to purchase new equipment to comply with regulations adopted to assure food safety quickly become familiar with other aspects of LHD work, as do homeowners required to drill new drinking water wells or to replace their septic system with a connection to public sewer. LHD staff may also help residents or school children identify appropriate clinical care or ease access to it.

There are approximately 2,800 LHDs operating in the country.[1] Every state except Rhode Island and Hawaii either has LHDs or units of the state health agency that serve portions of the state. Across the nation, the workforce, technology, and programs of LHDs vary not only based on the availability of federal, state, local, or private funding, but also because state or local law describing their authority and responsibilities varies. The creativity of department staff, the work performed by other community organizations, or the priorities established or freedoms tolerated by the LHD governing board or the courts also influence the work of the department.

LHDs coordinate their work vertically, outside their jurisdiction, with state and federal government agencies and horizontally with religious groups, private and nonprofit businesses, organizations delivering clinical care, schools, community residents, and the media.[5] Some may imagine a hierarchical view of powers or duties which gives more authority to a state or the federal government than to local government. While this may be true where local public health authorities have been preempted by state or federal law, in some local jurisdictions the authorities and powers of an LHD parallel those of state and federal government (see, for example, the grant of authority to Michigan's LHDs, in part 24 of P.A. 368 of 1978, Michigan Compiled Law).[6]

The activities of an LHD are important elements in the collective action required for health to be either easy or difficult and by design: LHDs save lives and money.[7] The 1988 *The Future of Public Health* report from the Institute of Medicine articulated the critical role of LHDs stating: "…no citizen from any community, no matter how small or remote should be without identifiable and realistic access to the benefits of public health protection, which is possible only through a local component of the public health delivery system."[2]

A BRIEF HISTORICAL PERSPECTIVE ON LOCAL HEALTH DEPARTMENTS

The first LHDs were established in urban areas in response to health issues related to dense populations and because these population centers were often the disembarkation point for travelers from other parts of the world. LHDs, or a local health "official," localized responsibility for health and community protection. Paul Revere chaired a board which adopted regulations to reduce the pollution of Boston's harbor in which all manner of offal and detritus from city life collected. By the late 1800s, LHDs were operating in Baltimore, Charleston, Philadelphia, Providence, Cambridge, New York City, Chicago, Louisville, Indianapolis, and Boston, largely for the purposes of monitoring and addressing contagious diseases, enforcing quarantine and isolation rules, and reducing environmental hazards through sanitation measures.[8] As science informed the understanding of disease causation, treatment, and prevention, additional responsibility for the population's health shifted to the public realm and influenced the work of LHDs. Early in the twentieth century, more LHDs emerged, including the first in rural areas.

Throughout the twentieth century, additional LHDs were established across the country. By 1953, 1,239 LHDs served local jurisdictions.[9] In 1989, 2,888 had been identified.[10] The number and scope of services delivered by LHDs changed in response to state and local law and politics, funding, evidence of effectiveness, and the evolving needs identified by communities. In the late twentieth century, LHDs gave increasing attention to the causes and prevention of chronic disease. In the early twenty-first century, in response to the events of 9/11 (2001) and, especially, the anthrax attacks of 10/11 (2001), LHDs turned their attention to the identification, response, mitigation, and follow-up to man-made and natural disasters, particularly those which have a biological origin.

LHDs have helped to accomplish, and sometimes played a major role in, the 10 great public health achievements of the twentieth century: immunization, motor-vehicle safety, workplace safety, control of infectious disease, declines in death from heart disease and stroke, safer and healthier foods, healthier mothers and babies, family planning, fluoridation of drinking water, and a reduced exposure to tobacco and tobacco smoke.[11] LHDs are the "boots on the ground" for response and interventions which media often identify with state and federal agencies.

Over time the component elements of assessment, policy development, and assurance have been described conceptually and practically.[12,13] Since 1988, publications of the Institute of Medicine (IOM), the National Association of County and City Health Officials (NACCHO), and the Centers for Disease Control and Prevention (CDC) have influenced the American understanding of the LHD's role.

The IOM introduced the influential rubric of assessment, policy development, and assurance[2] and has more recently shared opinion in multiple reports.[5,14,15] NACCHO first elaborated on the IOM's three core functions in the Blueprint.[16] The Blueprint coincided with earlier concerns about the problems of cost and quality of, and access to, medical care and the importance of recognizing the unique roles and capacities of LHDs. NACCHO's *Operational Definition* framed a set of 10 standards for "what everyone, regardless of where they live, should reasonably expect from the local governmental public health presence."[17] In this same period, CDC defined "a public health system" of which LHDs were a part;[18] standards and measures for the performance of that system were elaborated;[19] and, a set of national goals were established through the *Healthy People* framework, some of which eventually applied to LHDs themselves.[20]

LOCAL HEALTH DEPARTMENTS IN THE TWENTY-FIRST CENTURY

Study of the feasibility and desirability of LHD **accreditation** led to the establishment of the Public Health Accreditation Board (PHAB) in 2007.[21] The Board used the earlier definitional work from the IOM and NACCHO to develop its study domains, grounding these in a philosophy of continuous quality improvement as a means to standardize the work of LHDs. The first LHDs were accredited in 2013. Several state-based accreditation systems for LHDs complement the national accreditation process, although designed to accomplish different goals such as programmatic or contractual compliance,[22] workforce competency, or departmental function.[23] An initial review of the goals and process of PHAB indicate that it is operating in a manner consistent with the initial vision.[24]

In addition, organizations and processes have been established to assure competency for specific elements of the LHD workforce. See, for example, those established for nurses,[25] environmental health professionals,[26] health educators,[27] and for public health physicians.[28] The public health workforce receives its formal and continuing education from a variety of undergraduate, graduate, certificate, association, nonprofit, and private-sector organizations. The workforce is comprised of those with high school through postgraduate, residency, and fellowship credentials.

Missing from the earlier conceptual frameworks described above was an elaboration of the workforce, technology, and funding needed to adequately and sustainably support the future work of LHDs. A group has recently begun to explore the foundational capabilities and the funding, workforce, and technology needed for these capabilities to be exercised regardless of the specific programs which the LHD may deliver.[29] Proportionate cost-sharing arrangements among local, state, and federal governments and, perhaps, a tax or fees charged against the delivery of medical care services could be envisioned as possible sources of funding.[15]

The programs and practices of LHDs are now in flux as a result of funding and staff reductions during the Great Recession (2007–2009), passage of the Patient Protection and Affordable Care Act (ACA), technology changes, a growing understanding of the way in which power affects the likelihood of health, climate change, and the opposing partisan political philosophies adopted by elected officials of LHD jurisdictions. The Great Recession had a profound effect on the staffing and operations of LHDs. From 2008 to 2013, LHDs lost 48,300 jobs through layoff or attrition.[30]

The ACA introduced new experiments in organizational form and reimbursement including the idea that maintenance of health could be profitable, more so than treatment of disease. Experiments involving accountable care organizations and patient-centered medical homes were introduced. Reimbursement for "bundled care" and outcomes were meant to replace incentives for overuse of care. Nonprofit hospitals were required to engage in community health assessment and community health improvement planning to justify the financial benefit their tax status conveyed. These experiments incentivize closer relationships between providers of clinical services and LHDs but also raise questions about where the locus of this work should rest and whose priorities will dominate.

Assembly and control of "big data," democratization of access to it and to tools for analysis, enable any resident with the requisite skill and technology the ability to develop a population-wide perspective on a jurisdiction's health. Electronic medical records give clinical providers or their organizations and, in some communities, the LHD, an increasing ability to know more and more about health or disease status in real time.

Increasingly, the influence on health of race, gender, culture, lifestyle, housing, education, and systems of justice are elucidated, drawing LHDs into conversations with other local organizations about the means to make life and opportunity for quality of life more equitable. So, too, has a growing awareness of how power exercised by small minorities of people has helped shape community mores or design, which either facilitate or serve as barriers to the health of those without power.[31,32]

As climate change makes more visible to local residents threats not only to the public's health but to private property and business and to the assumed supply of safe food, air, and water, and to ecological diversity and the environment, the LHD's focus will increasingly be drawn to these issues. Climate change is already thought to be responsible for the introduction of new biological threats to health in some regions of the United States.

Partisan differences about the size of government are producing experiments in the jurisdictional configuration for LHDs and in the placement and relationships between LHDs and sister human services departments within local government. For example, some jurisdictions are exploring how to share staff and other resources across jurisdictions. Services formerly delivered by each jurisdiction are in some cases being regionalized. Smaller departments have in some cases combined into larger districts. In still others, LHDs are being merged with departments of mental and behavioral health or social services. LHD regulatory services are being transferred to local planning or licensing departments in order to centralize common functions or like tasks in one place. In a few instances, LHDs have become a component of a larger health and hospitals department.

In the following sections we examine more deeply the organization and work of LHDs.

LOCAL HEALTH DEPARTMENT ORGANIZATION AND GOVERNANCE

LHDs vary in several organizational characteristics, including jurisdictional type, relationship to their state health department, governance structure, governing bodies, and size.

Jurisdictional Type

LHDs are governmental entities serving jurisdictions comprised of towns, cities, or counties (see Figure 9-1).[1] Sixty-eight percent of LHDs serve a county jurisdiction. Eight percent of LHDs serve multiple counties, although regions consisting of multiple towns or cities are found in some states. In Idaho, for example, 44 counties are organized into 7 district health departments, each comprising 4 to 8 counties. The district structure creates a larger population and tax base for the health departments, which allows them to expand staff numbers and skills and provide a broader and more consistent range of services throughout the state.

Relationship to the State Health Agency

The **governance** of an LHD refers to where the ultimate authority for, or control of, its activities resides. Public health authority resides at the state level, but states differ in the extent to which they have delegated that authority

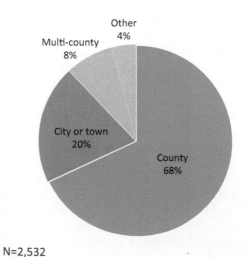

N=2,532

FIGURE 9-1 **Types of Jurisdictions of Local Health Departments**

DATA SOURCE: 2013 National Profile of Local Health Departments

to the local level. Four categories are most often used to describe the relationship between state and LHDs according to how the LHDs are governed: state-governed (authority rests with the state health department, sometimes referred to as centralized), locally governed (authority rests with a single or combined local government, sometimes referred to as decentralized), shared (authority rests with both state health department and local government), and mixed (state includes LHDs with more than one kind of governance).[33]

Figure 9-2 shows states by governance type and the number of LHDs in each state.[1] Significant variation exists across U.S. census geographic regions, such that Southern states tend to be centralized, and those in the Midwest are more often decentralized.[34]

Decentralized Governance

In decentralized states, LHDs operate independently from their respective state health agencies. In these states, the local governing bodies for the LHDs typically develop and approve their budgets, set priorities, develop local health ordinances, and hire their directors/health officers.

Some important advantages of this model are better integration of local government and the community priorities into the health department's services

and stronger connections with other local government agencies. In addition, locally governed LHDs tend to receive more revenues from local sources, which have been shown to be most associated with improved performance.[35] Disadvantages can include a lack of communication among departments, noninvolvement of LHDs in state planning and decision making, and uneven service delivery across the state.

Centralized Governance

In centralized states, LHDs are units of the state health agencies, and the degree to which they work with local government and receive local tax dollars varies considerably. The local offices of the state health department are often organized into regions or districts.

Advantages of this model are more consistency with respect to resource allocation and service provision across the state, interoperable information and communications systems, a more coordinated approach to public health, and the ability to address priorities statewide. LHDs in centralized states are more likely to share resources (e.g., personnel, equipment) across jurisdictions than those in decentralized states.[36] Disadvantages include the limited ability of an LHD to focus on locally determined priorities, programs, and policies and typically lower revenues from local sources.

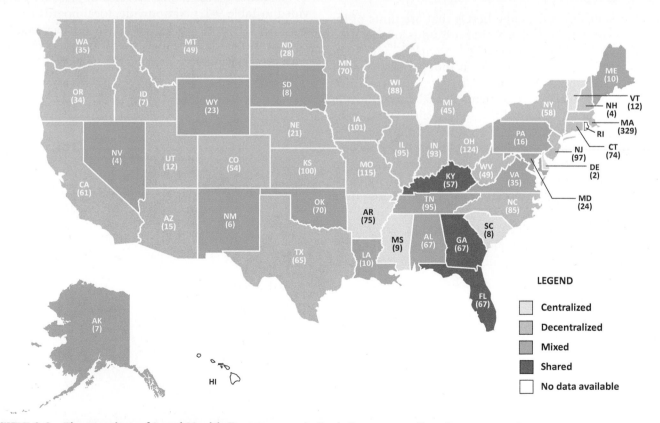

FIGURE 9-2   The Number of Local Health Departments in Each State, as well as Governance Type

DATA SOURCE: 2013 National Profile of Local Health Departments

Shared Governance

Shared governance means that state and local government agencies share authority over LHDs. In Florida, for example, LHDs are entities of state government and also have a direct reporting relationship to county government. The state health department approves the county health department budget, sets priorities, and determines the programmatic emphasis. The county usually contributes tax dollars to the state health department budget and, after developing the county budget, contracts with the state for services. The county makes only limited policy and programmatic decisions. The selection of a county health official is begun by the state health department, with review and appointment made by the county board of commissioners. The county health department staff is also made up of state employees.

Shared governance provides at least some degree of the advantages and disadvantages associated with both local governance (greater local revenue, greater attention to local priorities, better connections to other local government agencies) and state governance (more uniform resource allocation, better integration with state health priorities, and better communication among local units). LHDs with shared governance are typically well-funded relative to other LHDs.[1]

Mixed Governance

Several states include some LHDs that are units of local government and others that are units of the state health agency. In these states, the larger cities and counties typically organize their own independent health department (e.g., Oklahoma City-County and Tulsa City-County Health Departments in Oklahoma), while local or regional offices of the state health department serve the remaining cities or counties in the state. For example, Maryland and Wyoming include LHDs with both shared and local governance. Advantages of this variation include ensuring the availability of state-run public health services in smaller communities that have few resources, while giving broader authority and local control to the health departments serving larger communities. Disadvantages may include inconsistency in policy development and significant variation in services.

Governing Bodies

LHDs may be governed by a local board of health, local elected officials (e.g., county council or commission, city council, mayor), a state health agency, or a combination of these bodies.

Local Boards of Health

Local boards of health are present in most states with varying responsibilities and composition according to state statute.[37] Many local boards of health work with LHDs to establish public health priorities, approve LHD budgets, hire and fire LHD top executives, and have authority to propose, adopt, or enforce local public health regulations.[37] Members of local boards of health are most often appointed or designated by statute. Board of health members can be designated based on elected positions (e.g., county commissioner, mayor, township trustee) or nonelected positions (e.g., school superintendent, municipal administrator). Board of health members are elected in approximately one-quarter of jurisdictions. In some jurisdictions, a local governmental body (e.g., county board of commissioners) serves as the local board of health. The size of most local boards of health ranges between three and seven members, and they most often meet monthly or quarterly.[37]

Most local boards of health also serve as a link between LHDs and the communities they serve.[37] In this capacity, the board of health represents the community's interest in adopting priorities and establishing needed services, while also communicating with the community about health department goals and services available. Boards of health most often receive community input via elected officials or at public forums or hearings. Members of boards of health who are not elected officials may be able to advocate to legislators more directly than is possible for local health officials.[37]

Statistics on local board of health presence are provided in Table 9-1.[1] Nationwide, local boards of health are less likely to be present in larger jurisdictions. Local boards of health are much more common for LHDs with local governance than LHDs with state or shared governance.

TABLE 9-1   Presence of Local Board of Health by Local Health Department (LHD) Characteristics

	Percentage of LHDs with Local Board of Health
All LHDs	70%
Jurisdiction population	
<50,000	72%
50,000–499,999	70%
500,000–999,999	57%
1,000,000+	33%
Governance	
State	46%
Local	79%
Shared	52%

Other Forms of Governance

Approximately 30 percent of all LHD jurisdictions do not have local boards of health, and in some cases the board of health serves in an advisory capacity only.[1] Most of these LHDs are governed by either state health agencies or local elected officials, such as the county council, county commissioners, board of supervisors, mayor, or city or town council. Most locally governed LHDs that include multiple counties, cities, or towns are governed by a single governing body, but a few are governed by multiple local boards of health or other governing bodies.

Population Served by Local Health Departments

Populations served by LHDs range from very large—approximately 9.3 million for Los Angeles County and 8.2 million for New York City—to several communities of fewer than 1,000 people.[38] Figure 9-3 provides statistics on the percentage of LHDs in different size categories and the percentage of the U.S. population served by LHDs in each size category.[1] Most LHDs serve jurisdictions with relatively small populations. Jurisdictions with fewer than 50,000 residents account for 61 percent of the nation's LHDs; 41 percent of all LHDs serve jurisdictions with fewer than 25,000 residents. Remarkably, nearly half (49 percent) of people in the United States are served by large-jurisdiction LHDs (those serving 500,000 or more residents), which comprise only 5 percent of the nation's LHDs. The large number of LHDs with jurisdictions of less than 50,000

serves approximately 10 percent of the U.S. population. A number of studies have shown a positive relationship between jurisdiction population size and LHD performance, though some have shown that the apparent benefit of jurisdiction size on agency performance diminishes or disappears for LHDs serving very large populations (e.g., more than 500,000 people).[39]

As expected, LHD expenditures and number of staff increase as the size of the population served increases (see Table 9-2).[1]

TABLE 9-2 Local Health Department Expenditures and Staffing by Jurisdiction Population

Jurisdiction Population	Total Annual Expenditures (Median)	Total Staff Full-Time Equivalents (FTEs) (Median)
<25,000	$459,000	6.5
25,000–49,999	$1,180,000	15
50,000–99,999	$2,570,000	28
100,000–249,999	$5,910,000	64
250,000–499,999	$11,100,000	130
500,000–999,999	$28,100,000	251
1,000,000+	$60,500,000	453

SOURCE: National Association of County and City Health Officials. 2013 National Profile of Local Health Departments. Washington, DC: National Association of County and City Health Officials; 2013.

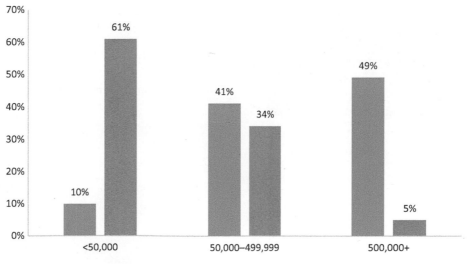

N=2,532   ■ Percentage of U.S. Population Served by LHDs   ■ Percentage of All LHDs

FIGURE 9-3   Size of Population Served by Local Health Departments

DATA SOURCE: 2013 National Profile of Local Health Departments

LOCAL HEALTH DEPARTMENT FINANCING

LHDs vary widely in budgets (both on total and per capita bases) and in the sources from which they derive their revenue.

Total Annual Expenditures

LHD total annual expenditures range over six orders of magnitude. The smallest annual LHD expenditure reported in 2013 was $10,855, whereas the largest was $1.577 billion.[38] Nearly half (43 percent) of LHDs have total annual expenditures of less than $1 million, while 22 percent have total annual expenditures of $5 million or greater (see Figure 9-4).[1]

Per Capita Local Health Department Expenditures

Because LHD annual expenditures are strongly related to the population size of their jurisdiction, computing per capita expenditures (total expenditures divided by jurisdiction population) is useful for examining differences in governmental local public health investments. Comparisons of spending by individual LHDs must be made cautiously, however, as the types of services they provide vary greatly. For example, some LHDs provide extensive clinical services, whereas others provide few or none. Some LHDs provide a wide range of environmental health services, while these services are provided

by another governmental agency in other jurisdictions. However, research has shown that great variation in public health spending remains, even after accounting for differences in population demographics and service mix.[35] Table 9-3 provides selected percentiles of per capita annual LHD expenditures.[38]

The mean and median per capita annual LHD expenditures show modest variations with agency characteristics such as jurisdiction population size and type of governance. Much larger variations are seen across states. Median per capita LHD expenditures vary more than tenfold across the states, and there is also considerable variation in per capita funding among LHDs within a state.

Local Health Department Revenue Sources

LHD revenues come from a variety of sources, including local government; state government; federal funds passed through to the LHD by state agencies (federal pass-through); direct funding from federal agencies (e.g., CDC, Health Resources and Services Administration, Substance Abuse and Mental Health Services Administration); reimbursement from Medicare, Medicaid, and other insurers; regulatory and patient personal fees; and other sources (e.g., grants from private foundations). Nationwide, revenues from local governments (county, city, or town) account for the largest percentage of LHD revenues (see Figure 9-5).

The amount of funding from these sources varies by governance type. Not surprisingly, local funds contribute to a greater percentage of total LHD revenues on average for agencies that are units of local government than for those that are units of the state health agency. The latter receive larger percentages of revenues from both state direct and federal pass-through sources. Large differences are also seen across states. Some

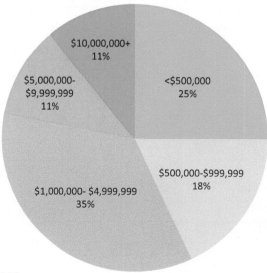

n=1,516

FIGURE 9-4   Total Annual Local Health Departments Expenditures

DATA SOURCE: 2013 National Profile of Local Health Departments

TABLE 9-3   Per Capita Annual Local Health Department Expenditures

	Total Expenditures (Median)
10th percentile	$11.72
25th percentile	$22.03
50th percentile	$38.80
75th percentile	$66.34
95th percentile	$150.75

SOURCE: National Association of County and City Health Officials. 2013 National Profile of Local Health Departments. Washington, DC: National Association of County and City Health Officials; 2013.

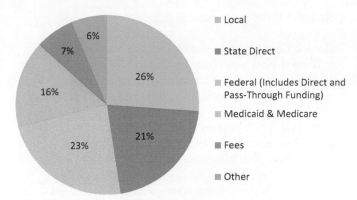

FIGURE 9-5   Local Health Departments Revenue Sources
DATA SOURCE: 2010 National Profile of Local Health Departments

- Local — 26%
- State Direct — 21%
- Federal (Includes Direct and Pass-Through Funding) — 23%
- Medicaid & Medicare — 16%
- Fees — 7%
- Other — 6%

TABLE 9-4   Local Health Departments Conducting Surveillance and Epidemiology

Area of Surveillance and Epidemiology	Percentage Conducting		
	2013	2005	1993
Communicable/ infectious disease	91%	86%	82%
Environmental health	78%	74%	*
Maternal and child health	61%	*	*
Syndromic surveillance	47%	32%	*
Chronic disease	44%	39%	42%
Behavioral risk factors	36%	34%	20%
Injury surveillance	27%	22%	15%

* No data available

states' revenues are balanced among local, state, federal, and other sources, whereas others are dominated by one or two sources.

LOCAL HEALTH DEPARTMENT FUNCTIONS AND SERVICES

The functions and services of LHDs vary based on the department's authority and resources, and by the needs of the community. LHD functions are described in this section organized around the 10 Essential Public Health Services, which are the basis for the first 10 domains of standards for PHAB accreditation and the 10 areas of the Operational Definition of a Functional Local Health Department (which informed the PHAB standards).[17] (A description of discrete activities and services is included at the end of this section.)

Monitor Health Status and Understand Health Issues Facing the Community

LHDs must understand the specific health issues confronting their community and how physical, behavioral, environmental, social, and economic conditions affect them. To accomplish this, LHDs both collect community health data and use data collected by other organizations (e.g., other state and local agencies, hospitals, or community-based organizations). Most LHDs conduct surveillance for communicable/infectious diseases and environmental health indicators; some LHDs also conduct surveillance for chronic diseases, behavioral risk factors, and injuries (Table 9-4).[1] Since 1993, the percentage of LHDs reporting conducting surveillance for behavioral risk factors and injuries has increased. Syndromic surveillance is the use of health-related data that precedes diagnosis of disease (e.g., school absence,

pharmaceutical use, emergency room visits) to identify potential outbreaks that may warrant a public health response. The utility of syndromic surveillance for identifying bioterrorism-related outbreaks is being explored in some local and state health departments. Since 2005, more LHDs have been conducting syndromic surveillance.

Many LHDs work collaboratively with their communities to collect and analyze a wide variety of information related to the community's health in a process known as *community health assessment* (see Chapter 13 for additional detail). Participation by a wide range of community stakeholders is essential to community health assessment. In 2013, 70 percent of LHDs reported that they had completed a community health assessment in the past five years and another 11 percent intended to complete one in the next year.[1]

Protect People from Health Problems and Health Hazards

LHDs are responsible for investigating health problems and health threats and for preventing, minimizing, and containing adverse health effects from communicable diseases, disease outbreaks from unsafe food or water, chronic diseases, environmental hazards, injuries, and risky health behaviors. This includes both activities focused on prevention (primary and secondary) and responding to health problems and hazards (see Exhibit 9-1). Some LHDs provide screening and testing for communicable and chronic diseases (Table 9-5), whereas others provide referrals to such services.[1] Since 1993, while there has

TABLE 9-5 Local Health Department Provision of Screening and Treatment Services

Disease or Condition	Percentage Providing		
	2013	2005	1993
Communicable Disease			
Tuberculosis screening	83%	82%	*
Tuberculosis treatment	76%	71%	*
STD screening	64%	60%	64%
STD treatment	60%	56%	59%
HIV/AIDS screening	61%	58%	62%
HIV/AIDS treatment	24%	20%	24%
Noncommunicable Disease or Condition			
Blood lead screening	61%	62%	*
High blood pressure screening	57%	69%	79%
Diabetes screening	36%	48%	55%
Cancer screening	36%	42%	47%
Cardiovascular disease screening	27%	34%	53%

* No data available

SOURCE: National Association of County and City Health Officials. 1993, 2005, and 2013 National Profiles of Local Health Departments. Washington, DC: National Association of County and City Health Officials; 2013.

TABLE 9-6 Local Health Departments Providing Select Environmental Health Services

Environmental Health Service	Percentage Providing		
	2013	2005	1993
Food safety education	72%	73%	*
Vector control	48%	52%	57%
Groundwater protection	40%	38%	58%
Surface water protection	33%	32%	52%
Indoor air quality	31%	27%	37%
Pollution prevention	22%	28%	*

* No data available

SOURCE: National Association of County and City Health Officials. 1993, 2005, and 2013 National Profiles of Local Health Departments. Washington, DC: National Association of County and City Health Officials; 2013.

EXHIBIT 9-1 Project Needle Smart

Greene County Public Health Department (GCPHD) in Catskill, New York, created Project Needle Smart to address the Greene County Solid Waste Department (GCSW) staff being exposed to a large amount of "home" sharps (such as insulin syringes) at GCSW transfer stations, putting many employees at risk for a blood-borne pathogen exposure. GCPHD worked to reduce the risk of blood-borne pathogen exposure by examining the protocol for disposal of home sharps and how they can be removed from transfer stations and landfills and safely disposed. GCPHD partnered with local pharmacies, long-term care facilities, county employees, local urgent care facilities, and the New York State Department of Health, to place needle disposal kiosks at convenient locations such as pharmacies, long-term care facilities, and the county office building. This project has removed hundreds of pounds of home sharps from transfer stations and landfills, reducing risks to GCSW staff.

been little change in communicable disease screening and treatment, fewer LHDs are now providing screening for noncommunicable diseases (such as screening for high blood pressure, diabetes, cancer, and cardiovascular disease).

Some LHDs have primary responsibility for many environmental health functions, whereas others have primary responsibility for only a few or none. Environmental health services provided most frequently by LHDs include food safety education and vector control (Table 9-6).[1] Overall, LHDs decreased most environmental health services reported since 1993, with groundwater and surface water protection showing the largest decrease over time. Regardless of what organization has primary responsibility for these environmental health services, the LHD is responsible for coordinating with that organization and ensuring that the public's health is protected.

LHDs have a primary responsibility for planning for and responding to public health emergencies, often working with state and federal public health agencies on large-scale events. LHDs also collaborate with other local responders to assist in other emergencies with public health significance, such as natural disasters. Emergency preparedness has continued to receive a high degree of attention in recent years, and nearly all LHDs are preparing to respond to a public health emergency by developing and exercising emergency response plans and by training staff to serve in specific capacities (often very different from their everyday jobs) in an emergency. Since September 2010, almost all LHDs have participated in an emergency response drill or exercise and more than half have responded to at least one all-hazards event, most commonly natural disasters and influenza outbreaks.[1] Planning occurs within the context of the National Incident Management System (part of the Federal Emergency Management Agency[40]) because although most emergency situations are handled locally, a major incident often necessitates involvement and assistance from other jurisdictions, the state, and the federal government.

Inform and Educate About Public Health Issues and Functions

LHDs provide a variety of health education and health promotion activities in their communities, working at both the individual and population levels. Table 9-7 shows the percentage of LHDs with population-based primary prevention programs in selected areas.[1] Many LHDs work with others in their communities to promote better health through policy, system, and environmental interventions (such as increasing access to smoke-free environments or healthy foods). LHDs work closely with members of the population to which a health education or promotion effort is directed to ensure that the program is culturally and linguistically appropriate (see Exhibit 9-2). LHDs use many different communication channels to reach their target population (including social media) and frequently work with community partners on health education and promotion

TABLE 9-7 Local Health Departments Providing Population-Based Primary Prevention Services

Primary Prevention Services	Percentage Providing
Nutrition	69%
Tobacco	68%
Physical activity	52%
Chronic disease programs	50%
Unintended pregnancy	49%
Injury	38%
Substance abuse	24%
Violence	21%
Mental illness	12%

SOURCE: National Association of County and City Health Officials. 2013 National Profile of Local Health Departments. Washington, DC: National Association of County and City Health Officials; 2013.

EXHIBIT 9-2 Building Economic Security Today (BEST)

The Contra Costa Health Services' Family, Maternal and Child Health Programs in Martinez, California, developed Building Economic Security Today (BEST), a project designed to teach families financial stability and economic self-sufficiency through the local WIC (Special Supplemental Nutrition Program for Women, Infants, and Children) program. BEST uses the life course framework, conceptualizing health and development within biological, social, and cultural contexts. BEST responds to the county's steadily rising rates of preterm and low birth weight and the substantial inequities in birth outcomes between racial/ethnic groups. Community partners engaged in BEST offer expertise related to asset-development and building sustainable economic security. Through educational classes offered at the Contra Costa WIC sites, WIC clients deepen their understanding of the connection between health and wealth, and adopt strategies to improve their financial behaviors.

efforts. Risk communication is another component of information dissemination. Skillful use of mass media has become increasingly important both for successful health education and promotion programs and for risk communication—a critical facet of providing people with information they need about public health events. Nearly all LHDs partner with their local media.[41]

Engage the Community to Identify and Solve Health Problems

LHDs develop partnerships with public and private health care providers and institutions, community-based organizations, and other government agencies engaged in services that affect health (e.g., housing, criminal justice, education) to collectively identify, alleviate, and act on the sources of public health problems. Over 90 percent of LHDs have a collaborative relationship with schools, emergency responders, hospitals, the media, physician practices/medical groups, other health care providers, and community-based organizations (see Exhibits 9-3 thru 9-5).[42]

Collective action for public health purposes may be generated through community-wide strategic planning for improving health. MAPP (Mobilizing for Action through Planning and Partnerships[43]) is one tool for such a process. Conducting a community health assessment is usually part of this process, and one of the products of strategic planning is a community health improvement plan, which identifies specific action steps to improve community health. More than half of LHDs have developed a community health improvement plan in the past five years, and the vast majority of these plans are based on a community health assessment.[1] Sixty-four percent

EXHIBIT 9-3 The Students Eat Locally Project

Cuyahoga County Board of Health in Parma, Ohio, established the Students Eating Locally Project (SEL) to address childhood obesity in the South Euclid Lyndhurst School District (SELSD) and promote healthy eating environments that support decreasing chronic disease rates in the county's most disadvantaged schools. This farm-to-school program uses produce from local growers for school meal programs, increasing both access to fresh produce and opportunities to educate students and families about the relationships between dietary choices, the food system, and health outcomes. The SEL project increased the number of students in the SELSD meal program, reduced school food waste, expanded farm growing space, increased dollars spent in the northeast Ohio food economy, and increased the number of experiential learning opportunities for students around agriculture and nutrition.

EXHIBIT 9-4 Fit City Challenge

The Northeast Texas Public Health District, in Tyler, Texas, developed the Fit City Challenge, a campaign to fight obesity and sedentary lifestyles. Joining forces with local media and community partners including hospitals, health clubs, local businesses, and others, the health department-led coalition works to educate the public through community member success stories, and to provide activities such as Fit City Day events and several fitness walk events to fight the obesity epidemic of Tyler and northeast Texas. Media buy-in has made this program successful. In support of the program, the Tyler Morning Telegraph added a new Health and Wellness section, and a local broadcaster (CBS 19TV) started a new series called Fit City Success.

EXHIBIT 9-5 Hospital Sugar-Sweetened Beverage Learning Network

The Boston Public Health Commission in Boston, Massachusetts, developed a sugar-sweetened beverage (SSB) hospital learning network to provide a forum for Boston-area hospitals to address access to SSBs in the health care setting. Hospital representatives participated in hospital learning network meetings, where they received technical assistance and resources on making SSB policy, systems, and environmental changes. Boston's hospital system employs over 50,000 people and provides care for over one million patients each year. Because of this substantial impact on the Boston community, the hospital setting represents a unique opportunity for promoting healthy behaviors. Over a 14-month period, 10 participating hospitals successfully employed a variety of strategies to reduce access to SSBs within their institutions.

Develop Public Health Policies and Plans

LHDs serve as a primary resource to their governing bodies and policy makers to establish and maintain public health policies, practices, and capacity. Nearly 80 percent of LHD leaders discuss proposed legislation, regulations, or ordinances with elected officials, and many develop issue briefs or public testimony to inform policy makers about important public health issues. In recent years, many LHDs have been involved in policy activities to address tobacco use, obesity, emergency preparedness, food safety, and other public health issues.[1] LHDs, as well as the federal and many state governments, are increasingly employing the innovative Health in All Policies approach to change the systems that determine how decisions are made and implemented by local, state, and federal governments to ensure that policy decisions have neutral or beneficial impacts on the determinants of health. The Health in All Policies approach emphasizes the need to collaborate across sectors to achieve common health goals.

Although the modern institution of public health arose as an organized response to the ill effects of industrialization, the focus on broad aspects of social and economic life has been de-emphasized in favor of categorically funded programmatic activities. Many local health officials are returning to these public health roots, with more than half of LHDs reporting that they use data to describe health inequities in their communities and support community efforts to change the root causes of health inequities (e.g., social or economic conditions, public policies).[1]

of LHD community health improvement plans are linked to statewide health improvement plans.[1] The identified action steps might be new programs, changes in existing programs at the LHD or another public or private organization, or collaborative efforts to secure funding for needed programs. The community health improvement plan should also include a mechanism to evaluate whether the action steps are achieving the desired goals.

In addition to community-wide processes such as MAPP, LHDs may also work on targeted efforts with a subset of community partners to generate interest in and support for new and emerging public health issues. Raising community awareness of public health needs and soliciting the community's concerns and perspectives about public health issues are important roles of LHD leaders. Most LHD leaders discuss public health issues on local radio and television programs and also have such discussions with local civic groups.[41]

Enforce Public Health Laws and Regulations

Various state and local government agencies, including LHDs, are responsible for enforcing public health laws and regulations. Table 9-8 lists the areas of regulation in which LHDs most frequently have responsibility.[1]

A primary role for LHD staff in this arena is to educate regulated individuals and organizations about the meaning, purpose, and benefit of regulatory compliance, and how to comply with public health laws, ordinances, and regulations (see Exhibit 9-6). They monitor the compliance of regulated entities and conduct enforcement activities when necessary.

Help People Receive Health Services

Although the ACA expanded access to health insurance, access to affordable, appropriate, culturally competent health care remains a serious problem in the United States. A 2014 Gallup poll estimated that 13.4 percent of Americans lack health insurance.[44] Although some LHDs provide a variety of personal health services, their role is not typically to provide primary health care services. Data on provision of personal health services by LHDs in 1993 and 2013 show a decrease in the number providing personal health services (see Table 9-9).[38,41] More frequently, LHDs work with health care providers and community organizations to identify gaps in access to personal health services, including preventive and health promotion services, and to develop strategies to close the gaps. LHDs partner with community organizations to increase access to health care and link individuals to personal health care providers in the community (see Exhibit 9-7).

TABLE 9-8   Local Health Department Regulation, Inspection, or Licensing Activities

Area of Regulation, Inspection, or Licensing	Percentage Providing
Food service establishments	78%
Schools/daycares	69%
Public swimming pools	68%
Septic systems	66%
Smoke-free ordinances	59%
Private drinking water	56%
Body art	55%
Hotels/motels	50%
Lead inspection	49%

SOURCE: National Association of County and City Health Officials. 2013 National Profile of Local Health Departments. Washington, DC: National Association of County and City Health Officials; 2013.

EXHIBIT 9-6   Reducing Hepatitis A Outbreaks

St. Louis County Department of Health, in Berkeley, Missouri, has jurisdiction for the largest, most urban county in the state. It was the first jurisdiction in Missouri to mandate hepatitis A vaccine for food handlers. This practice was novel and controversial at the time that the ordinance was enacted. Prior to the creation of the ordinance, St. Louis County had three hepatitis A outbreaks, each involving major food establishments, and responding to these outbreaks strained the county's resources. While food handlers are not more likely to get the virus, if infected they pose a major public health risk for spreading hepatitis A to hundreds of people. Once the ordinance was enacted, informational brochures were sent out to all licensed food service establishments. Information on locations providing the vaccine was posted on the health department website. Since the ordinance took effect, the rate of hepatitis A cases in St. Louis County has declined tenfold.

TABLE 9-9   Local Health Department Provision of Personal Health Services

Type of Health Service	Percentage Providing		
	2013	2005	1993
Early and periodic screening, diagnosis, and treatment	24%	46%	70%
Prenatal care	13%	42%	63%
Home health care	13%	28%	53%
Oral health care	10%	31%	44%
Obstetrical care	7%	16%	32%
Comprehensive primary care	6%	14%	30%
Behavioral/mental health services	4%	13%	*
Substance abuse services	3%	11%	*

* No data available

SOURCE: National Association of County and City Health Officials. 1993, 2005, and 2013 National Profiles of Local Health Departments. Washington, DC: National Association of County and City Health Officials; 2013.

EXHIBIT 9-7 Toothy 2 Brings Dental Care to Children

Central Florida's Lake County Health Department, with the support of the Lake County School District, tackled tooth decay, a common childhood disease, with "Toothy 2," a Mobile Dental Unit that brings preventive dental care and oral health education directly to children while at school. With this program, 7- and 8-year-old second grade students who are low-income, eligible for Medicaid, uninsured, or without access to regular dental care receive a visual exam, teeth cleaning, brushing and flossing instruction, fluoride varnish, and sealants on their permanent first molars. The sealants are checked and reapplied if needed to third graders who were seen the previous year.

EXHIBIT 9-8 Community Resources for Mass Fatality Management

Public Health Seattle & King County in Seattle, Washington, created the Community Resources for Mass Fatality Management practice to address the needs of the cities and health care facilities in the county during a catastrophic mass fatality incident. Through the use of tools, templates, and trainings, Public Health Seattle & King County was able to prepare cities and health care facilities to manage decedents when normal operations at King County Medical Examiner's Office are expected to be suspended or impacted due to a high number of fatalities. A major benefit of this practice is that the tools, including templates, forms, and instructions, can be quickly and easily adapted for use by other local health jurisdictions. This practice has gradually been implemented in King County with tools and templates being created and shared during trainings with health care organizations.

Maintain a Competent Public Health Workforce

An LHD must employ a competent and diverse staff (i.e., **workforce**) to achieve its goals. Core Competencies for Public Health Professionals define the set of skills, knowledge, and attitudes necessary for the broad practice of public health (see Appendix B).[45] The Core Competencies cover skills in eight domains (analytical/assessment, policy development/program planning, communication, cultural competency, community dimensions of practice, basic public health science, financial planning and management, and leadership and systems thinking) that are defined for three levels of public health professionals (frontline/entry-level staff, program management/supervisory level staff, and senior management/executive level staff). PHAB accreditation standards for LHDs require a formal workforce development plan that is based on nationally adopted core competencies and includes curricula and training schedules.

In addition, a recent literature review identified four new priority areas for the public health workforce, including in LHDs: (1) developing a diverse workforce; (2) planning for retirements and recruiting and retaining qualified employees; (3) increasing workforce capacity through education and training; and (4) establishing career advancement opportunities and providing competitive salaries.[46] An effective public health system relies on the capacity of its workforce, making it important for LHDs to work on these priority areas in order to recruit and retain qualified employees.

LHDs' contribution to the public health workforce does not end with their own agency staff. Most LHDs accept students from schools of public health and other academic institutions as trainees, interns, or volunteers. LHD leaders and staff may also serve as regular, adjunct, or guest faculty at academic institutions.[47] Further, because many others in the community are also engaged in public health interventions, LHDs often promote the use of effective public health practices by these practitioners (see Exhibit 9-8).

Evaluate and Improve Programs and Interventions

To maximize their effectiveness, LHDs must have a culture of continuous quality improvement that fosters ongoing, evidence-based evaluation efforts that drive performance improvement activities. They also need to review the effectiveness of public health interventions provided by others in the community. For example, to assess the effectiveness of immunization programs in the community, the LHD needs to evaluate not only its own immunization practices but also those of physicians, clinics, and other health care providers in the community. Fifty-six percent of LHDs report that they are engaged in formal agency-wide quality improvement activities or participate in formal quality improvement in specific program areas. Another 32 percent participate in informal or ad hoc quality improvement efforts.[1]

Contribute to and Apply the Evidence Base of Public Health

Using evidence-based public health approaches can help LHDs ensure the effectiveness of the strategies they implement to improve the health of their communities (see Exhibit 9-9). To assist in the evidence-based processes, a number of federal agencies have developed resources to help LHDs identify evidence-based public health practices (see Chapter 11). The CDC's *Guide to Community*

Preventive Services summarizes what is known about the effectiveness, economic efficiency, and feasibility of interventions to promote community health and prevent disease.[48] The Agency for Healthcare Research and Quality publishes the *Guide to Clinical Preventive Services*, which provides recommendations on screening, counseling, and preventive medication topics and includes clinical considerations for each topic.[49]

Building an evidence base for public health requires practitioners to share information about effective public health practices and programs. Reciprocally, academicians must effectively utilize their skills and time in partnership with LHDs. LHD staff members do not have the kinds of incentives for publication that academicians do, but their experiences are a critical part of the public health evidence base. The National Association of County and City Health Officials sponsors the Model Practices program, which recognizes effective programs and allows LHD staff to benefit from their colleagues' experiences, to learn what works, and to ensure that resources are used wisely on effective programs that have been implemented with good results. Both model and promising practices are available in a web-based toolkit.[50]

Academic Health Departments and Practice-Based Research Networks (PBRNs) are models that encourage collaboration between public health practitioners and researchers to build the evidence base for public health practice. In the Academic Health Department model, LHD staff become involved in the academic roles of teaching, service, and research with either formal or informal affiliations with academic institutions.[51] A PBRN brings public health agencies together with academic research partners to identify pressing research questions of interest, design rigorous and relevant studies, execute research effectively, and translate findings rapidly into practice.[52] In several recent surveys, responding health departments report that a majority are involved in some way with academic institutions.[47]

Overview of Specific Programmatic Areas

Another way to consider the work of the LHD is to look at specific program areas. Despite the variation among LHD organization and structure, some specific program areas are nearly universal. Table 9-10 lists the 10 most frequently provided by LHDs.[1] The most frequently provided services have remained similar since 2005.

THE LOCAL HEALTH DEPARTMENT WORKFORCE

Like most areas of public health practice, the LHD workforce comprises individuals with a wide variety of academic and professional training. In addition, the

TABLE 9-10   Activities and Services Provided Most Frequently by Local Health Departments

Activity or Service	Percentage Providing	
	2013	2005
Communicable/infectious disease surveillance	91%	89%
Adult immunization provision	90%	91%
Childhood immunization provision	90%	90%
Tuberculosis screening	83%	85%
Environmental health surveillance	78%	75%
Food service establishments inspection	78%	76%
Tuberculosis treatment	76%	75%
Food safety education	72%	75%
Population-based nutrition services	69%	*
Schools/daycare center inspection	69%	*

* No data available

DATA SOURCE: National Association of County and City Health Officials. 2005 and 2013 National Profiles of Local Health Departments. Washington, DC: National Association of County and City Health Officials; 2013.

EXHIBIT 9-9 The Program Summary Tool

Cobb and Douglas Public Health (CDPH) in Marietta, Georgia, created a comprehensive program evaluation and performance measurement tool called The Program Summary Tool. It not only measures performance but also includes a logic model, a "stories from the field" component, a performance scorecard, and a quality improvement section. The template captures performance across 30 diverse public health programs offered by the department. The Tool provides a snapshot of program performance in relation to achieving desired goals, which has been beneficial to raising new funds through grants. Completion of the Program Summary Tool has increased program awareness, facilitated discussion among CDPH program managers, clinical staff, center directors, and leadership team members. Comparable evaluation across programs has enabled the CDPH Leadership Team and District Health Director to make informed decisions to maximize use of limited resources.

number of staff and types of occupations vary according to the size of the population served by the LHD and the functions and services provided.

Size and Composition of the Local Health Department Workforce

LHDs in the United States employ a total of approximately 146,000 full-time equivalent (FTE) staff.[1] The estimated size of the LHD workforce has decreased considerably since 2008 (approximately 12 percent).[1] In 2012, the U.S. Census Bureau estimated approximately 243,000 governmental health workers (in FTEs) at the local level, which includes not only workers at LHDs but also workers at other local agencies providing health-related services, including emergency medical, mental health, substance abuse, animal control, and environmental health services.[53]

Table 9-11 illustrates the proportions of the LHD workforce in selected occupations.[1] The occupations that make up the largest percentages of this workforce are administrative and clerical personnel (24 percent), registered nurses (19 percent), environmental health workers (9 percent), and public health managers (7 percent). The category "other occupation categories" includes emergency preparedness staff, public health physicians, licensed practical or vocational nurses,

TABLE 9-11   Local Health Department Workforce Composition

Occupation	Percentage of Total Full-Time Equivalents
Administrative or clerical personnel	24%
Registered nurse	19%
Environmental health worker	9%
Public health manager	7%
Community health worker	5%
Nursing aide and home health aide	4%
Health educator	3%
Nutritionist	3%
Other occupation categories	15%
Not categorized	15%

SOURCE: National Association of County and City Health Officials. 2013 National Profile of Local Health Departments. Washington, DC: National Association of County and City Health Officials; 2013.

epidemiologists, information systems specialists, public information specialists, oral health care professionals, laboratory workers, behavioral health professionals, and animal control workers (each of which account for less than 3 percent of the LHD workforce). The occupations included in the "not categorized" group are not known, but they likely include mostly nonprofessional or paraprofessional positions. This group also includes some professional occupations (e.g., attorneys, planners) that are employed in relatively small numbers by LHDs.

Typical Staffing Patterns for Local Health Departments

The types of functions and services LHDs provide also affect their staffing patterns. LHDs that provide environmental health services employ environmental scientists, specialists, or technicians. LHDs that provide a wide range of clinical services employ many types of health professionals. LHDs that provide health promotion programs may employ health educators and community health workers.

Despite these differences in employment based on services provided, it is instructive to compare typical staffing patterns for LHDs serving different jurisdictional sizes. Table 9-12 lists the median numbers of total LHD staff and selected occupations (expressed in FTEs) employed by LHDs serving three different jurisdiction sizes.[1] This analysis shows that LHDs serving small populations typically employ only a few different occupations: a public health manager, registered nurses, an environmental health worker, administrative or clerical personnel, and emergency preparedness staff. In these small LHDs, a single employee may serve in many roles (e.g., a nurse who provides clinical services, conducts disease investigation, and conducts health education and promotion). Certain specialized occupations (nutritionists and health educators) are common in LHDs serving 25,000 to 50,000 people. Additional specialized occupations (physicians, epidemiologists, and community health workers) are common in LHDs serving 100,000 or more.

Recruitment and Retention of Local Health Department Staff

Like other sectors of public health, LHDs are faced with challenges in recruiting and retaining a competent and diverse workforce. LHDs compete with many other employers for specialized occupations such as registered nurses and information management specialists. A 2012 survey showed that most LHD leaders are concerned with both finding and retaining high-quality employees and retaining currently funded positions.[54] This study identified some promising practices for motivating and

TABLE 9-12   Typical Staffing Patterns for Local Health Departments Serving Jurisdictions within Selected Population Size Categories

Serving <25,000	Serving 25,000–49,999	Serving 100,000–499,999
6.5 FTEs, including: 1 public health manager 2 registered nurses 0.9 environmental health workers 2 administrative or clerical personnel 0.1 emergency preparedness staff	15 FTEs, including: 1 public health manager 4 registered nurses 1.8 environmental health workers 4 administrative or clerical personnel 0.6 nutritionist 0.6 health educator 0.5 emergency preparedness staff	81.1 FTEs, including: 5 public health managers 14 registered nurses 9 environmental health workers 16 administrative or clerical personnel 3 nutritionists 2 health educators 1 emergency preparedness staff 0.5 public health physicians 1 epidemiologist 1 community health worker

SOURCE: National Association of County and City Health Officials. 2013 National Profile of Local Health Departments. Washington, DC: National Association of County and City Health Officials; 2013.

retaining employees, such as recognizing employee contributions through both nonmonetary and monetary rewards and providing opportunities for leadership and professional development, flexibility, and autonomy.[54]

In addition, LHDs and public health in general face credentialing challenges.[55] Many professional staff are trained as specialists in their primary occupation rather than receiving formal training in the theory or practice of public health (e.g., through a Master's in Public Health).[55] More specific information on the training of public health leaders is provided below.

PROFILE OF AGENCY TOP EXECUTIVES

The top executive of the LHD usually is also the health official, but in some departments, these responsibilities reside in two different individuals (i.e., manager and health official). The top agency executive bears responsibility for administrative issues and management of their agencies, and if they lack public health or medical training, they may rely on appropriately trained and licensed health officials or medical advisors to make health or medical decisions.

Selected Characteristics of Agency Top Executives

Most health departments (90 percent) are served by a full-time agency executive.[1] Not surprisingly, as the population of the jurisdiction served increases, the likelihood that the job of agency executive will be a full-time position also increases, from 84 percent in the smallest agencies to 100 percent in the largest.[38] Sixty percent of local health directors are female, and 93 percent of local health directors are white. Approximately 4.4 percent are African American, 2.5 percent are other races, and 2 percent are of Hispanic ethnicity.[1]

LHD directors are aging: in 2013, 25 percent of LHD top executives were 60 years or older, compared to 16 percent in 2005.[1] This indicates that retirement rates among top executives will likely increase in the coming years. Without appropriate succession planning, top executive retirements can result in a loss of institutional knowledge and community connections.

Academic Degrees of Agency Top Executives

Most agency top executives have earned graduate level degrees.[1] Twenty-two percent of local health directors have public health undergraduate or graduate degrees (BSPH, MPH, DrPH, or PhD in Public Health), and 12 percent have medical degrees (MD, DO, DVM, or DDS); these degrees are most common for leaders in large jurisdictions. Thirty-two percent of local health directors have nursing degrees (at associate, bachelors, masters, or doctoral levels), and nursing degrees are most common for leaders in small jurisdictions.

Tenure of Local Health Directors

In contrast to state health officials, many local health directors have been in their positions for many years. The mean tenure of a local health director in 2013 was almost 9 years.[1] Health directors serving large jurisdictions have shorter tenures on average than those serving small jurisdictions (6.4 years for jurisdictions over 500,000 versus 9.2 years for jurisdictions under 25,000). By contrast, the average tenure of state health department officials in 2012 was 3.4 years.[56] Many attribute the difference in tenure to a lesser degree of politicization of the health director positions at the local level.

Duties of Local Health Officials

Local health officials have cited leadership, communication, working with elected officials, and financial planning and management as the most important abilities for leading LHDs.[57]

Leadership can be defined as "an activity, not a skill set."[58] Local public health leaders must embrace their role to "mobilize, coordinate and direct broad collaborative actions within the complex public health system,"[5] and take advantage of the many leadership training opportunities that exist.

Communication, with an emphasis on risk communication, is an especially crucial duty in public health. LHDs, as the "backbone" of the local public health system,[2] need to have a leader who is skilled in communicating effectively with all entities that influence the public's health. Additionally, they need to cultivate trust and credibility with the public they serve, and deliver information about public health threats in an open, honest, and compassionate manner.

Local health officials also need to understand the political environment, and educate decision makers about the return on investments realized through public health practice. Messages must be well-timed and framed within the current political climate. The ability to communicate with these insights, in a concise and compelling fashion, is at the heart of successful relationships with policy makers.

Financial planning and management has become increasingly important over the past several years. A long trend of dwindling federal dollars continues, and many local health officials continually need to do more with less. It is important that the leaders of LHDs make or influence the financial decisions that have the greatest positive impact on maintaining and improving the health of their communities.

SUMMARY

As they have always been, in the foreseeable future, LHD organization, practices and programs will be subject to conceptual, political, social, economic, governance, leadership, financial, and technological forces.

Variability in LHD practice results from the uneven manner in which local governing bodies fund LHDs, but also from the jurisdiction size the LHD represents. States differ in how they appropriate their own resources and reallocate federal resources to LHDs. Variability in LHD practice is also due to the different choices jurisdictions make with respect to the collective resources available to them.

There is no single federal agency which funds LHDs or provides them with such a large proportion of their funding as to drive uniformity in practice nationwide. While uniform capabilities and competencies for LHD practice are desirable, there is difference of opinion about whether all LHDs should be providing exactly the same services. Local priorities and needs vary from jurisdiction to jurisdiction. LHDs need the same capabilities, instead, and to be able to apply them at the scale and to the needs of their jurisdiction.

LHDs have operated and will continue to operate at the nexus of evidence, theory, and politics using science, stories, and collective action to influence health in their jurisdictions. Future electoral cycles will determine whether increased attention to disease prevention and health promotion currently being stimulated by the ACA will continue and normalize. If it does, resources and attention will turn increasingly to the design of environments in which residents of local jurisdictions live, learn, earn, yearn, and play as a means of keeping people healthy and well longer and compressing the number of years for which expensive medical care is needed. A virtuous cycle of assessment, policy development, and assurance will result, with the role and resources for the LHD's work defined, practiced, and proportionate to the jurisdiction's needs. What will always be important is the trust of local residents in the work and authority of their LHD, their active mobilization on behalf of the department's work, effective leadership of LHDs and their governing entities, and the capabilities and competencies to perform their work well.

The twenty-first century will introduce new technologies to analyze and influence health and intensify interest in what is needed for health. The movement of people for business and pleasure from one part of the globe to another will speed up and become increasingly common. A local governmental presence to identify, organize, and participate in response to naturally occurring, mutational, and exotic biological threats will continue to be needed. Despite a more recent emphasis on chronic diseases due to prevalence and their personal and societal cost, new infectious diseases as well as ones faced earlier by LHDs are still present. Responses to Ebola, Sudden Acute Respiratory Syndrome (SARS), chikungunya, and influenza illustrate this. Action by LHDs in response to the constellation of biological, chemical, radiological, nuclear, or explosive threats will continue to be demanded.

The form, scope, and work of LHDs also depend upon the imagination and creativity of those who govern, manage, and interpret the grant of legal authority available. Law sets a framework. Imagination and training of those involved illuminate the permutations and combinations of work and process possible for them.

Personal fortitude of those in positions of leadership within and outside the department provides the endurance to persevere despite political, personal, and other pressures when science, experience, or instinct points in an uncommon direction that promises better health in the population served.

REVIEW QUESTIONS

1. What are some of the factors affecting local public health practice?

2. What are the advantages and disadvantages of the various types of governance for LHDs?

3. What are some of the factors contributing to the variation among services provided by LHDs?

4. Many people regard LHDs as publicly funded health care providers. What is a better description of the role of LHDs?

5. What considerations should drive a recruitment plan for the local public health workforce?

REFERENCES

1. National Association of County and City Health Officials. *2013 National Profile of Local Health Departments.* Washington, DC: National Association of County and City Health Officials;2013.

2. Institute of Medicine Committee for the Study of the Future of Public Health. *The Future of Public Health.* Washington, DC: National Academy Press;1988.

3. National Association of County and City Health Officials. Health in All Policies. http://www .naccho.org/topics/environmental/HiAP. Accessed September 7, 2014.

4. Centers for Disease Control and Prevention. Health Impact Assessment. http://www.cdc.gov/ healthyplaces/hia.htm. Accessed September 7, 2014.

5. Institute of Medicine Committee on Assuring the Health of the Public in the 21st Century. *The Future of the Public's Health.* Washington, DC: National Academy Press;2002.

6. Michigan Legislative Website. Public Health Code (Excerpt): Act 368 of 1978, Part 24, Local Health Departments. http://www.legislature.mi.gov/ (S(tgfalf2usceesz55ojynyx45))/mileg.aspx?page= getObject&objectName=mcl-368-1978-2-24& highlight=public%20AND%20health%20AND%20 code. Accessed October 24, 2014.

7. Brown TT. How effective are public health departments at preventing mortality? *Economics & Human Biology.* 2014;13:34–45.

8. Pickett G, Hanlon J. *Public Health: Administration and Practice.* St. Louis, MO: Times Mirror/Mosby College Publishing;1990.

9. Mountin J, Flook E. *Guide to Health Organizations in the United States.* Washington, DC: US Public Health Service;1953.

10. National Association of County and City Health Officials. *1990 National Profile of Local Health Departments.* Washington, DC: National Association of County and City Health Officials;1990.

11. Centers for Disease Control and Prevention. Ten Great Public Health Achievements in the 20th Century. http://www.cdc.gov/about/history/ tengpha.htm. Accessed September 4, 2014.

12. American Public Health Association. *Desirable minimum functions and organization principles for health activities.* 1940.

13. The Local Health Department, Services and Responsibilities. *Am J Public Health.* 1950;40(1):67–72.

14. Institute of Medicine. *Healthy Communities: New Partnerships for the Future of Public Health.* Washington, DC: National Academy Press; 1996.

15. Institute of Medicine. *For the Public's Health: Investing in a Healthier Future.* Washington, DC: Institute of Medicine;2012.

16. National Association of County and City Health Officials. *Blueprint for a Healthy Community: A Guide for Local Health Departments.* Washington, DC: National Association of County and City Health Officials;1994.

17. National Association of County and City Health Officials. *Operational Definition of a Functional Local Health Department.* Washington, DC: National Association of County and City Health Officials;2005.

18. Core Public Health Functions Steering Committee. *Public Health in America.* Washington, DC: Core Public Health Functions Steering Committee; 1994.

19. Centers for Disease Control and Prevention. National Public Health Performance Standards (NPHPS). http://www.cdc.gov/nphpsp/. Accessed December 15, 2007.

20. US Department of Health and Human Services. HealthyPeople.gov. www.healthypeople.gov. Accessed December 15, 2007.

21. Exploring Accreditation Steering Committee. *Final Recommendations for a Voluntary National Accreditation Program for State and Local Health Departments.* Washington, DC: Exploring Accreditation Steering Committee;2006.

22. Michigan Local Public Health Accreditation Program. The Michigan Local Public Health Accreditation Program: Creating a Better Public Health System in Michigan. http://www.accreditation .localhealth.net/. Accessed September 5, 2014.

23. Missouri Institute for Community Health. Accreditation Program: Missouri Voluntary Local Public Health Agency Accreditation Program. http:// www.michweb.org/accred.htm. Accessed September 5, 2014.

24. Pestronk RM, Benjamin GC, Bohlen SA, Drabczyk AL, Jarris PE. Accreditation: on target. *Journal of Public Health Management and Practice.* 2014;20(1):152–155.

25. American Association of Colleges of Nursing. Commission on Collegiate Nursing Education: CCNE Accreditation. 2014; http://www.aacn .nche.edu/ccne-accreditation. Accessed September 5, 2014.

26. National Environmental Health Association. National Environmental Health Association. 2014; http://www.neha.org/index.shtml. Accessed September 5, 2014.

27. National Commission for Health Education Credentialing. National Commission for Health Education Credentialing: Credentialing Excellence in Health Education. 2008; http://nchec.org/. Accessed September 5, 2014.

28. American Board of Preventive Medicine. Board Certification. 2014; https://www.theabpm.org/ certification.cfm. Accessed September 5, 2014.

29. RESOLVE Health. Public Health Leadership Forum. 2014; http://www.resolv.org/site-health leadershipforum. Accessed September 6, 2014.

30. National Association of County and City Health Officials. *Local Health Department Budget Cuts and Job Losses: Findings from the 2014 Forces of Change Survey.* Washington, DC: National Association of County and City Health Officials;2014.

31. National Association of County and City Health Officials. *Exploring the Roots of Health Inequity: Essays for Reflection.* Washington, DC: National Association of County and City Health Officials;2014.

32. National Association of County and City Health Officials. *Expanding the Boundaries: Health Equity and Public Health Practice.* Washington, DC:

National Association of County and City Health Officials;2014.

33. Association of State and Territorial Health Officials. *State Public Health Agency Classification: Understanding the Relationship between State and Local Public Health.* Arlington, VA: Association of State and Territorial Health Officials;2012.

34. Beitsch L, Brooks R, Menachemi N, Libbey P. Public health at center stage: New roles, old props. *Journal of Health Affairs.* 2006;25(24):12.

35. Mays GP, Smith SA. Geographic variation in public health spending: correlates and consequences. *Health Services Research.* 2009;44(5):1796–1817.

36. National Association of County and City Health Officials. *Cross-Jurisdictional Sharing of Services among Local Health Departments: Findings from the 2013 and 2010 Profile Studies.* Washington, DC: National Association of County and City Health Officials;2014.

37. National Association of Local Boards of Health. *2011 Local Board of Health National Profile.* Bowling Green, OH: National Association of Local Boards of Health;2011.

38. National Association of County and City Health Officials. Unpublished Data: 2013 National Profile of Local Health Departments. Washington, DC: National Association of County and City Health Officials; 2013.

39. Hyde JK, Shortell SM. The structure and organization of local and state public health agencies in the US: a systematic review. *American Journal of Preventive Medicine.* 2012;42(5 suppl 1): S29–S41.

40. Federal Emergency Management Agency. National Incident Management System. http://www .fema.gov/national-incident-management-system. Accessed July 11, 2014.

41. National Association of County and City Health Officials. *2005 National Profile of Local Health Departments.* Washington, DC: National Association of County and City Health Officials;2005.

42. National Association of County and City Health Officials. *2008 National Profile of Local Health Departments.* Washington, DC: National Association of County and City Health Officials;2008.

43. National Association of County and City Health Officials. *Mobilizing for Action through Planning and Partnerships.* Washington, DC: National Association of County and City Health Officials;2000.

44. Levy J. *U.S. Uninsured Rate Holds Steady at 13.4 Percent.* Washington, DC: Gallup;2014.

45. The Council on Linkages Between Academia and Public Health Practice. *Core Competencies for Public Health Professionals.* Washington, DC: The Council on Linkages;2014.

46. Hilliard TM, Boulton ML. Public health workforce research in review: a 25-year retrospective. *American Journal of Preventive Medicine.* 2012;42(5):S17–S28.

47. National Association of County and City Health Officials. *The Local Health Department Workforce: Findings from the 2008 National Profile of Local Health Departments.* Washington, DC: National Association of County and City Health Officials;2008.

48. Community Preventive Services Task Force. The Community Guide: The Guide to Community Preventative Services. http://www.thecommunityguide.org/. Accessed December 15, 2007.

49. US Preventive Services Task Force. *The Guide to Clinical Preventive Services.* Rockville, MD: Agency for Healthcare Research and Quality;2014.

50. National Association of County and City Health Officials. Model Practices. http://www.naccho.org/topics/modelpractices/. Accessed December 15, 2007.

51. Erwin PC, Keck CW. The Academic Health Department: the process of maturation. *Journal of Public Health Management and Practice.* 2014;20(3):270–277.

52. Mays GP, Hogg RA, Castellanos-Cruz DM, Hoover AG, Fowler LC. Public health research implementation and translation: evidence from practice-based research networks. *American Journal of Preventive Medicine.* 2013;45(6):752–762.

53. US Census Bureau. Government Employment & Payroll. https://www.census.gov/govs/apes/. Accessed October 30, 2014.

54. Darnell J, Cahn S, Turnock B, Becker C, Franzel J, Wagner DM. *Local Health Department Workforce Recruitment and Retention: Challenges and Opportunities.* Center for State & Local Government Excellence, UIC School of Public Health;2013.

55. Gebbie K, Turnock B. The public health workforce, 2006: new challenges. *Health Affairs.* 2006;25(4): 923–933.

56. Association of State and Territorial Health Officials. *ASTHO Profile of State Public Health: Volume Three.* Arlington, VA: Association of State and Territorial Health Officials;2014.

57. National Association of County and City Health Officials. Unpublished Data: New Local Health Official Environmental Scan. Washington, DC: National Association of County and City Health Officials; 2007.

58. National Public Health Leadership Institute. http://www.phli.org. Accessed December 15, 2007.

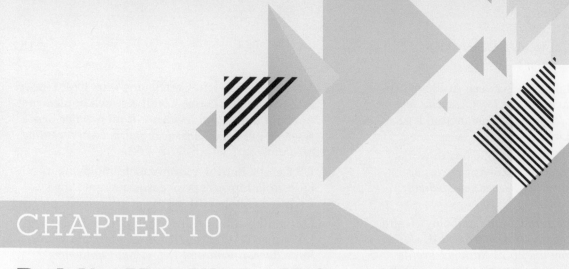

CHAPTER 10

Public Health in U.S.-Affiliated Tribes, Territories, and Freely Associated States

A. Mark Durand, MD, MPH • Joseph Seahquia Finkbonner, MHA • José F. Cordero, MD, MPH • Gregory Dever, MD • Emi Chutaro, MSc

LEARNING OBJECTIVES

Upon completion of this chapter, the reader will be able to:

1. Describe the historical context of the health systems of the U.S.-associated tribal and insular areas.

2. Describe how public health services are organized and linked to the U.S. public health system.

3. Understand the health status and disparities in the U.S.-associated tribal and insular areas.

4. Explain geographic and population factor challenges that affect the practice of public health in tribal and insular areas.

5. Identify specific opportunities and advantages for public health practice in tribal and insular areas.

KEY TERMS

Amerindians
Compacts of Free Association
dengue
Freely Associated States (FAS)
government-to-government relationships
Indian health system
insular jurisdictions
I/T/U (Indian Health Service, Tribally Operated Programs, Urban Indian Clinics)
tribal sovereignty
trust responsibility

INTRODUCTION

The mainstream of public health practice in the United States takes place at the federal, state, and local levels. However, there are communities within the scope of the U.S. public health system that lie beyond this norm, including American Indian/Alaska Native (AI/AN) and Caribbean and Pacific island insular jurisdictions. There are 566 American Indian/Alaska Native (AI/AN) tribes that are recognized as sovereign nations within the exterior boundaries of the United States. Among the U.S.-associated jurisdictions are tropical island groups in the Caribbean and Pacific (known collectively as the U.S. insular areas) which are comprised of three sovereign Freely Associated States (FAS)—the Federated States of Micronesia, Republic of Palau, and Republic of the Marshall Islands—and five territories—Puerto Rico, U.S. Virgin Islands, Guam, American Samoa, and the Commonwealth of the Northern Mariana Islands.

These communities vary widely in history, culture, geography, and political status, and offer instructive insights into public health practice applied across varying contexts.

GEOGRAPHY, HISTORY, AND PUBLIC HEALTH SYSTEMS

American Indians/Alaska Natives

The federal government has recognized tribal sovereignty since the beginning of U.S. history. Tribal sovereignty means that each tribe is treated as a nation within a nation, the status of which is recognized either through a formal treaty or an executive order. Numerous additional presidential executive orders have reinforced the relationship of the federal government with AI/AN nations, and have provided the policy framework for the creation of a separate health system for addressing AI/AN health care needs. Of particular note was President Bill Clinton's Executive Order issued on April 29, 1994 that directed the heads of each executive department to operate within a government-to-government relationship with federally recognized tribal governments, to consult with tribes prior to taking actions that affect the tribes, and assess the impacts of federal activities on tribal trust resources and to take steps to remove barriers that impede working directly with tribal governments.[1] The cession of most of the lands in the United States by the Indians, codified in hundreds of treaties, forms the basis for the U.S. government's provision of health care to Indians. Many treaties identified health services as part of the U.S. government's payment for Indian land. Indian treaties are contracts between the federal and tribal governments. In essence, Indian tribes gave up their land in return for payments and/or services from the U.S. government. The result is a trust responsibility on behalf of the federal government to provide services to AI/AN persons.

In *Worcester v. Georgia*[2] the U.S. Supreme Court established that the federal government has authority over and responsibility for matters relating to members of Indian tribes; because it assumes the authority, it also assumes the responsibility of protecting the tribes.[1] This expanded the ruling of *Cherokee Nation v. Georgia*[3] in establishing tribes as "domestic dependent" nations and was the foundation of the "trust relationship," that is, the special relationship between tribes and the U.S. government. It established the responsibility of the well-being for tribes and its membership in the hands of the federal government and not the individual states.[2]

In addition to the aforementioned Supreme Court cases, there are key legislative acts that are the foundation of public health services within the Indian health system:

▶ *The 1921 Snyder Act* provided permanent authorization for the allocation and expenditure of resources to provide health care to AI/AN populations. Language within the Act codified the long-standing emphasis on public health principles and the general population's movement toward wellness and health promotion programs.[4]

▶ *The Transfer Act of 1954* shifted the responsibility of the provision of health care services from the Bureau of Indian Affairs to the Indian Health Services.[5]

▶ *The Self-Determination Act of 1975* was enacted after Congress recognized the importance of tribal decision making in tribal affairs and the primacy of the nation-to-nation relationship between the United States and tribes through the passage of the Indian Self-Determination and Education Assistance Act (ISDEAA) (Public Law 93–638) in 1975.[6] Subsequent amendments to the ISDEAA strengthened the federal policies supporting tribal self-determination and self-governance. In 1992, Congress amended the ISDEAA to authorize a Tribal Self-Governance Demonstration Project within the Indian Health Services (IHS), giving federally recognized tribes the option of entering into self-governance compacts to gain more autonomy in the management and delivery of their health care programs. By 2000, Congress permanently authorized the IHS Tribal Self-Governance Program by creating Title V of the ISDEAA through Public Law 106–260.

The transformation brought about by the ISDEAA has led to the definition of the Indian health system, also called the "I/T/U," inclusive of the three models for delivering health services. The "I" represents services provided by the IHS, "T" represents the programs and services operated by the tribes under ISDEAA authorization, and "U" represents urban centers as authorized under Title V in the Indian Health Care Improvement Act.[7]

Organizational Structure

The 1954 Transfer Act[5] moved responsibility for Indian health to the U.S. Public Health Service, which was a division of the Department of Health, Education, and Welfare. (The Department of Health, Education, and Welfare was renamed the Department of Health and Human Services in 1980.) Previous to the IHS, the Bureau of Indian Affairs (BIA, U.S. Department of Interior) provided health care for the AI/AN population. The BIA primarily used contracts with local physicians as their means for delivering health care. This has contributed to some of the issues that make the funding of the IHS complex.

The IHS is divided into 12 administrative regions, each with an Area Office, and further subdivided into Service Units that are the facilities that provide the delivery of services, primary personal care, and public health services (see Figure 10-1).

The 12 administrative Areas of the IHS are Portland, Billings, California (not labeled on the map), Phoenix, Albuquerque, Northern Plains (formerly Aberdeen), Bemidji, Nashville, Oklahoma, Navajo, Tucson, and Alaska (not labeled on the map).

Presently, there are two basic structures that are available to federally recognized tribes: they can receive their health care directly operated through the IHS (also called Direct Service), or they can receive the funding that would have been appropriated for the IHS to provide care and operate their own health care system (tribally operated). However, it is not an all-or-nothing proposition. The majority of tribes have selected to receive the funding to operate specific programs within the overall health system, while

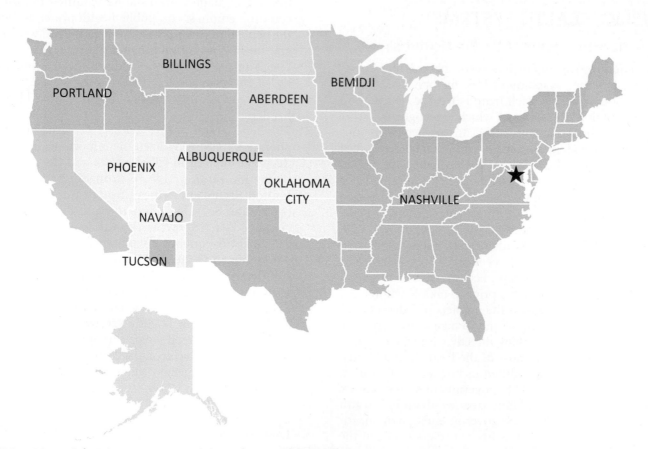

FIGURE 10-1   Administrative Areas of the Indian Health Services

the IHS maintains the primary care portion of the health system.

Currently, tribal health programs manage $2.5 billion dollars of the IHS budget.[8] The primary advantage for a tribe to exercise its right to contract with the IHS to operate the health programs is greater flexibility to adjust resources and programs to address local priorities. While the ability to completely eliminate programs is inherent in contracting the health services, tribes have largely continued to operate the same programs. Thus, the AI/AN health system includes programs and facilities run by the U.S. government through the IHS as well as those run by the tribes. Both the IHS as well as the tribes also run a number of urban health centers that are located off of tribal reservations.

Because IHS was developed in a public health context rather than a medical model, the IHS budget and programs contain items that are usually not part of insurance programs or managed care plans. These include environmental programs, such as water and sewer system construction, health promotion, injury prevention, school health, epidemiology, and health promotion units.

A description of the typical public health programs included in the IHS line item budgets for hospitals and clinics is provided in Table 10-1.

Insular Areas in the Caribbean

The Caribbean U.S. territories (Figure 10-2) include Puerto Rico and the U.S. Virgin Islands (USVI), both located southeast of Florida. Puerto Rico includes the uninhabited Mona Island to the west, the island of Puerto Rico, the island municipalities of Vieques and Culebra to the east, and a number of surrounding cays. The USVI includes the islands of St Thomas, St. Croix, St. John, Water Island, and several cays.

Amerindians originally inhabited Puerto Rico and the USVI; following Columbus's landing in 1493, these Caribbean islands became European colonies for several centuries. After nearly four centuries as a Spanish colony, Puerto Rico was ceded to the United States in the Treaty of Paris of 1898, which ended the

TABLE 10-1 Public Health Programs Within the Indian Health Services

Public Health Program Category	Description
Behavioral Health	Serious behavioral health issues such as substance use disorders, mental health disorders, suicide, violence, and behavior-related chronic diseases have a profound impact on the health of American Indian/Alaska Native (AI/AN) individuals, families, and communities.
Environmental Health	This program monitors and investigates disease and injury related to children's environment, safe drinking water, food safety, vector-borne and communicable diseases, and healthy homes.
Health Communications	Develops cultural and linguistic trainings and materials for health providers to enhance the health messages delivered to AI/AN population.
Health Promotion	Selects a small subset of the *Healthy People* indicators to establish Primary Prevention Focus Areas and leads the Agency in emphasizing programs to address the Focus Areas.
Injury Prevention	Promotes building the capacity of tribes and communities by increasing understanding about the injury problem, sharing effective solutions, and assisting communities in implementing programs.
School Health	Collaborates with local schools that educate AI/AN students on subjects related to nutrition, physical activity, oral health, and injury prevention.
Sustainability	Works with I/T/U on water conservation, energy management, pollution prevention, and sustainable communities.
Visualizing Data	Using Geographic Information Systems (GIS) tools to help with health messaging to the public and providers.

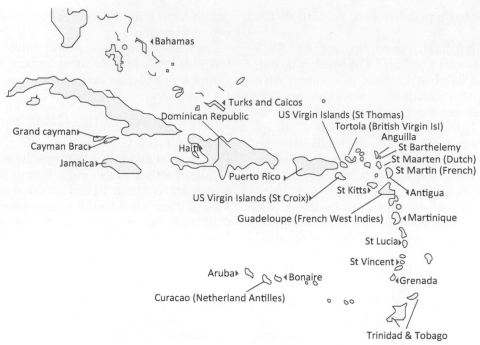

FIGURE 10-2 Caribbean Islands

Spanish-American War. The islands of the current USVI were under intermittent control of the British, French, and Dutch throughout the same time. In 1917, the USVI became a U.S. territory through a purchase from the Dutch.

Puerto Ricans and Virgin Islanders are U.S. citizens and have representation in Congress through an elected delegate that has voice, but no vote. Each jurisdiction has an elected governor and legislature. The local state government has most of the same functions as states in the continental United States, but federal funding for some public health programs vary and in some cases, territories are excluded. A recent example is the Patient Protection and Affordable Care Act (ACA). It includes the territories under most of the provisions of the Public Health Act, but there are specific exclusions. Other components of the ACA, such as those linked to the U.S. Internal Revenue Service and related to tax incentives under the Exchanges, exclude the territories as well.

The Puerto Rico and USVI Health Departments are responsible for the execution of the essential public health functions and work closely with federal agencies, such as the Centers for Disease Control and Prevention (CDC), the Health Resources and Services Administration, the Centers for Medicare and Medicaid Services, the Environmental Protection Agency (EPA), and others. Both Puerto Rico and USVI receive funding from the U.S. government for public health programs through grants and also receive federal technical assistance. The U.S. Department of Health and Human Services regional office provides a single point of contact for federal assistance and coordination to these jurisdictions.

Public health practice in Puerto Rico is mostly conducted by the Puerto Rico Department of Health and by municipalities. These municipalities have governance structures similar to counties in the U.S. mainland and their public health functions are coordinated with the Department of Health. The Department of Health has regional offices that assist in the coordination of public health activities. San Juan, the capital of Puerto Rico, has an independent health department, similar to the relationship between the New York State and New York City Health Departments.

According to the U.S. Census, Puerto Rico had an estimated health care workforce of 59,580 in 2012, mostly employed in direct health care activities. For the USVI the estimate for the same period is 2,370. In Puerto Rico, the total number of health department employees was estimated at nearly 2,700 in 2011, and underscores the strong emphasis on health care delivery versus prevention and wellness programs. Most of the public health workforce has an associate or college degree (88 percent), but a recent needs assessment survey identified training needs related to most public health competencies, ranging from outbreak investigation to laws and policies in public health. There are no comparable published data on the public health workforce in the USVI.

Regarding training of the public health workforce, Puerto Rico has an accredited School of Public Health in San Juan with nearly 500 students enrolled, and offers 15 Master's level degrees, three doctoral degrees, and five graduate certificates. The Ponce Health Sciences University has an accredited public health program with an estimated 135 students and offers a Master of Public Health and a PhD in Epidemiology. The USVI does not have a public health program or school, but the University of Virgin Islands has a Nursing School that trains nurses to become engaged in public health functions, and has an exploratory Center for Excellence on Health Disparities, funded by the U.S. National Institutes of Health, that offers opportunities for training and research on health disparities, a major public health issue.

Insular Areas in the Pacific

The United States-Affiliated Pacific Islands (USAPI) comprise the six jurisdictions of the Territory of Guam, the Territory of American Samoa, the Commonwealth of the Northern Mariana Islands (CNMI), the Republic of Palau, the Republic of the Marshall Islands, and the Federated States of Micronesia (FSM). With the exception of American Samoa located in the southern Pacific between Hawaii and New Zealand, the rest of the jurisdictions are located in the northwestern part of the Pacific between Hawaii and the Philippines. Together they have a total population of about 500,000 in a land area equivalent to that of the state of Rhode Island, comprised of thousands of scattered and isolated volcanic islands and coral atolls, spanning five time zones within an ocean area as large as the continental United States (Figure 10-3).

Guam was ceded under the Treaty of Paris to the United States in 1898, following the Spanish American War. Samoa was divided into two parts by the Treaty of Berlin in 1898 with the eastern islands of Tutuila and Manoa ceded by Germany to the United States, and the western islands staying under German administration. The other USAPI were put under U.S. administration within the Trust Territory of the Pacific Islands by the United Nations in 1947 in the aftermath of World War II. In the 1980s and 1990s the island groups within the Trust Territory negotiated their present political status with the U.S. government. The Commonwealth of the Northern Mariana Islands became a flag territory of the United States, while Palau, the Marshall Islands, and the FSM (comprised of the districts of Pohnpei, Kosrae, Yap, and Chuuk) negotiated treaties known as

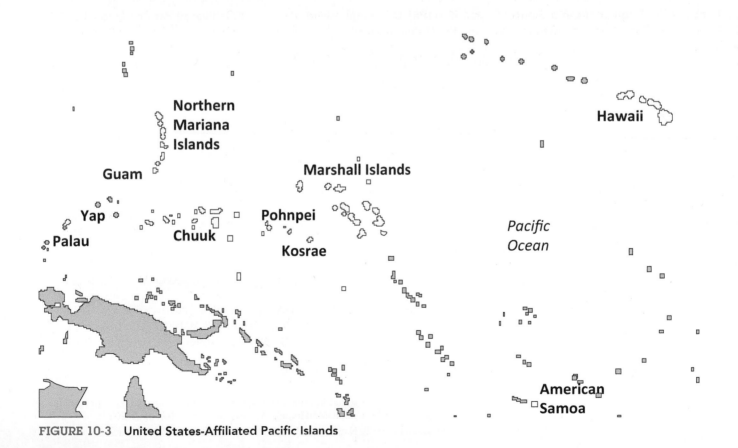

FIGURE 10-3 United States-Affiliated Pacific Islands

the **Compacts of Free Association**. These three countries are now known as the Freely Associated States (FAS). The compact agreements include protection under and hegemony by the U.S. military, free migration of citizens to and from the United States, the provision of American development "compact funding," and eligibility for many domestic, federally funded programs and technical assistance from the U.S. Department of Health and Human Services agencies. The territories, but not the FAS, have nonvoting representatives in the U.S. Congress.

Though the FAS have access to a range of U.S. federal programs and associated technical assistance support, because of their independent and sovereign status they are not required to fully comply with a number of federal regulations outside of specific conditions stipulated within eligible federal funding programs and grants. Unlike the FAS, the territories of Guam, CNMI, and American Samoa must comply with all federal regulations in order to continue to access and be eligible for a limited range of federal program funding and technical assistance. The U.S. government, therefore, has greater federal oversight over health systems development, maintenance, and public health service delivery in the territories than in the FAS. Currently,

key provisions of the ACA, such as mandatory enrollment and creation of health exchanges, do not apply in the USAPI.

Hospital services in all of the jurisdictions are delivered through local government agencies. With the exception of Guam, the majority of ambulatory health services are also delivered within the public sector. In all jurisdictions except Guam and American Samoa, public health, hospital, and ambulatory services are all administered by single local agencies. This presents opportunities for health services integration and innovation across public health and hospital services.

POPULATION, CULTURE, AND HEALTH INDICATORS

Tribal and insular areas have adverse health and economic disparities compared with the general population of the United States. These populations are younger, with lower incomes, higher poverty prevalence, higher infant mortality, and similar causes of death compared with the United States as a whole. Among these areas, the USAPI have the highest poverty prevalence and the poorest health status (Table 10-2).

TABLE 10-2   Populations at a Glance: Puerto Rico (PR), U.S. Virgin Islands (USVI), U.S.-Affiliated Pacific Islands (USAPI), American Indians/Alaska Natives (AI/AN), and the United States*

	PR	USVI	USAPI	AI/AN	US
Population	3,600,000	104,000	498,000	5,200,000	309,000,000
Life Expectancy at Birth (years)	79	79	70–76	74	79
Infant Mortality Rate (per 1000 live births, 2012)	7.9	6.7	11–29	8.4	6.1
Per Capita GDP	$13,800	$13,100	$7300-$28,500	$21,200	$52,800
% of population living below U.S. federal poverty level	41	33	25–91	19	15
% population <18 years of age	24	32	24–44	29	23
% population >=65 years of age	16	18	3–7	7	14

SOURCES: U.S. Census, 2010. United States. Census Bureau. Washington: Government Printing Office, 2010. Accessed March 25, 2015 at http://www.census.gov/2010census/data/

CIA Fact Book: https://www.cia.gov/library/publications/the-world-factbook/geos/aq.html (Accessed March 26, 2015)

Centers for Disease Control and Prevention. CDC Health Disparities and Inequalities Report- United States, 2013. MMWR 2013;62(Suppl 3):16.

Health, United States, 2013. National Center for Health Statistics. Health, United States, 2013: With Special Feature on Prescription Drugs. Hyattsville, MD. 2014

U.S. Department of Commerce Census Bureau (2012). *The 2012 Statistical Abstract.* Washington, DC.

Table 104 - Expectation of Life at Birth, 2010.

Secretariat for the Pacific, Community - Statistics for Development Pacific Regional Information System: National Minimum Development Indicators Database. Noumea, New Caledonia. Website: http://www.spc.int/nmdi/MdiHome.aspx. Accessed on 1 November 2014.

U.S. National Center for Health Statistics (2014). Deaths: Final Data for 2012 - National Vital Statistics Reports, Volume 63 #9. Hyattsville, MD.

American Indians and Alaska Natives

American Indians and Alaska Natives experience significant health disparities. Death rates are significantly higher in many areas for AI/ANs compared to the U.S. general population, including chronic liver disease and cirrhosis (368 percent higher), diabetes mellitus (177 percent higher), unintentional injuries (138 percent higher), assault/homicide (82 percent higher), suicide (65 percent higher), and chronic lower respiratory disease (59 percent higher).[9] These contribute to life expectancy which is four years less than for the general U.S. population.[10] As compared with other groups, AI/AN adults are more likely to report poorer health, have unmet medical needs due to cost, have diabetes, activity limitations, preterm birth, have experienced feelings of psychological distress in the past 30 days, and to be current smokers and binge drinkers.[11] Drug-induced death rates and preterm birth rates are also higher for AI/ANs than for the general U.S. population, though several disparities related to behavioral risk (smoking and binge drinking prevalence), infectious diseases (hepatitis A and B, new AIDS cases, tuberculosis incidence), and chronic diseases (diabetes-related deaths and end-stage renal disease incidence) have been decreasing over time.[12–14]

Table 10-3 lists the 10 leading causes of death for AI/AN for 2010, contrasting this with the 10 leading causes for the total U.S. population. The National Center for Health Statistics estimates that deaths for the AI/AN population are underreported by 30 percent,[11] and this degree of underreporting is not accounted for in the table.

Insular Areas of the Caribbean

Puerto Rico is the most populous of the U.S. territories, estimated in 2014 by the U.S. Census at nearly 3.6 million people. Since 2006, the U.S. Census has estimated that more Puerto Ricans reside in the continental United States than in Puerto Rico. That trend is likely the result of the massive migration of Puerto Ricans in the 1940s and 1950s to New York, Chicago, and other Northeast cities seeking better economic opportunities. The profile of migrants at that time were young adults, some migrating with their young children, most of a low educational level (less than 12 years of education), and seeking blue collar and agricultural employment. Puerto Rico experienced marked economic growth in the 1960s and migration slowed to the United States at that time. A new migratory wave has emerged in the last 15 years to Southeastern cities, in particular to Orlando, Florida. The profile of these new migrants is different from the 1960s in that they are mostly middle-aged, well-educated (university degrees), and many bring their businesses to the new area. These groups, in addition to seeking better economic opportunities, also consider personal safety as an additional factor to migrate. This recent migration trend has resulted in a net population loss for Puerto Rico of nearly 177,000 from 2010 to 2014.[15]

TABLE 10-3 Ten Leading Causes of Deaths for American Indians and Alaskan Natives, Compared to Total U.S. Population, 2010

American Indians and Alaskan Natives		Total U.S. Population	
Rank	Cause	Rank	Cause
1.	Cancer	1.	Heart Disease
2.	Heart Disease	2.	Cancer
3.	Unintentional Injuries	3.	Chronic Lower Respiratory Diseases
4.	Diabetes	4.	Stroke
5.	Chronic Liver Disease & Cirrhosis	5.	Unintentional Injuries
6.	Chronic Lower Respiratory Diseases	6.	Alzheimer's disease
7.	Stroke	7.	Diabetes
8.	Suicide	8.	Nephritis, Nephrotic Syndrome & Nephrosis
9.	Nephritis, Nephrotic Syndrome & Nephrosis	9.	Influenza and pneumonia
10.	Influenza & Pneumonia	10.	Suicide

SOURCE: National Vital Statistics Reports 2013[11]

The USVI has a population for 2014 estimated at nearly 104,000 and it is distributed mainly within the islands of St. Thomas and St Croix. The USVI has also been experiencing a population loss, but to a lesser extent than that seen in Puerto Rico. Most of the migration from the USVI to the U.S. mainland is to Northeastern states.[16]

While the leading causes of death for the insular areas of the Caribbean are similar to the United States in general (see below), the gap in life expectancy between males and females is almost eight years in the Caribbean areas, compared with four years in the United States.[17] This difference is driven by the high level of homicides and vehicular injuries among adolescents and young adult males in Puerto Rico.[18]

The age distribution in Puerto Rico and the USVI is typical of an older population. In Puerto Rico 16 percent of the population is 65 years and older, and in USVI it reaches 18 percent, compared to 14 percent in the United States. The racial distribution in Puerto Rico appears similar to the United States, but hides the fact that 99 percent of the Puerto Rican population described themselves as Hispanic, compared to 16 percent in the United States (Table 10-4). The Hispanic ethnicity in Puerto Rico also reflects the predominant language at home, school, business, and government, and it is nearly 95 percent Spanish.

Some key health indicators offer a window into the health status of the Puerto Rico and the USVI populations and some of their public health challenges. Leading causes of death in Puerto Rico and the USVI are similar to those of middle and high-income countries in the world. Ischemic heart disease, cancer, cerebrovascular disease, and diabetes are leading causes of mortality. Another important leading cause of mortality in the region is injuries, either resulting from violence or vehicular crashes.[18]

Preterm birth is a leading cause of neonatal and perinatal mortality in most countries in the world, and Puerto Rico and the USVI are no exception. Compared to the 2012 U.S. preterm birth rate of 11.5 percent, Puerto Rico is at 16.3 percent, and the USVI at 15.3 percent. Puerto Rico's preterm birth rate began to increase in 2006, and reached 19.9 percent in 2009, becoming the highest preterm birth rate in the Caribbean and the Americas. Some decline in this rate has been observed, but it remains one of the higher rates in the world.[19,20] A study conducted by the Institute of Medicine found that key risk factors for preterm births include lack of prenatal care, maternal smoking, maternal age (<19 and >35 years), assisted reproductive technology, and maternal pregnancy complications, such as eclampsia, uncontrolled diabetes, and maternal hypertension.[21] The study added that addressing those factors could potentially have an important impact in reducing the rate of preterm births, but that has not been the case in Puerto Rico.[21] While many of those risk factors improved over a period of two decades, the rate of preterm births continued to increase, suggesting that other factors, such as environmental exposures and clinical factors, may have a role in the observed increase.

HIV/AIDS is a major public health issue in Puerto Rico and the USVI. Intravenous drug use is a major source of infection in Puerto Rico and represents nearly 44 percent of all cases, compared to approximately 5 percent in the mainland U.S.[22] On the other hand, in the USVI, heterosexual contact and "other" account for nearly 67 percent of the HIV/AIDS cases, while men having sex with men account for about 18 percent of the cases.[23]

Infectious diseases have a large impact in Puerto Rico and USVI, with endemic dengue fever and tuberculosis being especially prevalent.[24] As tropical islands, Puerto Rico and USVI are endemic areas for emerging vector-borne diseases, including (most recently) chikungunya. The same vectors, the mosquitoes *Aedes aegypti* and *Aedes albopictus*, transmit both dengue and chikungunya. Dengue has been endemic for many decades in Puerto Rico and the USVI, with all four dengue types being reported in Puerto Rico.[25] In recent years chikungunya arrived in the Caribbean, with small clusters appearing in the USVI and a large epidemic of over 30,000 cases in Puerto Rico since 2014.[26,27]

Other environmental exposures in Puerto Rico and the USVI include frequent hurricanes and the large dust clouds that travel to the Caribbean from the Sahara desert. These dust clouds can reach a size of 200 miles wide and over 30,000 feet high. These clouds contain

TABLE 10-4   Race and Hispanic Ethnicity Distribution for Puerto Rico, U.S. Virgin Islands, and the United States, U.S. Census, 2010

Race and Ethnicity	Puerto Rico	USVI	United States
Racial Distribution	%	%	%
White	76	16	72
Black	12	76	13
American Indian/ Alaskan Native	1	0	1
Asian	0	0	5
Mixed	11	8	3
Hispanic	99	17	16

small particles, less than 10 μm, that can reach small airways in the lung and may have adverse health effects. Much needs to be learned about the health effects of this environmental phenomenon that can bring pollen, insects, bacteria, and chemicals, representing an opportunity for public health research and practice.[28,29]

Insular Areas of the Pacific

Both health and economic status are much worse in the USAPI compared with the United States as a whole, with the FAS being substantially worse off than the Pacific territories, in general (see Table 10-2). Per capita health spending in the USAPI is much lower than that in the United States as a whole ($300–1000 in the USAPI versus $8200 per year in the United States).[17]

In addition to economic disadvantages, the disparities of health seen in the USAPI can be related to urbanization, the shift in nutrition from local foods to low quality imports, social pathology due to breakdown of systems of traditional leadership in some areas, and environmental factors (lack of developed sewer systems, shortages of potable drinking water, environmental pollution, and increasingly, effects of climate change on in-shore fisheries and low-lying garden areas). Parts of the region are challenged by infectious diseases rarely seen in first world countries such as leprosy, epidemics of dengue fever and Zika virus, measles, and occasional outbreaks of cholera and typhoid fever. Recently, the World Health Organization (WHO) declared the tuberculosis (TB) rate in the Marshall Islands to be 900/100,000, one of the highest in the world. Multi-Drug Resistant Tuberculosis (MDR TB) has been found in the FSM and Marshall Islands, with a serious outbreak of MDR TB in FSM. The Marshall Islands also has one of the highest syphilis incidence rates globally.[30]

Micronutrient deficiencies, obesity rates, and related diseases in the Pacific are among the highest in the world.[31-35] Consumption of imported processed foods high in sugar and fat, and a loss of traditional food practices coupled with a decrease in physical activity, has led to significant increases in obesity rates in both sexes, and at increasingly younger ages. On the WHO's 2011 World's Fattest Countries List, seven Pacific countries are on the top 10 list, including the FSM and Palau. American Samoa has one of the highest adult diabetes prevalence rates (47 percent) in the world.[31] Chronic conditions overall are on the rise, including hypertension and related cardiovascular diseases and certain cancers.

Additionally, the Marshall Islands was the site for the U.S. nuclear weapons testing program, with the Bikini, Rongelap, and Enewetak atolls still unsafe for human habitation. Entire island communities of Marshallese were exposed to radioactive fallout and radiation levels equivalent to 7,000 Hiroshima-sized nuclear explosions from 67 test blasts conducted between 1946 and 1958.

The region is also among the most disaster-prone areas in the world, being especially subject to tsunamis, typhoons, drought, rising sea levels, and other effects of climate change.[36] Limited surge capacity of health and relief services, together with supply lines that are logistically difficult and expensive over long distances, compound the vulnerability of these scattered communities. The USAPI thus suffer from a "triple health burden," leading the world in obesity-related illness, while combating high rates of infectious diseases and frequent disasters.

PUBLIC HEALTH CHALLENGES AND OPPORTUNITIES

American Indians and Alaska Natives

AI/ANs have a unique relationship with the federal government due to historic conflict and subsequent treaties. Tribes exist as sovereign entities, but federally recognized tribes are entitled to health and educational services provided by the federal government. Geographic isolation and economic factors are examples of upstream factors that contribute to poorer health outcomes for AI/ANs. Though the Indian Health Service is charged with serving the health needs of these populations, more than half of AI/ANs do not permanently reside on a reservation, and therefore have limited or no access to IHS services.

The 1921 *Snyder Act* authorized Congress and the Bureau of Indian Affairs (BIA), under the supervision of the Department of Interior, to expend moneys for the benefit, care, and assistance of the Indians throughout the United States. The first documented appropriation of federal resources for Indian health was in 1832 for a vaccination program to combat the devastating effects of smallpox on the AI/AN populations. A second appropriation was made in 1839 to also combat the smallpox epidemic.

The IHS has been limited in its ability to provide care and services to AI/AN populations because it has been chronically resource-starved from congressional appropriations.[8] Between 1993 and 1998, IHS appropriations increased by a total of 8 percent, while medical inflation increased by 20.6 percent. This quickly led to diminishing services in order to pay for the rising cost of providing health care services. This trend continues to this day. President Obama's request for an increase of the 2015 budget is $199.7 million, which is a 4.5 percent increase over the previous year's enacted level. Current estimates forecast that it will take at least $450 million in fiscal year (FY) 2015 to maintain the current levels of health care provided by the Indian health system.[37] Anything less will result in Indian health programs having to absorb the mandatory costs of inflation on administration and salaries, within the context of population growth, which will lead to an erosion of services.

Chronic underfunding of a health system has long-term effects leading to greater disparities and lack of health improvement. Currently the appropriations for IHS are in the Department of Interior, while administratively IHS is an agency within the Department of Health and Human Services (DHHS). Tribal leaders are actively discussing if moving the appropriations for IHS into the DHHS would help improve the potential for budget increases annually.

Many AI/AN communities have the advantage of strongly shared cultural identity and unified curative and public health services. Many of the improvements relating to public health in the AI/AN populations are likely related to community health programs that are integrated into the fabric of the Indian health system, including injury prevention, a special diabetes project for Indians, school health, suicide prevention, substance abuse programs, and health communications.

Insular Areas of the Caribbean

The Caribbean region is well-known as the region where many hurricanes originate or come through on the way to the Gulf of Mexico and the eastern region of United States. Many hurricanes that impact Puerto Rico continue on to the mainland. For example, Hurricane Hugo landed in Puerto Rico in 1989, continued to the mainland and hit Charleston, South Carolina, causing major damage. Preparing for incoming hurricanes has been the platform to prepare for other natural and human-generated disasters.

Puerto Rico and USVI's location close to the eastern United States, with ample travel opportunities, has resulted in a bridge of transmission of HIV with major cities in the United States and will require combined efforts between jurisdictions to address this challenge.[38] On a positive note, Puerto Rico experienced great success in the prevention of perinatal HIV transmission. For nearly 15 years its program reduced perinatal transmission risk to nearly zero.[39] In the USVI, HIV perinatal transmission continues to be a challenge. There is an important opportunity in public health practice in understanding effective interventions for reduction and control of intravenous drug use-associated HIV transmission, including collaboration across public health departments in the United States and Puerto Rico.

Puerto Rico and the USVI have a considerable burden of toxic waste sites recognized by the U.S. Environmental Protection Agency under the National Priorities List (NPL) program.[40] Puerto Rico has the distinction of having more sites on the NPL per square mile than any other jurisdiction in the United States and includes large land areas such as the Atlantic Fleet Weapons Training Area in the island of Vieques. In comparison, the USVI has one site on the NPL.

A challenge for surveillance as well as clinical management is that the clinical symptoms of dengue, chikungunya, and other diseases presenting with a febrile illness, such as influenza and leptospirosis, have several features in common that often makes a specific diagnosis challenging. There are laboratory tests that can specifically diagnose these conditions, but they are not available for clinical diagnosis at the time patients present with the initial symptoms. This represents a challenge, particularly during the high tourist season, when infected tourists return home and develop symptoms that may be the onset of one of these emerging diseases.

As in most of the United States, curative health care services in Puerto Rico are organizationally separate from public health. Health care coverage is a key public health issue, particularly in addressing the needs of people living with chronic diseases, and for the elderly. Based on the Behavioral Risk Factor Surveillance System (BRFSS), 92.1 percent of adults in Puerto Rico report having some health care coverage, and in the USVI it is 69.4 percent. These estimates reflect the level of health care coverage before the implementation of the ACA and represent an opportunity to assess the impact of ACA in increasing health care coverage in these two jurisdictions.[41]

Insular Areas of the Pacific

The wide dispersion and remote location of populations in the Pacific pose major challenges to the delivery of health services. Keeping clinics and dispensaries that are located outside of the main population areas adequately staffed and supplied is a significant challenge. Telecommunications for training and education is generally weak and unreliable but improving in select areas. Long-distance phone rates are expensive, and phone/Internet service is often unavailable or low quality due to limited bandwidths. Many outer islands still rely on single side-band radios to communicate to the main islands. Even in the main hospitals, equipment and supplies for radiology, laboratory, and surgery are often unavailable in most of the USAPI.

This problem is compounded by the epidemic of non-communicable diseases. Cancers, ischemic heart disease, and renal failure require specialized diagnostic and treatment infrastructure which is very difficult to establish and sustain in small communities lacking economies of scale. Traditionally, these patients have been referred out of the region for specialized treatment. This practice has been a serious drain on health budgets, and shrinks the dollar amount remaining for other basic public health and social services. Less than 1 percent of the Pacific population accesses tertiary care, but 10 to 30 percent of total health budgets are spent on tertiary care and associated costs. In some years, American Samoa, Marshall Islands, and the FSM have spent between 20 to 30 percent of their health care budgets on off-island referrals. As health budgets have shrunk in the FAS in recent years, referral budgets have been cut and many unsponsored, low-income patients are now migrating from smaller islands to Guam and Hawaii to seek care for these conditions. This has caused friction between migrant and host communities in Guam and Hawaii.

Chronic shortages of fully trained health workers are also a serious barrier to the delivery of primary and secondary health care. Sending students outside the region for other health professions training is expensive and often unsuccessful due to weak academic skills of students, and even when successful, often results in out-migration of the newly trained health professional to higher paying jobs elsewhere. The use of local community colleges as platforms for formal nursing and public health degree programs provides versatile generalists who can do much of the work of public health at a basic but competent level. Other approaches that are being implemented in the region include setting up temporary health professions training programs within the region to train a cohort of needed health professions students, embedding faculty from regional health professions colleges and universities across jurisdictions to deliver curricula within local health agencies, and establishing distance learning platforms offering accredited university-level courses.[42–46]

The geography of the region has several other implications for health. The large distances that separate populations in the islands once protected them from the spread of cosmopolitan epidemics. Populations in the outer islands continue to be quite isolated. Children growing up in outer islands may have no contact with some common infectious diseases. When they migrate as young adults to district centers for employment they can be particularly vulnerable to diseases such as varicella, which is more severe in adults than in young children, and result in mortality rates that are higher than in cosmopolitan populations.[47] Also, in contrast to larger countries where diseases such as dengue fever, chikungunya, and measles are endemic, in the USAPI these diseases are only present during epidemics. The absence of a disease for several decades may allow large numbers of susceptible individuals to accumulate, resulting in epidemics with much higher attack rates than typically seen in larger countries. In addition, population densities may be very high on small islands. This, together with poor sanitation in many of the islands

has resulted in very high rates of tuberculosis, lymphatic filariasis, leprosy, rheumatic heart disease, leptospirosis, intestinal helminthes, and diarrheal diseases.[48–53]

While geography presents challenges, it also offers opportunities. The well-circumscribed boundaries and manageable size of Pacific island populations, combined with the limited number of health service providers, creates a favorable situation for integration of preventive services with curative services. It is easier to establish health information systems that can augment the success of community-wide approaches to deliver secondary preventive services for control of blood pressure, blood glucose, and cholesterol to patients with chronic diseases, for example. Islands with a single agency administering public health and curative services are in especially good positions to integrate services. Traditional village and leadership structures also lend themselves to organizing community health workers and outreach services both for follow-up of clinical services, and for delivery of preventive services (e.g., immunizations).

In 2010, through the Pacific Islands Health Officers Association, health leaders in the region issued a formal Declaration of Health Emergency for Non-Communicable Diseases (NCDs), a declaration which has since been endorsed by regional traditional leaders, legislators, and chief executives through the Pacific Traditional Leaders Council, the Association of Pacific Islands Legislators, and the Micronesian Chief Executive Summit group.[54] Pacific communities are relatively insulated from the influence of commercial interests that sometimes impede effective government policy toward chronic diseases. Their lawmakers can be more nimble and responsive in small communities than are those in large states having much more complex constituencies. Strong church communities and traditional leadership structures favor the establishment of effective community coalitions that can catalyze rapid change in government policies that have dramatic impact. Through a highly effective community coalition in Guam which is addressing chronic diseases, for example, the community, health agencies, and receptive legislators have worked together to facilitate passage of a number of tobacco bills, resulting in a reduction in the prevalence of youth smoking by half, from 50 percent to 25 percent, within a decade. Traditional and church leadership structures also present additional mechanisms for the establishment of policies at village and congregation levels. For example, in 2010, the Catholic Church in the CNMI changed the longstanding practice of families providing 10 days of feasts during rosary gatherings following funerals so that dinner is now only provided on the first day. Several traditional chiefs in Pohnpei in the FSM have also outlawed the serving of soft drinks and other prepared foods at all traditional ceremonies in their communities, while chiefs in the outer islands of Yap have successfully made their islands alcohol-free. On a regional level, the USAPI are pioneering a comprehensive approach, the USAPI NCD Regional Road Map and Policy Commitment Package, to the four principle chronic disease risk factors—tobacco, problem alcohol use, and obesity-related physical activity and nutritional patterns. This approach is patterned after the Framework Convention for Tobacco Control.[55] The USAPI are excellent places to pilot test important public health innovations such as this.

Other examples of pilot tests of important innovations in the islands include the proof of effectiveness of recombinant hepatitis B vaccine for reduction of chronic infections in highly affected populations, and the proof of effectiveness of the use of quinolone prophylaxis for MDR TB-exposed contacts.[56,57] Travel restrictions can be applied with relative ease in small island nations to protect populations from especially dangerous infectious disease outbreaks. During the 1918 influenza pandemic, the *Talune*, a steamship sailing from New Zealand and carrying influenza-infected passengers, was allowed to enter port in Apia, Western Samoa. Within a few weeks 22 percent of the population had died in what is thought to be the most deadly epidemic per capita within any country in the twentieth century. American Samoa was unaffected: its governor, John Hoyer, barred entry to the *Talune* and other ships carrying ill passengers.[58] Recommendations from authoritative bodies based in large countries may fail to address the feasibility of this approach for small island states. In the SARS outbreak of 2007, for example, the use of travel restrictions as a strategy for health protection was dismissed as unfeasible, though it may have been possible to implement successfully in the Pacific if the threat had escalated.

The USAPI avail themselves of the resources and expertise available through U.S. federal agencies and other international development organizations. However, there is often a mismatch between the assistance available from these agencies (which tend to operate through highly specialized, vertically organized programs that are geared toward much larger and more specialized constituents) and the needs and absorptive capacities of small island, low-resource communities. There are often overlapping and conflicting frameworks for assessment, programming, clinical guidelines, and policy development, creating inefficiencies and impairing effectiveness and impact. Harmonization and effective coordination of external technical assistance is therefore an important health systems function.

SUMMARY

Together, American Indian/Alaska Native communities and insular areas of the Caribbean and Pacific face adverse economic and health disparities compared with the general U.S. population. Their distinctive and varying histories, geography, patterns of migration, and population characteristics present special challenges for public health. These communities face triple burdens of infectious disease, noncommunicable diseases, and environmental vulnerability that are large compared with the United States as a whole. U.S. federal policy has a large impact on the ability of these communities to address their public health challenges. On the other hand, many of these jurisdictions also have advantages of close-knit communities and less complex health services environments, which all lend themselves to community-oriented, integrated models of care. Their distinctive features should be taken into account in public health practice. These features make these jurisdictions good places to test innovations that have value for informing the development of national public health practice and policy.

REVIEW QUESTIONS

1. Compare the health status of American Indians/Alaska Natives and people living in the Caribbean and Pacific insular areas with that of the continental United States.

2. Describe how migration plays a role in the epidemiology of HIV and other conditions in Puerto Rico and the USVI.

3. Describe the "triple health burden" faced by Caribbean and Pacific islands health systems.

4. Give two examples of health problems related to the tropical island geography of the Caribbean and Pacific.

5. Give three examples of how isolation and population dispersion affect the health of Pacific island communities.

6. Describe three advantages that Pacific islands jurisdictions have in combating the epidemic of noncommunicable diseases in the region.

7. Name two pieces of legislation that are key to the public health structure in the Indian health system.

REFERENCES

1. Executive Order No. 13175, 65 Reg. No 218. http://www.nps.gov/nagpra/AGENCIES/EO_13175.HTM. Accessed July 4, 2015.

2. *Worcester v. Georgia*, 31 U.S. (6 Pet.) 515. 1832.

3. *Cherokee Nation v. Georgia*, 21 U.S. (5 Pet.) 1.

4. Snyder Act, 25 U.S.C. 13.

5. Transfer Act (P.L. 83–568), 42 U.S.C. 2001.

6. Indian Self Determination and Education Assistance Act of 1975 (P.L. 93–638), 24 U.S.C. 450.

7. Indian Health Care Improvement Act (IHCIA) (P.L. 94–437) (later becoming an addendum to P.L. 111–148).

8. U.S. Commission of Civil Rights. A Quiet Crisis: Federal Funding and Unmet Needs in Indian Country. *US Commission on Civil Rights.* 2003:15.

9. Indian Health Services Factsheets Page. http://www.ihs.gov/newsroom/factsheets/quicklook/. Accessed December 27, 2014.

10. U.S. Department of Commerce Census Bureau. The 2012 Statistical Abstract. 2012.

11. National Vital Statistics Reports. December 20, 2013;62(6).

12. U.S. Department of Health and Human Services. Healthy People 2010 Database. 2010; http://wonder.cdc.gov/data2010/focraceg.htm. Accessed July 4, 2015.

13. National Center for Health Statistics. *Health, United States, 2013: With Special Feature on Prescription Drugs.* U.S. Government Printing Office Washington, DC

14. Garcia T, Keppel K, Hallquist S. Healthy People 2010 snapshot for the American Indian or Alaska Native population: Progress toward targets, size of disparities, and changes in disparities. www.cdc.gov/nchs/data/hpdata2010/aian_snapshot.pdf Accessed July 4, 2015.

15. U.S. Department of Commerce Census Bureau. US Census, Intercensal Estimates by year, sex. 2014.

16. U.S. Census. U.S. Virgin Islands. 2010; http://factfinder.census.gov/faces/tableservices/jsf/pages/productview.xhtml?src=bkmk. Accessed July 4, 2015.

17. U.S. Central Intelligence Agency. The World Factbook. 2013; https://www.cia.gov/library/publications/the-world-factbook/. Accessed December 27, 2013.

18. Murphy S, Xu J, Kochanek K. Deaths: Final data for 2010. *National Vital Statistics Reports.* 2013;61(4).

19. Centers for Disease Control and Prevention. CDC Reproductive Health Statistics. 2011; http://www.cdc.gov/reproductivehealth/maternalinfanthealth/infantmortality.htm. Accessed July 4, 2015.

20. Lee A, Katz J, Blencowe H, et al. RE: CHERG SGA-Preterm Birth Working Group. National and Regional Estimates of Term and Preterm Babies Born Small for Gestational Age in 138 Low-income and Middle-income Countries in 2010. *Lancet Global Health.* 2013;1(1):11.

21. Cordero J, Mattei H. Risks for Increase of Preterm Births in Puerto Rico: Not the Usual Suspects. Birth Defects Research Part A. *Clinical and Molecular Teratology.* 2009;85(5).

22. Puerto Rico Departmento de Salud, Sistema de Vigilancia, VIH. 2014; http://www.salud.gov.pr/Programas/OficEpidemiologia/Estadisticas%20Generales/Puerto%20Rico%20HIV%20not%20AIDS%20Surveillance%20Summary%20enero%202014.pdf. Accessed July 4, 2015.

23. Hobson A. Virgin Islands Dept of Health HIV Surveillance 2010 Annual Data Report. http://www.healthvi.com/assets/documents/2010/2010-hiv-surveillance%20report.pdf Accessed July 4, 2015.

24. Puerto Rico Deparamento de Salud. Tasa de incidencia de tuberculosis en Puerto Rico. 2012–2013; http://www.salud.gov.pr/Estadisticas-Registros-y-Publicaciones/Pages/Tuberculosis.aspx Accessed July 4, 2015.

25. Centers for Disease Control and Prevention Dengue Branch and Puerto Rico Dept of Health. Dengue Surveillance Weekly Report. 2015; http://www.cdc.gov/dengue/resources/wklyrpt_eng/wklyrpt_eng.pdf. Accessed July 4, 2015.

26. Centers for Disease Control and Prevention. Chikungunya virus surveillance summary. 2015; http://www.cdc.gov/chikungunya/geo/americas.html. Accessed July 4, 2015.

27. Puerto Rico Deparamento de Salud. Chikungunya en Puerto Rico. 2015; http://www.salud.gov.pr/Estadisticas-Registros-y-Publicaciones/Pages/Chikungunya.aspx Accessed July 4, 2015.

28. Monteil M. Saharan Dust Clouds and Human Health in the English-speaking Caribbean: What We Know and Don't Know. *Environmental Geochemistry and Health* 2008;30(4):5.

29. Griffin DW. Atmospheric movement of microorganisms in clouds of desert dust and implications for human health. *Clin Microbiol Rev.* 2007;20(3):459–477.

30. Wanyeki I. HIV Surveillance in Pacific Island Countries and territories, 2012 report. *Secretariat of the Pacific Community. Noumea, New Caledonia, 2012.* http://www.aidsdatahub.org/dmdocuments/2012_HIV_Epidemiological_Update_for_PICTs.pdf. Accessed July 4, 2015.

31. Maga A, DeCourten M, Dan L. American Samoa NCD Risk Factors STEPS Report, 2004. 2007;

http://www.who.int/chp/steps/Printed_STEPS_Report_American_Samoa.pdf. Accessed July 4, 2015.

32. Ng M, Fleming T, Robinson M. Global, Regional, and National Prevalence of Overweight and Obesity in Children and Adults during 1980–2013: A Systematic Analysis for the Global Burden of Disease Study 2013. *Lancet.* 2014;384(9945):176.

33. Pobocik R, Boudreau N. Nutrient Analysis of the Guamanian Diet: Acceptable Energy Distribution with Inadequate Nutrient Quality. *Pacific Health Dialogue.* 2005;2:13.

34. Palafox N, Gamble M, Dancheck B. Vitamin A Deficiency, Iron Deficiency, and Anemia Among Preschool Children in the Republic of the Marshall Islands. *Nutrition.* 2003;19(5):4.

35. Durand A. Progress in the Fight Against NCDs in the US-Affiliated Pacific Islands: 2000–2013. http://www.pihoa.org/fullsite/newsroom/wp-content/uploads/downloads/2015/02/Progress-in-the-Fight-against-NCDs-in-the-US-affiliated-Pacific-Islands-2000–2013-11–13.pdf. Accessed July 4, 2015.

36. Jeschonnek L. World Risk Report, 2012. 2013; http://www.ehs.unu.edu/article/read/worldriskreport-2012. Accessed November 1, 2014.

37. Roberts J. NPAIHB Policy Brief. 2014; http://www.npaihb.org/policy/current_policy_briefs. Accessed July 4, 2015.

38. Deren S, Gelbi-Acosta C, Albizu-Garcia C, Gonzalez A, Des Jarlais D, Santiago-Negron S. Addressing the HIV/AIDS Epidemic Among Puerto Rican People Who Inject Drugs: The Need for a Multiregion Approach. *Am J Public Health.* 2014;104(11):7.

39. Zorrilla C, Tamayo A, Febo I, et al. Reduction in the Perinatal HIV Transmission: the Experience at the Maternal Infant Studies Center and Gamma Projects at the University of Puerto Rico School of Medicine. *Puerto Rico Health Sciences Journal.* 2007;26(4):7.

40. US Environmental Protection Agency. Final National Priorities List (NPL) Sites- by State. 2015; http://www.epa.gov/superfund/sites/query/query-htm/nplfin.htm#PR Accessed July 4, 2015.

41. Centers for Disease Control and Prevention. Behavioral Risk Factor Surveillance System, Puerto Rico. 2013; http://apps.nccd.cdc.gov/brfss/page.asp?yr=2013&state=PR&cat=HC#HC. Accessed July 4, 2015.

42. Dever G. JABSOM's Legacy in the Pacific: Linking the PBMOTP and Pacific Basin AHEC Programs:

A Palau Perspective. *Pacific Health Dialogue.* 2005;12(1):5.

43. Durand A, Boliy A, Tamag L. DC-OS: Decentralized, On-site Training: A Sadly Neglected Option for Building the Pacific Islands Health Workforce. *Pacific Health Dialogue.* 2007;14(1):3.

44. Rao K, Giluli C. Reaching REMOTE Learners: Successes and Challenges for Students in an Online Graduate Degree Program in the Pacific Islands. *The International Review of Research in Open Distance and Learning.* 2010;11(1):10.

45. Dever G, McCormick R, Durand A. In-Country and Community-Based Postgraduate Family Practice Training for Micronesian Physicians: The Palau AHEC - A Collaborative Effort. *Pacific Health Dialogue.* 2002;9(1):5.

46. Buenconsejo-Lum L, Maskarinec G, Palafox N. Pacific Association for Clinical Training (PACT): Lessons Learned and Next Steps in Developing a Sustainable Continuing Health Professional Education System in the United States-Affiliated Pacific Island (USAPI) Jurisdictions. *Pacific Health Dialogue.* 2007;14(1):10.

47. Office of Vital Statistics, Commonwealth Healthcare Corporation. Mortality Records 1990–2000.

48. Carapetis J, Steer A, Mulholland E. A Global Burden of Group A Streptococcal Diseases. *Lancet Infectious Diseases.* 2005;5(11):10.

49. Berlioz-Arthaud A, Kiedrzynski T, Singh N. Multicentre Survey of Incidence and Public Health Impact of Leptospirosis in the Western Pacific. *Transactions of the Royal Society of Tropical Medicine and Hygiene.* 2007;101(7):8.

50. Haddock R. Disease Surveillance in Guam: A Historical Perspective. *Pacific Health Dialogue.* 2005;12(2):6.

51. Workshop on the Prevention of Leprosy. Proceedings of the Workshop on the Prevention of Leprosy, Pohnpei, Federated States of Micronesia. *International Journal of Leprosy and Other Mycobacterial Diseases.* 1999;67(4 Supplement):82.

52. Kirk M, Kiedrzynski T, Johnson E. Risk Factors for Cholera in Pohnpei during an Outbreak in 2000: Lessons for Pacific Countries and Territories. *Pacific Health Dialogue.* 2005;12(2):6.

53. Liang J, King J, Ichimori K. Impact of Five Annual Rounds of Mass Drug Administration with Diethylcarbamazine and Albendazole on Wuchereria Bancrofti Infection in American Samoa. *American Journal of Tropical Medicine and Hygiene.* 2008;78(6):5.

54. Pacific Islands Health Officers Association. PIHOA NCD Regional Emergency Declaration Resolution 48–01. http://www.pihoa.org/initiatives/policy/ncds.php. Accessed November 1, 2014.

55. Pacific Islands Health Officers Association. PIHOA NCD Regional Emergency Response. http://www.pihoa.org/initiatives/policy/ncds.php. Accessed November 1, 2014.

56. Durand A, Sabino HJ, Mahoney F. Success of Mass Vaccination of Infants Against Hepatitis B. *Journal of the American Medical Association.* 1996;276(22):2.

57. Bamrah S, Brostrom R, Dorina F. Treatment for LTBI in Contacts of MDR-TB Patients, Federated States of Micronesia, 2009–2012. *International Journal of Tuberculosis and Lung Disease.* 2014;18(8):7.

58. Tomkins S. The Influenza Epidemic of 1918–19 in Western Samoa. *Journal of Pacific History.* 1992;27(2):17.

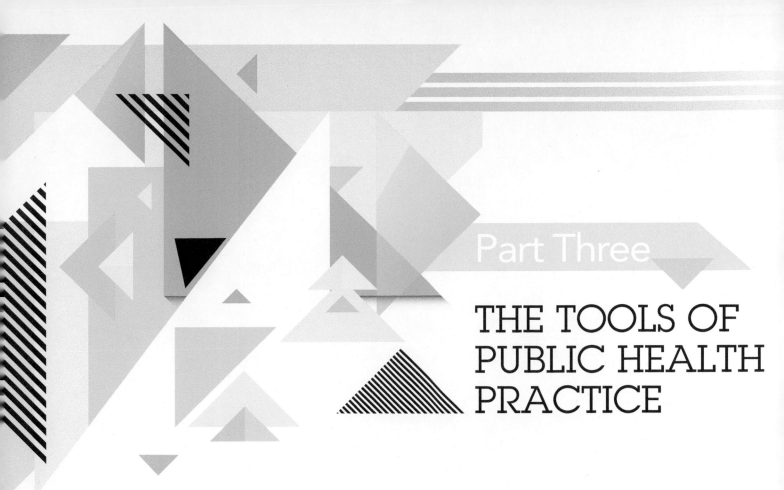

Part Three

THE TOOLS OF PUBLIC HEALTH PRACTICE

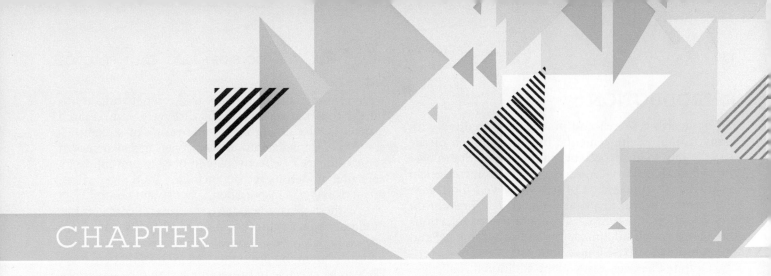

CHAPTER 11

Evidence-Based Public Health

Ross C. Brownson, PhD • Paul C. Erwin, MD, DrPH

LEARNING OBJECTIVES

Upon completion of this chapter, the reader will be able to:

1. Describe the principles of evidence-based public health (EBPH), including types of evidence, the role of transdisciplinary problem solving, and similarities and differences from clinical practice.

2. Define six key characteristics of EBPH.

3. Recognize analytic tools that assist in the EBPH process by describing the size of a problem, effective interventions, contextual conditions, and relative value of various approaches.

4. Describe a seven-stage framework for EBPH that, if implemented, has the potential to improve public health decision making.

5. Describe several barriers to implementing principles of EBPH in practice and some potential approaches for overcoming these challenges.

KEY TERMS

disease prevention
evidence-based medicine (EBM)
evidence-based public health (EBPH)
intervention
population-based

INTRODUCTION

Public health research and practice are credited with many notable achievements, including much of the 30-year gain in life expectancy in the United States over the twentieth century.[1] A large part of this increase can be attributed to provision of safe water and food, sewage treatment and disposal, tobacco use prevention and cessation, injury prevention, control of infectious diseases through immunization and other means, and other population-based interventions.[2]

Despite these successes, many additional challenges and opportunities to improve the public's health remain. To achieve state and national objectives for improved public health, more widespread adoption of evidence-based strategies has been recommended.[3–8] Increased focus on evidence-based public health (EBPH) has numerous direct and indirect benefits, including access to more and higher quality information on what works, a higher likelihood of successful programs and policies being implemented, greater workforce productivity, and more efficient use of public and private resources.[5,9,10]

Ideally, public health practitioners should always incorporate scientific evidence in selecting and implementing programs, developing policies, and evaluating progress. Society pays a high opportunity cost when interventions that yield the highest health return on an investment are not implemented (i.e., in light of limited resources, the benefit given up by implementing less effective interventions).[11] In practice, intervention decisions are often based on perceived short-term opportunities, lacking systematic planning and review of the best evidence regarding effective approaches. Still apparent today,[12] these concerns were noted nearly three decades ago when the Institute of Medicine determined that decision making in public health is too often driven by "…crises, hot issues, and concerns of organized interest groups" (p. 4).[13] Barriers to implementing EBPH include the political environment (including lack of political will), and deficits in relevant and timely research, information systems, resources, leadership, organizational culture, and the required competencies.[14–18]

Nearly every public health problem is complex,[19] requiring attention at multiple levels and among many different disciplines. Partnerships that bring together diverse people and organizations have the potential for developing new and creative ways of addressing public health issues.[20] Transdisciplinary research provides valuable opportunities to collaborate on interventions to improve the health and well-being of both individuals and communities.[21,22] For example, tobacco research efforts have been successful in facilitating cooperation among disciplines such as advertising, policy, business, medical science, and behavioral science. Research activities within these multidisciplinary tobacco networks try to fill the gaps between scientific discovery and research translation by engaging a wide range of stakeholders.[23–25] A transdisciplinary approach has also shown some evidence of effectiveness in obesity prevention by engaging numerous sectors including food production, urban planning, transportation, schools, and health.[26,27]

As these disciplines converge, several concepts are fundamental to achieving a more evidence-based approach to public health practice. First, we need scientific information on the programs and policies that are most likely to be effective in promoting health (i.e., undertake evaluation research to generate sound evidence).[5,9,28,29] An array of effective interventions is now available from numerous sources including the *Guide to Community Preventive Services*,[30,31] the *Guide to Clinical Preventive Services*,[32] Cancer Control PLANET,[33] and the National Registry of Evidence-based Programs and Practices.[34] Second, to translate science to practice, we need to marry information on evidence-based interventions from the peer-reviewed literature with the realities of a specific real-world environment.[35,36] To do so, we need to better define processes that lead to evidence-based decision making.[37] Finally, wide-scale dissemination of interventions of proven effectiveness must occur more consistently at state and local levels.[38,39]

This chapter includes five major sections that describe: (1) relevant background issues, including a brief history, definitions, an overview of evidence-based medicine, and other concepts underlying EBPH; (2) several key characteristics of an evidenced-based process that crosses numerous disciplines; (3) analytic tools to enhance the uptake of EBPH and the disciplines responsible; (4) a brief sketch of a framework for EBPH in public health practice; and (5) a summary of barriers and opportunities for widespread implementation of evidence-based approaches. A major goal of this chapter is to move the process of decision making toward a proactive approach that incorporates effective use of scientific evidence and data, while engaging numerous sectors and partners for transdisciplinary problem solving.

HISTORICAL BACKGROUND AND CORE CONCEPTS

Formal discourse on the nature and scope of EBPH originated about a decade ago. Several authors have attempted to define EBPH. In 1997, Jenicek defined EBPH as the "…conscientious, explicit, and judicious use of current best evidence in making decisions about the care of communities and populations in the domain of health protection, disease prevention, health maintenance and improvement (health promotion)."[40] In 1999, scholars and practitioners in Australia[6] and the United States[41] elaborated further on the concept of EBPH. Glasziou and colleagues posed a series of questions to enhance uptake of EBPH (e.g., "Does this intervention help alleviate this problem?") and identified 14 sources of high-quality evidence.[6] Brownson and colleagues described a six-stage process by which practitioners are able to take a more evidence-based approach to decision making.[5,41] Kohatsu and colleagues broadened earlier definitions of EBPH to include the perspectives of community members, fostering a more population-centered approach.[35] Rychetnik and colleagues summarized many key concepts in a glossary for EBPH.[42] There appears to be a consensus that a combination of scientific evidence, as well as values, resources, and context should enter into decision making (Figure 11-1).[3,5,42,43] A concise definition emerged from Kohatsu: "Evidence-based public health is the process of integrating science-based interventions with community preferences to improve the health of populations." (p. 419).[35] In addition, Satterfield and colleagues examined evidence-based practice across five disciplines (public health, social work, medicine, nursing, and psychology) and found many common challenges including: (1) how evidence should be defined; (2) how and when the patient's and/or other contextual factors should enter the decision-making process; (3) the definition and role of the experts or key stakeholders; and (4) what other variables should be considered when selecting an evidence-based practice (e.g., age, social class).[43]

Defining Evidence

At the most basic level, evidence involves "the available body of facts or information indicating whether a belief or proposition is true or valid."[44] The idea of evidence often derives from legal settings in Western societies. In law, evidence comes in the form of stories, witness accounts, police testimony, expert opinions, and forensic science.[45] Our notions of evidence are defined in large part by our professional training and experience. For a public health professional, evidence is some form of data—including epidemiologic (quantitative) data, results of program or policy evaluations, and qualitative data—for uses in making judgments or decisions (Figure 11-2).[46] Public health evidence is usually the result of a complex cycle of observation, theory, and experiment.[47,48] However, the value of evidence is in the eye of the beholder (e.g., usefulness of evidence may vary by stakeholder type).[49] Medical evidence includes not only research but characteristics of the patient, a patient's readiness to undergo a therapy, and society's values.[50] Policy makers seek out distributional consequences (i.e., who has to pay, how much, and who benefits)[51] and in practice settings, anecdotes sometimes trump empirical data.[52] Evidence is usually imperfect and, as noted by Muir Gray: "The absence of excellent evidence does not make evidence-based decision making impossible; what is required is the best evidence available not the best evidence possible."[3]

Several authors have defined types of scientific evidence for public health practice (see Table 11-1).[5,41,42] Type 1 evidence defines the causes of diseases and the magnitude, severity, and preventability of risk factors and diseases. It suggests that *something should be done* about a particular disease or risk factor. Type 2 evidence describes the relative impact of specific interventions that do or do not improve health, adding *"specifically*, this should be done."[5] It has been noted that adherence to a strict hierarchy of study designs may reinforce an "inverse evidence law" by which interventions most likely to influence whole populations (e.g., policy change) are least valued in an evidence matrix emphasizing randomized designs.[53,54] A recent study from Sanson-Fisher and colleagues showed the relative

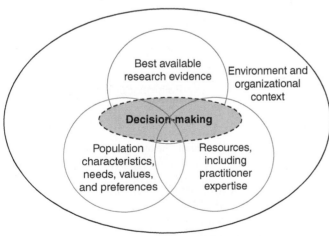

FIGURE 11-1   Domains that Influence Evidence-Based Decision-Making

Adapted from Satterfield et al.

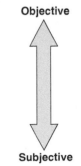

- Scientific literature in systematic reviews
- Scientific literature in one or more journal articles
- Public health surveillance data
- Program evaluations
- Qualitative data
  - Community members
  - Other stakeholders
- Media/marketing data
- Word of mouth
- Personal experience

Objective

Subjective

FIGURE 11-2   Different Forms of Evidence

Adapted from Chambers and Kerner

TABLE 11-1   Comparison of the Types of Scientific Evidence

Characteristic	Type One	Type Two	Type Three
Typical Data/ Relationship	Size and strength of preventable risk—disease relationship (measures of burden, etiologic research)	Relative effectiveness of public health intervention	Information on the adaptation and translation of an effective intervention
Common setting	Clinic or controlled community setting	Socially intact groups or community-wide	Socially intact groups or community-wide
Example	Smoking causes lung cancer.	Price increases with a targeted media campaign reduce smoking rates	Understanding the political challenges of price increases or targeting media messages to particular audience segments
Quantity	More	Less	Less
Action	Something should be done.	This particular intervention should be implemented	How an intervention should be implemented

lack of intervention research (Type 2) compared with descriptive/epidemiologic research (Type 1). In a random sample of published studies on tobacco use, alcohol use, and inadequate physical activity, their team found that in 2005–2006, 14.9 percent of studies reported on interventions whereas 78.5 percent of articles were descriptive or epidemiologic research. There is likely to be even less published research on Type 3 evidence—which shows how and under what contextual conditions interventions were implemented and how they were received, thus informing "*how* something should be done."[42] Studies to date have tended to overemphasize internal validity (e.g., well controlled efficacy trials) while giving sparse attention to external validity (e.g., the translation of science to the various circumstances of practice).[55,56]

Understanding the Context for Evidence

Type 3 evidence derives from the context of an intervention.[42] While numerous authors have written about the role of context in informing evidence-based practice,[9,42,49,57–61] there is little consensus on its definition. When moving from clinical interventions to population-level and policy interventions, context becomes more uncertain, variable, and complex.[62] One useful definition of context highlights information needed to adapt and implement an evidence-based intervention in a particular setting or population.[42] The context for Type 3 evidence specifies five overlapping domains (see Table 11-2). First, there are characteristics of the target population for an intervention such as education level and health history.[63] Next, interpersonal

TABLE 11-2   Contextual Variables for Intervention Design, Implementation, and Adaptation

Category	Examples
Individual	Education level Basic human needs[a] Personal health history
Interpersonal	Family health history Support from peers Social capital
Organizational	Staff composition Staff expertise Physical infrastructure Organizational culture
Sociocultural	Social norms Values Cultural traditions History
Political and economic	Political will Political ideology Lobbying and special interests Costs and benefits

[a]Basic human needs include food, shelter, warmth, safety.[63]

variables provide important context. For example, a person with a family history of cancer might be more likely to undergo cancer screening. Third, organizational variables should be considered. For example, whether an agency is successful in carrying out an evidence-based program will be influenced by its capacity (e.g., a trained workforce, agency leadership).[9,64] The important role of capacity building (e.g., more training toward prevention, increase the skills of professionals) has been noted as a "grand challenge" for public health efforts.[65] Fourth, social norms and culture are known to shape many health behaviors. Finally, larger political and economic forces affect context. For example, a high rate for a certain disease may influence a state's political will to address the issue in a meaningful and systematic way. Particularly for high-risk and understudied populations, there is a pressing need for evidence on contextual variables and ways of adapting programs and policies across settings and population subgroups. Contextual issues are being addressed more fully in the new "realist review," which is a systematic review process that seeks to examine not only whether an intervention works but also *how* interventions work in real-world settings.[66]

Challenges Related to Public Health Evidence

Evidence for public health has been described as underpopulated, dispersed, and different.[67,68] It is underpopulated because there are relatively few well-done evaluations of how well evidence-based interventions apply across different social groups (Type 3 evidence). Information for public health decision making is also more dispersed than evidence for clinical interventions. For example, evidence on the health effects of the built environment might be found in transportation or planning journals. Finally, public health evidence is different, in part because much of the science base for interventions is derived from nonrandomized designs or so-called "natural experiments" (i.e., generally takes the form of an observational study in which the researcher cannot control or withhold the allocation of an intervention to particular areas or communities, but where natural or predetermined variation in allocation occurs.)[69]

Triangulating Evidence

Triangulation involves the accumulation of evidence from a variety of sources to gain insight into a particular topic[70] and often combines quantitative and qualitative data.[5] It generally involves the use of multiple methods of data collection and/or analysis to determine points of commonality or disagreement.[71] Triangulation is often beneficial because of the complementary nature of information from different sources. Though quantitative data provide an excellent opportunity to determine how variables are related for large numbers of people, these data provide little in the way of understanding why these relationships exist. Qualitative data, on the other hand, can help provide information to explain quantitative findings, or what has been called

"illuminating meaning."[71] There are many examples of the use of triangulation of qualitative and quantitative data to evaluate health programs and policies, including AIDS prevention programs,[72] occupational health programs and policies,[73] and chronic disease prevention programs in community settings.[74] These examples also illustrate the roles of numerous disciplines in addressing pressing public health problems.

Cultural and Geographic Differences

The tenets of EBPH have largely been developed in a Western, European-American context.[75] The conceptual approach arises from the epistemological underpinnings of logical positivism,[76] which finds meaning through rigorous observation and measurement. This is reflected in a professional preference among clinicians for research designs such as the randomized controlled trial. In addition, most studies in the EBPH literature are academic-based research, usually with external funding for well-established investigators. In contrast, in developing countries and in impoverished areas of developed countries, the evidence base for how best to address common public health problems is often limited even though the scope of the problem may be enormous. Cavill compared evidence-based interventions across countries in Europe, showing that much of the evidence base in several areas is limited to empirical observations.[77] Even in more developed countries (including the United States), information published in peer-reviewed journals or data available through web sites and official organizations may not adequately represent all populations of interest.

Key Role of EBPH in Accreditation Efforts

A national voluntary accreditation program for public health agencies was established through the Public Health Accreditation Board (PHAB) in 2007.[78] As an effort to improve both the quality and performance of public health agencies at all levels, the accreditation process is structured around 12 domains which roughly coincide with the 10 Essential Public Health Services, with additional domains on management and administration (domain 11) and governance (domain 12).[79] The accreditation process intersects with EBPH on at least three levels. First, the entire process is based on the predication that if a public health agency meets certain standards and measures, quality and performance will be enhanced. The evidence for such a predication, however, is incomplete at best, and often relies on the type of best evidence available that can only be described as sound judgment, based on experience in practice. Second, domain 10 of the PHAB process is "Contribute to and Apply the Evidence Base of Public Health."

Successfully accomplishing the standards and measures under domain 10 involves using EBPH from such sources as the *Guide to Community Preventive Services*, having access to research expertise, and communicating the facts and implications of research to appropriate audiences. Third, the prerequisites for accreditation – a community health assessment, a community health improvement plan, and an agency strategic plan – are key elements of EBPH, as will be described later in this chapter.

A critical aspect of PHAB's early implementation is the development of an evaluation and research agenda, based on a logic model for accreditation, which can serve as a guide for strengthening the evidence base for accreditation. In many ways the accreditation process is coeval with the development of EBPH: the actual use of standards and measures presents opportunities to strengthen the evidence base for accreditation, and, as EBPH evolves, new findings will help inform the refinement of standards and measures over time. One example of this is the recent identification of evidence-based administrative practices,[37] which can be used to enhance the standards and measures for domain 11 on management and administration.

Audiences for EBPH

There are four overlapping user groups for EBPH as defined by Fielding.[80] The first includes public health practitioners with executive and managerial responsibilities who want to know the scope and quality of evidence for alternative strategies (e.g., programs, policies). In practice, however, public health practitioners frequently have a relatively narrow set of options. Funds from federal, state, or local sources are most often earmarked for a specific purpose (e.g., surveillance and treatment of sexually transmitted diseases, inspection of retail food establishments). Still, the public health practitioner has the opportunity, even the obligation, to carefully review the evidence for alternative ways to achieve the desired health goals. The next user group is policy makers at local, regional, state, national, and international levels. They are faced with macro-level decisions on how to allocate the public resources for which they are stewards. This group has the additional responsibility of making policies on controversial public issues. The third group is composed of stakeholders who will be affected by any intervention. This includes the public, especially those who vote, as well as interest groups formed to support or oppose specific policies, such as the legality of abortion, whether the community water supply should be fluoridated, or whether adults must be issued handgun licenses if they pass background checks. The final user group is composed of researchers on population health issues, such as those who evaluate the impact of a specific policy or program. They both develop and use evidence to answer research questions.

Similarities and Differences between EBPH and Evidence-Based Medicine

The concept of evidence-based practice is well established in numerous disciplines including psychology,[81] social work,[82,83] and nursing.[84] It is probably best established in medicine. The doctrine of **evidence-based medicine (EBM)** was formally introduced in 1992.[85] Its origins can be traced back to the seminal work of Cochrane, who noted that many medical treatments lacked scientific effectiveness.[86] A basic tenet of EBM is to de-emphasize unsystematic clinical experience and place greater emphasis on evidence from clinical research. This approach requires new skills, such as efficient literature searching and an understanding of types of evidence in evaluating the clinical literature.[87] There has been a rapid growth in the literature on EBM, contributing to its formal recognition. Using the search term "evidence-based medicine" there were 254 citations in PubMed in 1990, rising to 7,331 citations in 2008, and to 101,288 in 2014. Even though the formal terminology of EBM is relatively recent, its concepts are embedded in earlier efforts such as the Canadian Task Force for the Periodic Health Examination[88] and the *Guide to Clinical Preventive Services*.[89]

There are important distinctions between evidence-based approaches in medicine and public health. First, the type and volume of evidence differ. Medical studies of pharmaceuticals and procedures often rely on randomized controlled trials of individuals, the most scientifically rigorous of epidemiologic studies. In contrast, public health interventions usually rely on cross-sectional studies, quasi-experimental designs, and time-series analyses. These studies sometimes lack a comparison group and require more caveats in interpretation of results. Over the past 50 years, there have been over one million randomized controlled trials of medical treatments.[90] There are far fewer studies of the effectiveness of public health interventions[5,91] because they are difficult to design and often results derive from natural experiments (e.g., a state adopting a new policy compared to other states). EBPH has borrowed the term "intervention" from clinical disciplines, insinuating specificity and discreteness. However, in public health, there is seldom a single "intervention" but, rather, a program that involves a blending of several interventions within a community. Large community-based trials can be more expensive to conduct than randomized experiments in a clinic. **Population-based** studies generally require a longer time period between intervention and outcome. For example, a study on the effects of smoking cessation on lung cancer mortality would require decades of data collection and analysis. Contrast that with treatment of a medical condition (e.g., an antibiotic for symptoms of pneumonia) that is likely to produce effects in days or weeks, or even a surgical trial for cancer with endpoints of mortality within a few years.

The formal training of persons working in public health is much more varied than that in medicine or other clinical disciplines.[92] Unlike medicine, public health relies on a variety of disciplines; no single academic credential "certifies" a public health practitioner, although efforts to establish credentials (via an exam) are now in place for those with formal public health training (e.g., the National Board of Public Health Examiners Certified in Public Health exam).[93] This higher level of heterogeneity means that multiple perspectives are involved in a more complicated decision-making process. It also suggests that effective public health practice places a premium on routine, on-the-job training.

KEY CHARACTERISTICS OF EVIDENCE-BASED DECISION MAKING

It is useful to consider several overarching, common characteristics of an evidence-based approach to public health practice. These notions are expanded upon in other chapters. Described below, these various attributes of EBPH and key characteristics include:

▹ Making decisions based on the best available peer-reviewed evidence (both quantitative and qualitative research);
▹ Using data and information systems systematically;
▹ Applying program planning frameworks (that often have a foundation in behavioral science theory);
▹ Engaging the community in assessment and decision making;
▹ Conducting sound evaluation; and
▹ Disseminating what is learned to key stakeholders and decision makers.

Accomplishing these activities in EBPH is likely to require a synthesis of scientific skills, enhanced communication, common sense, and political acumen.

Decisions Are Based on the Best Available Evidence

As one evaluates Type 2 evidence, it is useful to understand where to turn for the best available scientific evidence. A starting point is the scientific literature and guidelines developed by expert panels. In addition, preliminary findings from researchers and practitioners are often presented at regional, national, and international professional meetings.

Data and Information Systems Are Used

A tried-and-true public health adage is "what gets measured, gets done."[94] This has typically been applied to long-term endpoints (e.g., rates of mortality) and data for many public health endpoints and populations are not readily available at one's fingertips. Data are being developed more for local level issues (e.g., the Selected Metropolitan/Micropolitan Area Risk Trends of the Behavioral Risk Factor Surveillance System [SMART BRFSS]) and a few early efforts are underway to develop public health policy surveillance systems (see Chapter 32).

Systematic Program Planning Approaches Are Used

When an approach is decided upon, a variety of planning frameworks and theories can be applied. As an example, ecological or systems models are increasingly used in which changes in the social environment will produce changes in individuals and the support of individuals in a population is essential for implementing environmental changes.[95] These models point to the importance of addressing problems at multiple levels and stress the interaction and integration of factors within and across all levels—individual, interpersonal, community, organizational, and governmental. The goal is to create a healthy community environment that provides health-promoting information and social support to enable people to live healthier lifestyles.[96] Effective interventions are most often grounded in health behavior theory.[48,97]

Community Engagement Occurs

Community-based approaches involve community members in research and intervention projects and show progress in improving population health and addressing health disparities.[98,99] As a critical step in transdisciplinary problem solving, practitioners, academicians, and community members collaboratively define issues of concern, develop strategies for intervention, and evaluate the outcomes. This approach relies on "stakeholder" input,[100] builds on existing resources, facilitates collaboration among all parties, and integrates knowledge and action that seeks to lead to a fair distribution of the benefits of an intervention for all partners.[99,101]

Sound Evaluation Principles Are Followed

Too often in public health, programs and policies are implemented without much attention to systematic evaluation. In addition, even when programs are ineffective, they are sometimes continued because of historical or political considerations. Evaluation plans must be laid early in program development and should include both formative and outcome evaluation (as further described in Chapter 15). For example, an injury control program was appropriately discontinued after its effectiveness was evaluated. This program evaluation also illustrates the use of both qualitative and quantitative data in framing an evaluation.[102]

Results Are Disseminated to Others Who Need to Know

When a program or policy has been implemented, or when final results are known, others in public health can rely on findings to enhance their own use of evidence in decision making. Dissemination may occur to health professionals via the scientific literature, to the general public via the media, to policy makers through personal meetings, and to public health professionals through training courses. It is important to identify appropriate targets for dissemination, since public health professionals differ in where they seek information, e.g., public health practitioners prefer peer leaders in practice, while academicians prefer peer-reviewed journals.[103] Effective interventions are needed in a variety of settings, including schools, worksites, health care settings, and broader community environments.

ANALYTIC TOOLS AND APPROACHES TO ENHANCE THE UPTAKE OF EBPH

Several analytic tools and planning approaches can help practitioners in answering questions such as:

▸ What is the size of the public health problem?
▸ Are there effective interventions for addressing the problem?
▸ What information about the local context and this particular intervention is helpful in deciding its potential use in the situation at hand?
▸ Is a particular program or policy worth doing (i.e., is it better than alternatives) and will it provide a satisfactory return on investment, measured in monetary terms or in health impacts?

Public Health Surveillance

Public health surveillance is a critical tool for those using EBPH (as will be described in much more detail in Chapter 12). It involves the ongoing systematic collection, analysis, and interpretation of specific health data, closely integrated with the timely dissemination of these data to those responsible for preventing and controlling disease or injury.[104] Public health surveillance systems should have the capacity to collect and analyze data, disseminate data to public health programs, and regularly evaluate the effectiveness of the use of the disseminated data.[105] For example, documentation of the prevalence of elevated levels of lead (a known toxicant) in blood in the U.S. population was used as the justification for eliminating lead from paint and then gasoline and for documenting the effects of these actions.[106]

Systematic Reviews and Evidence-Based Guidelines

Systematic reviews are syntheses of comprehensive collections of information on a particular topic. Reading a good review can be one of the most efficient ways to become familiar with state-of-the-art research and practice on many specific topics in public health.[107–109] The use of explicit, systematic methods (i.e., decision rules) in reviews limits bias and reduces chance effects, thus providing more reliable results upon which to make decisions.[110] One of the most useful sets of reviews for public health interventions is the *Guide to Community Preventive Services* (the *Community Guide*),[31,111] which provides an overview of current scientific literature through a well-defined, rigorous method in which available studies themselves are the units of analysis. The *Community Guide* seeks to answer:

▸ What interventions have been evaluated and what have been their effects?
▸ What aspects of interventions can help *Community Guide* users select from among the set of interventions of proven effectiveness?
▸ What might these interventions cost and how do they compare with the likely health impacts?

A good systematic review should allow the practitioner to understand the local contextual conditions necessary for successful implementation.[112]

Economic Evaluation

Economic evaluation is an important component of evidence-based practice.[113] It can provide information to help assess the relative value of alternative expenditures on public health programs and policies. In cost-benefit analysis, all of the costs and consequences of the decision options are valued in monetary terms. More often, the economic investment associated with an intervention is compared with the health impacts, such as cases of disease prevented or years of life saved. This technique, known as cost-effectiveness analysis, can suggest the relative value of alternative interventions (i.e., health return on dollars invested).[113] Cost-effectiveness analysis has become an increasingly important tool for researchers, practitioners, and policy makers. However, relevant data to support this type of analysis are not always available, especially for possible public policies designed to improve health.[52,114] Additional information on economic evaluation is provided in Chapter 15.

Health Impact Assessment

Health impact assessment (HIA) is a relatively new method that seeks to estimate the probable impact of a policy or intervention in nonhealth sectors, such as agriculture, transportation, and economic development, on the health of the population.[115] Some HIAs have focused on ensuring the involvement of relevant stakeholders in the development of a specific project. This latter approach, the basis of environmental impact assessment required by law for many large place-based projects, is similar to the nonregulatory approach that has been adopted for some HIAs. Overall, HIA, in both its forms, has been gaining acceptance as a tool because of mounting evidence that social and physical environments are important determinants of health and health disparities in populations. It is now being used to help assess the potential effects of many policies and programs on health status and outcomes.[116-118] This approach dovetails with the conceptualization and application of Health in All Policies (see Chapter 32).

Participatory Approaches

Participatory approaches that actively involve community members in research and intervention projects[98,99,119] show promise in engaging communities in EBPH.[35] Practitioners, academicians, and community members collaboratively define issues of concern, develop strategies for intervention, and evaluate the outcomes. This approach relies on "stakeholder" input,[100] builds on existing resources, facilitates collaboration among all parties, and integrates knowledge and action that hopefully will lead to a fair distribution of the benefits of an intervention or project for all partners.[99,101] Stakeholders, or key players, are individuals or agencies that have a vested interest in the issue at hand.[120] In the development of health policies, for example, policy makers are especially important stakeholders.[121] Stakeholders should include those who would potentially receive, use, and benefit from the program or policy being considered. Three groups of stakeholders are relevant: people developing programs, those affected by interventions, and those who use results of program evaluations. Participatory approaches may also present challenges in adhering to EBPH principles, especially in reaching agreement on which approaches are most appropriate for addressing a particular health problem.[122]

Addressing Administrative Evidence-Based Practices

Fostering EBPH requires a combination of applying evidence-based interventions from scientific sources (e.g., the *Community Guide*,[31] the Cochrane Collaboration[123]) along with performance in carrying out effective organizational practices in health departments or other agencies. This process of EBPH can include so-called "administrative evidence-based practices," which are structures and activities occurring at the agency (health department) and the work unit level that are positively associated with performance measures (e.g., achieving core public health functions, carrying out evidence-based interventions).[37] These administrative evidence-based practices often fit under the umbrella of public health services and systems research,[124,125] and cover five major domains of workforce development: leadership, organizational climate and culture, relationships and partnerships, and financial processes. These practices were recently articulated via a literature review[37] and are potentially modifiable within a few years, making them useful targets for quality improvement efforts.[126-129] Recent studies have begun to measure and track these administrative evidence-based practices.[130,131]

AN APPROACH TO INCREASING THE USE OF EVIDENCE IN PUBLIC HEALTH PRACTICE

Strengthening EBPH competencies needs to take into account the diverse education and training backgrounds of the workforce. The emphasis on principles of EBPH is not uniformly taught in all the disciplines represented in the public health workforce. For example, a public health nurse is likely to have had less training in how to locate the most current evidence and interpret alternatives than an epidemiologist. A recently graduated health educator with an MPH is more likely to have gained an understanding of the importance of EBPH than an environmental health specialist holding a bachelor's degree. Probably fewer than half of public health workers have any formal training in a public health discipline such as epidemiology or health education.[132] An even smaller percentage of these professionals have formal graduate training from a school of public health or other public health program. Currently, it appears that few public health departments have made continuing education about EBPH mandatory.

While the formal concept of EBPH is relatively new, the underlying skills are not. For example, reviewing the scientific literature for evidence or evaluating a program intervention are skills often taught in graduate programs in public health or other academic disciplines and are building blocks of public health practice. The most commonly applied framework in EBPH is probably that of Brownson and colleagues (Figure 11-3), which uses a seven-stage process[5,64,133] that is nonlinear and entails numerous iterations.[134] Competencies for more effective public health practice are becoming clearer.[135–137] For example, to carry out the EBPH process, the skills needed to make evidence-based decisions require a specific set of competencies (see Table 11-3).[138] Many of the competencies on this list illustrate the value of developing partnerships and engaging diverse disciplines in the EBPH process.

To address these and similar competencies, EBPH training programs have been developed to train public health professionals,[64,139–143] local health departments, and community-based organizations,[17,144] and similar programs have been developed in other countries.[133,145,146] Some of these training programs show evidence of effectiveness.[17,64,141] The most common format uses didactic sessions, computer labs, and scenario-based exercises, taught by a faculty team with expertise in EBPH. The reach of these training programs can be increased by emphasizing a train-the-trainer approach.[133,147] Other formats have

been used including Internet-based self-study,[144,148] CD-ROMs,[149] distance and distributed learning networks, and targeted technical assistance. Training programs may have greater impact when delivered by "change agents" who are perceived as experts yet share common characteristics and goals with trainees.[150] A commitment from leadership and staff to lifelong learning is also an essential ingredient for success in training[151] and is itself an example of evidence-based decision making.[37]

Implementation of training to address EBPH competencies should take into account principles of adult learning. These issues were recently articulated by Bryan and colleagues,[152] who highlighted the need to: (1) know why the audience is learning; (2) tap into an underlying motivation to learn by the need to solve problems; (3) respect and build upon previous experience; (4) design learning approaches that match the background and diversity of recipients; and (5) actively involve the audience in the learning process.

In this section, a seven-stage, sequential framework to promote greater use of evidence in day-to-day decision making is briefly described (Figure 11-3).[41] It is important to note that this process is seldom a strictly

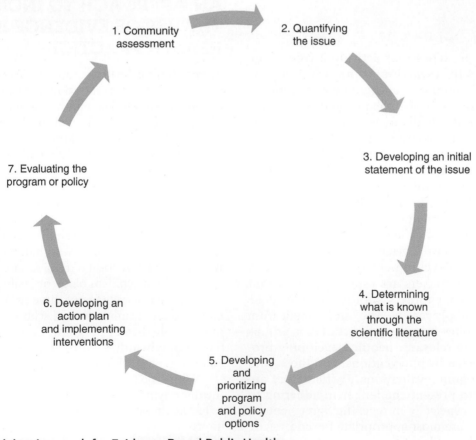

FIGURE 11-3   Training Approach for Evidence-Based Public Health

SUMMARY

The successful implementation of EBPH in public health practice is both a science and an art. The science is built on epidemiologic, behavioral, and policy research showing the size and scope of a public health problem and which interventions are likely to be effective in addressing the problem. The art of decision making often involves knowing what information is important to a particular stakeholder at the right time. Unlike solving a math problem, significant decisions in public health must balance science and art, since rational, evidence-based decision making often involves choosing one alternative from among a set of rational choices. By applying the concepts of EBPH outlined in this chapter, decision making and, ultimately, public health practice, can be improved.

REVIEW QUESTIONS

1. If one is seeking to find more Type 3 (contextual) evidence, what are the methods for obtaining this information?

2. In understanding the seven-stage framework for EBPH, what are the core public health disciplines that might be most useful or informative within each of the seven stages?

3. Choose an important current public health problem. In addressing this problem, think about which disciplines outside of the health sector might be important for addressing the issue.

4. For the same problem, how might participatory approaches help you in engaging these various disciplines or sectors?

5. In addition to the barriers to EBPH covered in this chapter, consider additional barriers that might limit your ability to implement a transdisciplinary approach to evidence-based decision making. How might you begin to overcome these barriers?

ACKNOWLEDGMENTS

Parts of this chapter were adapted with permission from the **Annual Review of Public Health**, Volume 30 ©2009 by Annual Reviews http://www.annualreviews.org. The authors are also grateful for the input of Jonathan Fielding and Christopher Maylahn.

REFERENCES

1. National Center for Health Statistics. *Health, United States, 2000 with Adolescent Health Chartbook*. Hyattsville, MD: Centers for Disease Control and Prevention, National Center for Health Statistics; 2000.

2. Centers for Disease Control and Prevention. *Public Health in the New American Health System. Discussion Paper*. Atlanta, GA: Centers for Disease Control and Prevention; March, 1993.

3. Muir Gray JA. *Evidence-Based Healthcare: How to Make Health Policy and Management Decisions*. New York and Edinburgh: Churchill Livingstone; 1997.

4. Brownson RC, Fielding JE, Maylahn CM. Evidence-based public health: A fundamental concept for public health practice. *Annu Rev Public Health*. April 21, 2009;30:175–201.

5. Brownson RC, Baker EA, Leet TL, Gillespie KN, True WR. *Evidence-Based Public Health*. 2nd ed. New York: Oxford University Press; 2011.

6. Glasziou P, Longbottom H. Evidence-based public health practice. *Australian and New Zealand Journal of Public Health*. 1999;23(4):436–440.

7. McMichael C, Waters E, Volmink J. Evidence-based public health: what does it offer developing countries? *J Public Health (Oxf)*. June 2005;27(2):215–221.

8. Fielding JE, Briss PA. Promoting evidence-based public health policy: can we have better evidence and more action? *Health Aff (Millwood)*. July–August 2006;25(4):969–78.

9. Hausman AJ. Implications of evidence-based practice for community health. *Am J Community Psychol*. June 2002;30(3):453–67.

10. Kohatsu ND, Melton RJ. A health department perspective on the Guide to Community Preventive Services. *Am J Prev Med*. January 2000;18(1 Suppl):3–4.

11. Fielding JE. Where is the evidence? *Annu Rev Public Health*. 2001;22:v–vi.

12. Committee on Public Health Strategies to Improve Health. *For the Public's Health: Investing in a Healthier Future*. Washington, DC: Institute of Medicine of The National Academies; 2012.

13. IOM. Committee for the Study of the Future of Public Health. *The Future of Public Health*. Washington, DC: National Academy Press; 1988.

14. Dobbins M, Cockerill R, Barnsley J, Ciliska D. Factors of the innovation, organization, environment, and individual that predict the influence five systematic reviews had on public health decisions. *Int J Technol Assess Health Care*. Fall 2001;17(4):467–78.

15. Dodson EA, Baker EA, Brownson RC. Use of evidence-based interventions in state health departments: a qualitative assessment of barriers and solutions. *J Public Health Manag Pract*. November–December 2010;16(6):E9–E15.

16. Jacobs JA, Dodson EA, Baker EA, Deshpande AD, Brownson RC. Barriers to evidence-based decision making in public health: a national survey of chronic disease practitioners. *Public Health Rep*. September–October 2010;125(5):736–742.

17. Maylahn C, Bohn C, Hammer M, Waltz E. Strengthening epidemiologic competencies among local health professionals in New York: teaching evidence-based public health. *Public Health Rep*. 2008;123(Suppl 1):35–43.

18. Frieden TR. Six components necessary for effective public health program implementation. *Am J Public Health*. January 2013;104(1):17–22.

19. Murphy K, Wolfus B, Lofters A. From complex problems to complex problem-solving: Transdisciplinary practice as knowledge translation. In: Kirst M, Schaefer-McDaniel N, Hwang S, O'Campo P, eds. *Converging Disciplines: A Transdisciplinary Research Approach to Urban Health Problems*. New York: Springer; 2011:111–29.

20. Roussos ST, Fawcett SB. A review of collaborative partnerships as a strategy for improving community health. *Annu Rev Public Health*. 2000;21:369–402.

21. Harper GW, Neubauer LC, Bangi AK, Francisco VT. Transdisciplinary research and evaluation for community health initiatives. *Health Promot Pract*. October 2008;9(4):328–37.

22. Stokols D. Toward a science of transdisciplinary action research. *Am J Community Psychol*. September 2006;38(1–2):63–77.

23. Kobus K, Mermelstein R. Bridging basic and clinical science with policy studies: The Partners with Transdisciplinary Tobacco Use Research Centers experience. *Nicotine Tob Res*. May 2009;11(5):467–474.

24. Kobus K, Mermelstein R, Ponkshe P. Communications strategies to broaden the reach of tobacco use research: examples from the Transdisciplinary Tobacco Use Research Centers. *Nicotine Tob Res*. November 2007;9 Suppl 4:S571–582.

25. Morgan GD, Kobus K, Gerlach KK, et al. Facilitating transdisciplinary research: the experience of the transdisciplinary tobacco use research centers. *Nicotine Tob Res*. December 2003;5 Suppl 1:S11–19.

26. Byrne S, Wake M, Blumberg D, Dibley M. Identifying priority areas for longitudinal research in childhood obesity: Delphi technique survey. *Int J Pediatr Obes*. 2008;3(2):120–122.

27. Russell-Mayhew S, Scott C, Stewart M. The Canadian Obesity Network and interprofessional practice: members' views. *J Interprof Care*. March 2008;22(2):149–65.

28. Black BL, Cowens-Alvarado R, Gershman S, Weir HK. Using data to motivate action: the need for high quality, an effective presentation, and an action context for decision-making. *Cancer Causes Control*. October 2005;16 Suppl 1:15–25.

29. Curry S, Byers T, Hewitt M, eds. *Fulfilling the Potential of Cancer Prevention and Early Detection*. Washington, DC: National Academies Press; 2003.

30. Briss PA, Brownson RC, Fielding JE, Zaza S. Developing and using the Guide to Community Preventive Services: lessons learned About evidence-based public health. *Annu Rev Public Health*. January 2004;25:281–302.

31. Zaza S, Briss PA, Harris KW, eds. *The Guide to Community Preventive Services: What Works to Promote Health?* New York: Oxford University Press; 2005.

32. Agency for Healthcare Research and Quality. Guide to Clinical Preventive Services, 3d Edition, Periodic Updates. 3d: http://www.ahrq.gov/clinic/gcpspu.htm Accessed October 11, 2005, 2005.

33. Cancer Control PLANET. Cancer Control PLANET. Links resources to comprehensive cancer control. http://cancercontrolplanet.cancer.gov/index.html Accessed May 26, 2008.

34. SAMHSA. SAMHSA's National Registry of Evidence-based Programs and Practices. http://www.nrepp.samhsa.gov/. Accessed August 16, 2008.

35. Kohatsu ND, Robinson JG, Torner JC. Evidence-based public health: an evolving concept. *Am J Prev Med*. December 2004;27(5):417–421.

36. Green LW. Public health asks of systems science: to advance our evidence-based practice, can you help us get more practice-based evidence? *Am J Public Health*. March 2006;96(3):406–409.

37. Brownson RC, Allen P, Duggan K, Stamatakis KA, Erwin PC. Fostering more-effective public health by identifying administrative evidence-based practices: a review of the literature. *Am J Prev Med*. September 2012;43(3):309–319.

38. Kerner J, Rimer B, Emmons K. Introduction to the special section on dissemination: dissemination research and research dissemination: how can we close the gap? *Health Psychol.* September 2005;24(5):443–446.

39. Rychetnik L, Bauman A, Laws R, et al. Translating research for evidence-based public health: key concepts and future directions. *J Epidemiol Community Health.* December 2012;66(12):1187–1192.

40. Jenicek M. Epidemiology, evidence-based medicine, and evidence-based public health. *J Epidemiol Commun Health.* 1997;7:187–197.

41. Brownson RC, Gurney JG, Land G. Evidence-based decision making in public health. *J Public Health Manag Pract.* 1999;5:86–97.

42. Rychetnik L, Hawe P, Waters E, Barratt A, Frommer M. A glossary for evidence based public health. *J Epidemiol Community Health.* July 2004;58(7):538–545.

43. Satterfield JM, Spring B, Brownson RC, et al. Toward a transdisciplinary model of evidence-based practice. *Milbank Q.* June 2009;87(2):368–390.

44. McKean E, ed. *The New Oxford American Dictionary.* 2d ed. New York, NY: Oxford University Press; 2005.

45. McQueen DV. Strengthening the evidence base for health promotion. *Health Promot Int.* September 2001;16(3):261–268.

46. Chambers D, Kerner J. Closing the gap between discovery and delivery. *Dissemination and Implementation Research Workshop: Harnessing Science to Maximize Health.* Rockville, MD; 2007.

47. McQueen DV, Anderson LM. What counts as evidence? Issues and debates. In: Rootman, ed. *Evaluation in Health Promotion: Principles and Perspectives.* Copenhagen, Denmark: World Health Organization; 2001:63–81.

48. Rimer BK, Glanz DK, Rasband G. Searching for evidence about health education and health behavior interventions. *Health Educ Behav.* 2001;28(2):231–248.

49. Kerner JF. Integrating research, practice, and policy: what we see depends on where we stand. *J Public Health Manag Pract.* March–April 2008;14(2):193–198.

50. Mulrow CD, Lohr KN. Proof and policy from medical research evidence. *J Health Polit Policy Law.* April 2001;26(2):249–266.

51. Sturm R. Evidence-based health policy versus evidence-based medicine. *Psychiatr Serv.* December 2002;53(12):1499.

52. Brownson RC, Royer C, Ewing R, McBride TD. Researchers and policymakers: travelers in parallel universes. *Am J Prev Med.* February 2006;30(2):164–172.

53. Nutbeam D. How does evidence influence public health policy? Tackling health inequalities in England. *Health Promot J Aust.* 2003;14:154–158.

54. Ogilvie D, Egan M, Hamilton V, Petticrew M. Systematic reviews of health effects of social interventions: 2. Best available evidence: how low should you go? *J Epidemiol Community Health.* October 2005;59(10):886–892.

55. Glasgow RE, Green LW, Klesges LM, et al. External validity: we need to do more. *Ann Behav Med.* April 2006;31(2):105–108.

56. Green LW, Glasgow RE. Evaluating the relevance, generalization, and applicability of research: issues in external validation and translation methodology. *Eval Health Prof.* March 2006;29(1):126–153.

57. Castro FG, Barrera M, Jr., Martinez CR, Jr. The cultural adaptation of prevention interventions: resolving tensions between fidelity and fit. *Prev Sci.* March 2004;5(1):41–45.

58. Kerner JF, Guirguis-Blake J, Hennessy KD, et al. Translating research into improved outcomes in comprehensive cancer control. *Cancer Causes Control.* October 2005;16 Suppl 1:27–40.

59. Rychetnik L, Frommer M, Hawe P, Shiell A. Criteria for evaluating evidence on public health interventions. *J Epidemiol Community Health.* February 2002;56(2):119–127.

60. Glasgow RE. What types of evidence are most needed to advance behavioral medicine? *Ann Behav Med.* January–February 2008;35(1):19–25.

61. Kemm J. The limitations of "evidence-based" public health. *J Eval Clin Pract.* June 2006;12(3):319–24.

62. Dobrow MJ, Goel V, Upshur RE. Evidence-based health policy: context and utilisation. *Soc Sci Med.* January 2004;58(1):207–217.

63. Maslov A. A theory of human motivation. *Psychological Review.* 1943;50:370–96.

64. Dreisinger M, Leet TL, Baker EA, Gillespie KN, Haas B, Brownson RC. Improving the public health workforce: evaluation of a training course to enhance evidence-based decision making. *J Public Health Manag Pract.* March–April 2008;14(2):138–143.

65. Daar AS, Singer PA, Persad DL, et al. Grand challenges in chronic non-communicable diseases. *Nature.* November 22 2007;450(7169):494–496.

66. Pawson R, Greenhalgh T, Harvey G, Walshe K. Realist review – a new method of systematic review

designed for complex policy interventions. *J Health Serv Res Policy.* July 2005;10 Suppl 1:21–34.

67. Millward L, Kelly M, Nutbeam D. *Public Health Interventions Research: The Evidence.* London: Health Development Agency; 2003.

68. Petticrew M, Roberts H. Systematic reviews – do they "work" in informing decision-making around health inequalities? *Health Econ Policy Law.* April 2008;3(Pt 2):197–211.

69. Petticrew M, Cummins S, Ferrell C, et al. Natural experiments: an underused tool for public health? *Public Health.* September 2005;119(9):751–757.

70. Tones K. Beyond the randomized controlled trial: a case for 'judicial review'. *Health Educ Res.* June 1997;12(2):i–iv.

71. Steckler A, McLeroy KR, Goodman RM, Bird ST, McCormick L. Toward integrating qualitative and quantitative methods: an introduction. *Health Education Quarterly.* 1992;19(1):1–8.

72. Dorfman LE, Derish PA, Cohen JB. Hey Girlfriend: An evaluation of AIDS prevention among women in the sex industry. *Health Education Quarterly.* 1992;19(1):25–40.

73. Hugentobler M, Israel BA, Schurman SJ. An action research approach to workplace health: Integrating methods. *Health Educ Q.* 1992;19(1):55–76.

74. Goodman RM, Wheeler FC, Lee PR. Evaluation of the Heart to Heart Project: lessons from a community-based chronic disease prevention project. *Am J Health Promot.* 1995;9:443–455.

75. McQueen DV. The evidence debate. *J Epidemiol Community Health.* February 2002;56(2):83–84.

76. Suppe F. *The Structure of Scientific Theories.* 2d ed. Urbana, IL: University of Illinois Press; 1977.

77. Cavill N, Foster C, Oja P, Martin BW. An evidence-based approach to physical activity promotion and policy development in Europe: contrasting case studies. *Promot Educ.* 2006;13(2):104–111.

78. Bender K, Halverson PK. Quality improvement and accreditation: what might it look like? *J Public Health Manag Pract.* January–February 2010;16(1):79–82.

79. Public Health Accreditation Board. Public Health Accreditation Board Standards and Measures, version 1.5. 2013. http://www.phaboard.org/wp-content/uploads/SM-Version-1.5-Board-adopted-FINAL-01-24-2014.docx.pdf. Accessed December 7, 2014.

80. Fielding JE. Foreword. In: Brownson RC, Baker EA, Leet TL, Gillespie KN, eds. *Evidence-Based Public Health.* New York: Oxford University Press; 2003:v–vii.

81. Presidential Task Force on Evidence-Based Practice. Evidence-based practice in psychology. *Am Psychol.* May–June 2006;61(4):271–285.

82. Gambrill E. Evidence-based practice: Sea change or the emperor's new clothes? *J Social Work Educ.* 2003;39(1):3–23.

83. Mullen E, Bellamy J, Bledsoe S, Francois J. Teaching evidence-based practice. *Research on Social Work Practice.* 2007;17(5):574–582.

84. Melnyk BM, Fineout-Overholt E, Stone P, Ackerman M. Evidence-based practice: the past, the present, and recommendations for the millennium. *Pediatr Nurs.* January–February 2000;26(1):77–80.

85. Evidence-Based Medicine Working Group. Evidence-based medicine. A new approach to teaching the practice of medicine. *JAMA.* 1992;17:2420–2425.

86. Cochrane A. *Effectiveness and Efficiency: Random Reflections on Health Services.* London: Nuffield Provincial Hospital Trust; 1972.

87. Guyatt G, Cook D, Haynes B. Evidence based medicine has come a long way. *BMJ.* October 30, 2004;329(7473):990–991.

88. Canadian Task Force on the Periodic Health Examination. The periodic health examination. Canadian Task Force on the Periodic Health Examination. *Can Med Assoc J.* November 3, 1979;121(9):1193–254.

89. US Preventive Services Task Force. *Guide to Clinical Preventive Services: An Assessment of the Effectiveness of 169 Interventions.* Baltimore: Williams & Wilkins; 1989.

90. Taubes G. Looking for the evidence in medicine. *Science.* 1996;272:22–24.

91. Oldenburg BF, Sallis JF, French ML, Owen N. Health promotion research and the diffusion and institutionalization of interventions. *Health Educ Res.* February 1999;14(1):121–130.

92. Tilson H, Gebbie KM. The public health workforce. *Annu Rev Public Health.* 2004;25:341–356.

93. National Board of Public Health Examiners. Certified in Public Health. http://www.nbphe.org/examinfo.cfm. Accessed November 24, 2014.

94. Thacker SB. Public health surveillance and the prevention of injuries in sports: what gets measured gets done. *J Athl Train.* April–June 2007;42(2):171–172.

95. McLeroy KR, Bibeau D, Steckler A, Glanz K. An ecological perspective on health promotion programs. *Health Education Quarterly.* 1988;15:351–377.

96. Stokols D. Translating social ecological theory into guidelines for community health

promotion. *American Journal of Health Promotion.* 1996;10(4):282–298.

97. Glanz K, Bishop DB. The Role of Behavioral Science Theory in the Development and Implementation of Public Health Interventions. *Annu Rev Public Health.* January 4.

98. Cargo M, Mercer SL. The value and challenges of participatory research: Strengthening its practice. *Annu Rev Public Health.* April 21, 2008;29:325–350.

99. Israel BA, Schulz AJ, Parker EA, Becker AB. Review of community-based research: assessing partnership approaches to improve public health. *Annual Review of Public Health.* 1998;19:173–202.

100. Green LW, Mercer SL. Can public health researchers and agencies reconcile the push from funding bodies and the pull from communities? *Am J Public Health.* December 2001;91(12):1926–1929.

101. Leung MW, Yen IH, Minkler M. Community based participatory research: a promising approach for increasing epidemiology's relevance in the 21st century. *Int J Epidemiol.* June 2004;33(3):499–506.

102. Land G, Romeis JC, Gillespie KN, Denny S. Missouri's Take a Seat, Please! and Program Evaluation. *Journal of Public Health Management and Practice.* 1997;3(6):51–58.

103. Brownson R. Research Translation and Public Health Services & Systems Research. *Keeneland Conference: Public Health Services & Systems Research.* Lexington, KY; 2013.

104. Thacker SB, Berkelman RL. Public health surveillance in the United States. *Epidemiol Rev.* 1988;10:164–190.

105. Thacker SB, Stroup DF. Public health surveillance. In: Brownson RC, Petitti DB, eds. *Applied Epidemiology: Theory to Practice.* 2nd ed. New York, NY: Oxford University Press; 2006:30–67.

106. Annest JL, Pirkle JL, Makuc D, al e. Chronological trend in blood lead levels between 1976 and 1980. *N Engl J Med.* 1983;308:1373–1377.

107. Hutchison BG. Critical appraisal of review articles. *Can Fam Physician.* 1993;39:1097–1102.

108. Milne R, Chambers L. Assessing the scientific quality of review articles. *J Epidemiol Community Health.* 1993;47(3):169–170.

109. Mulrow CD. The medical review article: state of the science. *Ann Intern Med.* 1987;106(3):485–488.

110. Oxman AD, Guyatt GH. The science of reviewing research. *Ann N Y Acad Sci.* December 31 1993;703:125–133; discussion 133–124.

111. Mullen PD, Ramirez G. The promise and pitfalls of systematic reviews. *Annu Rev Public Health.* 2006;27:81–102.

112. Waters E, Doyle J. Evidence-based public health practice: improving the quality and quantity of the evidence. *J Public Health Med.* September 2002;24(3):227–229.

113. Gold MR, Siegel JE, Russell LB, Weinstein MC. *Cost-Effectiveness in Health and Medicine.* New York: Oxford University Press; 1996.

114. Carande-Kulis VG, Maciosek MV, Briss PA, et al. Methods for systematic reviews of economic evaluations for the Guide to Community Preventive Services. Task Force on Community Preventive Services. *Am J Prev Med.* January 2000;18 (1 Suppl):75–91.

115. Harris P, Harris-Roxas B, Harris E, Kemp L. *Health Impact Assessment: A Practical Guide.* Sydney: Australia: Centre for Health Equity Training, Research and Evaluation (CHETRE). Part of the UNSW Research Centre for Primary Health Care and Equity, UNSW; August 2007.

116. Cole BL, Wilhelm M, Long PV, Fielding JE, Kominski G, Morgenstern H. Prospects for health impact assessment in the United States: new and improved environmental impact assessment or something different? *J Health Polit Policy Law.* December 2004;29(6):1153–1186.

117. Kemm J. Health impact assessment: a tool for healthy public policy. *Health Promot Int.* March 2001;16(1):79–85.

118. Mindell J, Sheridan L, Joffe M, Samson-Barry H, Atkinson S. Health impact assessment as an agent of policy change: improving the health impacts of the mayor of London's draft transport strategy. *J Epidemiol Community Health.* March 2004;58(3):169–174.

119. Green LW, George MA, Daniel M, et al. *Review and Recommendations for the Development of Participatory Research in Health Promotion in Canada.* Vancouver, British Columbia: The Royal Society of Canada; 1995.

120. Soriano FI. *Conducting Needs Assessments. A Multidisciplinary Approach.* Thousand Oaks, CA: Sage Publications; 1995.

121. Sederburg WA. Perspectives of the legislator: allocating resources. *MMWR Morb Mortal Wkly Rep.* 1992;41(Suppl):37–48.

122. Hallfors D, Cho H, Livert D, Kadushin C. Fighting back against substance abuse: are community coalitions winning? *Am J Prev Med.* November 2002;23(4):237–245.

123. The Cochrane Public Health Group. The Cochrane Collaboration; 2013. http://ph.cochrane.org/. Updated Last Updated Date. Accessed July 13, 2013.

124. Mays GP, Scutchfield FD. Advancing the science of delivery: public health services and systems research. *J Public Health Manag Pract.* November 2012;18(6):481–484.

125. Scutchfield FD, Patrick K. Public health systems research: the new kid on the block. *Am J Prev Med.* February 2007;32(2):173–174.

126. Baker SL, Beitsch L, Landrum LB, Head R. The role of performance management and quality improvement in a national voluntary public health accreditation system. *J Public Health Manag Pract.* July–August 2007;13(4):427–429.

127. Beitsch LM, Leep C, Shah G, Brooks RG, Pestronk RM. Quality improvement in local health departments: results of the NACCHO 2008 survey. *J Public Health Manag Pract.* January–February 2010;16(1):49–54.

128. Drabczyk A, Epstein P, Marshall M. A quality improvement initiative to enhance public health workforce capabilities. *J Public Health Manag Pract.* January–February 2012;18(1):95–99.

129. Erwin PC. The performance of local health departments: a review of the literature. *J Public Health Manag Pract.* March–April 2008;14(2):E9–18.

130. Brownson RC, Reis RS, Allen P, et al. Understanding administrative evidence-based practices: findings from a survey of local health department leaders. *Am J Prev Med.* January 2013;46(1):49–57.

131. Erwin PC, Harris JK, Smith C, Leep CJ, Duggan K, Brownson RC. Evidence-Based Public Health Practice Among Program Managers in Local Public Health Departments. *J Public Health Manag Pract.* November 18, 2013.

132. Turnock BJ. *Public Health: What it is and How it Works.* Fourth ed. Sudbury, MA: Jones and Bartlett Publishers; 2009.

133. Brownson RC, Diem G, Grabauskas V, et al. Training practitioners in evidence-based chronic disease prevention for global health. *Promot Educ.* 2007;14(3):159–163.

134. Tugwell P, Bennett KJ, Sackett DL, Haynes RB. The measurement iterative loop: a framework for the critical appraisal of need, benefits and costs of health interventions. *J Chronic Dis.* 1985;38(4):339–351.

135. Birkhead GS, Davies J, Miner K, Lemmings J, Koo D. Developing competencies for applied epidemiology: from process to product. *Public Health Rep.* 2008;123 Suppl 1:67–118.

136. Birkhead GS, Koo D. Professional competencies for applied epidemiologists: a roadmap to a more effective epidemiologic workforce. *J Public Health Manag Pract.* November–December 2006;12(6):501–504.

137. Gebbie K, Merrill J, Hwang I, Gupta M, Btoush R, Wagner M. Identifying individual competency in emerging areas of practice: an applied approach. *Qual Health Res.* September 2002;12(7):990–99.

138. Brownson RC, Ballew P, Kittur ND, et al. Developing competencies for training practitioners in evidence-based cancer control. *J Cancer Educ.* 2009;24(3):186–93.

139. Baker EA, Brownson RC, Dreisinger M, McIntosh LD, Karamehic-Muratovic A. Examining the role of training in evidence-based public health: a qualitative study. *Health Promot Pract.* July 2009;10(3):342–348.

140. Jansen MW, Hoeijmakers M. A masterclass to teach public health professionals to conduct practice-based research to promote evidence-based practice: a case study from The Netherlands. *J Public Health Manag Pract.* January–February 2012;19(1):83–92.

141. Gibbert WS, Keating SM, Jacobs JA, et al. Training the workforce in evidence-based public health: an evaluation of impact among us and international practitioners. *Prev Chronic Dis.* 2013;10:E148.

142. Pettman TL, Armstrong R, Jones K, Waters E, Doyle J. Cochrane update: building capacity in evidence-informed decision-making to improve public health. *J Public Health (Oxf).* December 2013;35(4):624–627.

143. Yost J, Ciliska D, Dobbins M. Evaluating the impact of an intensive education workshop on evidence-informed decision making knowledge, skills, and behaviours: a mixed methods study. *BMC Med Educ.* 2014;14:13.

144. Maxwell ML, Adily A, Ward JE. Promoting evidence-based practice in population health at the local level: a case study in workforce capacity development. *Aust Health Rev.* August 2007;31(3):422–429.

145. Oliver KB, Dalrymple P, Lehmann HP, McClellan DA, Robinson KA, Twose C. Bringing evidence to practice: a team approach to teaching skills required for an informationist role in evidence-based clinical and public health practice. *J Med Libr Assoc.* January 2008;96(1):50–57.

146. Pappaioanou M, Malison M, Wilkins K, et al. Strengthening capacity in developing countries for evidence-based public health: the data for decision-making project. *Soc Sci Med.* November 2003;57(10):1925–1937.

147. Jacobs JA, Duggan K, Erwin P, et al. Capacity building for evidence-based decision making in local health departments: scaling up an effective training approach. *Implement Sci.* September 24, 2014;9(1):124.

148. Linkov F, LaPorte R, Lovalekar M, Dodani S. Web quality control for lectures: Supercourse and Amazon.com. *Croat Med J.* December 2005;46(6):875–878.

149. Brownson RC, Ballew P, Brown KL, et al. The effect of disseminating evidence-based interventions that promote physical activity to health departments. *Am J Public Health.* October 2007;97(10):1900–1907.

150. Proctor EK. Leverage points for the implementation of evidence-based practice. *Brief Treatment and Crisis Intervention.* September 2004;4(3):227–242.

151. Chambers LW. The new public health: do local public health agencies need a booster (or organizational "fix") to combat the diseases of disarray? *Can J Public Health.* September–October 1992;83(5):326–328.

152. Bryan RL, Kreuter MW, Brownson RC. Integrating Adult Learning Principles Into Training for Public Health Practice. *Health Promot Pract.* April 2, 2008.

153. Ginter PM, Duncan WJ, Capper SA. Keeping strategic thinking in strategic planning: macro-environmental analysis in a state health department of public health. *Public Health.* 1992;106:253–269.

154. Florin P, Stevenson J. Identifying training and technical assistance needs in community coalitions: a developmental approach. *Health Education Research.* 1993;8:417–432.

155. Kaplan GE, Juhl AL, Gujral IB, Hoaglin-Wagner AL, Gabella BA, McDermott KM. Tools for identifying and prioritizing evidence-based obesity prevention strategies, Colorado. *Prev Chronic Dis.* 2013;10:E106.

156. Robeson P, Dobbins M, DeCorby K, Tirilis D. Facilitating access to pre-processed research evidence in public health. *BMC Public Health.*10:95.

157. Ramanadhan S, Crisostomo J, Alexander-Molloy J, et al. Perceptions of evidence-based programs among community-based organizations tackling health disparities: a qualitative study. *Health Educ Res.* August 2011;27(4):717–728.

158. IOM. Committee on Public Health. *Healthy Communities: New Partnerships for the Future of Public Health.* Washington, DC: National Academy Press; 1996.

159. Wright K, Rowitz L, Merkle A, et al. Competency development in public health leadership. *Am J Public Health.* August 2000;90(8):1202–1207.

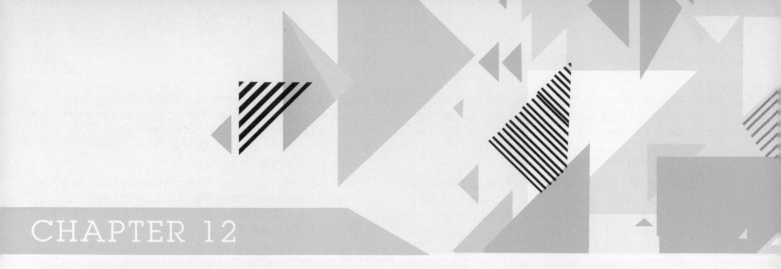

CHAPTER 12

Quantitative Sciences: Epidemiology, Biostatistics, and the Use of Public Health Data

Margaret Shih, MD, PhD • Steven M. Teutsch, MD, MPH • Ross C. Brownson, PhD

LEARNING OBJECTIVES

Upon completion of this chapter, the reader will be able to:

1. Understand and apply basic epidemiologic methods.

2. Understand the basic definition and components of public health surveillance.

3. Recognize and apply ethical principles to the conduct of public health surveillance.

4. Identify and evaluate relevant public health data sources.

5. Recognize how epidemiologic and public health surveillance data can contribute to public health policy decisions.

6. Understand the role of systematic reviews in public health practice.

7. Describe the uses of Geographic Information Systems in public health practice.

KEY TERMS

analytic epidemiology
descriptive epidemiology
Geographic Information Systems (GIS)
health impact assessment (HIA)
prevention effectiveness
surveillance
systematic review

EPIDEMIOLOGY AND BIOSTATISTICS—FOUNDATIONAL TOOLS FOR PUBLIC HEALTH PRACTICE

A solid grounding in the quantitative sciences is essential for every public health practitioner. Epidemiology and biostatistics provide the necessary foundations for measuring and understanding populations, defining health problems, quantifying risks, and identifying policies and programs that work. The practice of epidemiology is the study of the distribution and determinants of health-related states or events and the application of this study to the control of health problems.[1] Alexander Langmuir expressed that the "...basic operation of the epidemiologist is to count cases and measure the population in which they arise," so that rates can be calculated and the occurrence of a health problem can be compared among different groups of people.[2] Biostatistics is the application of statistics to biological problems, health, and medicine. Its importance to public health is in its application to finding and characterizing underlying patterns, comparing populations, distinguishing randomness from nonrandomness, measuring, controlling, and communicating uncertainty, and addressing variation in data to reach meaningful and reliable conclusions.[3]

Descriptive Epidemiology

Descriptive epidemiology concerns the study of the distribution of health-related outcomes or events. In descriptive epidemiology, data (or observations) at the population level are organized and summarized quantitatively by person, place, and time. This important initial step allows epidemiologists to gain a better understanding of the data and population of interest, look for patterns and trends, and generate hypotheses for further study.

Measuring Populations

In epidemiology, a comprehensive understanding of the population of interest is essential. People can be described in terms of their inherent characteristics (age, sex, race), acquired characteristics (marital status, vaccination status), behaviors and activities (occupation, leisure activities, use of medications/tobacco/seat belts), and the circumstances under which they live (socioeconomic status, access to health care). These characteristics, activities, and conditions determine to a large degree who is at increased or decreased risk for different diseases and other adverse health outcomes. With the development of sophisticated molecular techniques, descriptive epidemiology now extends to assessing the role of individual genetic risk for disease.[4] More complex methods to assess patterns in personal characteristics include logistic regression, classification and regression tree analysis,[5] and categorical methods.[6]

Graphs, tables, and descriptive statistics are useful for organizing and summarizing the data once collected or acquired. A useful first step is to summarize the data graphically. Histograms, stem-and-leaf plots, and box plots are used to examine the frequency distribution to help identify outliers and the shape of the distribution. The data can also be described numerically using measures of central tendency and measures of spread. Measures of central tendency such as the mean, median, and mode, indicate the center, or middle of a distribution of observations. Measures of spread such as the range, standard deviation, and variance, are important for describing the variability, or dispersion of the data.[7]

Measures of Disease Frequency and Burden

The most common health outcomes measured by public health agencies are those related to morbidity (illness, injury, and disability), mortality (death), and natality (birth). Morbidity measures include disease incidence and prevalence. Mortality measures include crude, specific, and standardized mortality rates as well as years of potential life lost.

Morbidity measures quantify a population's likelihood of developing or having an illness, injury, disability, or other adverse health condition. An incidence rate is the rate at which new events (e.g., new cases of disease) occur among a population during a specified period. The numerator is the number of persons who experience new cases of illness among a population during the stated period. The denominator is either a sum of the time during which all persons were observed (person-time rate) or the average or midperiod size of the population at risk.

An attack rate or cumulative incidence is a measure of incidence calculated most commonly during the investigation of an acute outbreak of disease. This number is simply the proportion of the population that experienced illness during a specified period. The numerator is the number of new cases. The denominator is the size of the population at risk at the beginning of the observation period. The attack rate is a measure of the probability or risk of experiencing illness.

The prevalence is the proportion of persons among a population who have a particular disease or attribute at a specific point in time or during a specified period. Prevalence differs from incidence in that prevalence includes all cases, both old and new, whereas incidence is limited to new cases only. Point prevalence refers to prevalence measured at a particular point in time (i.e., the proportion of persons with a particular disease or attribute on a particular date). Period prevalence refers to prevalence measured over an interval of time (i.e., the proportion of persons who had a particular disease or attribute at any time during the interval). Prevalence is most often measured by cross-sectional surveys of a population.

The mortality rate, or death rate, estimates the frequency of occurrence of death among a defined population during a specified period. The crude death rate (or crude mortality rate) is the number of deaths from all causes for the entire population, divided by the population. In the United States in 2010, a total of 2,468,435 deaths were recorded. The 2010 estimated midyear population was 308,745,538. The crude mortality rate, therefore, was 799.5 deaths/100,000 population.[8]

Epidemiologists are often interested in comparing mortality rates among different populations or the same population across time. However, if these populations differ by factors such as age, gender, or race, these comparisons may be confounded, and the crude death rates must be adjusted. For example, because death rates increase with age, a higher crude death rate among one population than another might simply reflect that the first population is older, on average, than the second. When the underlying age distribution of two (or more) populations varies, practitioners can either compare age-specific death rates or compute age-standardized (or age-adjusted) death rates. An age-specific death rate is a death rate limited to a particular age group. Similarly, a gender-specific or race-specific death rate is limited to one gender or one racial group, respectively. Age-standardized death rates are based on statistical techniques that eliminate the effects of different age distributions among different populations. This is accomplished by applying the observed age-specific rates from each population to a standard population.[9]

Death rates can also be calculated for a specified cause for a population. The numerator is the number of deaths attributed to a specific cause. The denominator is the same as the crude death rate (i.e., an estimate of the entire population). Cause-specific death rates are usually expressed per 100,000 population. In the United States, diseases of the heart and malignant neoplasms have had the two highest cause-specific death rates since at least 1950, but the gap between the two has narrowed considerably.[8]

The infant mortality rate, a type of age-specific death rate, is used by all nations as a key public health indicator. The numerator is the number of deaths among infants who die before 1 year of age during a specific

period, usually a calendar year. The denominator is the number of live births reported during the same period. The infant mortality rate is usually expressed per 1,000 live births. In 2010, the U.S. infant mortality rate was 6.14 infant deaths/1,000 live births.[10]

Years of potential life lost (YPLL) is a measure of the impact of premature mortality on a population. For a person who dies "prematurely" (usually defined as either before age 75 years or before the average life expectancy is reached), YPLL is calculated as the difference between that defined end point and the actual age at death. For an entire population, the YPLL is the sum of the individual YPLLs (Figure 12-1). The YPLL rate represents years of potential life lost per 1,000 population who are aged less than the specified end point. YPLL rates are used to compare premature mortality among different populations, because YPLL alone does not involve consideration of differences in population size. Furthermore, YPLL rates can be standardized by age to adjust for differences in the underlying age distribution of populations.

Another approach to estimating overall burden of disease is to use health-adjusted life years (HALYs). These are population health measures which allow morbidity and mortality to be described by a single number. They can be particularly useful for comparing the relative impact of specific illnesses and conditions on communities, and in economic analyses. Quality-adjusted life years (QALYs) and disability-adjusted life years (DALYs) are types of HALYs.

Quality-adjusted life years (QALYs) is the standard unit of measure in a cost-utility analysis that reflects the quality of life, or desirability of living, as well as the duration of survival. Quality of life is integrated with length of life by using a multiplicative formula and discounting length of life by the quality of life expected.[11] The measures are based on surveys of individual persons, where they are asked to weigh a particular health state against perfect health and against death by using methods such as person tradeoff, time tradeoff, and standard gamble.[11]

Disability-adjusted life years (DALYs) is a variant of QALYs used by the World Health Organization (WHO) that measures the burden of disease, not only from premature mortality, but also from disability. It is a composite measure (sum) of time lost as a result of premature mortality (Years of Life Lost, or YLL), and time lived with a disability, adjusted for the severity of the disability. An expert panel weights the severity of disability by using methods similar to those used for QALYs. Also included in the calculation of DALYs are age weights (different values of life for each age) and discounted future years of life.[12] Critics of using DALYs have examined the heuristic nature of the value

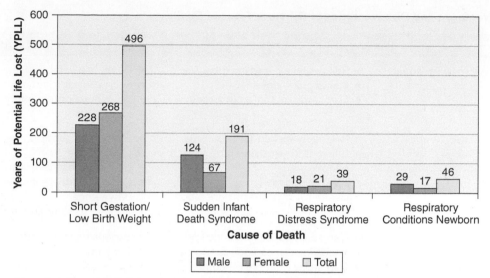

FIGURE 12-1 **Smoking Attributable Years of Potential Life Lost (YPLL) for Infants Born in Massachusetts, 2001**

SOURCE: Published in American Journal of Preventive Medicine, Vol 4, Livengood et al., pp 268-73, Copyright Elsevier (1988).

judgments and the fact that the components do not allow a distinction between use for measuring burden and allocating resources and the fact that age-weighting and discounting methods minimize the importance of conditions affecting older persons, younger persons, and those living with a disability.[13]

Analytic Epidemiology

Descriptive epidemiology often suggests where to look more closely at the data and leads to the generation of hypotheses that can be analyzed using inferential methods. **Analytic epidemiology** is concerned with the study of the determinants—the causes and risk factors—or the "why" or "how" of a health-related outcome. Determinants of health-related outcomes refer to both the direct causes of the health outcome and the factors that determine the risk for the outcome. Analytic epidemiology makes use of inferential statistics to evaluate the data, assess the strength of the evidence for or against a hypothesis, make comparisons, and generalize conclusions from a representative sample of data to the whole population.

A key feature of analytic epidemiology is the use of a comparison group. With a case report or case series, apparently unusual features can be described for one or more persons with disease, but this information cannot answer the question about how unusual those features really are. In an analytic epidemiologic study, the comparison group explicitly provides such information. If persons with a particular characteristic are more likely than those without the characteristic to

experience a certain disease, then the characteristic is said to be associated with the disease. The characteristic can be a demographic factor (e.g., age or gender), a constitutional factor (e.g., blood group or immune status), a behavior (e.g., smoking or having eaten potato salad), or a circumstance (e.g., living in a poor neighborhood). These factors help to identify populations at increased risk for disease, which can lead to appropriate targeting of public health prevention and control activities, as well as to ideas for future etiologic research.

Contingency Tables and Measures of Association

Many different types of studies can be used to generate data and to examine the relationships between risk factors and outcomes. These can be broadly categorized into observational (e.g., case-control and cohort studies) and experimental (e.g., laboratory and animal studies, randomized controlled trials).[14] Each has specific strengths and weaknesses that are described in Table 12-1. A contingency table is a common way to cross-classify study data in tabular form and to test for associations between variables. The simplest contingency table is the two-by-two table, which is illustrated in Table 12-2. Each cell contains the number of study subjects with the exposure status as indicated in the row heading to the left and with the disease status indicated in the column heading above. For example, c represents the number of persons in the study who were not exposed, but who became ill (or case subjects) nonetheless.

TABLE 12-1 Advantages and Disadvantages of Different Types of Studies

	Type of Study	Advantages	Disadvantages
Observational	Cross-Sectional	• Relatively fast and inexpensive • Yields prevalence • Can study multiple outcomes	• Unable to establish causal sequence • Self-reported data can result in bias • Difficult to obtain information on rare conditions
	Case-Control	• Relatively fast and inexpensive • Efficient for studying rare conditions • Yields odds ratio • Useful for hypothesis generation	• Cases and controls may not be comparable • Unable to establish causal sequence • Cannot estimate incidence or prevalence • Subject to sampling and recall bias
	Cohort	• Can study causal relationships • Yields incidence and relative risk • Can study multiple outcomes	• Expensive to conduct • Time-intensive • Not feasible for rare outcomes • Attrition of cohort over time
Experimental	Laboratory and Animal Studies	• Provides strong evidence for causal relationships • High internal validity	• Results difficult to extend to humans • Ethical concerns • Does not reflect 'real world' conditions
	Randomized Controlled Trials (RCTs)	• May be less expensive and faster than cohort studies • Provides strong evidence for causal relationships • Reduces or eliminates important sources of bias • High internal validity	• Expensive to conduct • Ethical constraints • Limited generalizability and external validity
	Nonrandomized, Quasi-experimental Studies	• Can make use of 'natural experiments' • High external validity • Avoids some of the ethical constraints of RCTs	• Unable to allocate subjects randomly • Reduced internal validity

TABLE 12-2 Data Layout and Notation for a Standard Two-by-Two Table

	Ill/Case-patients	Well/Control subjects	Total	Attack rate
Exposed	a	b	a + b	a/(a + c)
Unexposed	c	d	c + d	c /(c + d)
Total	a + c	b + d	a + b + c + d	(a + c)/(a + b + c + d)

Data from the investigation of an outbreak of gastro-enteritis following an Easter Sunday dinner are presented in Table 12-3. The table provides a cross-tabulation of ham consumption (exposure) by presence or absence of gastroenteritis (outcome). Attack rates (59.3 percent for those who ate ham; 14.3 percent for those who did not) are provided to the right of the table.

A measure of association quantifies the strength or magnitude of the association between the exposure and the disease or health outcome of interest. In cohort studies, where a defined population is usually followed over a long period of time, the measure of association used is the risk ratio or rate ratio (also referred to as relative risk). In case-control studies, where the past history of exposure

TABLE 12-3 Consumption of Ham and Risk for Gastroenteritis After an Easter Sunday Dinner, State A

	Ill	Well	Total	Attack rate
Ate ham	16	11	27	59.3%
Did not eat ham	1	6	7	14.3%
Total	17	17	34	50.0%

SOURCE: Cassius Lockett, California Department of Health Services, personal communication, 2000

TABLE 12-4 Legionnaires' Disease and Exposure to Hospital A, State B

	Case-patients	Control subjects	Total
Visited hospital	12	4	16
Did not visit hospital	1	18	19
Total	13	22	35

SOURCE: Joel Ackelsberg, New York City Department of Health, personal communication, 2000

to a risk factor of interest is compared between groups of individuals with (cases) and without (controls) the disease, the measure of choice is the odds ratio.

A risk ratio or relative risk compares the risk for disease or other health outcome between two groups (e.g., an exposed and unexposed group). It is calculated as the ratio of two risks, as follows:

$$\text{Risk ratio} = \frac{\text{risk}_{\text{exposed}}}{\text{risk}_{\text{unexposed}}} = \frac{a/h_1}{c/h_0}$$

The risk ratio based on the data presented in Table 12-3 is 59.3 / 14.3 = 4.1. That is, persons who ate ham were 4.1 times more likely to experience gastroenteritis than those who did not eat ham. The risk ratio will be > 1.0 when the risk among the exposed group is greater than the risk among the unexposed group. The risk will be equal to 1.0 if both groups have the same risk for disease (i.e., if exposure is unrelated to risk for disease). The risk will be < 1.0 if the risk for disease among the exposed group is less than the risk among the unexposed group, as would be expected when the exposure is a protective one such as vaccination or prophylactic antibiotic use.

In the majority of case-control studies, the sizes of the exposed and unexposed groups are unknown and the investigator decides the number of controls. Without true denominators, risks (e.g., attack rates) cannot be calculated; therefore, risk ratios cannot be calculated directly. However, the odds ratio can be calculated as its own measure of association, and when the disease is relatively rare, the odds ratio approximates the risk ratio. The odds ratio is calculated as:

$$\text{Odds ratio} = \frac{ad}{bc}$$

During an outbreak of Legionnaires' disease, 13 cases occurred among residents of a small community. Control subjects were selected from local physician logs. Ironically, visiting the local hospital appeared to be associated with illness, as displayed in Table 12-4. The odds ratio, calculated as 12 × 18/ (4 × 1), was

54.0. That is, cases (those with Legionnaires' disease) were 54 times more likely than controls (those without Legionnaires' disease) to have visited the hospital. This odds ratio indicates a strong association. Subsequent cultures of the cooling tower atop the hospital grew *Legionella pneumophila* with patterns indistinguishable from clinical samples from the patients.

Causal Inference, Bias, and Confounding

Not every elevated risk ratio or odds ratio indicates a significant or causal association between exposure and disease. Particularly when the risk ratio or odds ratio is only slightly different from 1.0, or when a study has a small number of subjects, the apparent association might simply be a chance finding. While tests of statistical significance and confidence intervals can be used to quantify the statistical likelihood of an observed measure of association,[7] potential explanations for the apparent association should be assessed first. In addition to chance, possible reasons include bias (e.g., selection bias, information bias), confounding, and investigator error.

Bias is a systematic error in how the study was conducted, and cannot be "corrected" by post hoc analytical methods. There are several types of bias which can result in errors of association. Selection bias is a systematic flaw in how participants were selected, enrolled, or categorized, which results in an erroneous estimate of the association between exposure and disease. Information bias is a systematic flaw in the information collected from or about the participants in the study that results in an erroneous estimate of the association between exposure and disease. If cases are more likely to recall an exposure than control subjects, then that exposure will appear to be associated with illness. If interviewers probe more thoroughly when interviewing cases than control subjects, or data abstractors review hospital charts of cases more vigorously than charts of control subjects, the exposure will appear to be associated with illness.

Another possible explanation for an observed association is "confounding." Confounding is a mixing of two effects, specifically when an unstudied risk factor is associated with both the exposure and outcome under study. Consider a hypothetical, poorly randomized clinical trial in which more cancer patients with early-stage disease receive investigational drug A than tried-and-true drug B, and more cancer patients with late-stage disease receive tried-and-true drug B than investigational drug A. Assume that persons with early-stage disease survive longer than persons with late-stage disease. Even if investigational drug A is no better than tried-and-true drug B, drug A will appear to be associated with improved survival, compared with drug B, because drug A was preferentially administered to persons with early-stage disease. In this example, the unstudied risk factor is stage of disease, resulting in an apparent association between drug A and improved survival when no such effect truly exists. Unlike bias, however, confounding (if identified) can be "corrected" analytically through adjustment or stratification—in the above example, the effects of drug A versus B can be measured separately in patients with early-stage disease and again in patients with late-stage disease.

Another explanation for an observed association is **investigator error**. Investigator error can result from erroneous data entry or manipulation, inappropriate analysis, or misinterpretation. This might be unintentional or intentional.

Assuming that an observed association does not appear to be attributable to chance, bias, confounding, or investigator error, a causal relationship might well be the explanation. Multiple criteria have been proposed for helping an investigator decide whether an association should be considered causal. These criteria include the magnitude of association (the larger the risk ratio or odds ratio, the more plausible), biologic plausibility, consistency with other studies, dose-response effect (increasing exposure associated with increased risk for disease), and exposure preceding disease.[15] These criteria involve judgment, and reasonable people can disagree about whether the available evidence is sufficient to demonstrate causality.

SURVEILLANCE

Surveillance is the ongoing collection, analysis, and interpretation of data and dissemination to those who need to know; it is the informational nervous system for public health practice. Embedded within that simple statement are key concepts that make surveillance a critical piece of assessment, one of the three Core Functions of public health.[16,17] Public health surveillance grew out of a long history of use of data to assess the health of populations. Public health surveillance dates to William Farr's *Articles of Mortality*, which described the salient health problems of nineteenth century London, but was most notably described by Alexander Langmuir as applied to infectious disease control out of which the basic concepts of public health surveillance evolved.[18]

Control of infectious disease requires timely identification of cases, characterizing the mode of transmission, and implementing appropriate control strategies. The more rapidly and accurately the cases are reported and analyzed, the more rapidly and precisely those strategies can be implemented; hence the need for effective surveillance systems. The National Notifiable Disease Surveillance System (NNDSS) (http://www.cdc.gov/nndss) lays out the case definitions and requirements for reporting of individual cases of notifiable diseases (largely infectious diseases) by laboratories, physicians, and health care institutions. Local, tribal, territorial, or state health authorities have their own lists of reportable diseases; they communicate information on cases of reportable diseases to the Centers for Disease Control and Prevention (CDC) each week. Each reportable condition has specific requirements for reporting. For example, meningococcal meningitis, a serious, but treatable bacterial disease with a high case fatality rate, must be reported by physicians and laboratories immediately to local (or state) public health departments because identification of contacts and administration of prophylactic medication must be done urgently to prevent life-threatening disease. States report those cases to CDC weekly. Influenza, on the other hand, is monitored to identify whether influenza cases are occurring, the types of influenza occurring, and the number and severity of cases. To accomplish this, laboratories report the types of viruses found in specimens submitted by physicians for influenza-like illness (ILI), sentinel physicians report ILI and submit specimens, and 122 cities monitor deaths from pneumonia and influenza. These systems rapidly present a picture of influenza that public health officials can use to guide prevention activities (e.g., flu vaccine campaigns, use of prophylactic medications, determine which viral strains to include in vaccines, or even encourage social distancing).

Routine surveillance activities facilitate the identification of potential outbreaks which, in turn, require epidemiologic investigation. The NNDSS is a passive surveillance system. It relies on health care providers to report cases. For most common conditions, it is rarely complete. Nonetheless, trends can be monitored since the proportion of cases actually reported remains reasonably constant for most conditions. However when problems are publicized, such as increasing numbers of pertussis (whooping cough) cases, increased attention often leads to greater recognition and reporting of cases. Perhaps equally important, though, the NNDSS establishes a mechanism whereby health care providers can report unusual conditions or clusters to public health agencies. These reports, which are commonly by phone, are critical for rapid identification of potentially serious conditions in the community and enable public health officials to take appropriate action.

Notifiable diseases are monitored and reported to those who need to take action. Local authorities analyze the data on an ongoing basis, look for patterns, and take appropriate actions, whether watchful waiting, further investigations, taking control measures, (e.g., removing contaminated foods from shelves), or informing clinicians of changing patterns and advising them on prevention and management strategies. At the state and national levels, data are compiled and broader trends become more readily apparent. Patterns that were undetectable at a local level may be detectable with surveillance of larger populations. For example, a single particularly virulent type of *E. coli* infection led to 33 cases among individuals exposed to contaminated spinach. That could only be detected with laboratory testing of specimens from multiple jurisdictions and investigations to identify the source.[19]

The same principles of surveillance apply to other conditions of public health importance. While the frequency of analysis and reporting may vary, surveillance reports provide critical information on the magnitude of problems, which populations are affected, where they are located, and trends. These are the essential person, place, and time components basic to epidemiologic analysis.

The specific data needed for surveillance varies widely. Surveillance of many conditions can be accomplished with commonly available databases. For example, childhood obesity can be monitored through school-based assessments of students' heights and weights. Infant mortality is universally reported on death certificates. Emergency room visits and hospitalizations can be monitored to assess asthma. Teen substance abuse can be assessed from the Youth Behavioral Risk Factor Survey much as risk factors in the general population can be monitored using the Behavioral Risk Factor Surveillance System.

Planning a Surveillance System

Surveillance systems should serve a practical purpose. They are not data collection for data collection's sake. Among the most common uses are to quantify and understand the distribution of a health problem, detect changes in the natural history of a condition or changes in infectious agents, detect outbreaks, facilitate studies, evaluate interventions, detect changes in health practices, and facilitate planning. Priority for establishing surveillance systems is generally based on

- Importance (frequency, severity, and cost of the condition)
- Preventability (what can be done)
- Communicability (risk to others)
- Public interest

A surveillance system needs clear objectives, case definitions, data sources, an analytic approach, routine interpretation and dissemination of findings, and a mechanism for assuring the results are used. The list of nationally notifiable diseases is determined by the Council of State and Territorial Epidemiologists. Because states, not the federal government, have the primary responsibility for health in the United States, each state maintains its own list. Each jurisdiction typically conducts surveillance of the nationally notifiable conditions as well as additional conditions.

Basic surveillance should inform every public health programmatic area. After all, how does one manage a program, if the problem is not clearly understood in terms of trends, who is affected, and where the greatest problems are located? The same principles apply whether one is trying to prevent and control infectious diseases, improve health behaviors, control chronic diseases, reduce injuries and their consequences, improve mental health and substance use, or to improve maternal and child health. Ongoing surveillance is important to monitor how well interventions are working, understand changes, and to enable the development of new initiatives and modify existing ones.

Data Collection and Sources

The process for securing data for surveillance requires a balance between the need for data with the burden for securing it. It needs to consider the urgency of the need, the level of detail and completeness required, and the availability of existing data systems that can be used or modified. Rapid changes in the availability of data from electronic devices, the Internet, and elsewhere (often called big data) will transform the types of data that may become available. (See the section on data sources below.)

Evaluation of Surveillance Systems

Surveillance systems should not be static. They should be regularly evaluated to assess whether they are still meeting important health needs. Evaluations should include an assessment of the

- Importance of the problem (is it still important?)
- Characteristics of the system (how does it operate, what are the case definitions?)

▸ Attributes of the system (Is it simple? Flexible? Acceptable to participants? Does it have the necessary epidemiologic characteristics, e.g., sensitivity, positive predictive value, representativeness? Is it sufficiently timely for action to be taken?)

▸ Cost

The evaluation should look at examples of how the system has been used and whether it met its basic purposes. Based on the evaluation, there should be a set of recommendations about the system—should it be continued? How can the system be made more effective or more efficient? How will necessary improvements be made?

Ethical Issues

Public health surveillance is a public trust. It has been authorized and supported because society, through its elected legislators and officials, believes that the benefits substantially outweigh the harms, and particularly the potential harms to individuals. Nonetheless, those responsible for surveillance systems must adhere to high standards of professional conduct, assure that benefits exceed harms, minimize risks to individuals and communities, assure that benefits are provided, and protect confidentiality and privacy. Surveillance differs from research which generates knowledge for its own sake and has additional protections.

Privacy and Data Protection

Surveillance data often contain protected health information (PHI). The Health Information Portability and Accountability Act (HIPAA) contains many provisions for the use and protection of PHI by public health officials. PHI is essentially any data that can be used to personally identify an individual and health information about that individual. HIPAA lays out 18 measures which constitute PHI. In addition, results of analyses must be presented in such a way that an individual is not identifiable. Maps of cases must not inadvertently disclose an individual's identity. In practice, this means publishing the number of cases only when they exceed a certain number of cases (typically five or more in any one category) in a geographic area. In particularly sensitive conditions, such as was the case for HIV in the 1980s, identifiers may not be collected to reduce concerns about identifying individuals. More typically, identifiers are collected where required to conduct investigations or take action. On the other hand, for many surveillance purposes, identifiable information is neither required nor obtained. For example, to monitor adolescent obesity, height, weight and age or grade are needed, and other information, such as other behaviors

or characteristics, may be useful, but specific identifiable information is not needed. When surveillance data are used for research purposes, it is incumbent to secure Institutional Review Board (IRB) approval or exemption as it is for any other health research study.

Future Challenges

While the basic principles of public health surveillance remain the same, the health landscape continues to evolve. New information and technologies provide new opportunities for prevention and control, increasing the salience of different conditions. Information management and analysis technologies are changing as well. As complex social and environmental problems are addressed across public health systems, there will be an increased need to apply more sophisticated analytic and modeling methodologies. All these require individuals with new skills in already stretched local and state health departments. Transitioning from traditional models of reporting diseases and conducting surveys to a future where the vast data pools being created from electronic health records, personal electronic devices, business data systems, social media, and the Internet will require new skills and great creativity to transform those data streams into meaningful, timely, and actionable information. Public health departments will need teams of epidemiologists, data managers, social scientists, and communication experts to develop the future surveillance systems, manage the information, analyze and interpret it, and communicate it effectively to drive action by those who need to do so.

DATA SOURCES

Recent years have seen a proliferation of data sources for surveillance, monitoring health conditions, and identifying and characterizing public health problems and health determinants. Traditional data sources used by public health practitioners include demographic data from the U.S. Census Bureau, vital records systems, morbidity and laboratory reporting systems, epidemic investigations, sentinel providers, syndromic surveillance, health- and non-health-related surveys, and health care data systems (e.g., administrative data, electronic health records, or registries). Other sources, such as those related to the physical and social environments, are becoming increasingly important as public health agencies work more closely with partners in other sectors such as transportation and education. The data landscape has undergone rapid transformation, with federal, state, and local governments and other public agencies moving toward open data frameworks (see http://www.healthdata.gov), and with immense volumes of data now available from social media, the Internet, mobile devices, other remote electronic devices, genomic databases, and business databases. We describe selected examples of these sources here.

Demography

The central importance of accurate and timely population data is frequently underestimated. The various analytic, programmatic, and planning activities carried out by public health practitioners are conducted based on the assumption that the basic demographic data being utilized are accurate and reliable. For example, in interpreting health-related data, analysts frequently use rates rather than counts to assess health trends since they provide a common basis for comparing events between different groups of people at different times, places, and situations. Demographic data provide the denominators for these rate-based assessments. Sources of demographic data include the U.S. Census, the American Community Survey, and state and local population estimates.

Vital Statistics

One of the oldest and most complete public sources of health information for the United States and the majority of economically developed countries is the documentation of vital events (births and deaths). **Vital records** establish a permanent legal record of birth and death and provide an essentially complete and continuous source of data for health assessment and policy making. William Farr, considered one of the founders of modern vital statistics, collected, analyzed, and interpreted vital statistics and disseminated the information in weekly, quarterly, and annual reports. To standardize vital statistics data, the first international list of causes of death was developed in 1893.[18] The *International Classification of Diseases* (ICD), which undergoes revision approximately every 10 years, is currently in its 10th Revision, and is the standardized coding system used for mortality analyses.[20]

In the United States, each birth or death certificate contains individual identifiers (e.g., Social Security number, name), geographic location, date, and personal characteristics (e.g., gender, race, and education for death certificates [see http://www.cdc.gov/nchs]). Birth certificate data are generally more complete than data from death certificates and include length of pregnancy, birth weight, time and place of birth, and selected information on maternal characteristics (e.g., prenatal care and smoking during pregnancy).[21] Mortality data are commonly used to examine trends in leading causes of death and for surveillance of mortality associated with acute events (e.g., heat waves [22] and influenza[23])

(see Figure 12-2). Analyses of death certificates in the United States have highlighted racial differences in mortality rates over time and preventable premature mortality specific to different populations. Birth data have been used to assess utilization of prenatal care and trends in methods of delivery and in birth weight. Use of birth data was essential to examining the impact of folic acid supplementation on neural tube defects.[24] Linked birth-death files can be used for maternal and infant mortality studies (http://www.cdc.gov/nchs/linked.htm).

Despite these uses, data from vital statistics systems pose certain challenges for public health decision making. For example, not all characteristics are reported with full accuracy. Reporting of socioeconomic information related to health (e.g., race, education, and income) may be misreported or reported incompletely.[25] In addition, using coding schemes developed for underlying cause versus multiple causes of death requires careful consideration and statistical examination.[26,27,28] In all countries, the accuracy and specificity of certain diagnoses is limited as a result of changes in the use of diagnostic categories and codes over time and the variation in the quality of information.

Finally, in the United States, there are long delays of two to three years in the availability of national birth and death files. However, the development of electronic birth and death registration systems and automated systems for coding mortality information has improved timeliness, both in the United States and internationally. At the local level, vital records are available on a more timely basis and have been important for surveillance of mortality associated with acute events such as influenza.

Health Care Systems

Health care data from physicians, hospitals, pharmacies, and registries have long been used for surveillance and monitoring of health trends. As discussed earlier in the chapter, physicians, laboratory officials, and other health care providers in the United States are required by state law to report all cases of health conditions that are notifiable, the majority of which are infectious diseases. Data from health care systems can also be useful for syndromic surveillance, which is focused on early recognition of syndromes, i.e., patterns of symptoms or behavior (e.g., emergency calls for medical assistance, sales of antiflu medications), rather than specific diseases (see Chapter 20 on Communicable and Infectious Diseases and Chapter 26 on Public Health Preparedness). Discharge diagnoses and other information from hospital administrative data is useful for monitoring trends in disease occurrence, examining comorbid conditions, characterizing risk groups, and calculating hospital related costs. However, as health care data become

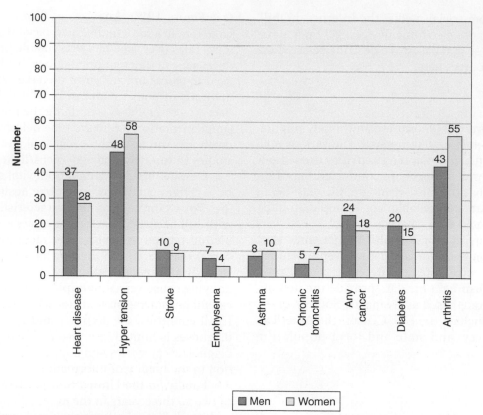

FIGURE 12-2   Number of Heat-related Deaths,* by Sex and Age Group—United States, 1999–2003

*Exposure to extreme heat is reported as the underlying cause of or a contributing factor to death (N 3,442).

SOURCE: Centers for Disease Control and Prevention. Heat-related deaths United States, 1999-2003. Morb Mortal Wkly Rep MMWR. 2006;55:796–798.

increasingly integrated and accessible with the wide-spread adoption of electronic health records (EHRs), this presents new opportunities for innovative public health applications and closer coordination between public health and health care providers. Improved collaboration between public health and health care is desirable not only for supporting surveillance for disease outbreaks and health threats, but also for moving toward more community-based efforts to address the increasing burden of disease from multifactorial chronic diseases such as obesity and diabetes.

Public health and health care professionals are increasingly realizing the potential of EHRs in their work. Some managed care organizations have established research activities based on the records of their patient populations.[29] In 2003, the New York City Department of Health and Mental Hygiene partnered with the Institute for Family Health to implement an EHR that facilitates data exchange to meet the needs of both primary care providers and public health. The demonstrated uses of this public health-oriented EHR include conducting syndromic surveillance, facilitating notifiable disease reporting, disseminating health alerts, enabling the exchange of information regarding immunizations and screening, and providing data on health disparities, high-risk populations, and gaps in care.[30]

Medical records, which can include detailed information about diagnostic classifications, treatments, and outcomes, are also a key source of data for registries. The purpose of registries is to obtain a comprehensive, longitudinal listing of all persons with a particular condition.[31] At the national level, Medicare data, which covers hospitalization expenses for approximately 95 percent of the elderly population, have been used as a registry for some conditions among the elderly. Registries have also been used to ensure the provision of appropriate care and to evaluate changing patterns of medical care; unlike other disease information systems, registries cut across the different levels of severity of illness and can provide information across time about individual persons. Longstanding noncommunicable disease registries exist for cancer, birth defects, occupational diseases, and lead poisoning.

Population-based cancer registries typically have relied on multiple sources of data, most importantly, clinical pathology laboratories and hospital diagnoses

(Figure 12-3). Death certification is also critical to these registries, as are other records, such as those from oncology or radiotherapy units, where available. In the United States, the National Cancer Institute's Surveillance, Epidemiology, and End Results (SEER) program, tracks long-term trends in cancer incidence and mortality, and the data are used to prioritize allocation of resources for cancer research and control. The idea of recording data for all cases of cancer in communities began in the first half of the twentieth century, with the original purpose being to describe patterns and trends.[32] The growth in the number of cancer registries and their use in following patients and analyzing quality of care and survival with comparability across different locations and distinct racial/ethnic groups has led to internationally recognized data collection and reporting standards.[33] In the United States, the National Coordinating Council for Cancer Surveillance was organized in 1995 to facilitate a collaborative approach among the involved organizations and to ensure maximal efficiency.[34]

Surveillance for birth defects was initiated in certain parts of the world in response to the thalidomide tragedy in the early 1960s; registries were established to provide reliable baseline rates for specific birth defects and to detect increases in the prevalence of birth defects as a means of rapidly identifying human teratogens.[35] The CDC has conducted birth defects surveillance in metropolitan Atlanta since 1967 by using multiple sources of ascertainment of all serious birth defects observed in stillborn and live-born infants or recognized by signs and symptoms apparent during the first year of life. This birth defects registry system has been a valuable resource for monitoring rates of change of specific

defects and for conducting numerous genetic and epidemiologic investigations of risk factors for birth defects.[36] The data from these state registries are also used to evaluate the effectiveness of prevention activities and to refer children for health services and early intervention programs.[37]

With the continuing shift in disease burden from communicable diseases to noncommunicable diseases, registries have also been developed to improve the quality of care for the treatment of chronic diseases. For example, in 2006, New York City began mandated reporting of hemoglobin A1C laboratory results, in essence creating the first population-based registry to track blood glucose control in people with diabetes.[38] While the purpose of this novel mandate is to provide improved surveillance and monitoring of trends in diabetes control and to more effectively direct interventions to improve patient outcomes, it has generated controversy largely in relation to privacy concerns.

Population Surveys

Population-based surveys are one of the most important sources of health data. The CDC's National Center for Health Statistics (NCHS) (see www.cdc.gov/nchs) conducts several national surveys, including the National Health Interview Survey (NHIS), an ongoing, nationwide, in-person survey of approximately 40,000 households (approximately 100,000 persons) of the civilian noninstitutionalized population. This survey includes a set of basic health and demographic questions, as well as one or more sets of supplemental questions on specific health topics. NCHS also conducts the National Health and Nutrition Examination Survey (NHANES),

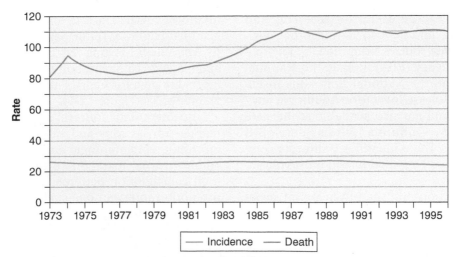

FIGURE 12-3 Incidence Rate and Death Rate of Invasive Breast Cancer, by Year—United States, 1973–1998

SOURCE: National Cancer Institute. SEER: Surveillance, Epidemiology, and End Results [homepage on the internet]. Bethesda, MD: US Department of Health and Human Services, National Institutes of Health; 2006. Available at: http://seer.cancer.gov/. Accessed October 5, 2006.

which collects physical examination and laboratory data in addition to information from in-person interviews from a nationally representative sample of the U.S. population. In England and Wales, the General Household Survey provides information on risk behaviors and disparities.[39] In the People's Republic of China, sentinel sites, known as disease surveillance points, are chosen through a statistical sample of provincial areas. Health care professionals at these sites collect mandated information on acute infectious conditions and data on health events and medical encounters for the entire population within their jurisdiction.[40]

Such nationwide surveys efficiently generate national estimates of the prevalence of diseases, injuries, behaviors, etc., but local jurisdictions can benefit from involvement in data collection and the flexibility to adapt the process to their particular needs.[41] Telephone-based interview surveys such as the Behavioral Risk Factor Surveillance System (BRFSS) can obtain self-reported health information with only minor differences from in-person interviews in the reported prevalence of health conditions.[42]

Additionally, surveys of hospitals and office-based medical care providers can provide information on medical treatments, surgical procedures, and prescribed medications. In the United States, the CDC's National Hospital Discharge Survey has been useful for surveillance of medical care technologies, such as trends in the use of hysterectomies (particularly by geographical region), in the rate of medical procedures by gender and race, and in the assessment of quality of care; and the National Ambulatory Medical Care Survey provides information on the use of medical care services, diagnoses, drug therapies, and other services.

Environmental Data

Environmental data can be useful for assessing and investigating hazards and exposures and other environmental threats. Data sources from the U.S. Environmental Protection Agency (EPA) include the National Air Toxics Assessment, the National Emissions Inventory, and the Toxics Release Inventory. Additional environmental hazards data are also available at the state level. For example, the California EPA has developed CalEnviroScreen, a tool that identifies California communities most burdened by pollution and most vulnerable to its effects.[43]

With the recognition that the physical and social environments where people live, work, play, and attend school have the greatest impacts on health,[44] there has been a renewed focus in public health on not only evaluating neighborhood hazards and exposures, but also in addressing the underlying social and economic determinants of health in communities. These upstream

health determinants, discussed further in Chapters 3 and 21, include other health determinants in the physical environment such as the design of our cities and transportation systems, as well as social determinants such as education, poverty, housing, and social cohesion. These data are important for assessing the health of communities, evaluating policies, and engaging cities, communities, community-based organizations, and policymakers in creating healthy communities.

Examples of data sources related to the physical environment include national and regional transportation data from the U.S. Department of Transportation's National Household Transportation Survey, climate data from the National Oceanic and Atmospheric Association, and commercial business databases which can be used to identify the number, location, and types of food retailers and recreational facilities within a community. Sources of data related to the social environment are further discussed in Chapter 3 and include the U.S. Census and American Community Survey, as well as data from the U.S. Bureau of Economic Analysis, Bureau of Labor Statistics, Department of Justice and other law enforcement agencies, and state and national surveys.

Other Administrative Systems

Other agencies involved in collecting data useful for public health include the U.S. Food and Drug Administration (FDA), which conducts postmarketing surveillance of drugs and devices and recently launched Mini-Sentinel (see http://mini-sentinel.org) as part of the FDA's Sentinel Initiative to improve the agency's ability to more actively identify and assess safety issues.[45,46] The Consumer Product Safety Commission conducts surveillance on product-related injuries through the National Electronic Injury Surveillance System; data on motor-vehicle crash fatalities are available from the National Highway Traffic Safety Administration's Fatality Analysis Reporting System; and insurance records and workers' compensation claims are useful sources of morbidity data for injuries and illnesses in specific geographic areas (Figure 12-4).

Business data sources, such as those that record market transactions and sales can also be useful for informing epidemiologic and policy analyses. For example, grocery market data can provide insights into food consumption patterns and the impacts of health promotion interventions such as economic incentives on food purchasing;[47] and data on cigarette sales can be used to assess the impacts of cigarette taxes on revenue generation and cigarette consumption.[48] Data systems in other sectors are also becoming increasingly utilized. Crime data from the Department of Justice and local law enforcement agencies provide information on

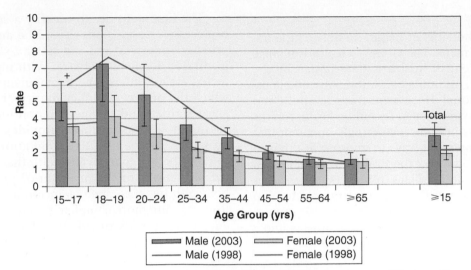

FIGURE 12-4 **Estimated Rates of Nonfatal Occupational Injuries and Illnesses Among Workers Treated in Hospital Emergency Departments, by Age Group and Sex of Worker—United States, 1998 and 2003**

SOURCE: Centers for Disease Control and Prevention. Nonfatal occupational injuries and illnesses among workers treated in hospital emergency departments United States, 2003. Morb Mortal Wkly Rep MMWR, 2006; 55: 449–452.

neighborhood crimes and safety, and educational data can be used to monitor trends in youth physical fitness and obesity.[49] Data on calls to telephone hotlines or help lines can be useful both for surveillance[50] and for assessing the impact of interventions.[51]

New Data Opportunities

As electronic devices and communication technologies become pervasive and increasingly mobile, massive quantities of data are being generated from Internet sites, social media, commercial transactions, GPS locators, cameras, and networked sensors which now exist on everything from cars to appliances to pacemakers – the so-called "Internet of Things." These present new and intriguing opportunities for research in medicine and public health, including public health surveillance, drug safety monitoring, identification of high-risk groups, assessing the effectiveness of interventions, social network analysis, and modeling of disease transmission.[52,53,54]

As an example, public health departments have begun to investigate the utility of social media for foodborne illness surveillance. The New York City Department of Health and Mental Hygiene examined the potential for identifying unreported foodborne illnesses through an online restaurant review website;[55] and the Chicago Department of Public Health along with civic partners implemented Foodborne Chicago, an effort that mines Twitter feeds for foodborne illness complaints and responds by providing links to a website, http://www.foodbornechicago.org, which serves as an online surveillance and response tool.[56] Studies have also examined the utility of using Google Flu Trends,

which uses anonymized, aggregated Internet search data and social media data from Twitter for early detection of influenza.[57,58] These new sources of data present tremendous opportunities and advantages in timeliness, low cost, and scalability, while the challenges include inherent biases, nonrepresentativeness, and difficulty in separating "signal" from "noise." These also present serious analytic and privacy concerns that challenge existing paradigms in how data are analyzed, stored, accessed, and used—which are at various stages of being addressed.[59,60]

OTHER QUANTITATIVE METHODS FOR PUBLIC HEALTH PRACTICE

Prevention Effectiveness and Quantitative Policy Analysis

Prevention effectiveness is the systematic approach to understanding the effectiveness and value of interventions (policies and programs) and includes a variety of quantitative policy analysis tools including economic evaluation (cost-effectiveness, cost utility, and cost-benefit analysis); systematic evidence reviews and meta-analysis; methods for developing evidence-based guidelines; decision analysis; and **health impact assessment**. Many of these are addressed elsewhere (see Chapter 15 on Evaluation and Chapter 11 on Evidence-Based Public Health). Here we address two particular aspects: health impact assessment and systematic evidence reviews.

Health Impact Assessment

The greatest determinants of health lie outside the traditional health domains. The County Health Rankings estimates 40 percent of health is determined by the social environment, including education, jobs, and housing, and an additional 10 percent from the built and natural physical environments. As public health returns to its roots,[61] it has become increasingly apparent that among the most important ways to improve health is to integrate information about the health consequences of projects, programs, and policies into decision processes in other sectors. One of the primary tools to develop and communicate the information is a **health impact assessment (HIA)**. HIAs systematize the process into a discrete set of steps[62] as shown in Figure 12-5.

The first steps are to identify a suitable policy or project to assess. There should be an active decision process underway and the activity should have high likelihood for health effects. With input from the affected stakeholders, the mechanisms (pathways) by which the project or policy intervention affects health are described and the most important selected for assessment. The assessment provides baseline health measures for the affected populations and proceeds to describe the changes in health that would likely occur as a result of the program or policy. Those may be health benefits, such as increased physical activity from creating more complete streets that provide pleasant places to walk or ride bicycles, or harms, such as harms from displacement of occupants of low-income

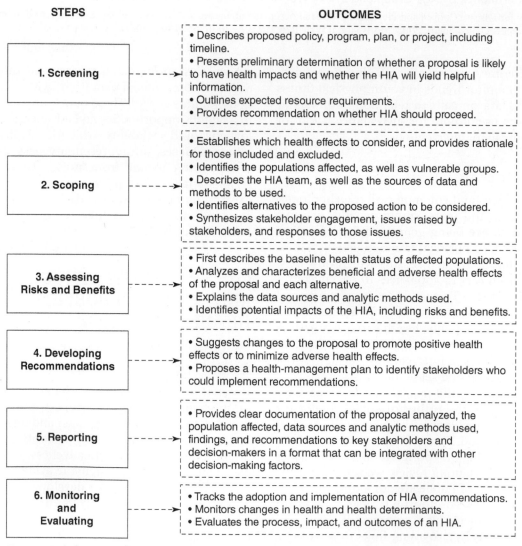

STEPS

OUTCOMES

1. Screening
- Describes proposed policy, program, plan, or project, including timeline.
- Presents preliminary determination of whether a proposal is likely to have health impacts and whether the HIA will yield helpful information.
- Outlines expected resource requirements.
- Provides recommendation on whether HIA should proceed.

2. Scoping
- Establishes which health effects to consider, and provides rationale for those included and excluded.
- Identifies the populations affected, as well as vulnerable groups.
- Describes the HIA team, as well as the sources of data and methods to be used.
- Identifies alternatives to the proposed action to be considered.
- Synthesizes stakeholder engagement, issues raised by stakeholders, and responses to those issues.

3. Assessing Risks and Benefits
- First describes the baseline health status of affected populations.
- Analyzes and characterizes beneficial and adverse health effects of the proposal and each alternative.
- Explains the data sources and analytic methods used.
- Identifies potential impacts of the HIA, including risks and benefits.

4. Developing Recommendations
- Suggests changes to the proposal to promote positive health effects or to minimize adverse health effects.
- Proposes a health-management plan to identify stakeholders who could implement recommendations.

5. Reporting
- Provides clear documentation of the proposal analyzed, the population affected, data sources and analytic methods used, findings, and recommendations to key stakeholders and decision-makers in a format that can be integrated with other decision-making factors.

6. Monitoring and Evaluating
- Tracks the adoption and implementation of HIA recommendations.
- Monitors changes in health and health determinants.
- Evaluates the process, impact, and outcomes of an HIA.

FIGURE 12-5   Framework for HIA, Illustrating Steps and Outputs

housing that might occur as a result of a development project. Based on the findings, a set of recommendations is provided about how benefits might be augmented or harms mitigated with modifications to the proposed approach. Most importantly, the findings are actively communicated to stakeholders and decision makers.

HIA has been extensively used abroad,[63] and its use is becoming more widespread in the United States. The Health Impact Project (see http://www.thehealthimpactproject.org) has excellent resources and examples of HIAs that have been conducted.

Systematic Reviews

A review can be thought of as a more comprehensive, modern-day equivalent of the encyclopedia article. Traditionally, an encyclopedia article was written by a person knowledgeable in a subject area, who was charged with reviewing the literature and writing a summary assessment of the current state of the art on that particular topic.

A **systematic review** uses a formal approach to identify and synthesize the existing knowledge base and prespecifies key questions of interest in an attempt to find all of the relevant literature addressing those questions (see Exhibit 12-1). It also systematically assesses the quality of identified papers (often based on the design and execution of component studies). Systematic reviews can address any number of problems and have recently been used in advertising, astronomy, criminology, ecology, entomology, and parapsychology. In this chapter the focus is on reviews of the effectiveness of interventions to improve health (as shown in Exhibit 12-1). The goal of a systematic review is an unbiased assessment of a particular topic, such as interventions to improve vaccination rates or to reduce smoking rates, that summarizes a large amount of information, identifies beneficial or harmful interventions, and points out gaps in the scientific literature. Reading a good review can be one of the most efficient ways to become familiar with state-of-the-art research and practice on many specific topics in public health, as well as a way to inform health policy.[64,65,66,67]

EXHIBIT 12-1 Guidelines for Interventions in Community Settings.

In 2000, an expert panel (the Task Force on Community Preventive Services), supported by the Centers for Disease Control and Prevention, began publishing *The Guide to Community Preventive Services: Systematic Reviews and Evidence-Based Recommendations* (the *Community Guide*).[73] The underlying reasons for developing the *Community Guide* were as follows: (1) practitioners and policy makers value scientific knowledge as a basis for decision making; (2) the scientific literature on a given topic is often vast, uneven in quality, and inaccessible to busy practitioners; and (3) an experienced and objective panel of experts is seldom locally available to public health officials on a wide range of topics.[74] This effort evaluates evidence related to community, or "population-based," interventions and is intended as a complement to the *Guide to Clinical Preventive Services*. It summarizes what is known about the effectiveness and cost-effectiveness of population-based interventions designed to promote health, prevent disease, injury, disability and premature death as well as reduce exposure to environmental hazards.

Sets of related systematic reviews and recommendations are conducted for interventions in broad health topics, organized by behavior (tobacco product use prevention), environment (the sociocultural environment) or specific diseases, injuries, or impairment

(vaccine-preventable diseases). A systematic process is followed that includes forming a review development team, developing a conceptual approach focused around an analytic framework, selecting interventions to evaluate, searching for and retrieving evidence, abstracting information on each relevant study, and assessing the quality of the evidence of effectiveness. Information on each intervention is then translated into a recommendation for or against the intervention or a finding of insufficient evidence. For those interventions where there is insufficient evidence of effectiveness, the *Community Guide* provides guidance for further prevention research. In addition, the *Community Guide* takes a systematic approach to economic evaluation, seeking out cost-effectiveness information for those programs and policies deemed effective.[75]

To date, Community Guide reviews and recommendations are available for 24 different public health topics, including reducing risk factors (tobacco control), promoting early detection (cancer screening), addressing sociocultural determinants (housing), and promoting health in settings (worksites). Based on dissemination of an early evidence review in the *Community Guide*, health policy has already been positively influenced at the national and state levels.[76]

The use of explicit, systematic methods in reviews limits bias and reduces chance effects, thus providing more reliable results upon which to make decisions.[68,69] Numerous approaches are used in developing systematic reviews. All systematic reviews have important common threads as well as important differences. General methods used in a systematic review as well as several types of reviews and their practical applications are available elsewhere. [64,70-72]

Modeling for Public Health Action

As public health practitioners address increasingly complex social and environmental problems, they need to apply more sophisticated analytic and modeling methodologies that involve multiple disciplines.[77] These include modeling of complex systems and **systems science** approaches. Systems science methodologies allow researchers to incorporate data from multiple sources and disciplines,[78] and use of these modeling approaches in public health has been increasing as changes in computational processing speed and the development of software applications for modeling has made these methodologies much more accessible.

Systems Dynamics Modeling

Systems dynamics modeling is well suited to modeling many public health issues.[79] These models express causal relationships and model systems of interacting variables at the population level, but not individual agents. They have been used, for example, in modeling tobacco policies,[80] health systems,[81] and chronic diseases.[82,83] They have also been widely used in modeling infectious diseases such as influenza to conduct outbreak planning and simulate countermeasures.[84] One of the main disadvantages of systems dynamics models is that they are unable to model heterogeneous populations.

Microsimulation Modeling

Microsimulation models are useful for modeling the health and economic impacts of policies over time.[85] Modeling begins with a sample of individuals or households and follows them through time, constraining them with a set of assumptions and parameters. The advantages of these models include beginning with a real rather than a hypothetical sample and allowing the flexibility to incorporate changing assumptions and parameters over the time period. The disadvantages include the inability for modeled individuals to interact and the need to create complex transition matrices, often using published estimates from the peer-reviewed literature. For example, microsimulation models have been used to look at the health and economic benefits

of preventing common risk factors in older adults,[86] to estimate the impacts of changes in physical activity and calorie intake on obesity prevalence,[87] to model the impacts of tobacco control measures on cardiovascular deaths,[88] and to estimate the impact of federal policies on childhood obesity prevalence.[89]

Agent-based Modeling

Agent-based models are another type of modeling approach that begins with a simulated population of individuals and follows these individuals (or agents) over time. Agents interact with each other and with their environments, and can be simulated in different scenarios and geographic areas.[78] These models can aid in better understanding the effects of social and environmental factors on health behaviors such as walking[90] or diet,[91] and can be used to examine the impacts of different policies while incorporating feedback mechanisms and nonlinear relationships. The drawbacks to agent-based models include the possibility of oversimplifying the dynamic complexity occurring within systems and overreliance on simplifying assumptions.

Small Area Estimation

Local level data that demonstrate local health impacts are vitally important for local and state health departments, cities and communities, community-based organizations, and local decision makers. Local data can aid in better understanding how community-level factors influence health, in prioritizing resources to areas with higher disease burden, and in developing prevention-oriented policies. While there are many rich sources of national data such as the NHIS and NHANES, there are often few data available at the local level. Small area analysis techniques can be used to address this need.

Several different statistical approaches are commonly used to create small area estimates: direct estimation, indirect estimation using synthetic methods, spatial data smoothing, and small area modeling.[92,93] Small area modeling approaches are becoming more common with the improvements in computational processing and the availability of modeling tools and spatial analysis software.[94,95] Challenges in small area estimation include defining geographic boundaries, the need to draw on multiple data sources, and the potentially large variability in estimates for areas with small numbers of cases.

Geographic Information Systems

It has long been recognized that place matters to health. Spatial analyses have evolved considerably since John Snow's map of the London Cholera outbreak of 1854. Nearly all data have geographic attributes, and a **Geographic Information System (GIS)** is a tool for capturing, managing, analyzing, and presenting geographically referenced data. A GIS facilitates the examination of spatial relationships, the identification of spatial and temporal patterns and trends, and the display of complex relationships in a more intuitive form. This can advance the understanding of complex systems, support better communication and collaboration, and improve decision making by integrating and analyzing geo-referenced data from different sources.

Although geospatial technologies have not been adopted as quickly in public health practice compared to other sectors, GIS is increasingly used for disease surveillance, environmental health monitoring, emergency preparedness and response, assessing service needs, and prioritizing the allocation of health resources. Place is a key component in epidemiologic investigations, and spatial analysis methods are being increasingly employed.[96] Examples of the application of spatial epidemiologic methods include examinations of obesity in relation to neighborhood environments,[97] identification of children at high risk for lead exposure and assessing the need for neighborhood-level blood lead testing,[98] spatial analyses of childhood asthma and traffic exposure,[99] and detection of cancer clusters.[100]

SUMMARY

Epidemiology and biostatistics provide the necessary scientific foundation for public health practitioners to measure and understand how disease and illness occur in populations, to quantify health risks, and to assess and evaluate the impacts of policies and programs. Public health surveillance, high-quality data, and quantitative analyses are essential for assessing the health of populations at risk for diseases, injury, and disability and for translating data into meaningful public health action. As new information and technologies afford new data and analysis opportunities, new skills and methodologies will be needed to translate these opportunities into public health practice.

REVIEW QUESTIONS

1. Define three common measures of disease frequency used by public health practitioners.

2. What are the primary reasons for conducting public health surveillance?

3. Describe biases that commonly occur in epidemiologic analyses and suggest ways to manage them.

4. Assume you are working in a state health department in which none of the following conditions is on the state list of reportable diseases. For each condition, what sources of data might be available if you wished to conduct surveillance? What factors make one source of data more appropriate than another?

   a. Preterm births
   b. *E. coli*
   c. Diabetes
   d. Lung cancer

5. Describe how health impact assessments can be used by public health practitioners to inform policy decisions.

6. For a public health practitioner, provide two advantages of using a systematic review such as the Community Guide.

ACKNOWLEDGMENTS

We sincerely thank Richard C. Dicker, Donna F. Stroup, and the late Stephen B. Thacker, the authors of some of the material which we have retained from earlier editions.

REFERENCES

1. Last JM, ed. *A Dictionary of Epidemiology.* 4th ed. New York: Oxford University Press; 2001.

2. Langmuir AD, Andrews JM. Biological warfare defense. The Epidemic Intelligence Service of the Communicable Disease Center. *Am J Public Health Nations Health.* March 1952;42(3):235–238.

3. Davidian M, Louis TA. Why statistics? *Science.* April 6, 2012;336(6077):12.

4. Culler D, Grimes SJ, Acheson LS, Wiesner GL. Cancer genetics in primary care. *Prim Care.* September 2004;31(3):649–683, xi.

5. Lemon SC, Roy J, Clark MA, Friedmann PD, Rakowski W. Classification and regression tree analysis in public health: methodological review and comparison with logistic regression. *Ann Behav Med.* December 2003;26(3):172–181.

6. Preisser JS, Koch GG. Categorical data analysis in public health. *Annu Rev Public Health.* 1997;18:51–82.

7. Rosner B. *Fundamentals of biostatistics.* 6th ed. Belmont, CA: Thomson-Brooks/Cole; 2006.

8. Murphy SL, Xu J, Kochanek KD. Deaths: final data for 2010. *Natl Vital Stat Rep.* May 8 2013;61(4):1–117.

9. Hoyert DL, Heron MP, Murphy SL, Kung HC. Deaths: final data for 2003. *Natl Vital Stat Rep.* April 19, 2006;54(13):1–120.

10. Mathews TJ, MacDorman MF. Infant mortality statistics from the 2010 period linked birth/infant death data set. *Natl Vital Stat Rep.* January 24, 2013;62.

11. Haddix AC, Teutsch SM, Corso PS. *Prevention effectiveness: a guide to decision analysis and economic evaluation.* 2d ed. Oxford; New York: Oxford University Press; 2003.

12. McKenna MT, Michaud CM, Murray CJ, Marks JS. Assessing the burden of disease in the United States using disability-adjusted life years. *Am J Prev Med.* June 2005;28(5):415–423.

13. Anand S, Hanson K. Disability-adjusted life years: a critical review. *J Health Econ.* December 1997;16(6):685–702.

14. Jewell NP. *Statistics for Epidemiology.* Boca Raton: Chapman & Hall/CRC; 2004.

15. Steenland K, Armstrong B. An overview of methods for calculating the burden of disease due to specific risk factors. *Epidemiology.* September 2006;17(5):512–519.

16. Institute of Medicine. *The Future of Public Health.* Washington, DC: National Academy Press; 1988.

17. Lee LM, Teutsch SM, Thacker SB, St. Louis ME, eds. *Principles & Practice of Public Health Surveillance* 3d ed. New York: Oxford University Press; 2010.

18. Langmuir AD. William Farr: founder of modern concepts of surveillance. *Int J Epidemiol.* March 1976;5(1):13–18.

19. Multistate Outbreak of Shiga Toxin-producing Escherichia coli O157:H7 Infections Linked to Organic Spinach and Spring Mix Blend (Final Update) http://www.cdc.gov/ecoli/2012/O157H7–11–12/index.html. Accessed August 25, 2014.

20. Mathers CD, Fat DM, Inoue M, Rao C, Lopez AD. Counting the dead and what they died from: an assessment of the global status of cause of death data. *Bull World Health Organ.* March 2005;83(3):171–177.

21. Schoendorf KC, Branum AM. The use of United States vital statistics in perinatal and obstetric research. *Am J Obstet Gynecol.* April 2006;194(4):911–915.

22. Centers for Disease Control and Prevention. Heat-related deaths–United States, 1999-2003. *MMWR Morb Mortal Wkly Rep.* July 28, 2006;55(29):796–798.

23. Simonsen L, Reichert TA, Viboud C, Blackwelder WC, Taylor RJ, Miller MA. Impact of influenza vaccination on seasonal mortality in the U.S. elderly population. *Arch Intern Med.* February 14, 2005;165(3):265–272.

24. Honein MA, Paulozzi LJ, Mathews TJ, Erickson JD, Wong LY. Impact of folic acid fortification of the US food supply on the occurrence of neural tube defects. *JAMA.* June 20, 2001;285(23):2981–2986.

25. National Research Council. In: Ver Ploeg M, Perrin E, eds. *Eliminating Health Disparities: Measurement and Data Needs.* Washington (DC)2004.

26. Williams DR, Jackson PB. Social sources of racial disparities in health. *Health Aff (Millwood).* March–April 2005;24(2):325–334.

27. Wall MM, Huang J, Oswald J, McCullen D. Factors associated with reporting multiple causes of death. *BMC Med Res Methodol.* January 17, 2005;5(1):4.

28. Redelings MD, Sorvillo F, Simon P. A comparison of underlying cause and multiple causes of death: US vital statistics, 2000-2001. *Epidemiology.* January 2006;17(1):100–103.

29. Weiner M, Stump TE, Callahan CM, Lewis JN, McDonald CJ. A practical method of linking data from Medicare claims and a comprehensive electronic medical records system. *Int J Med Inform.* August 2003;71(1):57–69.

30. Calman N, Hauser D, Lurio J, Wu WY, Pichardo M. Strengthening public health and primary care collaboration through electronic health records. *Am J Public Health.* November 2012;102(11):e13–18.

31. Gladman DD, Menter A. Introduction/overview on clinical registries. *Ann Rheum Dis.* March 2005;64 Suppl 2:ii101–102.

32. Parkin DM. The evolution of the population-based cancer registry. *Nat Rev Cancer.* August 2006;6(8):603–612.

33. Brewster DH, Coebergh JW, Storm HH. Population-based cancer registries: the invisible key to cancer control. *Lancet Oncol.* April 2005;6(4):193–195.

34. Swan J, Wingo P, Clive R, et al. Cancer surveillance in the U.S.: can we have a national system? *Cancer.* October 1, 1998;83(7):1282–1291.

35. Holtzman NA, Khoury MJ. Monitoring for congenital malformations. *Annu Rev Public Health.* 1986;7:237–266.

36. Kirby RS, Seaver LH. Birth defects research: improving surveillance methods and addressing epidemiologic questions and public health issues. *Birth Defects Res A Clin Mol Teratol.* October 2005;73(10):645.

37. Edmonds LD. Birth defect surveillance at the state and local level. *Teratology.* July–August 1997;56(1-2):5–9.

38. Chamany S, Silver LD, Bassett MT, et al. Tracking diabetes: New York City's A1C Registry. *Milbank Q.* September 2009;87(3):547–570.

39. Richards L, Fox K, Roberts C, Fletcher L, Goddard E. *Living in Britain No. 31: Results from the 2002 General Household Survey.* London, England: Office of National Statistics, Stationery Office;2002.

40. Yang G, Hu J, Rao KQ, Ma J, Rao C, Lopez AD. Mortality registration and surveillance in China: History, current situation and challenges. *Popul Health Metr.* March 16, 2005;3(1):3.

41. Simon PA, Wold CM, Cousineau MR, Fielding JE. Meeting the data needs of a local health department: the Los Angeles County Health Survey. *Am J Public Health.* December 2001;91(12):1950–1952.

42. Nelson DE, Powell-Griner E, Town M, Kovar MG. A comparison of national estimates from the National Health Interview Survey and the Behavioral Risk Factor Surveillance System. *Am J Public Health.* August 2003;93(8):1335–1341.

43. California Environmental Protection Agency. *California Communities Health Screening Tool, Version 2.0.* August 2014.

44. Institute of Medicine. *The Future of the Public's Health in the 21st Century.* Washington, DC: National Academies Press; 2002.

45. Psaty BM, Breckenridge AM. Mini-Sentinel and regulatory science–big data rendered fit and functional. *N Engl J Med.* June 5, 2014;370(23):2165–2167.

46. Southworth MR, Reichman ME, Unger EF. Dabigatran and postmarketing reports of bleeding. *N Engl J Med.* April 4 2013;368(14):1272–1274.

47. Sturm R, An R, Segal D, Patel D. A cash-back rebate program for healthy food purchases in South Africa: results from scanner data. *Am J Prev Med.* June 2013;44(6):567–572.

48. Sung HY, Hu TW, Ong M, Keeler TE, Sheu ML. A major state tobacco tax increase, the master settlement agreement, and cigarette consumption: the California experience. *Am J Public Health.* June 2005;95(6):1030–1035.

49. Aryana M, Li Z, Bommer WJ. Obesity and physical fitness in California school children. *Am Heart J.* February 2012;163(2):302–312.

50. Bogevig S, Hogberg LC, Dalhoff KP, Mortensen OS. Status and trends in poisonings in Denmark 2007–2009. *Dan Med Bull.* May 2011;58(5):A4268.

51. Centers for Disease Control and Prevention. Impact of a national tobacco education campaign on weekly numbers of quitline calls and website visitors–United States, March 4-June 23, 2013. *MMWR Morb Mortal Wkly Rep.* September 20, 2013;62(37):763–767.

52. Brownstein JS, Freifeld CC, Madoff LC. Digital disease detection–harnessing the Web for public health surveillance. *N Engl J Med.* May 21, 2009;360(21):2153–2155, 2157.

53. Freifeld CC, Brownstein JS, Menone CM, et al. Digital drug safety surveillance: monitoring pharmaceutical products in twitter. *Drug Saf.* May 2014;37(5):343–350.

54. Wojcik OP, Brownstein JS, Chunara R, Johansson MA. Public health for the people: participatory infectious disease surveillance in the digital age. *Emerg Themes Epidemiol.* 2014;11:7.

55. Harrison C, Jorder M, Stern H, et al. Using online reviews by restaurant patrons to identify unreported cases of foodborne illness - New York City, 2012-2013. *MMWR Morb Mortal Wkly Rep.* May 23 2014;63(20):441–445.

56. Harris JK, Mansour R, Choucair B, et al. Health department use of social media to identify foodborne illness - Chicago, Illinois, 2013-2014. *MMWR Morb Mortal Wkly Rep.* August 15, 2014;63(32):681–685.

57. Cook S, Conrad C, Fowlkes AL, Mohebbi MH. Assessing Google flu trends performance in the United States during the 2009 influenza virus A (H1N1) pandemic. *PLoS One.* 2011;6(8):e23610.

58. Broniatowski DA, Paul MJ, Dredze M. National and local influenza surveillance through Twitter: an analysis of the 2012-2013 influenza epidemic. *PLoS One.* 2013;8(12):e83672.

59. President's Council of Advisors on Science and Technology. *Report to the President. Big Data and Privacy: A Technological Perspective.* Executive Office of the President; May 2014.

60. Lane JI. *Privacy, big data, and the public good: frameworks for engagement.* New York, NY: Cambridge University Press; 2014.

61. Teutsch SM, Fielding JE. Rediscovering the core of public health. *Annu Rev Public Health.* 2013;34:287–99.

62. National Research Council. *Improving Health in the United States: The Role of Health Impact Assessment.* Washington (DC)2011.

63. Kickbusch I, Buckett K, eds. *Implementing Health in All Policies.* Adelaide: Department of Health, Government of South Australia; 2010.

64. Bambra C. Real world reviews: A beginner's guide to undertaking systematic reviews of public health policy interventions. *J Epidemiol Community Health*. September 18, 2009.

65. Lavis JN. How can we support the use of systematic reviews in policymaking? *PLoS Med*. November 2009;6(11):e1000141.

66. Waters E, Doyle J, Jackson N. Evidence-based public health: improving the relevance of Cochrane Collaboration systematic reviews to global public health priorities. *J Public Health Med*. September 2003;25(3):263–266.

67. Oliver K, Innvar S, Lorenc T, Woodman J, Thomas J. A systematic review of barriers to and facilitators of the use of evidence by policymakers. *BMC Health Serv Res*. 2914;14:2.

68. Petticrew M, Roberts H. *Systematic Reviews in the Social Sciences: A Practical Guide*. Oxford: Blackwell Publishing; 2006.

69. Murad MH, Montori VM, Ioannidis JP, et al. How to read a systematic review and meta-analysis and apply the results to patient care: users' guides to the medical literature. *JAMA*. July 2014;312(2):171–179.

70. Galsziou P, Irwig L, Bain C, Colditz G. *Systematic Reviews in Health Care: A Practical Guide*. New York: Cambridge University Press; 2001.

71. Guyatt G, Rennie D, eds. *Users' Guides to the Medical Literature. A Manual for Evidence-Based Clinical Practice*. Chicago, IL: American Medical Association Press; 2002.

72. Higgins J, Green S. *Cochrane Handbook for Systematic Reviews of Interventions*. New York: John Wiley and Sons; 2008.

73. Zaza S, Briss PA, Harris KW, eds. *The Guide to Community Preventive Services: What Works to Promote Health?* New York: Oxford University Press; 2005.

74. Truman BI, Smith-Akin CK, Hinman AR. Developing the guide to community preventive services - overview and rationale. *Am J Prev Med*. 2000;18(1S):18–26.

75. Carande-Kulis VG, Maciosek MV, Briss PA, et al. Methods for systematic reviews of economic evaluations for the Guide to Community Preventive Services. Task Force on Community Preventive Services. *Am J Prev Med*. 2000;18(1 Suppl):75–91.

76. Mercer SL, Sleet DA, Elder RW, Cole KH, Shults RA, Nichols JL. Translating evidence into policy: lessons learned from the case of lowering the legal blood alcohol limit for drivers. *Ann Epidemiol*. June 2010;20(6):412–420.

77. Mabry PL, Olster DH, Morgan GD, Abrams DB. Interdisciplinarity and systems science to improve population health: a view from the NIH Office of Behavioral and Social Sciences Research. *Am J Prev Med*. August 2008;35(2 Suppl):S211–224.

78. Maglio PP, Mabry PL. Agent-based models and systems science approaches to public health. *Am J Prev Med*. March 2011;40(3):392–394.

79. Homer JB, Hirsch GB. System dynamics modeling for public health: background and opportunities. *Am J Public Health*. March 2006;96(3):452–458.

80. Tengs TO, Osgood ND, Chen LL. The cost-effectiveness of intensive national school-based anti-tobacco education: results from the tobacco policy model. *Prev Med*. December 2001;33(6):558–570.

81. Milstein B, Homer J, Briss P, Burton D, Pechacek T. Why behavioral and environmental interventions are needed to improve health at lower cost. *Health Aff (Millwood)*. May 2011;30(5):823–832.

82. Milstein B, Jones A, Homer JB, Murphy D, Essien J, Seville D. Charting plausible futures for diabetes prevalence in the United States: a role for system dynamics simulation modeling. *Prev Chronic Dis*. July 2007;4(3):A52.

83. Homer J, Milstein B, Wile K, Pratibhu P, Farris R, Orenstein DR. Modeling the local dynamics of cardiovascular health: risk factors, context, and capacity. *Prev Chronic Dis*. April 2008;5(2):A63.

84. Flahault A, Vergu E, Coudeville L, Grais RF. Strategies for containing a global influenza pandemic. *Vaccine*. November 10, 2006;24 (44–46):6751–6755.

85. Abraham JM. Using microsimulation models to inform U.S. health policy making. *Health Serv Res*. April 2013;48(2 Pt 2):686–695.

86. Goldman DP, Zheng Y, Girosi F, et al. The benefits of risk factor prevention in Americans aged 51 years and older. *Am J Public Health*. November 2009;99(11):2096–2101.

87. Basu S, Seligman H, Winkleby M. A metabolic-epidemiological microsimulation model to estimate the changes in energy intake and physical activity necessary to meet the Healthy People 2020 obesity objective. *Am J Public Health*. July 2014;104(7):1209–1216.

88. Basu S, Glantz S, Bitton A, Millett C. The effect of tobacco control measures during a period of rising cardiovascular disease risk in India: a mathematical model of myocardial infarction and stroke. *PLoS Med*. 2013;10(7):e1001480.

89. Kristensen AH, Flottemesch TJ, Maciosek MV, et al. Reducing Childhood Obesity through U.S. Federal Policy: A Microsimulation Analysis. *Am J Prev Med*. August 25, 2014.

90. Yang Y, Diez Roux AV, Auchincloss AH, Rodriguez DA, Brown DG. Exploring walking differences by socioeconomic status using a spatial agent-based model. *Health Place.* January 2012;18(1):96–99.

91. Zhang D, Giabbanelli PJ, Arah OA, Zimmerman FJ. Impact of different policies on unhealthy dietary behaviors in an urban adult population: an agent-based simulation model. *Am J Public Health.* July 2014;104(7):1217–1222.

92. Jia H, Muennig P, Borawski E. Comparison of small-area analysis techniques for estimating county-level outcomes. *Am J Prev Med.* June 2004;26(5):453–460.

93. Goodman MS. Comparison of small-area analysis techniques for estimating prevalence by race. *Prev Chronic Dis.* March 2010;7(2):A33.

94. Zhang X, Holt JB, Lu H, et al. Multilevel regression and poststratification for small-area estimation of population health outcomes: a case study of chronic obstructive pulmonary disease prevalence using the behavioral risk factor surveillance system. *Am J Epidemiol.* April 15, 2014;179(8):1025–1033.

95. Ha NS, Lahiri P, Parsons V. Methods and results for small area estimation using smoking data from the 2008 National Health Interview Survey. *Stat Med.* June 9, 2014.

96. Auchincloss AH, Gebreab SY, Mair C, Diez Roux AV. A review of spatial methods in epidemiology, 2000-2010. *Annu Rev Public Health.* April 2012;33:107–122.

97. Feng J, Glass TA, Curriero FC, Stewart WF, Schwartz BS. The built environment and obesity: a systematic review of the epidemiologic evidence. *Health Place.* March 2010;16(2):175–190.

98. Vaidyanathan A, Staley F, Shire J, et al. Screening for lead poisoning: a geospatial approach to determine testing of children in at-risk neighborhoods. *J Pediatr.* March 2009;154(3):409–414.

99. Gauderman WJ, Avol E, Lurmann F, et al. Childhood asthma and exposure to traffic and nitrogen dioxide. *Epidemiology.* November 2005;16(6):737–743.

100. Huang L, Pickle LW, Das B. Evaluating spatial methods for investigating global clustering and cluster detection of cancer cases. *Stat Med.* November 10, 2008;27(25):5111–5142.

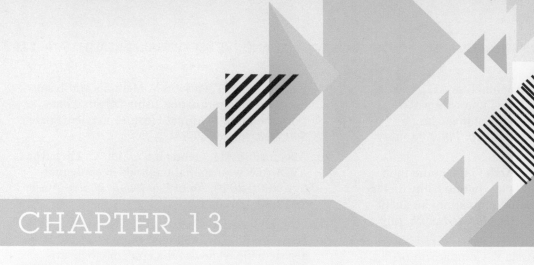

Community Health Assessment, Planning, and Implementation

Cynthia D. Lamberth, MPH, CPH • F. Douglas Scutchfield, MD

LEARNING OBJECTIVES

Upon completion of this chapter, the reader will be able to:

1. Express the importance of citizen engagement in public health assessment, planning, and implementation.

2. Identify and explain national and local models that can be used for community health assessment, improvement, and planning.

3. Understand the role of the Public Health Accreditation Board (PHAB) in directing national, state, and local health program planning.

4. Recognize how the national focus areas of PHAB and new Internal Revenue Service requirements under the Patient Protection and Affordable Care Act foster collaboration and prompt additional partnerships to achieve local health improvement.

5. Explain how coalitions serve as a particular type of community organization and describe the essential components for developing a coalition.

6. Describe how communities create action plans to achieve goals on priority issues identified by the community.

KEY TERMS

accreditation
action planning
assessments
civic engagement
coalitions
community
deliberation
Leading Health Indicators (LHIs)
population health
public deliberation
SMART objectives

INTRODUCTION

Community health assessment, planning, and implementation are core requirements for population health initiatives and public health practice.[1] Recent initiatives and specific mandates in community assessment, planning, and implementation encourage or require, in many cases, listening to the voice of the public to identify goals and initiatives to improve population health. These initiatives include the Patient Protection and Affordable Care Act of 2010 (ACA)[2] and the opportunity to pursue accreditation through the Public Health Accreditation Board (PHAB).[3] These programs and mandates provide incentives to governmental public health and their community health partners to engage the public in the assessment, planning, and implementation activities designed to identify and remediate major community health problems. As such, these mandates and requirements impact much of today's public health functions and responsibilities and specifically require a strong working relationship with citizens as community partners. Knowledge and skills in areas such as community participation, citizen engagement, and community empowerment are central to successful public health practice. This chapter focuses on describing the importance of building community interaction when focusing on public health programs, activities, linkages, and policy. In this chapter we have defined community as all who are affected by public health practice and research, generally thought of as confined to a specific geographical area, but in certain circumstances, not necessarily directly circumscribed by specific geographical boundaries.

Population health, described by either geography or other attributes, is profoundly influenced by the factors that influence the health outcomes of groups, including the distribution and equity of such health outcomes across various segments of society.[4] Therefore, listening to the population can and should focus our efforts on understanding the health needs of the community, involving the community in measuring and evaluating health status, and in developing collaborative programs that will improve health outcomes. A population health approach addresses the interrelatedness of biologic, environmental, and behavioral factors in addition to the social determinants of health, and results in a lowered risk for the entire population or subsets of that population that require special attention. It also can reduce inequalities in disease patterns particular to specific populations, such as racial minorities.[5]

A review of the social determinants of health as described in Chapter 3 reveals the necessity of working in new ways with communities to respond to and distill the etiologic risk factors responsible for disease and disability. Further, the community, given the nature of these social determinants, is not a passive entity but rather the "engine" that is necessary to achieve optimal health status for a community.[6] The nature of public health practice is evolving in ways that require more significant participation by concerned citizens, governmental or not-for-profit community organizations, and community organizations that provide the capacity for traditional public health practitioners to promote and protect the public's health.

FINDING THE COMMUNITY IN COMMUNITY HEALTH

The focus on public engagement with issues that are its proper purview is grounded in time-honored public deliberation approaches.[7] The historical approach to public health has not always included this emphasis on an empowered public, but rather public health authorities relying on data to design and implement programs and related evaluation measurements without input from community members.[6] Although public health uses the term "public," the traditional "public health" system, made up of various organizations, has been, and to a great degree remains, a very closed, professional group whose decision-making process is far removed from common citizens.[8–11] In fact, many of the organizations that historically guide the work of public health, notably boards of health, are comprised of medical professionals and high-level civic leaders.[12] This characteristic of public health governance bolsters the accusation that those such as Gittell has made, when he points out that community institutions or organizations fail to continually provide opportunities for citizen participation, particularly low-income citizens who lack the resources to join the political process.[13]

The underlying premise behind community engagement in dealing with community health problems mimics work in quality improvement, where we know that those closest to the problem often have the solutions to the problem.[14] People, given the opportunity to have a voice in their community, can bring positive change and help compensate for existing social determinants of health. If the problem is in the community, the solution is likely in the community. Kania and Kramer capture this approach in their work on collective impact, encouraging broad cross-sector coordination as a mechanism to achieve better outcomes in dealing with community health problems.[15]

Over the past 50 years, physicians, policy makers, researchers, and community organizers began to question the role of community and community involvement in public health.[16] In the words of Dr. E.G. McGavran, a public health leader in the 1950s, the issue is, "In scientific public health, we no longer treat the individual—the segment of the community—but the total body politic—mental, physical, social, and economic. We no longer treat individuals who have communicable disease, but we prevent, control, or eradicate the disease in the body politic."[17] This quote suggests recognition at the middle of the past century that communities should be the locus of concern in public health. The idea of the community as a patient created the community medicine movement of the 1950s and 1960s, with the emergence of medical school Departments of Community Medicine or Community Health during that period.[18] This history builds the foundation for the current call to integrate primary care and public health to achieve the triple aim of achieving improved patient-centered care, bend the cost curve, and improve population health. This further strengthens the population focus in community health assessment, planning, and implementation, and the need for expanding citizen involvement in matters related to health.[18]

EXPANDING CITIZEN ENGAGEMENT

Decisions about health problems in communities, the nature of public health programs designed to deal with those problems, and assessment of program effectiveness is a community responsibility. In fact, democratic traditions in America suggest that local citizens should be engaged with experts to make decisions about things that affect their communities, including those activities that relate to the public's health.[19,20]

The practice of public health seeks to inform decisions about the health of the population by engaging citizens in dialog and planning, implementation, and evaluation of public health interventions. The celebration and importance of deliberation by citizens has a long history with origins in Greek city-states. The ancient Athenian Assembly met on the hillside of Pynx where citizens gathered to discuss matters important to their city.[21] In the Colonies and later United States, this was replicated in town hall meetings in colonial New England and flows into present day deliberation, both formal and informal, that occur at county, city, village, and neighborhood levels. Building on the success of engaging the public to make wise health program decisions, public health has designed numerous ways to comprehensively develop these partnerships with the community. Today we see public health in face-to-face forums and community town hall type meetings as well as online deliberation through Twitter, Facebook, blogs, and Internet sites set up for the sole purpose of spirited debate.

With conceptual underpinnings in political philosophy, public deliberation is grounded in philosophies of the social contract and bonds among individuals and institutions that shape societies' political and social life. The philosophies of a number of both ancient and contemporary authors from Aristotle and Plato, to Jurgen Habermas, have shaped contemporary normative constructions of deliberation.[7] Public deliberation supports the area of political science whose proponents argue that members of the public should be thoughtfully engaged in and informed about the issues that shape their public life. Deliberation is viewed as a way to bolster democratic life, include the voices of underrepresented groups, and propel moral reasoning and mutual decision making.[20] Fishkin's definition of public deliberation—"The people, either directly or through their representatives should meet together to hear competing arguments and discuss the issues in preparation for collective decisions"—adds the idea of representation to a decision-making body and also specifies improving the completeness of public debate by including public engagement.[22] Bringing in relevant ideas and facts from all corners of the community where they can be aired, discussed, and weighed to make decisions enhances the completeness of the debate and the ultimate decisions about how best to address the health of the community. The practice of public health seeks to both engage citizens representative of the population and citizens themselves being served to achieve true "citizen voice." For the purpose of this chapter and an epistemic-based definition focused on the purpose of engaging citizens as it relates to their health, the following definition will be used for civic engagement: specifically; "Community-based preferences, opinions and decisions reached through public discourse." (Additional detail on the processes of community development—a related but distinct topic—is provided in Chapter 25.)

COMMUNITY HEALTH ASSESSMENT

Civic engagement is key to conducting community health assessments to fulfill essential public health services. Public health's core functions encompass the assessment of health needs and assets, policy development, and assurance of conditions for individuals to be healthy. Assessments can inform service provision, set and assess goals, and determine the direction of local initiatives. The Institute of Medicine (IOM) 2003 report *The Future of the Public's Health in the 21st Century*[23] established a framework for action for improving the health of the nation. It identified who must be involved, including state and local health departments, as well as other members of the broader public health system, and recommended a population approach be taken to improve the public's health. The report offered a rationale for multisectoral engagement in partnership with government and the roles that various community partners, members of the public health system, might play. To build and strengthen an effective, intersectional public health system, the IOM Committee identified the need for a new generation of partnerships to build consensus on health priorities and support community and individual actions that are evidence-based.[23]

Community Benefit

Local and state health departments are increasingly being called on to lead, facilitate, or engage in conducting community health assessments (CHAs). Several transecting events have led to this situation. The national public health voluntary accreditation program for state, local, and tribal health departments, administered by PHAB, requires CHAs as a prerequisite for applying for accreditation.[3] Concomitantly, as part of the ACA, the Internal Revenue Service has recently revised the community benefits requirements for nonprofit hospitals to conduct Community Health Needs Assessments (CHNAs).[24] Specifically, provisions of the ACA require each nonprofit hospital facility in the United States to conduct a CHNA and adopt an implementation strategy to meet identified community health needs.[25] In conducting the CHNA, nonprofit hospitals are required to take into account input from persons who represent the broad interests of the community served, including those with special knowledge of or expertise in public health.

This requirement builds on the community benefit practices of hospitals and hospital systems to strategically invest resources and build partnerships with community groups to improve community health.[26] Every three years, hospitals must conduct CHNAs in collaboration with local health departments (LHDs) and community partners. Furthermore, this assessment, along with an implementation strategy and evaluation plan to track progress, must be reported to the Internal Revenue Service (IRS) using Schedule H of Form 990[24] as an obligation for tax exemption. Through annual reporting to the IRS, nonprofit hospitals describe how they are meeting their community benefit requirements.[26]

PHAB—The Public Health Accreditation Board

An initiative focused on improving population health is the national voluntary public health accreditation program for local, state, territorial, and tribal health departments.[24,25] The Public Health Accreditation Board (PHAB), a nonprofit 501(c)3 entity, serves as the independent accrediting body.[26] PHAB established prerequisites for LHDs that wish to apply for national accreditation, including completing a CHA, a community health improvement plan (CHIP), and an agency-wide strategic plan within the past five years.

The standards for LHDs specify that they conduct or participate in a collaborative process to complete a comprehensive CHA.[29] In addition, health departments must conduct a comprehensive planning process resulting in a CHIP, assess health care service capacity, identify and implement strategies to improve access to health care, and use a performance management system to monitor achievement of objectives. The results of all of these prerequisites are heavily represented in the standards for accreditation by PHAB, so that an effective CHA and CHIP are not only spelled out in the prerequisites but also in the standards for accreditation. A consensus statement from numerous national organizations[30] underscores the significance of these assessments and implementation strategies to improve the health of communities and the importance of civic engagement in the process.

Partnerships

The convergence of the ACA policy that requires tax-exempt hospitals to conduct a CHNA for its catchment area and to build goals to address these needs,[25] combined with the voluntary public health accreditation efforts, have the potential to make significant inroads to improve population health. Mays and Scutchfield contend that collaborations of partners can lead to enhanced population health programs and policies, coordinated delivery of health care services and economies of scope, allowing each partner to pursue objectives not possible by acting alone.[27]

It is important to recognize that other components of the health care system may have either required CHAs, such as those required by Federally Qualified Health Centers,[28] or voluntary efforts to do community assessments, such as those undertaken by organizations such as the United Way, to focus their funding most appropriately. While substantial attention has focused on the hospital/health department collaboration in developing a CHA and CHIP, in the case of the health department, or for the CHNA, in the case of the hospital, there are other organizations that can and would benefit from cooperation in these planning and implementation exercises in any community.

TOOLS FOR COMMUNITY HEALTH ASSESSMENT, COMMUNITY HEALTH IMPROVEMENT PLANNING, AND IMPLEMENTATION

A number of planning and programming tools have been developed for use when working with communities. These include state-developed models, local community and consulting approaches, and national approaches. The following section includes a brief overview of several methods, instruments, and tools commonly used in community health assessment and improvement planning. Public health tools/planning models in this section include:

- CHA, CHIP, and CHNA approaches and templates
  - Association for Community Health Improvement's CHA Toolkit[29]
  - Centers for Disease Control and Prevention's CHANGE[30]
  - County Health Rankings Roadmaps Action Center[31]
- Mobilizing for Action through Planning and Partnerships (MAPP)[32]
- Map-it (Healthy People 2020)[33]
- Assessment Protocol for Excellence in Public Health (APEX/PH)[34]
- Healthy Cities: Healthy Settings[35]
- Community Asset Mapping[36]

Planning and programming tools have been developed for use when working with communities. The number and scope of these approaches and instruments have grown quickly following the IRS ruling for non-profit hospitals and the development of the PHAB prerequisite for a CHA and CHIP. The use of these planning tools and approaches is widely accepted, with most LHDs engaged in CHA (70 percent) and CHIP (56 percent) according to the 2013 Profile Study from the National Association of County and City Health Officials (NACCHO). The description of these methods, instruments, and tools will be brief, primarily intended to acquaint readers with some of the various models and approaches available. The interested reader should follow the summary presented in this section with more detailed investigation and exploration of assessment models. References provided in the descriptions of these models can provide insight into sources for a more detailed description and resources. The selection of framework, method, and approach should be based on the local community's experience and history of citizen engagement and health planning, as well as the experience and expertise of those who will lead and participate in this process.

Community Health Assessment (CHA), Community Health Improvement Plan (CHIP), and Community Health Needs Assessment (CHNA) Approaches and Templates

All the models discussed in this section share certain common attributes. A systems-based approach used by all models is represented by the Take Action model (Figure 13-1) where communities are guided to work together to assess needs and assets, focus on what is important, choose evidence-based programs and policies, act on what is important, and evaluate those actions and make adjustments and improvements. All approaches begin with the creation of a group of citizens empowered to lead a systematic approach to examining the community's health. This assemblage may be a prior constituted group with some responsibility to act on behalf of the community and deal with its health status, such as the local board of health. It may also be an ad hoc group. Frequently, such ad hoc groups include "stakeholders" who represent other agencies and organizations in the community with a concern about the community's wellbeing, including its health status, and are frequently the executive directors of those organizations, particularly in rural communities. Those who have resources and share concerns with public health departments are key to solutions that may be crafted in the process. In fact, some have suggested that a formal "stakeholder analysis" is useful to identify those in the community with common interests in problems identified and the resources that will be necessary to address them.[37,38] When such groups are constituted or identified, it is important to recognize that although they may have some credibility embedded in their mission or constitution, rarely do they represent or engage the ordinary citizens of the community in this process. These individuals and agencies are key, but their efforts should not substitute for citizen engagement. It is imperative to involve not only those who are "grasstops" but also "grassroots" individuals.

Collecting and analyzing data, that is, statistics or measures of community health, is necessary for assessing the health and wellbeing of community members. Data can be obtained through primary or secondary data collection. In some cases, primary or newly collected data from surveys, observations, hospital records, or other means will be used to document the health status and problems of community members. In other cases, secondary data or previously collected data are available to inform the assessment and planning process. Using secondary data can decrease the time and costs associated with data collection procedures. Utilization of geographic information systems (GIS) can also inform our understanding of core geographic concepts such as space, place, location, and distance, and core health statistics related to spatial data.[39]

Quantitative data might not capture all of the information needed to assess the health of a community, depending on the model being used; some of the models require qualitative information as well. This

TAKE ACTION

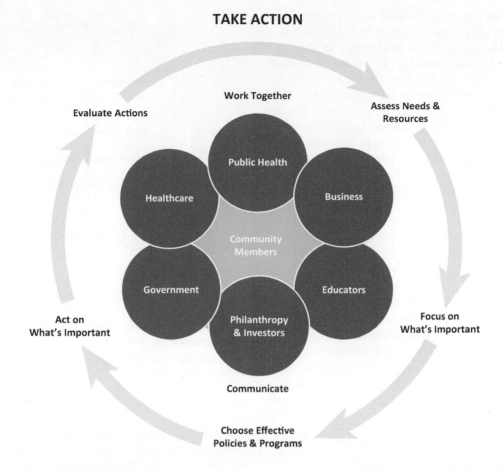

FIGURE 13-1 Take Action Systems Model

Courtesy of University of Wisonsin Population Health Institute. *County Health Rankings & Roadmaps* 2015. www.countyhealthrankings.org

information can be obtained in a variety of ways, including focus groups, nominal group processes with existing community groups, community surveys, or other mechanisms for tapping the perceptions of the community.[40] Again, this is an appropriate phase in the process for community deliberative forums to be convened so that a broad array of community members—representative of the community demographic—is involved in the assessment and planning for the community's health.

Next the group reviews the data to attempt to identify major community health issues that need to be addressed. They may also establish priorities or search for "root causes" of the problems that they have identified. The "snapshot" of the community may be viewed from three perspectives:—the data; the voice of the citizens from surveys, deliberative sessions, and focus groups; and the voices of those participating in the planning sessions. A fairly comprehensive and responsive assessment will result. Regardless of the

particular framework and steps used, a list of issues will also be developed.

The next step is to identify specific programs that can address these identified community needs. The basis for such programs can and should be scientific evidence of effectiveness (see Chapter 11). Although public health is a relative newcomer to evidence-based practice, significant strides have been made over the past decade thanks in great measure to the growth of public health services and systems research (PHSSR), covered in detail in Chapter 17.[5,41,42] The *Guide to Community Preventive Services* provides a list of programs that evidence indicates work for specific problems, those that do not, and where there is no evidence to ascertain the likelihood of a specific program working to solve the problem.[43] The Centers for Disease Control and Prevention (CDC) is currently planning the availability of a new reference, *Navigator*, to help communities identify evidence-based programs and approaches. The selected program should be oriented to specific outcomes that are focused on improving specific health status problems identified in the earlier part of this process. The most logical step in this regard is to link the initiative to objectives for improving health status, such as those contained in *Healthy People 2020*, its state counterpart, or subsequent iterations of that document.[44] Doing so provides program goals that can be used for both formative evaluations to make changes in the program, should it need adjustment along the way, and summative evaluations to assure the success of the program.

As is the case in quality improvement planning processes, the evaluation phase of this model ultimately returns to the point of the planning process, and the cycle is repeated following the "plan, do, check, act" cycle.[14] The various CHA, CHIP, and CHNA approaches and templates are provided in numerous organizational resources including the Association for Community Health Improvement's CHA Toolkit,[29] CDC's CHANGE,[30] County Health Rankings Roadmaps Action Center,[31] and state models such as the Illinois IPLAN approach.[45] All of these represent specific approaches to planning and program implementation, based on a systems approach to community health planning. The specific programs described next are variations on this theme.

Mobilizing for Action through Planning and Partnerships

Mobilizing for Action through Planning and Partnerships (MAPP) is the most widely used public health method of performing community health assessment and planning. MAPP, developed by NACCHO, with major help and support from CDC, involves not only the public health department but also all the components of the *local public health system*. Recollect that the Local Public Health System (LPHS) (see Chapter 9) includes all community organizations and agencies that contribute to the mission of public health, "assuring conditions in which people can be healthy."[11] Thus, it involves not only the health department but also other community components that contribute to the social determinants of health. These include, for example, school systems, the justice system, hospitals, community health centers, employers, insurers, managed care organizations, and not-for-profit organizations. The decision to undertake a MAPP process should include recognizing the amount of time and energy that is required to do the entire MAPP process. It requires a major investment, not only from the health department but also from others in the community. Figure 13-2 illustrates the key components of MAPP.

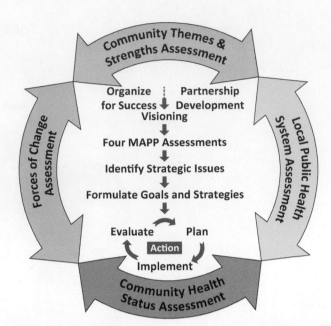

FIGURE 13-2   Mobilizing for Action through Planning and Partnerships (MAPP) Framework

Reprinted with permission from National Association of County and City Health Officials, MAPP Framework, Copyright © 2015.

The process includes several steps and four separate assessments. MAPP begins with organizing the community—its organizations, agencies, and stakeholders—into a group to proceed with the MAPP process.[46-48] This, in turn, is followed by a visioning process, which asks the group to describe how the community's health should look several years downstream. These steps are places where citizen-deliberative forums can be used to broaden the community's engagement with the process and benefit from their deliberation. This also allows for sharing and agreeing on values and strategic directions.

Next, four separate assessments are undertaken. The four assessments are community themes and strengths assessment, local public health system assessment, community health status assessment, and forces of change assessment. These assessments include both quantitative and qualitative data collection processes. Following those assessments, community members must identify strategic health issues in their community and then formulate goals and strategies to address them. This step can draw heavily on *Healthy People 2020* or its successor in establishing community health objectives consistent with a national set of objectives. This then is followed by an action cycle, involving planning, implementation, and evaluation. NACCHO provides more descriptions of the process of MAPP and tools that a community undertaking this process can use for leading the work in the correct direction. This process is time-intensive but ensures that elements in the community are committed to the process and the outcome of improved community health.[32]

MAP-IT

MAP-IT—Mobilize, Assess, Plan, Implement, Track—is a framework used to plan and evaluate health interventions to achieve *Healthy People 2020* objectives. Developed by the U.S. Department of Health and Humans Services Office of Disease Prevention and Health Promotion, the MAP-IT framework helps communities create a path to a healthy community and supports the *Healthy People 2020* comprehensive set of 10-year, national goals and objectives for improving the health of all Americans. *Healthy People 2020* contains 42 topic areas with over 1,200 objectives. A smaller set of *Healthy People 2020* objectives, called Leading Health Indicators, has been selected to communicate high-priority health issues and actions that can be taken to address them.

The series of *Healthy People* objectives has a history that stretches back to the original set of objectives for 1990 which have been updated every decade since then, as they have provided a national framework for states and communities to focus their health status goals, based on national data and objectives. Great strides have been made over the past three decades including an increase in life expectancy at birth and decreased rates of death from coronary heart disease and stroke.[49] The *Healthy People 2020* Leading Health Indicators place renewed emphasis on overcoming challenges and tracking progress over the course of the decade. The indicators are used to assess the health of the nation, facilitate collaboration across sectors, and motivate action at the national, state, and community levels to improve the health of the U.S. population. Progress Updates on the status of each of the 26 indicators are released at regular intervals on the *Healthy People* website.[49] It is likely that we will continue to see the development of sets of objectives for the U.S. health status for the next decade given its success in mobilizing efforts across the United States to achieve those health objectives. MAP-IT assists communities in developing and tracking their contributions to achieve these objectives.

Assessment Protocol for Excellence in Public Health (APEX/PH)

The Assessment Protocol for Excellence in Public Health (APEX/PH) was created by the National Association of County Health Officials (NACHO) before it merged with the U.S. Conference of Local Health Officers to form NACCHO (see Chapter 9). APEX/PH is still in use even though the approach has been greatly expanded through MAPP. More streamlined than MAPP, APEX/PH consists of three parts. The first part is an organizational assessment designed to facilitate an assessment by the LHD of its own capacities to address community health needs and problems. This is an inventory of LHD capacity done by senior staff at the agency. It assures that the issues that might prevent the LHD from being successful in its efforts at community health planning and programming are identified and addressed prior to any effort to engage the community. The notion is to make sure the LHD has the capacity to do a CHA and develop programs to address health problems identified in the assessment. This gives the LHD an opportunity to improve its internal capacity to support the process before the community is mobilized for action.

The second part of APEX/PH is the community assessment and planning activity, which requires the creation of a representative community group that examines community data indicators. Findings inform the choice of health status improvement objectives, frequently taken from those contained in the *Healthy People* series to apply locally. The third part of APEX/PH involves linking the organizational capacity of the health department, appropriately configured, to focus on the problems of the community and to work with a group of community representatives to address the problems identified. This process involves the LHD in assessing and addressing its strengths and weaknesses and then bringing that renewed health department forward to work with the community to improve health.[34]

Healthy Cities: Healthy Settings

The Healthy Cities projects developed from the World Health Organization's (WHO) focus on the "Global Strategy of Health for All by the Year 2000" that was described in the early 1980s.[50] The notion was to mobilize multisectoral approaches to city health problems and issues. This has some natural appeal because it recognizes the social determinants of health and how many community organizations, public and private, need to collaborate to address underlying sets of etiologies of poor health status. Healthy Cities also has a series of steps similar to the generalized scheme of previously described CHA models. The first step is organizing community relationships already in existence. Unlike other schemes, this community-organizing phase specifically focuses on including community leaders who control resources in various sectors. The public sector must be involved, but the private sector has much to contribute as well. The community must complete a community diagnosis or a similar process to identify major health issues in the city. The next step attempts to mobilize all sectors of a community to contribute to the solution of community health issues that have been identified.

An underlying theme is that many health problems have major contributions from outside the health sector, and that the health sector alone may not be successful in solving these problems. Issues such as obesity, safe neighborhoods, or unemployment for example, would benefit from a multisectoral approach. To tackle obesity issues, the parks department could contribute venues and support for physical activity, and the transportation sector could provide bike lanes for alternatives to car travel. The community-planning department could assure that restaurants, grocery stores, and schools are strategically located to allow individuals to walk to those facilities. Restaurants could offer healthy portions and heart-healthy options. The grocery stores of the community can participate

by providing more shelf space for healthier foods and using marketing techniques to facilitate healthy grocery shopping by residents of the community. The strength of this model is in recognizing that the health sector alone cannot create communities that produce healthy people. Finally, the Healthy City model is now enhanced to include Healthy Settings[35] to be more inclusive of other structures, yet continues to embrace the notion of mutual support and its effect on health. The process focuses on the entire city or community mobilizing around health, and each sector is in turn nurtured by others, creating a community culture committed to health.[51–54] Figure 13-3 illustrates the model and components.

Community Asset Mapping

Although these models and the generalized approach to community assessment and planning seem powerful and the appropriate tools for public health

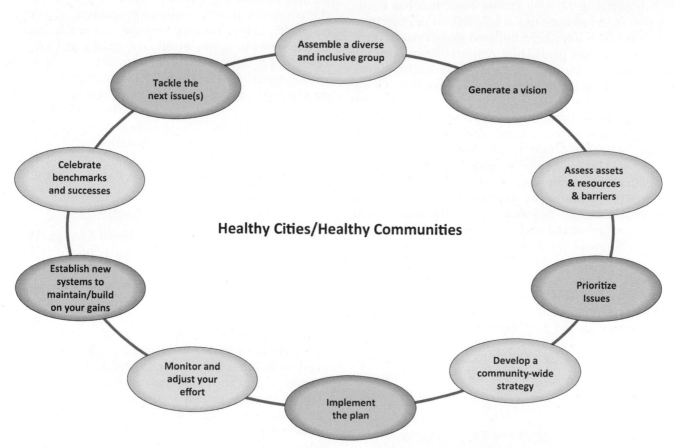

FIGURE 13-3   Healthy Cities/Healthy Communities Framework

KU Work Group for Community Health and Development. (2015). Chapter 3, Section 1: Developing a Plan for Assessing Local Needs and Resources. Lawrence, KS: University of Kansas. Retrieved January 9, 2015, from the Community Tool Box: http://ctb.ku.edu/en/table-of-contents/assessment/assessing-community-needs-and-resources/develop-a-plan/main

professionals to use in their efforts to work with the community, a major caveat has been raised about this process: as McKnight posits, no community was ever built by only defining needs. Instead, he and his colleagues suggest assessments should take a "half-full" as opposed to a "half-empty" approach for true community change. Needs-based surveys insist that residents focus on their emptiness and their insufficiencies. If a culture of deficiency-based assessment becomes the dominant paradigm, then communities could lose the power of wise citizens. Identifying local assets empowers citizens to tap into the capacity that is already available in their community.[36] Kretzmann and McKnight[36] describe three levels of assets that are available in all communities: individual, associations, and institutions (see Figure 13-4). Each level has resources that are necessary to address a problem, issue, or concern. Individuals living in communities possess significant and diverse gifts, skills, and capacities that can be used to improve community health. All residents have expertise and knowledge that can play an effective role in addressing important local matters. Similarly, when individuals gather as civic associations in pursuit of common goals, another level of collective assets is available to strengthen the community. Figure 13-4 compares the community needs map to the asset map, allowing matching up of what we have to what we need.[36] Whether through formal or informal associations, organized citizens provide additional monetary, service, and educational assets to a community. Local institutions, such as government agencies, school systems, cooperative extension, and hospitals, can increase the level of assets available for developing and sustaining community or neighborhood improvements.

At its core, asset mapping depends on community members having necessary resources for identifying and solving a community problem or issue, and identifying those assets already available to bring about change. This community-based approach can involve lay citizens as cocreators and colearners in identifying the desired community outcomes. Moreover, citizens and local organizations and institutions are fundamental to defining the issues to be addressed and creating and implementing the solutions to the issues of concern.

In contrast to traditional needs assessments that focus on mapping deficiencies, asset mapping focuses on the effectiveness of citizens identifying solutions to their own problems and addressing the issues that most affect their community. Community relationships, networks, and individual strengths can be responsive to local needs. Ultimately, asset mapping seeks to empower residents who might traditionally have a limited voice in local processes for addressing local concerns. This more equitable approach can and should be used in conjunction with traditional health assessment methods and tools.[55]

Tools Summary

In summary, there are a number of existing models for use by the public health practitioner in attempting to address community health issues. The most

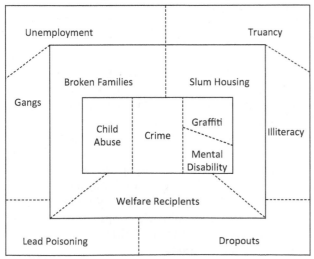

Neighborhood Needs Map

Community Assets Map

FIGURE 13-4 Asset Mapping

Building Communities from the Inside Out: A Path Towards Finding and Mobilizing a Community's Assets by John Kretzman and John McKnight

sophisticated is MAPP. This model developed as an evolution from earlier attempts to provide communities and professionals the tools they need to deal with major community health problems. As has been emphasized, two critical components—deliberative efforts among citizens (not just stakeholders) and asset mapping—could enhance the potential for effectiveness in any of the models described in this chapter. Incorporating these two elements into the assessment and planning phase can be a method for ensuring that the broader community is involved and that available community resources are used to address the issue(s) identified in the assessment and planning process. The addition of these two components is likely to increase the power of the process and its success.

Creating Action Plans for Priority Issues

Involving the public and community partners in the planning and implementation includes creating ownership leads or teams to implement the action plans. This bridging step of synthesizing all the data and determining issues to focus on and implement is challenging.[56] Numerous approaches are being used; however, most share similar elements. The following is a typical action planning cycle and is captured in Figure 13-5. Once priority issues are identified through one of the methods above, detailed action plans need to be implemented by community organizations or individuals who have agreed to take the lead on each initiative. While some of the planning approaches include implementation guidance, this part of the chapter summarizes these approaches and critical elements. Note that the steps outlined here continue to check, involve, and empower community partners to take the lead and guide this work.

The **action planning** process includes determining the stakeholders and public who represent the community who may have a stake in this issue, with consideration for shared ownership. This is followed by a more thorough analysis of the issue including the assets and strengths available within the community. Once the issue and potential root causes are clear, long- and intermediate-term goals and objectives are created using the **S.M.A.R.T. (Specific, Measurable, Achievable, Realistic, Time-bound)** objectives formula. Once the community knows where they want to head, then the identification of evidence-based practices and approaches are considered and planned along with process evaluation indicators and measures, culminating in detailed action plans for the strategies with specific actions, owners of action (accountability), timeline, and resources.

COLLABORATIONS TO IMPLEMENT COMMUNITY PUBLIC HEALTH PROGRAMS

The process of development, implementation, and evaluation of public health programs requires community involvement and participation at every step of the process. After the CHA, CHIP, CHNA, and asset mapping, establishing a new evidence-based public health program or approach remains a critical issue. Moving from planning to action—using one of the tools we describe—is a key step in the process of improving the public's health. In many cases, if not most, implementation of a new or revamped program requires new or reprogrammed resources. Rarely does the LHD, per se, have those resources, but they are likely to exist in a community, frequently in the hands or under control of other actors in the public health system. In any community, a mechanism for mobilizing partnerships and collaboration for program implementation is imperative if a program is to succeed. This notion is perhaps best expressed in the essential public health service of "mobilize community partnerships to identify and solve health problems."

One of the most promising recent developments is the formation of health coalitions including health providers such as hospitals, practitioners, public health officials, and other related community partners to address problems identified from CHAs or CHNAs. For many years coalitions that focused on a particular disease or populations have flourished and made strides toward reducing the burden of disease in their communities. Coalitions have been successfully used to address issues such as immunization, teen pregnancy, drug/alcohol abuse, and obesity and weight management;[57] however, a new type of consolidated coalition is emerging based on the resources and mandates discussed earlier in this chapter.

Coalitions are unions of people and organizations working to influence outcomes on a specific problem. Moreover, they involve multiple sectors of the community that come together to address community needs and solve community problems.[58,59] These groups join to collectively address a broad range of goals that are unattainable by one person or organization. Coalitions promote a critical mass behind social and health issues while conserving resources and reducing duplication of services. These networks cultivate cooperation between diverse sectors of the community that are striving for the same health-related goal.

Many of the local community partnerships aim to incorporate health considerations into decision

These are the steps after the priority issues have been identified through engagement, deliberation, assessments, CHA and CHNA.

1. **Determine stakeholders and public who represent the community who may have a stake in this issue.**
   a. Consider shared ownership.
   b. Define community and target populations.
   c. Identify any existing coalitions, groups or organizations working on priority issue.

2. **Analyze the priority issues within the local community context and the causes.**
   a. Review the data from assessments and gather any additional data on the issue.
   b. Identify any disparities with specific populations. Use small area analysis if possible.
   c. Use problem analysis tools to better understand the problem: underlying root causes including social determinants of health, risk factors, direct and indirect contributing factors, drivers, etc.

3. **Identify the assets, strengths, current efforts, and resources available to support efforts to address the problem.**
   a. Identify current efforts to address this issue.
   b. Define existing strengths and community readiness to address this issue.
   c. Identify any existing assets or resources related to addressing this issue.

4. **Define the long-term goal (outcome objective) for the priority issue.**

5. **Define the intermediate goals (impact objectives) for the priority issue.**
   a. Identify the HP 2020 related objectives. Use as a reference in developing long-term outcome objectives.
   b. Align with state based objectives.
   c. Define what the community wants/needs to achieve long-term on this issue.
   d. Develop SMART Objectives defining the degree of change, type of change, by whom, by when.

   > **S**pecific - What will change and for whom?
   >
   > **M**easurable – Is it quantifiable and can we measure it?
   >
   > **A**ttainable/**A**chievable – Can we accomplish this in the time-frame with the resources we have?
   >
   > **R**elevant - Is it directly related to the underlying causes or problem we are trying to change?
   >
   > **T**ime-Specific - Have we defined when this will be accomplished?

6. **Identify best practices and strategies to create the level of change required to achieve the intermediate and long-term goals.**
   a. Review evidence-based sites and literature to identify programs and approaches to achieve the level of change desired.
   b. Identify strategies at all levels of change (individual, workplace, school, community/environmental, etc.) using the social-ecological model of health.
   c. Identify strategies with a logical link to achieving the outcomes that can be implemented based on existing or planned resources.
   d. Define how, when and by whom progress and success will be measured (process and outcome evaluation) and reported.

FIGURE 13-5   Typical Process for Action Planning on Priority Issues

7. **Identify process evaluation indicators and measures. Process evaluation measures the work that you and your partners are doing.**

   a. Identify and develop an outcome evaluation plan. How will your outcomes be measured (methods), when and by whom? Outcome evaluation measures the impact of you and your partners' work . . . the level of change.

8. **Create detailed action plans for the strategies with specific actions, owners of action (accountability), time-line and resources.**

Terminology:

Outcome Objective(s): a goal for the level to which a health problem should be reduced within a specific time period. It is long term (within five years) and measurable. These are statements about how much and when the program should affect the health problem.

Risk Factors: Direct causes and determinants which, based on scientific evidence or theory, are thought to influence directly the level of a specific health problem.

Impact Objectives: a goal for the level to which a direct determinant or risk factor is expected to be reduced. An impact objective is intermediate (one to five years) in length of time and measurable. These are statements about how much and when the program should affect the determinant.

Contributing factor: a scientifically established factor that directly affects the level of a risk factor.

Indirect contributing factor: community-specific factor that directly affects the level of the direct contributing factors.

Health disparities: Health disparities are differences in health status between people that are related to social or demographic factors such as race, gender, income or geographic region. In general, health disparities are driven by a combination of social factors.

Potential Tools:

- Cause and Effect/Fishbone Diagram (Goal QPC)
- 5 Whys (Goal QPC)
- Change Tool: http://www.cdc.gov/healthycommunitiesprogram/tools/change.htm
- HP 2020 Objectives: http://www.healthypeople.gov/2020/topicsobjectives2020/
- Setting Targets: http://www.healthypeople.gov/2020/implementing/SettingTargets.pdf
- The Guide to Community Preventive Services http://www.thecommunityguide.org/index.html
- SAMHSA's National Registry of Evidence-based programs and practices: http://nrepp.samhsa.gov
- Cancer Control PLANET: http://cancercontrolplanet.cancer.gov/
- Beyond Healthcare: New Direction to a Healthier America: http://www.rwjf.org/pr/product.jsp?id=41008
- HP 2020 Interventions and Resources: http://www.healthypeople.gov/2020/topicsobjectives2020/default.aspx
- Coming attraction: CDC Navigator

FIGURE 13-5 *(Continued)*

Community Health Improvement:
A Framework to Promote Best Practices in
Assessment, Planning and Implementation

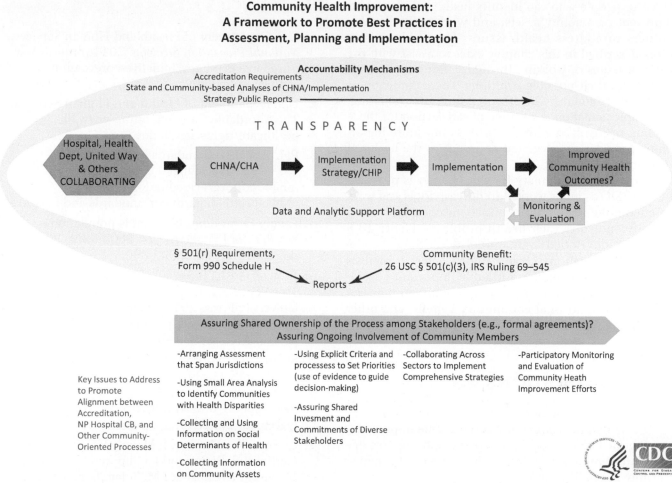

FIGURE 13-6   Community Health Improvement Logic Model
Courtesy of Centers for Disease Control and Prevention, Department of Health and Human Services

making across wide relevant policy areas. This is based on the recognition that policy and program decisions of "nonhealth" agencies impact health in significant and lasting ways. The collaborations initiated in Oregon and Washington to conduct CHAs and CHIPs are a good example of this integrated approach.[60] Their innovative partnership approach to create comprehensive, meaningful, and coordinated community health assessments and community health improvement plans fulfills the specific needs of the hospital systems, local public health agencies, and coordinated care organizations, including the IRS reporting requirements and the PHAB recommendations for assessment and planning by local health agencies. The members of the collaborative indicate that the establishment of a regional workgroup creates an effective, sustainable process and is the most efficient approach

to address their needs. A recent study has examined the specific nature and features of successful collaborations between health departments and hospitals, collaborations that started before the advent of IRS requirements or PHAB standards. These successful partnerships that focused on community health issues provide a set of recommendations for achieving the sort of collaborative that is likely to be successful in sustaining community commitment to achieving healthy community status.[61]

SUMMARY

Communities are the center of public health, indeed they are the "engine," and public health professionals must know how to work within their communities to listen to people who can identify health problems and represent community assets, and work with all stakeholders to address health issues. The public health tools described in this chapter exist to assist with the various stages of working through community health issues and their possible solutions. The completion of thorough community health planning, programming, and implementation is a source of satisfaction for those leading or involved with the process but more importantly provides an integrated approach to the health of the community.

An excellent summary for this chapter is provided by the CDC as it has worked to develop tools and ways to encourage and support efforts in communities to identify and solve their health problems. Figure 13-6 is a CDC-developed logic model describing the elements of Community Health Improvement initiatives described in this chapter and adds important considerations or key issues to promote alignment between accreditation, hospital community benefit, and other community processes.

REVIEW QUESTIONS

1. At the beginning of the chapter, the statement is made that the community is the engine in promoting the public's health. In a paragraph, support this statement by explaining the importance of community in public health.

2. Explain why a community-based approach is necessary for assessing and addressing current public health conditions.

3. Describe the importance of an asset approach to health assessment and program planning. Give particular attention to how asset mapping can be used in conjunction with more traditional public health assessment models.

4. Describe ways that PHAB accreditation and ACA requirements for CHNA encourage collaboration.

5. Identify key characteristics of community-based action planning and explain how this approach could enhance community health initiatives.

ACKNOWLEDGMENTS

The authors would like to acknowledge the contributions of Laura H. Downey, DrPH, coauthor of the Community Health Planning and Programming chapter in the third edition for laying the foundation for portions of this chapter.

REFERENCES

1. U.S. Department of Health and Human Services. *National Prevention Strategy*. 2011; http://www.surgeongeneral.gov/initiatives/prevention/strategy/index.html.

2. U.S. Department of Health and Human Services. The Affordable Care Act. http://www.hhs.gov/healthcare/rights/law/index.html.

3. PHAB. PHAB Standards and Measures 1.0.; 2011(December 1). http://www.phaboard.org/accreditation-process/public-health-department-standards-and-measures/.

4. Kindig D, Stoddart G. What is population health? *Am J Public Health*. 2003;93(3):380–383. doi:10.2105/AJPH.93.3.380.

5. Brownson RC, Baker EA, Leet TL, Gillespie KN, True WR. *Evidence-based public health*. Oxford University Press; 2010:312. http://books.google.com/books?hl=en&lr=&id=9fxzvhVoD2cC&pgis=1. Accessed December 27, 2014.

6. Sharma RK. Putting the Community Back in Community Health Assessment. 2008; http://www.tandfonline.com/doi/abs/10.1300/J045v16n03_03#.VJ8h8sAAHM. Accessed December 27, 2014.

7. Carman KL, Maurer M, Mallery C, Wang G, Garfinkel S, Richmond J, Gilmore D WA, Yang M, Mangrum R, Ginsburg M, Sofaer S, Fernandez J, Gold M, Pathak-Sen E, Davies T S, A, Fishkin J, Rosenberg M FA. *Community Forum Deliberative Methods Demonstration: Summary, Evaluating Effectiveness and Eliciting Public Views on Use of Evidence. Executive AHRQ, (Prepared by the American Institutes for Research Under Contract No. 290-2010-00005.) Publication No. 14-EHC007-1-EF November 2013*. Rockville, MD; 2013. www.effectivehealthcare.ahrq.gov/reports/final.cfm.

8. Heller R, Heller T, Pattison S. Putting the public back into public health. Part II. How can public health be accountable to the public? *Public Health*. 2003; http://www.sciencedirect.com/science/article/pii/S0033350602000082. Accessed December 28, 2014.

9. Northridge M. Putting the "public" back into public health. *Am J Public Health*. 2002; http://ajph.aphapublications.org/doi/pdf/10.2105/AJPH.92.11.1710. Accessed December 28, 2014.

10. Khoo S. Putting the "public" back into public health. *Commonw Heal Partnerships 2013*. 2013. http://www.commonwealthhealth.org/wp-content/

uploads/2013/07/Putting-the-public-back-in-public-health_CHP13.pdf. Accessed December 28, 2014.

11. Crowley P, Hunter D. Putting the public back into public health. *J Epidemiol Community Health.* 2005; http://jech.bmj.com/content/59/4/265 .short. Accessed December 28, 2014.

12. Hays S, Toth J, Poes M, Mulhall P, Remmert D, O'Rourke T. Public Health Governance and Population Health Outcomes. *Front Public Heal Serv Syst Res.* 2012;1(1). http://uknowledge.uky.edu/ frontiersinphssr/vol1/iss1/4. Accessed December 30, 2014.

13. Gittell M, Hoffacker B, Rollins E, Foster S. Limits to citizen participation: the decline of community organizations. 1980; http://library.wur.nl/WebQuery/ clc/136790. Accessed December 27, 2014.

14. Scholtes PR. *The Leader's Handbook.* McGraw-Hill; 1998:53–55. doi:10.1002/pfi.4140380110.

15. Kania J, Kramer M. Collective Impact. *Stanford Soc Innov Rev.* 2011;Winter(Winter 2011):36–41. http://www.capsonoma.org/downloads/ AgendaPacketV1.pdf.

16. Cook FL. The need for public deliberation: Giving the public a voice on affordable health insurance. *J Heal Polit Policy Law.* 2011;36(5):879–885. doi:10.1215/03616878–1407667.

17. McGavran E. Scientific diagnosis and treatment of the community as a patient. *J Am Med Assoc.* 1956; http://jama.jamanetwork.com/article.aspx? articleid=318625. Accessed December 28, 2014.

18. Deuschle K, Fulmer H. The Kentucky experiment in community medicine. *Milbank Meml Q.* 1966; http://www.jstor.org/stable/3349036. Accessed December 28, 2014.

19. Mathews D, McAfee N. *Making Choices Together: The Power of Public Deliberation.* Dayton, OH; 2002. Kettering Foundation archives.

20. Mathews D. *The Ecology of Democracy.* Dayton, OH: Kettering Foundation Press; 2014.

21. Carpini MXD, Cook FL, Jacobs LR. Public deliberation, discursive participation, and citizen engagement: A review of the empirical literature. *Annu Rev Polit Sci.* 2004;7(1): 315–344. doi:10.1146/annurev.polisci. 7.121003.091630.

22. Fishkin J. *The Voice of the People: Public Opinion and Democracy.* New Haven, CT: Yale Univ. Press; 1997. http://books.google.com/ books?hl=en&lr=&id=D2uh2dbM-YsC&oi= fnd&pg=PP11&dq=the+voice+of+the+people &ots=Zpl6dpKfrW&sig=pFsQpNt6iiCLYL 1kETVzOVqwNG8. Accessed September 15, 2013.

23. Committee for the Study of the Future of Public Health. *The Future of the Public's Health in the 21st Century.* 2003; http://www.nap.edu/catalog .php?record_id=10548.

24. Internal Revenue Service. *Form 990, Schedule H.*

25. Section 9007 of the Patient Protection and Affordable Care Act (26 USC § 501(r)(3)(B)).

26. Rosenbaum S, Margulies R. Tax-exempt hospitals and the Patient Protection and Affordable Care Act: implications for public health policy and practice. *Public Heal reports (Washington, DC).* 2011;126(2):283–286. http://www.pubmedcentral .nih.gov/articlerender.fcgi?artid=3056045&tool= pmcentrez&rendertype=abstract. Accessed December 27, 2014.

27. Mays GP, Scutchfield FD. Improving public health system performance through multiorganizational partnerships. *Prev Chronic Dis.* 2010;7(6):A116. http://www.pubmedcentral.nih.gov/articlerende r.fcgi?artid=2995603&tool=pmcentrez& rendertype=abstract. Accessed December 27, 2014.

28. *Section 330 of the Public Health Service Act (42 USCS § 254b) Authorizing Legislation of the Health Center Program.*

29. Association for Community Health Improvement. ACHI Community Health Assessment Toolkit. http://www.assesstoolkit.org/.

30. Centers for Disease Control and Prevention. Community Health Assessment and Group Evaluation (CHANGE) action guide: Building a foundation of knowledge to prioritize community needs. http://www.cdc.gov/nccdphp/dch/programs/ healthycommunitiesprogram/tools/change.htm.

31. County Health Rankings. County Health Rankings Roadmaps Action Center. http://www .countyhealthrankings.org/roadmaps/action-center.

32. NACCHO. *Mobilizing for Action through Planning and Partnership (MAPP).* Washington, DC; 2000. http://www.naccho.org/topics/infrastructure/ mapp/.

33. U.S. Department of Health and Human Services. Healthy People 2020. MAP-IT. https://www .healthypeople.gov/2020/tools-and-resources/ Program-Planning.

34. National Association of County & City Health Officials. Assessment Protocol for Excellence in Public Health (APEXPH). http://www.naccho.org/ topics/infrastructure/APEXPH/.

35. World Health Organization. Healthy Cities; Healthy Settings. http://www.who.int/healthy_settings/en/.

36. Kretzman JP, McKnight JL. Asset-based community development: Mobilizing an entire community. In: *Building Communities from the inside out.* ACTA Publications; 1993:345–354.

37. Schmeer K. *Guidelines for Conducting a Stakeholder Analysis.* 1999; http://www.who.int/entity/management/partnerships/overall/GuidelinesConductingStakeholderAnalysis.pdf. Accessed December 28, 2014.

38. Brugha R. Stakeholder analysis: a review. *Health Policy Plan.* 2000;15(3):239–246. doi:10.1093/heapol/15.3.239.

39. Scotch M, Parmanto B, Gadd CS, Sharma RK. Exploring the role of GIS during community health assessment problem solving: Experiences of public health professionals. *Int J Health Geogr.* 2006;5(1):39. doi:10.1186/1476–072X-5-39.

40. Payne M. Role of quantitative community health assessment data in selecting regional health priorities in a federally-required community health needs assessment. *141st APHA Annu Meet Expo.* 2013; https://apha.confex.com/apha/141am/webprogram/Paper288928.html. Accessed December 28, 2014.

41. Ingram R, Scutchfield F, Mays G, Bhandari M. The economic, institutional, and political determinants of public health delivery system structures. *Public Health Rep.* 2012;127.

42. Scutchfield FD, Bhandari MW, Lawhorn NA, Lamberth CD, Ingram RC. Public health performance. *Am J Prev Med.* 2009;36(3):266–272. http://www.ncbi.nlm.nih.gov/pubmed/19215852.

43. Community Preventive Services Task Force. *The Guide to Community Preventive Services (the Community Guide).* Atlanta, GA; 2012. http://www.thecommunityguide.org/. Accessed December 28, 2014.

44. U.S. Department of Health and Human Services. Healthy People 2020. 2010. https://www.healthypeople.gov/.

45. Illinois Department of Public Health. IPLAN. 2009; http://app.idph.state.il.us/.

46. Lenihan P. MAPP and the evolution of planning in public health practice. *J Public Heal Manag Pract.* 2005; http://journals.lww.com/jphmp/Abstract/2005/09000/MAPP_and_the_Evolution_of_Planning_in_Public.2.aspx. Accessed December 28, 2014.

47. Hodges J. Utilizing MAPP in Shelby County, TN: Process evaluation and preliminary results. *141st*

APHA Annu Meet Expo. 2013; https://apha.confex.com/apha/141am/webprogramadapt/Paper285391.html. Accessed December 28, 2014.

48. Hershey J. MAPP (Mobilizing for Action through Planning and Partnerships) in the New River Valley, Virginia: A Planning Approach to Improve the Community's Health and. 2011. http://scholar.lib.vt.edu/theses/available/etd-04082011-012806/. Accessed December 28, 2014.

49. U.S. Department of Health and Human Services. Healthy People 2020. Leading Health Indicators Progress Reports. www.healthypeople.gov/2020/leading-health-indicators/Healthy-People-2020-Leading-Health-Indicators%3A-Progress-Update.

50. World Health Organization. *Global Strategy for Health for All by the Year 2000.* Geneva; 1981.

51. Hancock T. The evolution, impact and significance of the health cities/healthy communities movement. *J Public Health Policy.* 1993; http://www.jstor.org/stable/3342823. Accessed December 28, 2014.

52. Norris T, Pittman M. The healthy communities movement and the coalition for healthier cities and communities. *Public Health Rep.* 115(2–3): 118–124. http://www.pubmedcentral.nih.gov/articlerender.fcgi?artid=1308699&tool=pmcentrez&rendertype=abstract. Accessed December 28, 2014.

53. Dooris M, Poland B, Kolbe L. *Healthy Settings.* 2007; http://link.springer.com/chapter/10.1007/978-0-387-70974-1_19. Accessed December 28, 2014.

54. Dooris M. Healthy settings: challenges to generating evidence of effectiveness. *Health Promot Int.* 2006; http://heapro.oxfordjournals.org/content/21/1/55.short. Accessed December 28, 2014.

55. Williams K. Modeling the principles of community-based participatory research in a community health assessment conducted by a health foundation. *Health Promot Pract.* 2009. doi:10.1177/1524839906294419.

56. Erwin P, Knight M, Graham J. Data synthesis in community health assessment: practical examples from the field. *J Public Heal Manag Pract.* 2013. doi:10.1097/PHH.0b013e31828000f7.

57. Butterfoss FD, Goodman RM, Wandersman A. Community coalitions for prevention and health promotion: factors predicting satisfaction,

participation, and planning. *Heal Educ Behav.* 1996;23(1):65–79. doi:10.1177/10901981 9602300105.

58. Berkowitz B. Studying the outcomes of community-based coalitions. *Am J Community Psychol.* 2001. doi:10.1023/A:1010374512674.

59. Wolff T. Community coalition building—contemporary practice and research: introduction. *Am J Community Psychol.* 2001;29(2):165–172. doi:10.1023/A:1010314326787.

60. Shirley L, Davidson A, Franc M, et al. Commentary: A public health and hospital system collaboration for conducting community health assessments and community health improvement plans: seven hospital systems in Oregon and Washington and four county public health departments in Oregon and on. *Front Public Heal Serv Syst Res.* 2013;2(2). http://uknowledge.uky.edu/frontiersinphssr/vol2/iss2/1. Accessed December 28, 2014.

61. Commonwealth Center for Governance Studies I. *Models of Collaboration Involving Hospitals, Public Health Departments and Others: Improving Community Health through Successful Partnerships.* http://www.uky.edu/publichealth/hospital/collaboration.

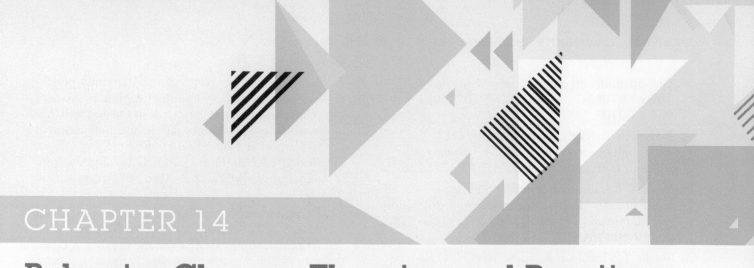

CHAPTER 14

Behavior Change Theories and Practices

John P. Elder, PhD • Ana Quiñones, PhD • Elizabeth Pulgarón, PhD • Daniel López-Cevallos, PhD

LEARNING OBJECTIVES

Upon completion of this chapter, the reader will be able to:

1. Become familiar with the most common health behavior theories.

2. List the elements of ONPRIME.

3. Understand the elements of the ONPRIME model as a structure for conducting effective health behavior change programs.

4. Apply the ONPRIME elements to current public health concerns.

5. Suggest roles of new public policies in the development of behavioral community health assessments.

KEY TERMS

behavioral risk factors
community empowerment
community health
community needs assessment
health behavior change
models
ONPRIME model

INTRODUCTION

The emphasis of the present chapter is on theories of public health behavior change as they are connected to the art and science of community needs assessment, with a special emphasis on behavioral risk factors and behavior change. Thus we present the more commonly used health communication and behavior change-related theories. This is followed by a model derived from these theories that links the various stages of the range of public health program development and implementation with the needs assessment that occurs early in this process. This chapter complements the contents of Chapters 13 and 25. In this particular effort, we compare and contrast the various theories, and then "drill down" into how needs assessment links with prior and subsequent processes both sequentially and recursively. With reference to the "ONPRIME" model, we provide a practical structure for conducting needs and resources (assets) assessment and for using critical data to implement and evaluate health behavior change programs. Examples of how ONPRIME can be used are taken from two distinct public health themes: childhood obesity control and falls prevention among seniors.

HEALTH BEHAVIOR THEORIES

Table 14-1 presents several health behavior and public health promotion theories and their respective emphases in terms of themes and content matter; others also are mentioned below. These are by no means completely representative of the entirety of relevant theories, which are too numerous to be presented in the present chapter. Instead, the theories discussed in this section are (1) among the most frequently cited in the health behavior field, and (2) are illustrative of the range of foci they represent, from the cognitive/intrapersonal to the community level. In turn, this range comprises the elements of the more inclusive socioecological model discussed below.

The relative emphases of each theory are visually represented by "***"-marked (darkly shaded) cells representing a central emphasis, to "*"-marked (lightly shaded) cells representing a moderate emphasis, to blank cells indicating little or no emphasis of that particular theory. With substantial overlap the emphases generally migrate from the upper to the lower rows as theories become more broadly focused.

TABLE 14-1 Health Behavior Theories

Variables Emphasized	Theory					
	TRA/TPB	HBM	SCT	TTM/SOC	Diffusion (Communication) of Innovations	Behaviorism
Intrapersonal (knowledge/attitude)	***	*	*	***		
Confidence/perceived control	***	***	***	***	*	
Perceived social norms	***	***	***	***	***	
Perceived environment (barriers/reinforcers)	***	***	***	*	*	
Social support/social networks			***		***	***
Objectively measured environment		*			*	***
Community applications			*		***	***

TRA/TPB: Theory of Reasoned Action and the Theory of Planned Behavior
HBM: Health Belief Model
SCT: Social Cognitive Theory
TTM/SOC: Transtheoretical Model/ Stages of Change

The Theory of Reasoned Action and the Theory of Planned Behavior

The Theory of Reasoned Action emphasizes the impact of attitudes and intentions on behavior.[1] These attitudes are driven by expectations or beliefs about the behavior, whether positive or negative, or of high or low cost. The TRA's primary constructs include "attitude" (expectations of consequences), subjective norms and normative beliefs, and the intention to behave in a particular way. The Theory of Planned Behavior (TPB) was later proposed to include the notion of control as an additional causal factor,[2] with the emphasis again on perceived control.[3,4]

Health Belief Model

The Health Belief Model (HBM) seeks to explain why people take action in preventing, screening, or controlling illness.[5] The HBM theorizes that individuals have a level of perceived threat regarding a particular disease. In order for action to be taken to lessen this threat, that person must believe that these actions will not result in an uphill battle (perceived barriers) and will have an advantageous outcome (perceived benefits).

Social Cognitive Theory

Social Cognitive Theory (SCT), which was earlier known as Social Learning Theory (SLT), emphasizes the interaction among the cognitive and environmental variables that influence and are influenced by human behavior. With its origins in behaviorism,[6] SCT has become popular in the field as it has drifted toward an intrapersonal focus. Central to SCT are two constructs: self-efficacy and outcome expectations. The former is essentially the confidence to perform a behavior, while the latter emphasizes the individual anticipation of "pain or gain" associated with the behavior.[7,8] SLT also established that behavior can be affected by vicarious learning and vicarious reinforcement via observing behavioral models, similar to the concept of "early adopters" (see below). Therefore, new behaviors and their potential consequences can be learned by an individual who has not previously engaged in the behavior.[7]

Diffusion (Communication) of Innovation and the Transtheoretical Model

The Diffusion (or "Communication") of Innovations theory[9,10] applies to how behavior change spreads through a community or some subset of it. Although referring to intrapersonal cognitive processes, Diffusion of Innovations (DOI) emphasizes the gradual spread of an innovative practice from one (an "innovator") to a few ("early adopters") to a majority ("early" and "late" adopters) of individuals. Eventually, even those resisting change ("laggards") may decide also to adopt the innovation. The speed by which the innovation will spread through a community depends on:

▸ the advantage of the innovation compared to previous practice,
▸ its compatibility with cultural norms,
▸ the complexity of the action,
▸ its trialability (i.e., whether one can experiment with the behavior before fully adopting it), and
▸ its observability (i.e., whether others can be observed engaging in the behavior, similar to SCT's modeling concept).

The DOI thus parallels Prochaska's "Stages of Change" (SOC) concept. The central theme of the "Transtheoretical Model" (TTM) holds that an individual progresses from not pondering behavior change (precontemplation), to beginning to consider (contemplation) and get ready for it (preparation), to embarking on a change (action), and finally to habitual practice of the behavior (maintenance). DOI instead applies to a collection of individuals (or in a sense, an individual community) rather than a single individual's thought processes, as does the SOC. Deriving initially from work in indigenous villages in South America,[9] DOI is arguably more applicable across cultures than are the more Western-oriented intrapersonal theories, discussed above. Along with McGuire's Communication-Persuasion[11] and Kotler's Social Marketing models,[12] DOI has been one of the most influential in the field of public health communication, emphasizing the need to identify opinion leaders and "champions" of a prevention program[13] who can proactively assist in promoting risk factor reduction efforts.

Behaviorism

Behaviorism* in its applied form has been central to mental health interventions and public health promotion for five decades.[6,14,15] Deriving from *positivism*

---

* The authors prefer this term over many other possibilities, even though "behaviorism," "behaviorists," etc., have a somewhat overly generalized application. Other possibilities are "operant psychology" but this connotes animal learning. "Behavior modification" and "contingency management" denote specific interventions rather than the broader field, and "applied behavior analysis" has evolved to refer specifically to interventions for autistic children. Thus, our term "behaviorism" refers specifically to the positivistic tradition of Skinner and before him Watson, Thorndike, and to a lesser extent, Pavlov.

and more recently Skinner's "operant psychology," behaviorism deviates from the aforementioned intrapersonal theories in holding that only phenomena that can be directly and reliably assessed through objective observation can be considered to be scientific.[16,17] Skinner described behavior-consequence relationships as "contingencies of reinforcement." "Positive reinforcement" is the contingency that strengthens a behavior, while "punishment" weakens it. Skinner's notion of "negative reinforcement" refers to the strengthening of behavior through avoiding or terminating an aversive condition.

For a variety of reasons unrelated to the scientific validity of behaviorism, behaviorism is not invoked as frequently as its more cognitive counterparts. Nevertheless, behaviorism is probably the most universally applicable and least culture-bound of all health behavior theories. Moreover, health interventions and especially those with a central policy component clearly employ behavior modification techniques. Clean indoor air rules, tobacco taxes, inexpensive public transportation, clean and safe parks, and DUI laws and their enforcement all directly apply contingency management procedures without any reference to individual cognitive processes. Internationally, contingency management is central to family planning, immunization, infant growth monitoring, and other national and even international programs.[18]

In summary, theories of **health behavior change** range from emphasizing individual intrapersonal factors to broad social and physical environmental forces. For example, most theories converge in the assumption that reinforcement plays a central role in strengthening health behavior, though positivist theories, especially behaviorism, examine the direct behavior-environment relationship whereas intrapersonal theories emphasize the individual's cognitive mediation of this relationship. In any case, few **community health** promotion programs rely on one specific theory to plan, implement, or evaluate a program, rather, a mix of theories blended within various multifaceted models guide these public efforts. The use of such models is presented below.

THE *ONPRIME* MODEL

Why do these theories matter? In a special issue of the *Lancet* dedicated to the promotion of physical activity, the Lancet Physical Activity Working Group notes that "the science of how to change individual behaviors has overshadowed efforts to understand true population change. Because of this unbalanced focus, the structural and systemic changes necessary to promote physical activity in populations across various sectors has not yet been addressed" (p. 72).[19]

In an implicit acknowledgment of the aforementioned concern regarding health behavior theories, the field has increasingly turned to more comprehensive models that are informed by the range of theories represented in Table 14-1 but are not specific to any one of them. **Models**, in contrast to theories, generally comprise representations of physical structures or processes and the interactions among these structures and processes, meant more to describe and logically link phenomena together than to imply broader meanings underlying these phenomena. These are often referred to as "ecological" or "socioecological" models, which accommodate a greater focus on the environment than do TRA, HBM, or SCT. Ecological models derive from biology and have recently been applied not only to public health promotion but even to social media and electronic information.[20]

Variables that had previously been the domain of intrapersonal theories, such as "self-regulation," are often extended to larger and more complex levels of society in socioecological models. In addition, the physical environment, and the social and cultural aspects of the community also need to be considered. Community organizing is a necessary process through which communities identify issues, establish goals, mobilize resources, and develop and implement strategies that have been collectively set.[21] In this approach, communities should be supported to embody the idea that they are (or need to be) at the center of health improvement initiatives. In other words, communities are not solely the passive recipients of external goodwill, but rather active participants on their collective path toward better health. Therefore, parallel to *self*-regulation, **community empowerment** is a critical component for community health programs. Empowering communities to take action for collective health is a key ingredient for success,[22,23] especially among disenfranchised, low-income, minority communities. Ultimately, our work toward improving community empowerment and organization has the added (and potentially longer lasting) effect of strengthening the social capital of our communities.[24] Social capital refers to trust, norms, and networks (features of social organization) that facilitate coordinated action.[25] In an increasingly interconnected world, public health practitioners must rely on coordinated action toward changing individual behaviors and improving population health.

Planning templates for changing individual and population health derive from broader ecological models rather than specific individual theories. The best-known pragmatic model used in health promotion planning is Lawrence Green's PRECEDE/PROCEED model,[26] most closely based on the Health Belief Model.[27] The RE-AIM (Reach Effectiveness-Adoption-Implementation-Maintenance) framework (RE-AIM, http://www.re-aim.org) also comprises a convenient framework for planning and evaluation.[28] The present chapter refers specifically to Elder and colleagues' ONPRIME model, which links needs and resources assessment (N/RA) and other planning, intervention, and evaluation steps and their specific elements into a singular staged, recursive process.[29] Based upon the standard approach to community health behavior change—planning, intervention, and evaluation (PIE) (see Chapter 13)—the ONPRIME model emphasizes the importance of seven process substeps: Organization, Needs/ Resources Assessment, Priority Setting, Research, Interventions, Monitoring, and Evaluation (see Figure 14-1). The N/RA process looks not only at behavioral problems and health needs of a community but also its assets and previous successes at tackling similar health and other problems.

The Elements of ONPRIME

"**O**rganization" refers to whether the program entails working within existing organizations, working through various community gatekeepers or out of the program planner's health office, or sometimes through grassroots community organizing in order to develop a sponsoring structure where no apparent candidate exists. Leadership Skills are essential here, as they are in the Priority Setting stage. Thus this step may already be established with programs sponsored by worksites, hospitals and clinics, health departments, or other entities. In some cases, however, grassroots organizing and true community-based participatory research (Chapter 25) may best fit an environment or funding mechanism. Alternatively, program developers may be called upon to make use of already existing resources and assets (Chapter 13) by linking them together and ensuring that concerned stakeholders work synergistically and not silo-fashion or even competitively.

The second element of ONPRIME is "**N**eeds and Resources Assessment (N/RA)," the primary emphasis of the present chapter. This phase may include key informant interviews, archival research, and surveys, with a special examination of the existing health and related environmental, economic, and social problems of the community. This is parallel to the Community Dimensions of Practice Skills, as described in Appendix B. In terms of needs and resources assessment, the community advisors can also point the program planner to types of activities that have been conducted in the past and how the community resources have been, or could be, used to address the existing health problem. Similar to "asset mapping" (Chapter 13), the successful health program looks at the community as one that has many strengths, abilities, and potential resources that can be employed to address a given problem, not as a community that needs outside help.

After data are collected, health officials, community advisory boards, or representative individuals within the community can then examine the health information to help establish health- and disease-related priorities. Generally speaking, communities that have been successful in selecting their own intervention or targeted health "**P**riorities" will be more likely to embrace a program over a longer period of time than those that do not. Communication skills are essential for the practitioner to develop these priorities in partnership with the community.

"**R**esearch" in this sense refers not to epidemiological or survey research to identify health problems (as in the "Needs/Resources Assessment phase") but instead to the formative and other qualitative/quantitative research needed to develop health behavior change, intervention concepts, and direct applications. Thus the qualitative and quantitative research is conducted specifically to develop new techniques and/or refine old ones. Focus groups and in-depth or brief intercept interviews are the most common examples of qualitative research formats that can assist the program developer in determining the target audience's perception of a health issue, whether and how they feel something could be done about this issue, and what types of target audiences and target audience segments might exist in the community. Program planners can identify individuals (or families, organizations, etc.) who have adopted a practice and compare and contrast them with those who have not. Again, focus group and other types of research with these individuals may be effective in revealing what has influenced some individuals to improve their health or has presented barriers so that others have not. Through such research, program planners can make substantial progress toward selecting and building on existing practices rather than developing others that might be considered somewhat alien to the target population.

Once the aforementioned phases are completed, the planner develops a set of "**I**ntervention" activities

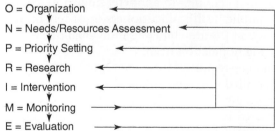

The ONPRIME Model and Interactions among Steps

O = Organization
N = Needs/Resources Assessment
P = Priority Setting
R = Research
I = Intervention
M = Monitoring
E = Evaluation

FIGURE 14-1   The ONPRIME Model

Adapted from Elder, JP et al.

that address the health issues through the most effective techniques available. Individual-level behavior change, skill building, and tailored communication, as well as mass communication, policy change, and changes in the physical environment can affect the behavior on the small or large scale, respectively. These intervention components derive from the diverse multilayered elements of "ecological models" (described in next section, below), comprising individual behavioral risk reduction embedded in family, organizational, environmental, or entire community change.

"Monitoring" is the penultimate step in the ON-PRIME sequence and a critical element of the planning-implementation-evaluation sequence (Chapter 13). It comprises both the monitoring of the implementation process (e.g., did television spots get aired when they were supposed to?) as well as responses to the intervention (e.g., once a grocery store promotion was undertaken, what sales changes if any were there?). Through regular collection of data sensitive to individual or community response to a program, the implementation team has an excellent feedback tool for themselves and the community. Thus, individuals who may or may not be attuned to statistical analyses and p-values may increase their awareness of how different trends of time-series data presented in a graphic format can represent their progress toward an existing health or behavior change criterion. These monitoring data may then be used in a variety of recursive processes to reinforce individual or community progress or to provide the implementation team with the information needed to conduct further N/RA and subsequently alter existing programs. This is relevant to Policy Development/Program Planning Skills.

Finally, "Evaluation" is used to determine whether a program was effective or which elements of the program were most effective. Evaluation information may be used to determine whether to extend a program and promote its generalization to other communities, or, conversely, whether to terminate the effort (also relevant to Policy Development/Program Planning Skills).

HEALTH BEHAVIOR AND ECOLOGICAL APPROACHES

Social ecological approaches to health promotion incorporate the interplay between behavioral and environmentally based interventions. This includes a combination of both active strategies (those which individuals must engage in) and passive strategies (that require no additional effort on behalf of the individual). The key determinant of health from a social ecological perspective is the successful match between an individual's biological, behavioral, and sociocultural needs and the environmental resources available to the individual.[30] One of the most prominent social ecological models is Bronfenbrenner's Social Ecological Theory.[31] This theory focuses on the environment's influence on an individual's development. The most influential environment is the microsystem, which is the environment most proximal to the individual (typically consisting of the home), extending to the macrosystem (an amalgamation of broad economic and public health-related forces). Bronfenbrenner's Social Ecological Theory has been applied to health behavior change in a variety of populations.[32,33] As applied to the present chapter, the Social Ecological Model with its various interacting, reciprocally influential layers is presented in Figure 14-2.

Community-Level Organization and Intervention Priorities

From an ecological perspective, communities where individuals and families live, play, and work, influence individual and family-level health outcomes.[34] In other words, physical, social, cultural, and political environments can have a strong influence in the health of individuals, families, and populations.[35] At a time when the majority of the world's population lives in urban environments, our homes, schools, workplaces, parks, and surroundings play an increasingly important role in human health.[36] The Institute of Medicine, Robert Wood Johnson Foundation, and other organizations have identified environmental and policy-level strategies as the most promising toward reducing the burden of chronic diseases (e.g., heart disease, stroke, cancer, diabetes, obesity, and arthritis) in the U.S. population.[37,38] The built environment includes all man-made entities that form the physical characteristics of a community, such as buildings, transportation networks, community layouts, and parks and trails.[38] Physical activity and food environments have been the two primary areas for research and intervention work thus far.[39,40]

In addition to the physical environment, the social and cultural aspects of the community also need to be considered. Organizing and mobilizing communities is a necessary process through which community health initiatives can be successful and sustainable.[21] Although funding mechanisms may not always be flexible, communities should be supported to embody the idea that they are (and need to be) at the center of health improvement initiatives. Therefore, as emphasized in Chapter 25, community empowerment is a critical component for organizational and priority-setting phases of ONPRIME, particularly among disenfranchised, low-income and/or diverse communities. Such communities stand to benefit substantially from the Patient Protection and Affordable Care Act (ACA), a major force in public health change at the national level.

and healthy eating. CATCH facilitators organized and attended committee meetings, facilitated CATCH presentations to school staff, provided in-service learning opportunities for teachers, and coordinated with school administration regarding implementation of CATCH.

Related to ONPRIME's monitoring phase, the degree of implementation was assessed with structured interviews of the CATCH Champions and teacher self-report questionnaires. Process data were collected, including the number of CATCH committee meetings held, perceptions of CATCH committee activities and composition, perceived principal support, implementation of CATCH Family Fun Night, and the number of health lessons taught to students. Student-related process data were also collected, including their report of CATCH lessons taught, correct identification of "Go" foods and CATCH characters, access to fruit at lunch, description of lunch as "usually healthy," and report of physical activity breaks led by teachers.

Results indicated significant differences between the two programs, with students in the CATCH BPC program demonstrating a significantly greater decrease in percent of overweight/obesity over time. Students in the CATCH BPC program also reported being more likely to consume breakfast, having a lower Unhealthy Food Index, and having a lower percentage of students spending more than two hours on the computer per day.

MOVE/me Muevo Extending interventions from the Family to the Community Level

Elder and colleagues' community-based parks and public recreation center childhood obesity intervention was conducted in every neighborhood of the city of San Diego.[48] The MOVE/me Muevo study recruited families to participate through direct phone calls and face to face at public locations (e.g., libraries, schools, fairs).

ONPRIME describes its research phase as having two components: a broad qualitative look at general perceptions and concepts, followed by a more specific qualitative + quantitative phase once initial intervention strategies were outlined that allowed the target audience to select among options or even include a pilot or efficacy test of an intervention. The initial formative research phase of MOVE/me Muevo yielded one critical finding that shaped all subsequent intervention and evaluation efforts. Parents (particularly mothers) all understood that childhood obesity was highly prevalent, especially in diverse and poorer communities. However, they tended not to see it in their own children: fully one-third of mothers of obese children rated them as normal weight. Subsequent formative research explored how best to correct misperceptions and underestimates, and this information evolved into a major element of the intervention.[48]

As part of the subsequent research phase of ONPRIME, a feasibility pilot study was conducted at a recreation center. The efficacy research included not only intervention (half-day training for the recreation center staff, family workshops, home visits with educational materials) but also monitoring and evaluation tools (process evaluation instruments and height and weight measurement protocols). Based on the experience and feedback from the pilot, various changes were implemented to the protocol. For example, the educational materials presented to parents in a folder were rarely used so those were changed to one- to two-page tip sheets that highlighted the most important information.

MOVE/me Muevo staff received extensive training on family and recreation center intervention procedures, motivational interviewing skills, and role-playing scenarios. Daily oversight and weekly meetings maintained intervention fidelity. The family intervention component of the intervention was customized for each family's needs. The intervention consisted of a 10-minute telephone survey about the family's use of the recreation center, a 90-minute orientation at the recreation center, and a one-hour home visit. Tip sheets were sent via mail to families and two more 10-minute follow-up phone calls were placed during the intervention. Motivational interviewing, self-monitoring, and goal setting techniques were used during the phone calls. Specific nutrition and physical activity behaviors were targeted.

A recreation specialist was hired by the study team to work with recreation center directors on increasing overall attendance at the centers and bolstering enrollment in children's physical activity programs. The recreation specialist met monthly with the recreation center staff to develop an action plan, monitor progress, and assist with health policies. During the initial months of the intervention, the recreation specialist learned from the recreation center staff how to promote the center as the prominent entity for physical activity in the community. In terms of broader community organizational strategies, the recreation specialist attended a recreation or city council meeting.

Monitoring data fed back into bolstering the intervention. Structured observations of the recreation centers and audits of physical activity programs were synthesized into a summary report that was shared with the recreation center director. The report included details on physical activity and healthy snack choices available for children at the center, the participants' experiences and perceptions of the center as a place for physical activity, and staff perceptions on the benefits of the MOVE/me Muevo resources and necessary supports to reach the physical activity targets. Based on these and broader community data (e.g., due to reductions in staff due to steep budget cuts) some of the initial plans were scrapped. Instead, actions plans were developed to promote and engage residents in existing and improved recreation center activities and services.

Monitoring and evaluation data were collected throughout the intervention trial. Outcome evaluation data showed significant differences on girls' BMI in favor of the intervention even though there was no overall (boy + girl) difference in BMI or waist circumference. Other promising changes included a reported decrease in fat and sugary beverages for those in the intervention condition compared to those in the control group.

Changing eating and physical activity habits has proved to be quite the challenge in the health behavior field, and interventions in the childhood obesity field have had limited results. Both the CATCH and MOVE/me Muevo interventions were large trials held at multiple community sites and included low socioeconomic status and minority families that were able to demonstrate some degree of change in obesogenic behaviors. These interventions are good examples of the importance of tailoring programs to the specific needs of a community and implementing the various stages of the ONPRIME model.

Falls Prevention

Falls are the leading cause of both fatal and nonfatal injuries for older adults.[49] Injuries resulting from falls have vast implications for the quality of life and functional independence of older Americans. Preventing falls from occurring is an important objective in order to promote the well-being of older adults.[50] Promoting public health efforts that result in fewer falls averts substantial health care costs associated with injuries and the often significant and lasting physical consequences of fall-related injuries. As a result, the implementation of evidence-based falls-prevention programs would vastly improve the lives of older adults and is an important public health goal for the growing numbers of older adults in the United States.

Population Aging

The proportion of older adults in the United States is increasing rapidly. In 2011, the first members of the large Baby Boom generation turned 65, corresponding to a rapid acceleration in the size of the aging population in the United States. In 1900, 4.1 percent of the population was 65 years or older, whereas in the latest U.S. Census figures collected in 2010, people aged 65 years or older represented 13 percent of the total population.[51] Within the first decade of the new century, the older population of persons aged 65 and older in the United States has grown from 34.99 million to 40.27 million. By 2050, U.S. Census figures estimate the population aged 65 and older will increase to 83.74 million, representing 20.9 percent of the projected total U.S. population (see Figure 14-3).

The racial and ethnic composition of the older population is also in a state of transition. In 2000, non-Hispanic whites comprised 86.9 percent of the

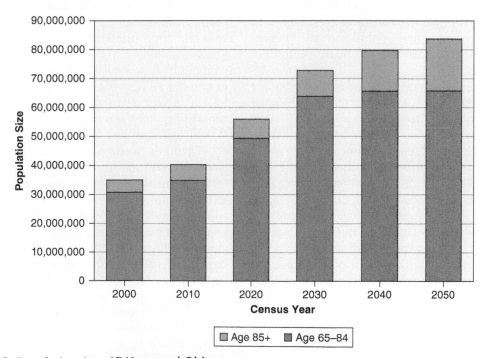

FIGURE 14-3 U.S. Population Age 65 Years and Older

SOURCE: U.S. Census Bureau, decennial census of population 2000 to 2010; 2010 Census Summary File 1

population aged 65 and older; however, in 2010 that proportion decreased to 84.8 percent as this age group became more ethnically and racially diverse with increases in African Americans (increasing their numbers by 5 percent), Asian Americans (by 35 percent) and Hispanics (by nearly 30 percent). Projections out to 2050 indicate that the older population, while still expected to be predominantly white/Anglo, will be increasingly racially and ethnically diverse—18.4 percent of the older population is expected to be Hispanic by 2050, more than twice what it was in 2010. Because of this changing demographic profile of older adults over the next 40 years, public health systems, public health professionals, and the communities where older adults live need to understand the needs and health priorities of a growing and diverse older population.

Health and Disease Priorities: Falls and Other Chronic Disease Trends

Population aging changes over the next few decades raise questions of how best to promote the health of older Americans who are increasingly living with chronic disease. For Americans 65 and older, the most common chronic conditions include arthritis, hypertension, diabetes mellitus, pulmonary disease, cancer, and osteoporosis.[52] Having multiple concurrent chronic diseases is associated with high health care utilization and costs, and more importantly, increases the likelihood of disability and mortality above and beyond the risk associated with an individual disease.[53] Because of the changing views of monitoring the well-being of older adults instead of specific disease rates, research and practice has been reformulated around care and prevention efforts that target improving the health and function of older adults.[54]

Multiple chronic conditions have been increasing for older Americans over the last 11 years.[55] In 2005, 45 percent of noninstitutionalized Americans 65–79 years of age and 54 percent of those 80 and older reported living with multiple chronic diseases.[56] Among older adults covered by Medicare, two-thirds of all beneficiaries had two or more chronic conditions, and one-third have four or more.[53] These chronic disease trends shift our thinking and public health practice away from examining individual diseases singly and instead favor health promotion programs that consider how multiple diseases interact to affect function and the quality of life for older adults.

For older adults, having more than one chronic disease at the same time is often accompanied by physiological declines, slower reflexes and frailty, and puts older adults at increased risk of suffering serious and debilitating falls.[52,54,57] Approximately 30 percent of Americans over age 65 will fall at least once every year, and 31–41 percent of those who fall will suffer injuries.[49,58–62] Direct medical costs for fall-related injuries

totaled $19 billion in 2000,[59] a figure that has grown in tandem with the burgeoning population of older adults.[60]

In response to this large and growing public health problem, *Healthy People 2020* targets a 10 percent reduction in the rate of fall-related emergency department visits and prevention of fall-related deaths among adults 65 and older as important objectives. (For more information, access http://www.healthypeople.gov/2020 and perform a search for the term "Older Adults.") Similarly, but more broadly, the National Center for Injury Prevention and Control (NCIPC) identified the prevention of falls in older adults as a priority focus area. Falls prevention is a national public health priority. Taking Oregon as a case state, the fall fatality rate from 2001–2005 among Oregon seniors, 65.5 per 100,000, was 71 percent greater than the national average. Additionally, while the national rate of fall fatalities decreased during this time period, the rate in Oregon remained the same.[63] Hence, falls-prevention programs represent an important public health *need* requiring effective interventions at all levels.

Community-Based Interventions for Falls Prevention

Fall-related injuries and mortality were previously seen as accidental in nature, and therefore unable to be intervened upon to prevent their occurrence and mitigate their effects; however, this attitude no longer predominates. Various projects have demonstrated that falls can be prevented and that intervention programs can be successfully implemented in community settings. Given the ease and appropriateness of making many of these programs available in the communities where seniors live, community-based falls-prevention programs have grown in number and have led the way for municipal and state health agency partnerships with community organizations to expand the reach of these falls-prevention efforts (ONPRIME's organizational aspect).

Through needs and resources assessment, effective interventions first identify older adults at risk of falling, and then connect these high-risk elders with falls-prevention programs that are appropriate for their specific needs and convenient for them. Needs assessment consists of an exploration of all risk factors, including a host of individual biological and behavioral factors—mobility problems, chronic health conditions, vision changes, inactivity, and alcohol use—as well as home and environmental hazards. The latter comprises clutter in the home, incorrectly sized or inappropriate footwear, incorrect assistive devices, and poorly designed public spaces. Primary care providers in health care settings have primarily conducted screenings for fall risk factors, but they can also be conducted by community organizations serving older adults. Regardless of the setting, the priority lies in identifying seniors at greater risk for falls in order to best intervene and prevent potentially devastating health outcomes. Effective interventions for reducing falls complement needs assessment and screening data, and have been demonstrated through exercise-based, home modification, and multifactorial interventions (interventions that do not rely on one approach alone but instead use a mixture of approaches to prevent falls). Promoting healthy lifestyle modifications, chronic disease self-management, and fall risk assessment—including home safety assessments, medication reviews, and vision screening—have all been shown to reduce falls among older adults.[64] The following section will describe two behavior change programs that aim to reduce the risk of falls and improve the health and function of older adults. The first program centers on delivering falls-prevention education and demonstration through an exercise-based program, Tai Chi Moving for Better Balance. The second program is an intervention to reduce falls using a multifactorial program, Stepping On, which combines health education, limited exercise-based activities and home safety checks, and encourages vision and medical assessments. Both of these programs illustrate the value of the ONPRIME model within the context of developing falls-prevention programs along Organization, Needs assessment, and Priority Setting elements for the population; implementation of falls-prevention programs with Research and Intervention activities targeting older adults; and finally, with the recursive improvements of the entire ONPRIME continuum through feedback during the Monitoring and Evaluation processes.

Tai Chi Moving for Better Balance

Tai Chi Moving for Better Balance is an eight-form Tai Chi program modified for seniors and consists of a twice-weekly sessions (60 minutes each) for a 12-week period. Each hour-long session includes a short warm-up period (5–10 minutes), the practice of Tai Chi movements, and a short cool-down period (5–10 minutes). In terms of ONPRIME's intervention, monitoring, and evaluation phases, participants were encouraged to practice at home, and were monitored through a home practice log. Evaluation (ONPRIME) of this Tai Chi program showed it to reduce falls in seniors by as much as 55 percent.[65] The program emphasizes weight shifting, postural alignment, and coordinated movements to improve balance and lower-extremity strength. Each session includes instructions in any new movements along with a review of movements presented in earlier sessions. Early pilot research demonstration projects noted that in Oregon, Tai Chi Moving for Better Balance resulted in significant improvements among participants in physical function tests, and reported improvements in physical and mental well-being.[66]

In initial evaluations of the Tai Chi Moving for Better Balance program, older adults (aged 70 years or older) who participated in the program had fewer falls and fewer fall-related injuries compared to older adults who conducted stretching activities. Evolving from the organizational and needs/resources assessment phases, Tai Chi Moving for Better Balance program was conducted in a variety of community-based settings, depending on community preferences and the resources available to conduct classes. Local senior centers, adult activity centers, and other community centers were typical settings where classes were held. Tai Chi, modified for the needs of seniors, has thus been shown to be a highly effective falls-prevention intervention with demonstrated translatability across community-based settings in the United States—this Tai Chi program is now widely distributed and conducted in senior centers across various states.

Generalization to Other Settings and Populations: "Stepping On"

Evolving from community outreach, in-depth interviews of older adults, and steps to develop and evaluate the Falls Behavioral Scale for Older People, the Stepping On program emerged as a multifactorial community-based program provided to small groups of older adults to engage in learning activities to improve fall prevention self-efficacy, encourage behavioral change, and reduce falls.[67,68] The intervention includes seven sessions over a 7-week period, a follow-up home visit within six weeks of the final program session, and a 3-month booster session. Stepping On employs a variety of strategies, such as raising awareness by informing seniors of factors that contribute to the risk of falls, targeting those behaviors that have the most effect on risk, and reinforcing their application to the individual's home environment and community setting. Stepping On also uses effective learning techniques such as storytelling, mastery experiences, and using the group setting as a dynamic learning environment.

During an initial evaluation of the program's effectiveness, Stepping On demonstrated a 31 percent reduction in falls for older, independent-living Australian adults (aged 70 and older) for a 14-month follow-up period.[69] The intervention focused on four key content areas and monitored subsequent activities of participants along these areas: (1) strength and balance exercises, (2) having a routine vision examination, (3) number of medications and psychotropic drugs used, and (4) recommendations arising from the follow-up home visit. Among participants in the initial monitoring and evaluation research, adherence was 59 percent for routine exercising, 72 percent for initiation of a vision assessment (compared to only 42 percent of the control group), only 8 percent for starting a new psychotropic drug (compared to 16 percent of the control group) and 70 percent for completing at least half of the home-visit recommendations. The program emerged from iterative processes of community needs assessment and outreach, research to help formulate what elements to include in the Falls Behavioral Scale for Older People, identifying and intervening on behavioral factors that lead to harmful falls in the intervention development phase, and employing monitoring and evaluation steps to ensure the program is appropriately administered and to assess its effectiveness. Since its inception, Stepping On has demonstrated itself to be an effective falls-prevention program that has been successfully implemented in community settings across various countries. These kinds of multifactorial falls-prevention programs are among the most highly effective programs evaluated thus far.

The role of public health in the face of population aging is critical. The aging of America's population will require greater dissemination and outreach of public health programs to prevent and control chronic health diseases and conditions that place people at risk for falls. Ongoing efforts in evaluation and implementation of effective programs will play a critical role in identifying best practices for educational and behavioral strategies to help older adults achieve good health-related quality of life.

SUMMARY

This chapter examines a range of health behavior theories in terms of their relative emphases on cognitive/intrapersonal factors versus direct behavior-environmental relationships. We conclude that no single theory is adequate to fully explain health behavior nor sufficient to plan community health promotion programs. Instead, models that are informed by theories while providing more practical planning-implementation-evaluation frameworks optimize the chances of success in the context of the social realities and resource limitations. ONPRIME is one such model, and examples of the relevance of ONPRIME are provided for childhood obesity control, the prevention of falls among older adults, and a range of other health challenges.

REVIEW QUESTIONS

1. What are the six main theories that inform health behavior and health change models?

2. What are the elements of the ONPRIME Model?

3. What are some potential implications of the ACA on community health behavior change programs?

4. What are some of the ways communities can facilitate health behavior change?

5. In your own words, discuss why a focus on obesity earlier in the lifespan is an important public health priority.

6. Again, in your own words, describe how two of the elements of the ONPRIME model apply to falls-prevention programs for seniors.

REFERENCES

1. Fishbein M. Attitude and the prediction of behavior. In: Fishbein M, ed. *Readings in attitude theory and measurement*. New York: Wiley; 1967.

2. Fishbein M, Ajzen I. *Belief, attitude, intention and behavior: An introduction to theory and research*. Reading, MA: Addison-Wesley; 1975.

3. Ajzen I. The Theory of Planned Behavior. In: Van Lange PAM, Kruglanski AW, Higgins ET, eds. *Handbook of Theories of Social Psychology*. Vol One. Thousand Oaks, CA: Sage; 2011:438–459.

4. Hagger MS, Chatzisarantis NL, Biddle SJ. The influence of autonomous and controlling motives on physical activity intentions within the Theory of Planned Behaviour. *British Journal of Health Psychology*. 2002;7(3):283–297.

5. Hochbaum GM. *Public participation in medical screening programs: a socio-psychological study*. Washington, DC: US Department of Health, Education, and Welfare, Public Health Service, Bureau of State Services, Division of Special Health Services, Tuberculosis Program; 1958.

6. Bandura A. *Principles of behavior modification*. Oxford, England: Holt, Rinehart, & Winston; 1969.

7. Bandura A. Social learning theory. Englewood Cliffs, NJ: Prentice-Hall; 1977.

8. Bandura A. *Social foundations of thought and action: A social cognitive theory*. Englewood Cliffs, NJ: Prentice Hall; 1986.

9. Rogers EM, Shoemaker FF. *Communication of Innovations; A Cross-Cultural Approach*. New York: The Free Press; 1971.

10. Rogers EM. *Diffusion of innovations*. 4th ed. New York: The Free Press; 1995.

11. McGuire WJ. Public communication as a strategy for inducing health-promoting behavioral change. *Preventive Medicine*. 1984;13(3):299–319.

12. Kotler P, Zaltman G. Social marketing: an approach to planned social change. *The Journal of Marketing*. 1971;35(July):3–12.

13. Goodman RM, Steckler A. A model for the institutionalization of health promotion programs. *Family & Community Health*. 1989;11(4):63–78.

14. Dishman R, Buckworth J. Increasing physical activity: a quantitative synthesis. *Medicine and Science in Sports and Exercise*. 1996;28(6):706–719.

15. Baer DM, Wolf MM, Risley TR. Some current dimensions of applied behavior analysis. *Journal of Applied Behavior Analysis*. 1968;1(1):91–97.

16. Skinner BF. *The behavior of organisms: An experimental analysis*. Oxford, England: Appleton-Century; 1938.

17. Skinner BF. How to teach animals. *Scientific American*. 1951;185:26–29.

18. Elder JP. *Behavior change and public health in the developing world*. Vol 4. Thousand Oaks, CA: Sage; 2001.

19. Kohl HW, Craig CL, Lambert EV, et al. The pandemic of physical inactivity: global action for public health. *The Lancet*. 2012;380(9838):294–305.

20. Spitzberg BH. Toward a model of meme diffusion (M3D). *Communication Theory*. 2014;24(3):311–339.

21. Minkler M. *Community organizing and community building for health*. New Brunswick, NJ: Rutgers University Press; 1997.

22. Laverack G, Labonte R. A planning framework for community empowerment goals within health promotion. *Health Policy and Planning*. 2000;15(3):255–262.

23. Laverack G, Wallerstein N. Measuring community empowerment: a fresh look at organizational domains. *Health Promotion International*. 2001;16(2):179–185.

24. López-Cevallos D, Dierwechter T, Volkmann K, Patton-López M. Strengthening rural Latinos' civic engagement for health: The Voceros de Salud project. *Journal of Health Care for the Poor and Underserved*. 2013;24(4):1636–1647.

25. Murayama H, Fujiwara Y, Kawachi I. Social capital and health: a review of prospective multilevel studies. *Journal of Epidemiology*. 2012;22(3):179–187.

26. Green LJ, Kreuter M. *Health Promotion Planning: An Educational Approach*. 3rd ed. Mountain View, CA: Mayfield Publishing Company; 1999.

27. Janz NK, Becker MH. The health belief model: a decade later. *Health Education & Behavior*. 1984;11(1):1–47.

28. Glasgow RE, Vogt TM, Boles SM. Evaluating the public health impact of health promotion interventions: the RE-AIM framework. *Am J Public Health*. 1999;89(9):1322–1327.

29. Elder JP, Geller E, Hovell M, Mayer J. *Motivating Health Behavior*. Albany, NY: Delmar Publishing; 1994.

30. Stokols D. Translating social ecological theory into guidelines for community health promotion. *American Journal of Health Promotion*. 1996;10(4):282–298.

31. Bronfenbrenner U. The ecology of human development: Experiments by design and nature. Cambridge, MA: Harvard University Press; 1979.

32. Feeg VD, Candelaria LM, Krenitsky-Korn S, Vessey J. The relationship of obesity and weight gain to childhood teasing. *Journal of Pediatric Nursing*. 2014:doi: 10.1016/j.pedn.2014.1008.1011.

33. Naar-King S, Podolski C-L, Ellis DA, Frey MA, Templin T. Social ecological model of illness management in high-risk youths with type 1 diabetes. *Journal of Consulting and Clinical Psychology*. 2006;74(4):785.

34. Smedley BD, Syme SL. Promoting health: intervention strategies from social and behavioral research. *American Journal of Health Promotion*. 2001;15(3):149–166.

35. Macintyre S, Ellaway A. Ecological approaches: rediscovering the role of the physical and social environment. In: Berkman LF, Kawachi I, eds. *Social Epidemiology*. New York: Oxford University Press; 2000:332–348.

36. Srinivasan S, O'Fallon LR, Dearry A. Creating healthy communities, healthy homes, healthy people: initiating a research agenda on the built environment and public health. *Am J Public Health*. 2003;93(9):1446–1450.

37. Institute of Medicine. *Does the Built Environment Influence Physical Activity? Examining the Evidence*. Washington, DC: The National Academies Press; 2005.

38. Sallis JF, Floyd MF, Rodríguez DA, Saelens BE. Role of built environments in physical activity, obesity, and cardiovascular disease. *Circulation*. 2012;125(5):729–737.

39. Glanz K, Sallis JF, Saelens BE, Frank LD. Healthy nutrition environments: concepts and measures. *American Journal of Health Promotion*. 2005;19(5):330–333.

40. Vernez Moudon A, Drewnowski A, Duncan GE, Hurvitz PM, Saelens BE, Scharnhorst E. Characterizing the food environment: pitfalls

and future directions. *Public Health Nutrition.* 2013;16(07):1238–1243.

41. Ogden CL, Carroll MD, Kit BK, Flegal KM. Prevalence of obesity and trends in body mass index among US children and adolescents, 1999–2010. *Journal of the American Medical Association.* 2012;307(5):483–490.

42. Centers for Disease Control and Prevention. Basics About Childhood Obesity. 2012; http://www.cdc.gov/obesity/childhood/basics.html. Accessed October 12, 2014.

43. Freedman DS, Khan LK, Serdula MK, Dietz WH, Srinivasan SR, Berenson GS. The relation of childhood BMI to adult adiposity: the Bogalusa Heart Study. *Pediatrics.* 2005;115(1):22–27.

44. Parcel GS, Perry CL, Kelder SH, et al. School climate and the institutionalization of the CATCH program. *Health Education & Behavior.* 2003;30(4):489–502.

45. Luepker RV, Perry CL, McKinlay SM, et al. Outcomes of a field trial to improve children's dietary patterns and physical activity: the Child and Adolescent Trial for Cardiovascular Health (CATCH). *Journal of the American Medical Association.* 1996;275(10):768–776.

46. Coleman KJ, Tiller CL, Sanchez J, et al. Prevention of the epidemic increase in child risk of overweight in low-income schools: the El Paso coordinated approach to child health. *Archives of Pediatrics & Adolescent Medicine.* 2005;159(3):217–224.

47. Hoelscher DM, Springer AE, Ranjit N, et al. Reductions in child obesity among disadvantaged school children with community involvement: the Travis County CATCH Trial. *Obesity.* 2010;18(S1):S36–S44.

48. Elder JP, Crespo NC, Corder K, et al. Childhood obesity prevention and control in city recreation centres and family homes: the MOVE/me Muevo Project. *Pediatric Obesity.* 2014;9(3):218–231.

49. National Center for Injury Prevention and Control. Falls Among Older Adults: An Overview. 2014; http://www.cdc.gov/HomeandRecreationalSafety/Falls/adultfalls.html. Accessed October 15, 2014.

50. DeVito C, Lambert D, Sattin RW, Bacchelli S, Ros A, Rodriguez J. Fall injuries among the elderly. Community-based surveillance. *Journal of the American Geriatrics Society.* 1988;36(11):1029–1035.

51. West LA, Cole S, Goodkind D, He W. *65+ in the United States: 2010.* Washington, DC: US Census Bureau; 2014.

52. Vogeli C, Shields AE, Lee TA, et al. Multiple chronic conditions: prevalence, health consequences, and implications for quality, care management, and costs. *Journal of General Internal Medicine.* 2007;22(3):391–395.

53. Fried LP, Ferrucci L, Darer J, Williamson JD, Anderson G. Untangling the concepts of disability, frailty, and comorbidity: implications for improved targeting and care. *The Journals of Gerontology Series A: Biological Sciences and Medical Sciences.* 2004;59(3):M255–M263.

54. Tinetti M, Fried T. The end of the disease era. *The American Journal of Medicine.* 2004;116(3):179–185.

55. Quiñones AR, Liang J, Bennett JM, Xu X, Ye W. How does the trajectory of multimorbidity vary across Black, White, and Mexican Americans in middle and old age? *The Journals of Gerontology Series B: Psychological Sciences and Social Sciences.* 2011;66(6):739–749.

56. Paez KA, Zhao L, Hwang W. Rising out-of-pocket spending for chronic conditions: a ten-year trend. *Health Affairs.* 2009;28(1):15–25.

57. American Geriatrics Society. Guideline for the prevention of falls in older persons. *Journal of the American Geriatrics Society.* 2001;49(5):664–672.

58. Masud T, Morris RO. Epidemiology of falls. *Age and Ageing.* 2001;30(Suppl 4):3–7.

59. Rubenstein LZ. Falls in older people: epidemiology, risk factors and strategies for prevention. *Age and Ageing.* 2006;35(Suppl 2):ii37–ii41.

60. Tinetti M. Preventing falls in elderly persons. *New England Journal of Medicine.* 2003;348(1):42–49.

61. Tinetti M, Kumar C. The patient who falls: "It's always a trade-off." *Journal of the American Medical Association.* 2010;303(3):258–266.

62. Rubenstein LZ, Josephson KR. The epidemiology of falls and syncope. *Clinics in Geriatric Medicine.* 2002;18(2):141–158.

63. Stevens JA, Corso PS, Finkelstein EA, Miller TR. The costs of fatal and non-fatal falls among older adults. *Injury Prevention.* 2006;12(5):290–295.

64. Stevens JA. *A CDC compendium of effective fall interventions: What works for community-dwelling older adults.* National Center for Injury Prevention and Control; 2010.

65. Li F, Harmer P, Mack KA, et al. Tai Chi: moving for better balance-development of a community-based falls prevention program. *Journal of Physical Activity & Health.* 2008;5(3):445–455.

66. Li F, Harmer P, Glasgow R, et al. Translation of an effective Tai Chi intervention into a community-based

falls-prevention program. *American Journal of Public Health*. 2008;98(7):1195.

67. Clemson AC, Carolyn Fozzard, Lindy. Managing risk and exerting control: determining follow through with falls prevention. *Disability & Rehabilitation*. 1999;21(12):531–541.

68. Clemson L, Cumming RG, Heard R. The development of an assessment to evaluate behavioral factors associated with falling. *American Journal of Occupational Therapy*. 2003;57(4):380–388.

69. Clemson L, Cumming RG, Kendig H, Swann M, Heard R, Taylor K. The effectiveness of a community-based program for reducing the incidence of falls in the elderly: a randomized trial. *Journal of the American Geriatrics Society*. 2004;52(9):1487–1494.

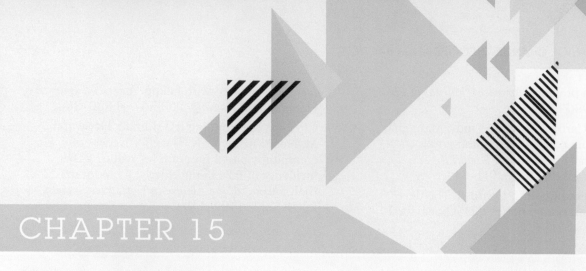

CHAPTER 15

Evaluation

Laura C. Leviton, PhD • Kerry A. McGeary, PhD

LEARNING OBJECTIVES

Upon completion of this chapter, the reader will be able to:

1. Describe and utilize the evaluation framework of the Centers for Disease Control and Prevention (CDC).

2. Explain why it is important to consult the various stakeholders when planning evaluation.

3. Choose appropriate evaluation questions for the purposes that stakeholders have in mind.

4. Choose and apply appropriate evaluation methods given available resources and information needs.

5. Distinguish between process and outcome evaluation and understand the importance of both types.

6. Explain where and when the various economic evaluation methods are needed.

7. Explain the typical alternative explanations for evaluations of program outcomes.

KEY TERMS

accountability
cost-benefit analysis
cost-effectiveness analysis
evaluation
implementation
objectives
stakeholders

WHAT IS EVALUATION?

Evaluation is the process of determining the merit, worth, or value of something.[1] Evaluation is data-based, systematic inquiry; it can use research methods, but not exclusively.[2] Although health professionals may try to draw a clear distinction between research and evaluation, in the areas of data collection, design, and analysis the two constantly blur together. For example, some of the most important evaluation studies across many human services are randomized experiments.[2] Like research, evaluations can sometimes build generalizable knowledge, though often limited in time and place.[2] The only consistent distinctions are that research does not necessarily have a focus on assessing value, and unlike research, evaluation is only justified if it is useful.[1]

Types and Focus

Types of evaluation include formative evaluation, which focuses on improvement ("forming" the program), and summative evaluation, which "summarizes" the value of the activity (e.g., the degree to which the activity met its objectives, had side-effects, was cost effective, or achieved population-wide "reach").[1] Evaluation can focus on implementation (monitoring activity or process), on outputs (the immediate results of an activity), or outcomes (how policies, environments, behaviors and population health are affected by an activity). Further, the evaluation may be focused on the cost of the activity, including cost-effectiveness (the cost relative to its outputs or outcomes), benefits (the dollar value of the output and outcomes), or cost-benefit analysis (benefits relative to the cost of the activity). Evaluation and economic evaluation have long been practiced in sectors such as education, social welfare, mental health, job training, criminal justice, and the military; however, public health led the way with the first book on evaluation.[3]

What to Evaluate

Most often in public health we evaluate:

▷ *Organizational performance*, as when a local health department reports on the extent to which it met stated objectives
▷ *Practices*, as when a health department evaluates whether it should modify its practices for environmental health or safety inspections
▷ *Programs*, as when the state or local health department evaluates participation in the Special Supplemental Nutrition Program for Women, Infants, and Children (WIC)
▷ *Policies*, as when a state health department assesses whether people are complying with a state seat belt law, or the effects of an active transportation law to encourage walking and biking
▷ *Products*, such as health education curriculum (did people understand the material? Did they change behavior?)
▷ *Systems*, which are increasingly a focus of public health evaluation, for example, assessing the degree to which diabetes treatment and prevention services are working together
▷ *Collaborations with other organizations and community leaders*, because they have the power and resources to bring about community improvements that lead to health

We will use "activity" or "program" as shorthand for all these objects of evaluation, except where there are special issues to describe. Evaluation of individual staff is very different and not a focus of this chapter.

WHY EVALUATE?

Program Improvement

Often, evaluations can show where there is need for improvement. While such formative evaluation is often considered only in the beginning phases of programs, in fact it is helpful at all points in the program life cycle. The primary audience is usually the organization and the practitioners who carry out the work. For example, a reproductive health organization discovered that it was not serving a community with a high rate of sexually transmitted infections (STIs) and unplanned pregnancies. Evaluation indicated that the community did not have easy access to the organization's offices and did not trust outsiders. The organization opened up a storefront office convenient for the community, worked with community leaders, and employed outreach workers from the community to spread the word about the importance of getting checked for STIs.

Accountability

Evaluations can also demonstrate accountability to decision makers and to the public. Accountability means accepting responsibility for activities and disclosing the results in a transparent manner. For example, a local health department recently set an objective that it would provide home visiting to all infants placed in foster homes in its jurisdiction by a specified date. By recording home visits and comparing the list of beneficiaries with the records of Child Protective Services, the health department demonstrated accountability to the city government and the public.

Input to Decisions

Evaluations can help to inform decisions about whether to expand, maintain, or change a practice or policy, although they are almost never the only consideration.[2] For example, practitioners and policy makers may have the choice among several programs, and they will want to consider cost per person, reach (how many people can be served or affected given the budget available), effectiveness (what is the outcome or benefit for the average individual), and cost-effectiveness (what amount of benefit or outcome per dollar spent). Evaluation can inform other aspects of the decision as well, including the feasibility of implementing a program locally, and the degree to which it is helping to eliminate disparities in services or health outcomes.

Sharpening Assumptions

Evaluations can give practitioners new insights about how a practice, program, or policy is supposed to happen and what is supposed to be the result. For example, once practitioners implement a program, it may become clear that it is just not working out as the planners assumed, or evaluation may reveal a critical bit of information that changes how policy makers and managers think about the underlying problem. This in turn can lead to important changes for the program.

Advocating on Behalf of Public Health and Its Policies

Evaluations can be used to justify advocacy efforts and persuade decision makers to change or maintain a policy, implement a program, or allocate more resources for a public health practice. For example, pregnant women need folic acid in their diet to prevent spina bifida, a serious birth defect. The federal government requires that grain products include folic acid to assure that women get enough of it. Evaluation indicates that the rate of spina bifida declined 31 percent since the federal policy was introduced. This information helps to sustain the federal requirement in case of political challenges.[4]

HOW TO EVALUATE?

Evaluation Guiding Principles and Standards

The discipline of evaluation has developed its own standards of ethics and quality, because the issues can become very tricky, or at least awkward, in many cases. Evaluations do not always come up with positive findings, and sooner or later evaluators will say something that the audience does not want to hear. The American Evaluation Association's *Guiding Principles for Evaluators* (found at http://www.eval.org) addresses technical standards, competence, integrity/honesty, respect for people, and responsibilities for general and public welfare. Several professional associations created the *Joint Program Evaluation Standards* (found at http://www.jcsee.org by clicking on the "Program Evaluation Standards Statement" link) which address issues of utility, feasibility, propriety, accuracy, and accountability. These standards help practitioners avoid or address many organizational, political, and methods problems. In what follows, several common and useful evaluation frameworks are described. These are meant as examples rather than an exhaustive list.

The Centers for Disease Control and Prevention (CDC) Evaluation Framework

The CDC created guidance on evaluation that is specific for public health practitioners. A self-study guide and many examples can be seen at http://www.cdc.gov/eval. The framework includes the following steps:[5]

- Engage **stakeholders**: people and groups with an interest in the evaluation or the program.
- Gain agreement on the program, its goals and objectives.
- Focus the evaluation on the right questions to ask, given the resources available.
- Gather evidence that is credible to the stakeholders and uses the best available measures and design to answer the question, given resources available.
- Justify conclusions using standards, analytic procedures, interpretation, and judgment.
- Ensure use and share lessons learned.

The RE-AIM Framework

Public health practitioners often need to translate research evidence for effective practices into real-world settings. Research on the effectiveness of a practice takes place under controlled conditions, but to achieve population health impact, we also want to know how to make the practice work in many different real-world situations. RE-AIM is an acronym that stands for:

- **R**each—*How do I reach the targeted population with the intervention?*
- **E**fficacy—*How do I know my intervention is effective?*
- **A**doption—*How do I develop organizational support to deliver my intervention?*

▸ **I**mplementation—*How do I ensure the intervention is delivered properly?*

▸ **M**aintenance—*How do I incorporate the intervention so that it is delivered over the long term?*

The RE-AIM website at http://www.re-aim.hnfe.vt.edu gives tools and advice, both for translating evidence-based practices and evaluating these questions.

Getting to Outcomes (GTO)

Practitioners do not automatically think in evaluative terms. GTO has great appeal for practitioners, because it offers them a way to build practical evaluation into planning and action, as seen in Figure 15-1.[6] Steps 1 through 6 are planning activities for a program or practice that guide practice toward specific evaluation measures. Steps 7 and 8 involve implementation and outcome evaluation, while steps 9 and 10 help the practitioner to use data for continuous quality improvement and to sustain programs. Manuals and workbooks are available for several public health programs.

The Community Tool Box

Public health practitioners need to engage communities and powerful outsiders in order to improve health. This can be a complex process! The Community Tool Box at http://ctb.ku.edu/en is a free resource that provides a wealth of advice side by side with evaluation tools. It offers detailed training and advice on best practices for community collaborations, such as creating and maintaining partnerships, assessing community needs and resources, analyzing problems and goals, and increasing participation and membership. At the same time, the Community Tool Box offers evaluation tools and training to measure progress in each of these activities. It also supports online workstations to document changes in communities and systems, uncovering factors affecting community change, tracking changes in health indicators, graphs and other help to interpret and make sense of the information. (Additional information on the Community Tool Box and its use is provided in Chapter 25.)

Finding the Resources for Evaluation

The two major costs of evaluation are person-power and data collection. Public health practitioners can do many forms of evaluation themselves, but to improve quality and lower the cost, it may be worthwhile to draw on the expertise of colleges and universities, whose faculty and students often need service-learning projects. A directory of professional evaluators by state and specialty can be found at the American Evaluation Association website (http://www.eval.org). Health departments, hospitals, and large nonprofits may also have expertise, resources, and information to share, such as surveillance data and community health needs assessments.

PLANNING AN EVALUATION

Engaging Stakeholders

Although evaluation can be useful for midcourse corrections and continuous quality improvements,

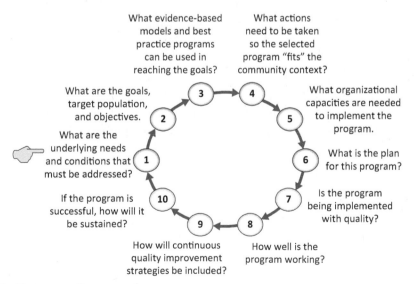

FIGURE 15-1 Getting to Outcomes Framework

Source: Wandersman, A., "Evidence Based Interventions are Necessary but not Sufficient for Outcomes: Empowerment Evaluation & Roles for Evaluators in an Evidence-based Intervention World." Speech delivered April 13, 2015 at the Eastern Evaluation Research Society conference, Absecon, New Jersey.

often the best time to plan an evaluation is before the program itself begins. Too often, evaluation is an afterthought, at which point its usefulness is greatly impaired. And the best way to get evaluation considered in advance is to engage the stakeholders as soon as possible, because the likelihood of a good process and outcome is greatly increased.[7] Involving stakeholders is consistent with public health practitioners' need to collaborate to achieve public health goals. Stakeholders for evaluation usually include program managers, practitioners, policy makers, and the beneficiaries of public health activities. Some evaluation approaches emphasize practitioner and community groups as having priority.[8,9] Depending on the evaluation, other stakeholders might include the business community (e.g., restaurants for evaluation of efforts to label menus with nutritional information); health care providers (e.g., hospitals to assess the value of their efforts for Community Benefit under the Affordable Care Act); or community associations (e.g., Hispanic churches for evaluation of outreach efforts on maternal and child health). It is best to consult stakeholders in advance about the questions and the likely implications of findings. If nothing will be done with findings, then evaluation is probably not justified.

Gaining Agreement on the Program, Its Goals and Objectives

In this step it is important to describe the program, its goals, and expected effects. This process is not as straightforward as it seems, because people have legitimate differences about what the program is supposed to accomplish, and they may have different information about activities or strategies, resources for implementation, and capacity to effect change. Also, programs can be at different stages of development and take place in different contexts. All of these factors need to be well understood, in the interest of fairness and transparency.

One tool that helps to gain agreement on these issues is the use of a logic model or theory of change. A logic model is a graphic representation of the rationale and expectations of the program, while a theory of change describes more about how and why the program's inputs and activities are thought to lead to the desired outcomes.[10] Logic models often take the form seen in Figure 15-2, using elimination of exposure to secondhand smoke in public places as an example. Reading from left to right, the logic model begins with inputs—such as resources and personnel—and activities. Outputs are the direct result of applying these resources,

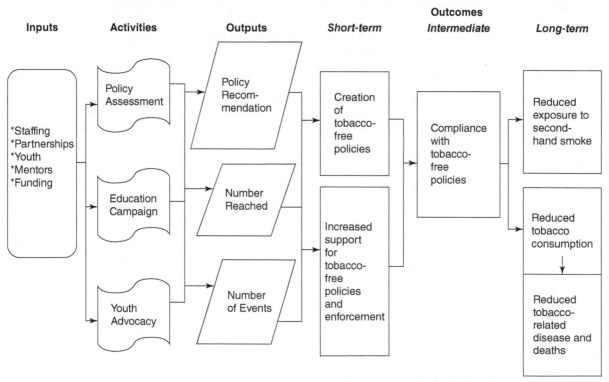

FIGURE 15-2   Logic Model for Eliminating Exposure to Secondhand Smoke in Public Places

Courtesy of the Missouri Department of Health and Senior Services. Adapted from Key Outcome Indicators for Evaluating Comprehensive Tobacco Control Programs. Centers for Disease Control and Prevention. 2005.

for example, in terms of numbers reached. The outputs are expected to lead to short-, intermediate-, and long-term outcomes or effects. One way to build a theory of change into a logic model is to think about "so that" statements: for example, "we will create compelling public communications so that the public increases support for tobacco-free policies." Logic models and theories of change do not have to be linear—they should take any form that people understand best. Use the simplest format and wording that gets the point across to stakeholders.

Another, longstanding tool of public health practice that greatly assists both evaluation and the management of practices and programs is creation of measurable objectives. Good objectives have several important features. Contrast the following two statements:

▶ *"We want to enhance infants' ability to thrive in [city]."* This is a wish, not an objective. What does enhance mean? Does "ability to thrive" imply that the babies are the ones that are responsible for progress? Actually, thriving could refer to several important things about infants, and perhaps they all deserve attention. But what are they? Who are "we" and what are "we" supposed to do, with what result?

▶ *"By September of 2015, the maternal and child health service will reduce the percentage of low birthweight infants in [city] from 11.6 percent to 11.2 percent."* This statement of objectives uses a **strong verb**, "reduce." It designates **who is responsible** and gives a **specific timeframe** for accomplishment. Low birthweight is **well-defined and measurable**: 2,500 g (5.5 pounds) regardless of gestational age. It is an **important indicator** of infant health, linked to a variety of problems. Public health objectives do not always need to include a numerical target (such as 11.2 percent) unless this is desired, but they need to be **feasible and realistic**.

Focusing the Evaluation

Not everything can be well-evaluated. Evaluations cost money, capacity may be limited, and some evaluation questions are more important than others. What are the priorities for evaluation, what are the credible measures, and what will likely be done with the results?

Evaluability assessment (EA) is a low-cost tool to assess the realism of programs, develop logic models, and select the right evaluation questions.[9] EA can surface disagreements about the program and what it is supposed to accomplish—a surprisingly common problem, especially for new programs, policies, and community collaborations. EA can also determine whether program resources and activities are consistent with

objectives, and whether stakeholders are likely to use the results. EA may indicate that an evaluation is premature, and further program development is needed. It can also help to select realistic and fair performance indicators and measures of effectiveness. EA begins with involving the end-users of evaluation, because if they do not intend to use the results, there is no point in doing evaluation. Through a review of program documentation and interviews with program managers and other key stakeholders, EA results in the creation of a logic model. Stakeholders review the model to see if it is correct from their viewpoint and the EA team revises the model. The EA team then "scouts" the program reality through observation and interviews, and reports on any needs for program development, whether an evaluation is feasible, and what the key questions might be.

Useful information flows from EA at every step. For example, an inner-city arts program underwent EA and discovered that key stakeholders held wildly different opinions about the program's goals, which was news to the program! Also EA revealed that only some of those goals were even feasible, given resources and activities: one goal was to keep kids out of trouble, but kids got to the arts studios on church buses; the churches did not want troublemakers to vandalize their buses, so the most troubled kids never got on the buses in the first place. The EA suggested that to help troubled kids, the program might want to find another way to connect them to the arts.

CHOOSING CREDIBLE MEASURES AND DATA COLLECTION

Balancing Cost against Credibility

An important principle is the idea of "good enough" evaluation: how good does the information have to be in order to achieve the evaluation purpose?[11] We want it to be an accurate reflection of program reality so that it will have credibility to stakeholders. But exquisite accuracy and detail are usually not justified if lesser detail would serve the evaluation purpose. To lower cost and provide "good enough" data, it is simply not necessary to measure entire populations or the entire universe of activities: random sampling can usually provide good statistical description. This principle is related to the concept of a confidence interval in statistics and epidemiology. Even when the evaluator can only afford small samples or available convenience samples, these can often give a qualitative idea of outputs and outcomes. For example, it is not necessary to monitor waiting time at a clinic every single day—sample the days and think about which days are likely to be busiest and slowest. Even a snapshot of waiting times may be sufficient for quality improvement or other decisions.

Information is less expensive when it is already available, or when it is a by-product of program activities, such as participation rosters or social media threads. Agencies may have service records that, with some review for reliability and validity, can serve the purpose. Local surveillance data have long been needed in public health and are difficult to come by, but states collecting national data for the Behavioral Risk Factor Surveillance System (BRFSS) and the Youth Behavioral Risk Factor Survey (YRBS) may sometimes oversample for state or even local analysis. Objectives for health outcomes from *Healthy People 2020*[12] and outcomes data from the County Health Rankings[13] may also be of value. The Center for Applied Research and Environmental Systems (CARES) at http://www.cares.missouri.edu gives practitioners the ability to map data geographically for thousands of publicly available data sets, sometimes down to the census tract or even the street location.

Evaluations cost more when data have to be collected from scratch. Qualitative data do not necessarily cost less than quantitative data—it depends on the circumstances and the methods of analysis. Surveys are often costly, although online surveys bring down the cost substantially—when we are confident that the respondents are a credible sample of the population we are interested in. Interviews are often costly, although they can sometimes be "batched" as focus groups. Collecting direct information on clinical health status is the most expensive of all. Electronic health records (EHRs) may eventually lower the expense of measuring population health; however, confidentiality can present obstacles, different EHRs may not measure things the same way, and information about preventive services and behavior changes is often missing from these records.

Reliability

Reliability means repeatability, consistency, or replicability of measurement. Reliability matters to the analysis of evaluative information because the lower the reliability, the more error in measurement. With more error, confidence intervals will be wider, and thus there will be less ability to find statistically significant differences or strong associations. *Any* measure and *any* data collection method will have at least some measurement error, so the choice of measures becomes a tradeoff between quality and cost/feasibility. For example, people have trouble remembering many health-related behaviors, so researchers have devised such methods as diaries (for diet), observation (plate waste in the school lunch program), biological markers (cotinine in saliva for smoking), and electronic measurement (accelerometers to measure physical activity). But these methods can be expensive and for many practitioners self-report may be satisfactory.

Validity

Validity means the extent to which "a measurement measures what it purports to measure."[14] This concept involves the extent to which there is bias in measurement, and also whether the measurement actually reflects the domain that the evaluation aims to assess. Bias is a problem in childhood obesity prevention, for example, when parents report their children's height and weight. They underestimate children's height, which means that Body Mass Index is overestimated. For youth and adults, self-reported height and weight are satisfactory for most purposes.[15] Validity of measurement is affected by missing data; for example, police crime statistics are notoriously lacking because many crimes are not reported, especially by the most vulnerable groups. Victimization surveys are a more valid resource for violence prevention efforts, although they are expensive.

Qualitative Measurement

Qualitative evaluations rely primarily on words, observations, and pictures to develop narratives and analyze themes.[16] They can use numbers as well, but in the service of those narratives and themes. Qualitative measurements are often done on small, convenient samples in order to get in-depth understanding of the "why" and "how" of programs. Open-ended interviews, maps, and pictures are common tools of qualitative measurement. Key informant interviews, focus groups, and photovoice are especially helpful for evaluation. Key informants are the people in a community who know what is going on: in many communities these include barbers, beauticians, and lay church leaders. Focus groups are group discussions that stimulate the participants to make thoughtful statements about the issue at hand.[17] Photovoice, as described in the Community Tool Box, is a method of eliciting how community members or service recipients are interpreting the meaning of a service or situation, and conveying their perceived reality to outsiders. Maps can often provide important qualitative information, using Geographic Information Systems (GIS). For example, public health practitioners can map cities in order to identify "food deserts" where healthy food is not readily available, or violent crime statistics in order to set priorities for violence prevention efforts. Such maps can also be highly effective for advocacy efforts. In Figure 15-3 a map of Philadelphia from 2003 overlays supermarket sales, income, and diet-related

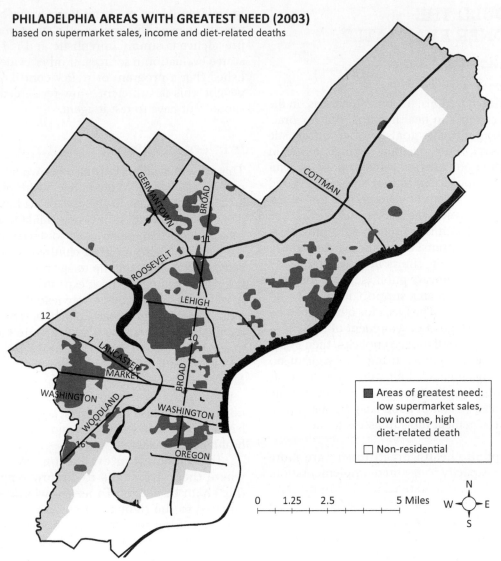

PHILADELPHIA AREAS WITH GREATEST NEED (2003)
based on supermarket sales, income and diet-related deaths

Areas of greatest need: low supermarket sales, low income, high diet-related death

Non-residential

0   1.25   2.5   5 Miles

FIGURE 15-3   Areas of Greatest Need Based on Supermarket Sales, Income, and Diet-Related Deaths, Philadelphia, 2003

Courtesy of the Food Trust

deaths to indicate areas of greatest need. Maps can also show qualitative changes over time; Philadelphia now has many new supermarkets located in these areas. Of course, such information can be quantified as well: for example, residents' average distance traveled to stores with healthy food.

The Importance of Mixed Methods

No single source of data represents the truth, and even if it did, it might not be credible to all the stakeholder groups. All data are flawed, but they do not have to share the same flaws. For these reasons, it is important to gather different kinds of data. If they point to the same conclusions, then it is more likely that the findings of evaluation are both correct and credible. Combining qualitative and quantitative information can be especially effective, because together they explain the evaluation results more completely. Telling a story and providing case examples is often more compelling to stakeholder audiences than dry statistics, and the examples make the numbers come alive. It sometimes happens that different kinds of data conflict with each other. At that point it is essential to look for the most likely and persuasive explanations. On that basis, additional information might guide us toward a better understanding of exactly what happened, or at least reach a better conclusion.

WHAT SHOULD THE PRACTITIONER EVALUATE?

Implementation and Short to Intermediate Outcomes

In posing evaluation questions, people often focus on the ultimate goal of changes in health status. But for practitioners, evaluating ultimate goals is often unrealistic and also unnecessary.* Look again at the logic model in Figure 15-2. Finding out whether tobacco policies actually *cause* reduced exposure to indoor smoke is beyond the capability of most practitioners, and it is not necessary anyway, because researchers have shown that the relationship exists.[18] Much more sensible for practice is to evaluate activities, outputs, and short- or intermediate-term outcomes. Have our efforts been well-targeted? Have they contributed to greater public support for clean indoor air policies? Is greater support leading to increased passage of policies? The focus for outcome evaluation depends on the stage of development of this effort: if there are not enough good tobacco policies, then evaluation should concentrate on measuring their enactment; if good ones have been enacted already, then the focus shifts to assessing compliance with the policies. The CDC website hosts a wealth of good suggestions and realistic, feasible measurement tools to assess tobacco control policies.[19]

In general, public health practitioners are more likely to have the capacity to evaluate implementation, that is, short- and intermediate-term outcomes, than the longer term health-related outcomes. There are at least four reasons for this. First, measuring long-term outcomes (such as health status or behavior change) generally costs more and takes longer than measuring short- and intermediate-term outcomes. Second, credible evaluation of long-term changes may require a statistician and expert in evaluation design. Third, observing a statistically significant change or difference in outcomes may require sample sizes that are beyond the resources of most practitioners. And finally, it may be unrealistic to expect health status and long-established behavior patterns to change because of one program or practice by itself. A case in point is evaluation of policies and programs to reduce the prevalence of obesity

in children. Many powerful forces contribute to healthy weight, so expecting one small change to reduce obesity prevalence is simply unrealistic and is likely to waste scarce evaluation resources. If other evidence has established that a program or policy contributes to healthy weight, this is sufficient—low-resourced practitioners should not have to test it again.

Implementation and Outputs

This type of evaluation is also known as monitoring or process evaluation. Many public health practices involve a chain of events, as in the case of lead exposure assessment and intervention in young children. Lead exposure causes intellectual impairment, so screening programs often start with screenings of children who are at risk, as early as 12 months and up to age 6 years. Children are at risk if their sibling has been exposed to lead or if they live in older neighborhoods where lead-based paint is common. Screening the general population of children is not recommended, because lead exposure has dropped so much in the United States.[20] A health department might screen for lead, or a health care provider might do so for Medicaid-eligible children. Finding lead exposure sparks several events as seen in Figure 15-4, including education of the parents or caregivers, assessment in the home, lead abatement in the home, and coordination with the health care provider.

Implementation evaluation can shed light on where there are needs for improvement, if any, in this chain of events. To assess whether screening is targeted to the right children, evaluators might compare screening reports to birth records by residence or demographics, or by eligibility for WIC or Medicaid. For example, providers may not be screening enough of the right children, or the children may not have a regular source of medical care. If so, then cases of lead exposure may go unrecognized. Providers may also be screening the general population, which is not cost effective. Even if screenings are actually taking place, providers may not report cases of lead exposure to the health department, impairing both services and accurate information. Once a case is identified, both the quality and completeness of follow-up can be assessed from service reports: whether parents and caregivers got education about lead; whether they understood the information; whether they acted on the information; whether the lead-exposed children were getting follow-up medical care; whether the home was assessed; and whether lead paint was removed from the home.

Many aspects of program activity could be measured, so it takes skill and discussion to focus the evaluation on the most useful information. Implementation monitoring can be simple checklists or detailed information from

---

* Other examples include seat belt campaigns, lead control efforts, and hypertension control. We know seat belts prevent injuries, so what we want to know is whether such campaigns increase seat belt use. (They do, in combination with laws requiring their use.) There is no need to assess the impact of exposure to lead on children's intellectual development, because we already know that lead impairs such development. And we know that hypertension medication works, so what prevention should focus on is early diagnosis, adherence to medication, and staying under a provider's care.

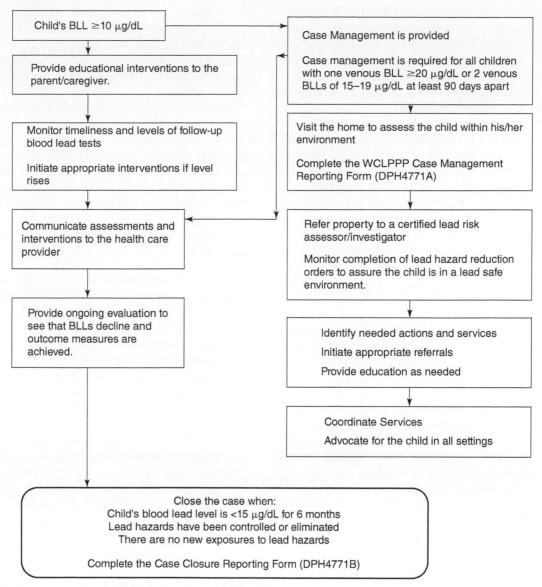

FIGURE 15-4 Assessment and Intervention for a Child with Lead Poisoning

Courtesy of Waushara County Wisconsin Department of Public Health

In January 2012 the Advisory Committee on Childhood Lead Poisoning Prevention recommended to the CDC that the "blood lead level of concern" be lowered to 5 micrograms per deciliter of lead in blood. The flow chart above was in use prior to this change in guidelines and is re-produced here only to represent steps in evaluation of a health department service.

practitioner notes. The amount of detail needs to be balanced against service providers' burden of time and energy to record the information. Practitioners have so much reporting and recording to do that any additional burden is likely to be resented or resisted. Is the needed information already available, and is the monitoring system duplicative? Think about each element that has to be recorded—is it really needed, and how will the information be used? It is much better to have more limited information that is complete and accurate, than to have detailed information that is incomplete and inaccurate. Also, monitoring systems are more complete and accurate if they have practitioner

buy-in, and the best way to get buy-in is to give useful feedback to the practitioners themselves.[15]

Evaluating Coalitions and Systems Changes

Working in coalitions requires special evaluation methods. Several tools are available to measure the quality of participation in coalitions, at different levels of detail. The Wilder Inventory (found at http://www.wilder.org by searching "Factors Inventory") is a free diagnostic tool that assesses coalitions in great detail and suggests ways to improve their functioning. But the Wilder Inventory requires a lot of effort from the partners and may not be necessary. Other tools can be as simple as a series of yes-no statements, although useful detail might be lost.[21] Still other tools are somewhere in between.[22] Picking the right evaluation tool is always a tradeoff between information versus evaluation capacity.

The Community Tool Box describes a strategy for measuring progress on systems changes. Community coalitions first agree together about what constitutes milestones or benchmarks, and then create a cumulative plot of these milestones over time. This information is helpful to give participants and outside stakeholders a sense of progress, to encourage continued participation, and for accountability to funders.[23] These milestone plots can also identify times when progress may have stalled, so that the coalition can search for causes and regain momentum. This information can also be overlaid against outcomes, as in Figure 15-5, which shows how changes in a community's environment for walking and biking were associated with increased physical activity.[24]

Evaluating Outcomes

The credibility of outcome evaluations often revolves around the issue of whether a program caused an outcome. Practitioners will not need to be concerned with cause for many evaluations they conduct. It may be enough simply to monitor trends and associations. If the trend is positive, then keep on course; if there is no change or a negative trend, then additional action may be necessary. However, practitioners will still want to be familiar with the criteria for establishing cause in order to appraise evaluation studies, and in case they need to defend the credibility of their own evaluations.

Assessing a causal relationship depends on several criteria: the cause has to precede the outcome in time; the association needs to be strong and consistent; and alternative explanations for the findings need to be ruled out. The interested reader can find a complete listing of alternative explanations and research designs to address them,[25] as well as a recent review of the advantages and disadvantages of designs to assess outcomes.[26] Some of the most common alternative explanations in evaluation include:

▸ *Self-selection bias*, in which people receiving the program are more likely (or less likely) to benefit from the program than a comparison group and thus show better outcomes.
▸ *Maturation bias*, in which outcomes are really caused, not by the program, but by people's normal changes over time. For example, children normally become more capable ("mature") over time; older adults normally become more frail and sick over time.
▸ *Attrition bias*, in which people drop out of data collection more often in the treatment or the control group. This pattern is often seen in treatment programs for alcohol, tobacco, and other drugs.

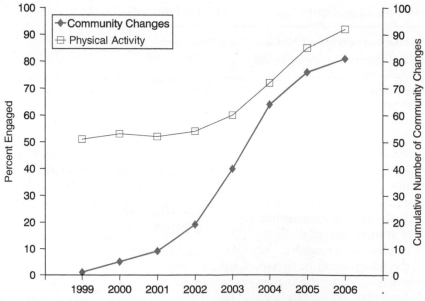

FIGURE 15-5   **Association of Community and System Changes with Increased Physical Activity**
DATA SOURCE: Institute of Medicine

- *Secular trends*, where outcomes may only be a reflection of the underlying societal trend. This is often a problem in prevention studies, as when society in general started eating less fat, giving up smoking, and practicing safer sex.
- *History*, where events having nothing to do with the program are causing outcomes. For example, when basketball player Magic Johnson announced he was HIV-infected, we saw people rush to get tested; when First Lady Betty Ford announced she had breast cancer, women rushed to get mammograms.
- *Regression to the mean*, where extreme measurements (highs and lows) tend to become less extreme when measured again. This can happen when community violence prevention addresses "hot spots" that represent a temporary spike in crime statistics.
- *Interactions of these factors.* For example, an interaction of selection bias with maturation bias is often a problem in evaluations of programs for disadvantaged children. Using more advantaged children as a comparison group introduces bias, because the children mature at different rates, making it seem as though the program is harming the children.

Randomized controlled trials (RCTs) are the most credible evaluation design to assess program outcomes because they generally rule out most alternative explanations. In RCTs, individuals, families, organizations, or communities are randomly assigned, thus relying on chance alone to determine which units receive the program or practice. RCTs are often not feasible for practitioners to conduct, and they can still be vulnerable to alternative explanations under some circumstances. For example, if measurement is unreliable, it may not be possible to establish a statistically significant difference between treatment and control groups, even if one exists. Secular trends can overwhelm large prevention RCTs, and local history can lead to problems in interpreting place-based randomized trials. Also, RCTs may have limited generalizability if outcomes were tested under ideal conditions (termed an efficacy trial), as opposed to real-world conditions (effectiveness trials).

Practitioners will most often utilize a simple before and after design, measuring a baseline of some kind, then beginning a program or practice, then measuring again. This design is vulnerable to many of the typical alternative explanations. It would be better to measure the baseline at several time points before introducing the program, which would help to rule out maturation, secular trends, history, and regression to the mean. Even better would be measuring outcomes at several time points after introducing the program, for the same reasons, and also to assure sustainability of the outcome. When many points are measured both before and after intervention, this design is termed an interrupted time series which under the right circumstances can approach the rigor and quality of an RCT.

Public health evaluations often utilize nonequivalent comparison groups, consisting of individuals or groups that are considered to be similar to those receiving the intervention. Any differences between groups may be adjusted statistically in an attempt to improve comparisons. Great caution must be used in interpreting such studies, because they can suffer from several of the typical alternative explanations, and statistical controls are prone to unpredictable over- and under-adjustments.[23] Such designs can be strengthened by adding measurement points both before and after intervention, thus making it less plausible that the real cause may involve local history, secular trends, regression to the mean, or selection bias. The passage of time can help in other ways, for example wait-listed participants can be a control group, or participation can be staggered over time.

The value of having several measurement points cannot be overstated. Take another look at Figure 15-5, in which community changes to promote walking and biking are plotted against citizens' reports of frequent physical activity during the same time period. We cannot be certain that this is a causal relationship, but it is very compelling. It is still possible that secular trends might be responsible both for the extent of community change and for increased physical activity, or that increased physical activity is actually increasing the demand for better walking and biking, thus leading to community changes. However, qualitative information should be readily available to support the idea that the community changes produced the increased physical activity. And the idea that this is a chance effect becomes less plausible with every passing year.

ECONOMIC EVALUATIONS

The various types of economic evaluation (EE) and the questions they answer are described in Table 15-1. In this chapter we can only provide an introduction to the most common types of EE which the practitioner is likely to either encounter or in which he/she may be a participant. Students should explore additional sources of more detailed information as referenced here.[27]

Cost Analysis

Analyzing costs and measuring them accurately are essential components to all other types of economic evaluation. When measuring costs consider carefully:

- What costs should be measured?
- How complete should the costs be?

TABLE 15-1   Economic Evaluations

Summarizing Economic Evaluation Types		
Type of Analysis	**Benefit (Outcome)**	**Measurement of Benefits**
Cost Minimization (CMA)	Identical, but costs are different *Can we do it for less?*	None
Cost Benefit (CBA)	Single, or multiple benefits (outcomes) standardized into a single monetary value (in present dollars) *Is there a reasonable return on investment?*	Dollars
Cost Effectiveness (CEA)	Single common benefit (or outcome) *Are the (natural) outcomes worth the cost?*	Natural units, e.g., life years gained, lower A1C levels, improved physical activity
Cost Utility (CUA)	1 or more benefits (outcomes) standardized into a single value *Are standardized outcomes worth the cost?*	QALYS DALYS

▷ Should the costs be nationally representative or generalizable?

▷ Does the information measured allow others to replicate the activity?

To answer the first question, cost measurement focuses on resource use, not pure accounting or financing. Focus your measurement by thinking of the resources needed to achieve an outcome or output as a special "recipe of ingredients" and steps that must be taken. The costs that need to be measured are the costs of all ingredients—all resources—used in each step of the recipe. This includes, for example, all the hours worked, all the travel expenses, all the office space and facilities used, and all the supplies and equipment purchased or rented. If a resource is used in the recipe then the value of that resource must be measured.

Second, a careful measurement of cost will implicitly measure the quantity (how much) and quality (how skilled) of the resource. The true value of the resources used to provide an activity is not necessarily the same as the actual funds or compensation given. For instance, if all staffing resources are provided by willing and able college-level volunteers, the resource use would be the number of hours worked by those volunteers. An accountant would value that resource use at zero since the volunteers were unpaid. However, the resources used are not truly zero. These students have an implicit value: since they are not yet skilled practitioners, they would be valued at the market compensation of those hours worked. If they are performing low-skilled cleaning, the minimum wage in the region would be the value of the service. If they are donating their time as computer programmers, you

would use the market value of a computer programmer's time. Keep in mind there are two concepts at play here. First, cost measurement values the resource regardless of the financing (donated or compensated). Second, there is a quality component to consider: if the resource is donated staffing, the skill level matters.

Once costs are measured, what do they mean? Market forces affect costs, so this is important to track and interpret. For example, consider nutrition Program X from Table 15-2, which costs $3,000 per year and serves 12,000 children. Now you are told that this program is in New York City, where the cost of living and wages are high (as opposed to, say, the rural South, where they are low). This total annualized cost could be considered against other similar programs of similar service numbers. However, the programs' locations should be considered, and to compare program costs, it would be appropriate to adjust the cost by regional or local area consumer price indices.

Cost-Effectiveness Analysis

This type of EE quantifies how many outputs, or how large of an outcome, a program achieves per dollar spent. This seems very similar to the average cost of a program that was just described, but it is something different. It is where program evaluation and cost analysis meet. Table 15-2 gives an example. A nutrition educator has a total budget of $3,000 a year to increase the amount of fruits and vegetables that children in low-income families eat. Program X serves 12,000 children per year at an average cost of $0.25. Because Program X aims to increase children's fruit and vegetable consumption, the outcome would be the average servings eaten per year: the total number of servings eaten per year, divided by 12,000. After investing for one year, the evaluator determines that the program increased vegetable consumption by one serving per child per week. The cost-effectiveness, described most commonly as a ratio, would be one serving per week per child, divided by $0.25 per child, or four servings per week per dollar spent. Program Y, following the same steps, yields an increase of 0.25 servings per week per child. While it is less effective than Program X, Program Y has a much lower cost per child at $0.05, and serves many more children (reach). So the cost-effectiveness of Program Y is 0.25 servings per week per child divided by $0.05 per child, or five servings per week per dollar spent.

Cost-Minimization Analysis

This type of EE involves two programs that have equal outcomes but different costs—imagine the nutrition education example, but with equal outcomes. Under those conditions, Program Y would also be the preferred choice in this scenario, based on cost-minimization. These analyses show how in a resource-scarce environment, decision makers may select one program over another. This is a typical scenario and it would be difficult to advocate for Program X based on either the cost-effectiveness or cost-minimization scenarios. However, this example also illustrates why the next type of economic evaluation is necessary.

Cost-Benefit Analysis

This type of EE offers a deeper level of understanding, because it describes the benefits of the activity relative to its costs. This level of economic evaluation is difficult in the best circumstances, as it requires those in public health to monetize benefits, that is, associate a dollar value with all outcomes of the program.

For instance, let us return to the nutrition education program in Table 15-2. What is the benefit of increased servings of vegetables? The news headline for Program Y might read "Nutrition Education Program Flops – Only ¼ More Healthy Servings per Week." But we might have more information, for instance, the vegetables might be replacing expensive cookies. In that case we might see a different headline "Nutrition Education Program Yields Total Economic Return." This headline is describing something important: there is an economic value to the program; it saves money. There might still be other questions about benefits that deserve to be answered:

▸ Is the return based on only one sector?
▸ Does it involve many other sectors?
▸ Who receives the economic benefits: participants, taxpayers, other nonparticipants?
▸ When does the return or savings occur?
▸ Is the benefit a projection into the future, or definite benefit right now?

Programs X and Y both had benefits. Y was more cost effective, increasing servings by 0.25, and there is a savings due to the substitution away from more expensive cookies. Program X is more effective at one serving per week per child, and let us assume for the moment that is enough to prevent obesity, but 0.25 servings is not. Then Program X has greater benefits compared to cost. Preventing obesity would have benefits for a variety of economic and societal sectors: reduced health care costs, increased wages, increased lifetime earnings due to increased life expectancy and increased human capital accumulation, reductions in mental and behavioral health care costs, increased maternal earnings, more physically fit military recruits, and others.

Currently there are no clear standards for valuing benefits or outcomes in terms of money, especially with preventive interventions. There are steps, however, that can be taken to help quantify benefits in other ways, and to monetize the outcomes that can be converted to dollars. First, when planning the economic evaluation,

TABLE 15-2   Comparing Effectiveness, Reach, and Cost-Effectiveness of Nutrition Education Programs for a Budget of $3,000 per Year

	Effectiveness: Increased Fruits and Vegetables Eaten per Week per Child	Cost per Child per Year	Reach: Children Served per Year	Cost-Effectiveness: Increased Fruits and Vegetables Eaten per Dollar Spent
Program X	+ 1.0	25 cents ($0.25)	$3,000 / 0.25 = 12,000	+ 1.0 / 0.25 = 4 per week
Program Y	+ 0.25	5 cents ($0.05)	$3,000 / 0.05 = 60,000	+ 0.25 / 0.05 = 5 per week

consider the reach and scope of the program. What are all the domains that could be affected by the program? How far in the future will these effects be felt? Who is affected now and in the future? Second, use the logic model. What are the best measures of the economic outcomes based on the intervention's logic model? You could consider the short-term, intermediate, and long-term effects. All outcomes, both those that are easily valued and those that are not, need to be determined.

Cost-Utility Analysis

All these benefits, while important, are difficult to monetize. How do you put a dollar value on a life, for example? Many stakeholders would revolt at doing this. For this reason, cost-utility analysis attempts to provide a unifying way to compare the benefits of widely different kinds of medical treatments and prevention activities. The quality-adjusted life year (QALY) measures the amount of life adjusted by people's perception of its quality, for example, a year of life with full function and health, versus a year of life in a vegetative state or with a painful chronic condition. A state of health that is higher in quality is viewed as more valuable. The disability-adjusted life year (DALY) is a way to value a year of healthy life lost to illness, disability, or premature death.

Further research in the area of economic evaluation may help alleviate the problem of valuing outcomes in terms of money. These difficulties illustrate why we have become more reliant on cost-effectiveness analysis. In the meantime, the benefits and the potential value of the outcomes should still be very clearly stated. When we do so, as the nutrition education program example suggests, we may fund programs with a much clearer shorter or longer term value. One example of quantifying potential benefits of programs is to ask, what is the cost of inaction? For instance, if we continue on the current path what would the costs be in the future? Then, if the costs are avoided by taking action, these avoided costs would be considered a benefit of the program. The lifetime costs of childhood obesity offer an example. Researchers estimate the lifetime medical cost of a child who becomes obese at age 10 at approximately $19,000 (when compared with a child of normal weight who maintains a normal weight throughout adult life). The cost falls to $12,900 per obese child when we take into account that many normal-weight children become overweight or obese at some point in their adult lives. For this example, a benefit of a program that maintains a normal weight over the lifetime rather than having the child become obese in adulthood would be approximately $19,000 in avoided costs.[28] Clearly this is an underestimate since no indirect medical, social, or emotional costs of obesity, nor the quality of life, are considered.

MAKING YOUR REPORTS USEFUL

Format

We do not want evaluation reports that just sit on the shelf. George Grob, former Deputy Inspector General of the U.S. Department of Health and Human Services, produced dozens of effective evaluation reports every year, and has a wealth of advice on this issue.[29] Write an executive summary first, that is no more than two pages. From that summary, develop a brief report, perhaps 10 pages, and put details in an appendix. Also develop a "killer paragraph" that is a compelling abstract of the report. This can be used as a cover letter to the evaluation stakeholders. Use verbal reports, PowerPoint, and other strategies. And most important, come up with a sentence or two that will pass "the Mom test": something that you could explain to your mother over the dinner table. If you cannot find a message that passes the Mom test, that probably means there is no message.

Timeliness and Relevance

We want evaluations to give information on a timely basis and retain their relevance. But data collection takes time. To meet this challenge, consider ongoing briefings and conversations with stakeholders, especially important when the evaluation's purpose is program improvement. Sometimes, programs and activities can present a moving target, so that the original evaluation plan is no longer relevant. Under those circumstances it is essential to return to the logic model and objectives, and carefully document the reasons for the changes. Also, use mixed methods that can change flexibly with program changes.

Fairness and Transparency

It is just as important to involve stakeholders in the interpretation of findings as it was in the planning of evaluation. It is even more important because of the need for fairness, as outlined in the evaluation *Guiding Principles*. For example, practitioners and community stakeholders may be able to explain findings differently than the evaluator does. There may be important corrections or additions to the report that need to be inserted. And if a negative evaluation is going to be presented, it is essential to notify people in advance and give them an opportunity to present a response. Under all circumstances, the key is "no surprises." A useful evaluation is often one that keeps stakeholders informed at all stages.

SUMMARY

Throughout this chapter, information on evaluations is provided within the context of public health practice, where the practitioner may be new to public health practice, unfamiliar with research and evaluation methods, and probably does not have many resources or the luxury of a long time for rigorous studies. Even under those conditions, however, practitioners can produce excellent, useful evaluations. The student will not go far wrong by following the CDC Evaluation Framework, focusing on implementation, outputs and short-term outcomes, and always bearing in mind the user's needs.

REVIEW QUESTIONS

1. Who are the likely stakeholders for the program on lead screening and treatment described under "Implementation and Outputs?" How would you go about finding this out?

2. What are some of the sources of cost for the lead screening and treatment program? Do you believe that screening the general population of children for lead exposure is cost effective? Why or why not?

3. What are the steps in the CDC Framework for Evaluation? Why do we need them?

4. What are some of the alternative explanations for the association between community-level changes and increased physical activity in Figure 15-5? Are they persuasive for you? Why or why not?

5. Pick a public health program you are familiar with. How would you focus the evaluation? What methods might you select, and why?

REFERENCES

1. Scriven M. Evaluation Thesaurus, 4th ed. Thousand Oaks, CA: Sage; 1991.

2. Shadish WR, Cook TD, Leviton LC. *Foundations of Program Evaluation: Theorists and Their Theories.* Thousand Oaks, CA: Sage; 1991.

3. Suchman, EA. *Evaluative Research: Principles and Practice in Public Service and Social Action Programs.* New York: Russell Sage Foundation; 1967.

4. Centers for Disease Control and Prevention. *Spina Bifida.* Atlanta, GA: author; 2014; http://www .cdc.gov/ncbddd/spinabifida/index.html. Accessed August 22, 2014.

5. Centers for Disease Control and Prevention. Framework for program evaluation in public health. MMWR 1999; 48 (No. RR-11):1–40. Accessed on September 2, 2014 at http://www .cdc.gov/mmwr/pdf/rr/rr4811.pdf.

6. RAND Corporation. *Getting To Outcomes®: Improving Community-Based Prevention.* Santa Monica, CA: author. http://www.rand.org/health/ projects/getting-to-outcomes.html. Accessed August 26, 2014.

7. Preskill H, Jones, N. *A Practical Guide for Engaging Stakeholders in Developing Evaluation Questions.* Princeton, NJ: Robert Wood Johnson Foundation; 2009; http://www.rwjf.org/en/ research-publications/find-rwjf-research/2009/12/ the-robert-wood-johnson-foundation-evaluation- series-guidance-fo/a-practical-guide-for-engaging- stakeholders-in-developing-evalua.html. Accessed August 22, 2014.

8. Fetterman, DM, Wandersman A, eds. *Empowerment Evaluation: Principles in Practice.* 2nd Edition. New York: The Guilford Press; 2014.

9. Cousins JB, Chouinard JA, eds. *Participatory Evaluation Up Close: An Integration of Research-Based Knowledge.* Charlotte, NC: IAP; 2012.

10. Leviton LC, Kettel-Khan L, Rog D, Dawkins N, Cotton D. Evaluability assessment to improve public health. *Annu Rev Publ Health* 2010; 31:213–34.

11. Rossi PH, Lipsey MW, Freeman HE. *Evaluation: A systematic approach.* Thousand Oaks, CA: Sage Publications; 2003.

12. US Department of Health Human Services, Office of Disease Prevention and Health Promotion. *Healthy People 2020.* Washington, DC. 2012.

13. Robert Wood Johnson Foundation. County Health Rankings. 2015; http://www.countyhealthrankings .org/. Accessed April/28, 2015.

14. Last JM. *A Dictionary of Epidemiology.* Oxford, England: Oxford University Press; 2001.

15. Dietz B, Story M, Leviton LC. *Pediatrics* 124 Supplement 1: Issues and Implications of Screening, Surveillance, and Reporting of Children's Body Mass Index; 2009.

16. Patton MQ. *Qualitative Research and Evaluation Methods* (4th Edition). Thousand Oaks, CA: Sage, 2014.

17. Krueger RA, Casey MA. *Focus Groups: A Practical Guide for Applied Research.* 4th ed. Thousand Oaks, CA: Sage; 2009.

18. McMullen K, Brownson R, Luke D, Chriqui J. Strength of clean indoor air laws and smoking related outcomes in the USA. *Tob Control* 2005; 14(1): 43–8.

19. Centers for Disease Control and Prevention. *Key Outcome Indicators for Evaluating Comprehensive Tobacco Control Programs*. Atlanta, GA. http://www.cdc.gov/TOBACCO/tobacco_control_programs/surveillance_evaluation/key_outcome/index.htm. Accessed August 22, 2014.

20. U.S. Preventive Services Task Force. Screening for Elevated Blood Lead Levels in Childhood and Pregnant Women: Recommendation Statement. *Pediatrics* 2006;118:2514–2518. http://www.uspreventiveservicestaskforce.org/uspstf06/lead/leadrs.htm. Accessed August 27, 2014.

21. Frey BB, Lohmeier JH, Lee SW, Tollefson N. Measuring collaboration among grant partners. *Am J Evaluation.* 2006; 27:383–92.

22. Marek LI, Brock DP, Savla J. Evaluating collaboration for effectiveness: Conceptualization and measurement. *Am J Evaluation*, 1098214014531068 Published online April 18, 2014; http://aje.sagepub.com/content/early/2014/04/18/1098214014531068.full. Accessed on August 27, 2014.

23. Fawcett SB, Schultz JA. Supporting participatory evaluation using the Community Tool Box online documentation system. In Minkler M, Wallerstein N, eds. *Community-Based Participatory Research for Health*. San Francisco, CA: Jossey-Bass, 2008, pp. 419–424.

24. Collie-Akers VL, Fawcett SB, Schultz JA, Carson V, Cyprus J, Pierle JE. Analyzing a community-based coalition's efforts to reduce health disparities and the risk for chronic disease in Kansas City, Missouri. *Prevent Chron Dis* 2007 4(3) http://www.cdc.gov/pcd/issues/2007/jul/06_0101.htm. Accessed August 28, 2014.

25. Shadish WR, Cook TD, Campbell, DT. Experimental and Quasi-Experimental Designs for Generalized Causal Inference. Boston, MA: Houghton Mifflin.

26. Mercer SL, DeVinney BJ, Fine LC, Green LW, Dougherty D. Study designs for effectiveness and translation research: Identifying trade-offs. *Am J Prev Med* 2007;33(2):139–154.

27. Three classics include: Drummond MF, Sculpher MJ, Torrance GW, O'Brien BJ, Stoddart GL. *Methods for the Economic Evaluation of Health Care Programmes*. 3rd ed. New York: Oxford University Press, 2005; Gold MR, Siegel JE, Russell LB, Weinstein MC. *Cost-Effectiveness in Health and Medicine*. New York: Oxford University Press, 1996; Haddix AC, Teutsch SM, Corso PS. *Prevention Effectiveness. A Guide to Decision Analysis and Economic Evaluation*. 2nd ed. New York: Oxford University Press; 2002.

28. Finkelstein EA, Graham WC, Malhotra R. Lifetime direct medical costs of childhood obesity. *Pediatrics*. 2014;133:854–862.

29. Grob G. Writing for impact. In Wholey JS, Hatry HP, Newcomer KE, eds. The Handbook of Practical Program Evaluation, 3rd ed. San Francisco, CA: Jossey-Bass, 2010, pp. 594–619.

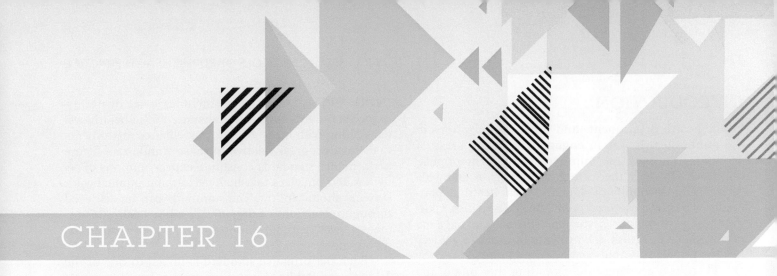

Performance Management and Quality Improvement

William Riley, PhD • Cecile Dinh, MPH • David Upjohn, BA • Paul Halverson, DrPH

LEARNING OBJECTIVES

Upon completion of this chapter, the reader will be able to:

1. Assess the need for performance management, quality improvement, and accreditation in public health organizations.

2. Describe how performance management systems, public health accreditation, and quality improvement methods can enhance the efficiency and effectiveness of public health organizations.

3. Apply cause and effect diagram, process map, and the Plan, Do, Study, Act (PDSA) cycle to public health.

4. Describe the five components of the Turning Point Performance Management Model for public health.

5. Critique the use of quality improvement collaboratives (QICs) in public health.

KEY TERMS

accreditation
National Public Health Performance Standards Program (NPHPSP)
PDSA cycle
performance management (PM)
quality improvement (QI)
quality improvement (QI) techniques
Turning Point Model

INTRODUCTION

Public health departments and other organizations in the public health system engage in a broad array of activities to protect and improve health at the population level. However, there are substantial gaps and wide variation in the ability of state and local health departments to perform essential public health activities. Closing these gaps requires systematic efforts to manage the performance of health departments in order to achieve healthy populations and healthy communities.

There is a growing understanding that one of the most effective ways to improve the health of the population is to improve the performance of public health departments and other organizations in the public health system (e.g., coalitions, voluntary health agencies). This chapter introduces performance management (PM) as a leading method to improve the results of health departments. Additionally, two prominent developments in public health are interconnected with performance management: the expanding application of quality improvement methods and techniques, and the creation of a national public health accreditation system to establish standards and ensure they are met.

BACKGROUND

Almost three decades ago, the seminal Institute of Medicine (IOM) report, *The Future of Public Health*, concluded that the public health system was in disarray, and introduced three core functions of a governmental public health department: Assessment, Policy Development, and Assurance.[1] Fourteen years later a subsequent IOM report, *The Future of the Public's Health in the 21st Century*, determined the public health infrastructure had systemic deficiencies due to outdated technologies and antiquated capacity.[2] More recently, however, attention has shifted to how health departments can achieve performance excellence through performance management systems based on the use of quality improvement methods and by achieving public health department accreditation.[3]

Developing Performance Standards in Public Health

The U.S. Centers for Disease Control and Prevention (CDC) sponsored an array of research and development efforts during the 1990s designed to identify the specific practice elements that comprise core public health functions and to develop ways of measuring the extent to which these elements are performed by local public health departments. The CDC launched the National Public Health Performance Standards Program (NPHPSP) in 2002, which includes a set of performance standards for local and state public health systems along with measures and surveillance instruments that track progress relative to these standards.[4] These performance standards constitute expert opinions of activities and practices that high-performing public health systems should follow. The standards can be achieved through the actions of the official public health department as well as other public and private organizations within the system.

Each performance standard is linked to one of the 10 Essential Public Health Services developed in 1994, with separate standards for local systems, state systems, and governing boards.[5] All public health departments are eligible to conduct a voluntary self-assessment using the National Public Health Performance Standards Program and submit their results to the national program for scoring and comparative reporting.

Based in part on these performance standards, a series of national health objectives related to public health infrastructure were included in the *Healthy People 2010* and *Healthy People 2020* planning documents developed by the U.S. Department of Health and Human Services.[6] A total of 17 infrastructure objectives were developed, including those related to public health data and information systems, the public health workforce, public health organizations, public health resources, and prevention research. Progress toward these objectives is monitored through a variety of national data sources including data collected through the CDC.

An example of how the NPHPS system works is shown in Table 16-1. The example shows the Essential Service 1, "Monitor Health Status to Identify Community Health Problems," and Standard 1.1, "Population-Based Community Health Profile." The table also shows examples of how local public health systems (LPHS) can work together, as well as discussion questions to assess how well they are performing to meet the standard, including topics on awareness, involvement, frequency, quality and comprehensiveness, and usability.

Public Health Quality

In the *National Framework for Public Health Quality*, the Department of Health and Human Services (HHS) defines quality in public health as "the degree to which policies, programs, services, and research for the population increase desired health outcomes and conditions in which the population can be healthy."[8] The HHS definition of quality includes nine aims to help guide public health practices for improving population health outcomes, establishing an important new direction for advancing population health metrics (Table 16-2).

TABLE 16-1 Example of a Performance Standard Used in the National Public Health Performance Standards Program[7]

Essential Service 1: Monitor Health Status to Identify Community Health Problems
Model Standard 1.1: Population-Based Community Health Profile
To accomplish this, members of the local public health system (LPHS) work together to: • Assess the health of the community regularly. • Continuously update the community health assessment (CHA) with current information. • Promote the use of the CHA among community members and partners.
Discussion Questions for Model Standard 1.1

Awareness

- Was everyone aware of the assessment?
- Does everyone have access to the CHA?

Involvement

- How many of you participated in the assessment?

Frequency

- How often is the CHA completed?
- How often do updates to the CHA occur?

Quality and Comprehensiveness

- Which data sets are included in the CHA?
- How is the CHA used to monitor progress toward:
  - o Local health priorities?
  - o State health priorities?
  - o *Healthy People 2020* national objectives?
- How well does the CHA examine data over time to track trends?
- How are the data helping identify health inequities?

Usability

- How accessible to the general public are the CHA results?
- How is the CHA distributed to the community?
- How is the CHA used to inform health policy and planning decisions?

SOURCE: Centers for Disease Control and Prevention

TABLE 16-2 National Framework for Public Health Quality: The Nine Aims[8]

Aim	Description
Population-Centered	Protecting and promoting healthy conditions and the health of the entire population.
Equitable	Working to achieve health equity.
Proactive	Formulating policies and sustainable practices in a timely manner, while mobilizing rapidly to address new and emerging threats and vulnerabilities.
Health Promoting	Ensuring policies and strategies that advance safe practices by providers and the population, and increase the probability of positive health behaviors and outcomes.
Risk Reducing	Diminishing adverse environmental and social events by implementing policies and strategies to reduce the probability of preventable injuries and illness or negative outcomes.
Vigilant	Intensifying practices and enacting policies to support enhancements to surveillance activities.
Transparent	Ensuring openness in the delivery of services and practices with particular emphasis on valid, reliable, accessible, timely, and meaningful data that is readily available to stakeholders, including the public.
Effective	Justifying investments by using evidence, science, and best practices to achieve optimal results in areas of greatest need.
Efficient	Understanding costs and benefits of public health interventions and facilitating the optimal use of resources to achieve desired outcomes.

SOURCE: U.S. Department of Health and Human Services

Public health departments and many other organizations collectively provide a range of programs and services directed toward improving the health of the population. While some public health programs dramatically succeed in improving health outcomes, many programs do not achieve their potential impact.[9] Indeed, very few local or national population health goals established by leading organizations have been met.[10,11] For example, as part of the Healthy People program, the CDC developed Leading Health Indicators (LHIs) to highlight certain high-priority targets. Table 16-3 shows that for *Healthy People 2020*, only four of the 26 LHIs have been met, while 19 indicators have not been met, and five indicators have worsened. Put another way, only 15 percent of the LHI target goals for *Healthy People 2020* have been met thus far.

Another example of the gaps in public health quality is reflected by the low rates of preventive practices in our nation. The Healthcare Effectiveness Data and

TABLE 16-3   Twenty-Six Leading Health Indicators, Targets, and Current Performance[10]

Leading Health Topic and Indicator	Baseline	Most Recent	Target
Access to Health Services			
Persons with medical insurance (percent, <65 years)	83.2% (2008)	83.1% (2012)	100%
Persons with a usual primary care provider (percent)	76.3% (2007)	77.3% (2011)	83.9%
Clinical Preventive Services			
Adults receiving colorectal cancer screening based on most recent guidelines (age adjusted, percent, 50–75 years)	52.1% (2008)	59.2% (2010)	70.5%
Adults with hypertension whose blood pressure is under control (age adjusted, percent, 18+ years)	43.7% (2005–2008)	48.9% (2009–2012)	61.2%
Persons with diagnosed diabetes whose A1c value is >9 percent (age adjusted, percent, 18+ years)	17.9% (2005–2008)	21.0% (2009–2012)	16.1%
Children receiving the recommended doses of DTaP, polio, MMR, Hib, hepatitis B, varicella and PCV vaccines (percent, aged 19–35 months)	44.3% (2009)	68.5% (2011)	80.0%
Environmental Quality			
Air Quality Index (AQI) exceeding 100 (number of billion person days, weighted by population and AQI value)	2.237 (2006–2008)	1.252 (2009–2011)	1.980
Children exposed to secondhand smoke (percent; nonsmokers, 3–11 years)	52.2% (2005–2008)	41.3% (2009–2012)	47.0%
Injury and Violence			
Injury deaths (age adjusted, per 100,000 population)	59.7 (2007)	57.1 (2010)	53.7
Homicides (age adjusted, per 100,000 population)	6.1 (2007)	5.3 (2010)	5.5
Maternal, Infant, and Child Health			
Infant deaths (per 1,000 live births, <1 year)	6.7 (2006)	6.1 (2010)	6.0
Total preterm live births (percent, <37 weeks gestation)	12.7% (2007)	11.5% (2012)	11.4%
Mental Health			
Suicides (age adjusted, per 100,000 population)	11.3 (2007)	12.1 (2010)	10.2
Adolescents with major depressive episodes (percent, 12–17 years)	8.3% (2008)	9.1% (2012)	7.5%
Nutrition, Physical Activity, and Obesity			
Adults meeting aerobic physical activity and muscle-strengthening federal guidelines (age adjusted, percent, 18+ years)	18.2% (2008)	20.6% (2012)	20.1%
Obesity among adults (age adjusted, percent, 20+ years)	33.9% (2005–08)	35.3% (2009–12)	30.5%

TABLE 16-3 (Continued)

Leading Health Topic and Indicator	Baseline	Most Recent	Target
Obesity among children and adolescents (percent, 2–19 years)	16.1% (2005–08)	16.9% (2009–12)	14.5%
Mean daily intake of total vegetables (age adjusted, cup equivalents per 1,000 calories, 2+ years)	0.8 (2001–04)	0.8 (2007–10)	1.1
Oral Health			
Persons who visited the dentist in the past year (age adjusted, percent, 2+ years)	44.5% (2007)	41.8% (2011)	49.0%
Reproductive and Sexual Health			
Sexually experienced females receiving reproductive health services in the past 12 months (percent, 15–44 years)	78.6% (2006–10)	n/a	86.5%
Knowledge of serostatus among HIV-positive persons (percent, 13+ years)	80.9% (2006)	84.2% (2010)	90.0%
Social Determinants			
Students awarded a high school diploma 4 years after starting 9th grade (percent)	74.9% (2007–08)	78.2% (2009–10)	82.4%
Substance Abuse			
Adolescents using alcohol or illicit drugs in past 3 days (percent, 12–17 years)	18.4% (2008)	17.4% (2012)	16.6%
Binge drinking in past 30 days—Adults (percent 18+ years)	27.1% (2008)	27.1% (2012)	24.4%
Tobacco			
Adult cigarette smoking (age adjusted, percent, 18+ years)	20.6% (2008)	18.2% (2012)	12.0%
Adolescent cigarette smoking in past 30 days (percent, grades 9–12)	19.5% (2009)	18.1% (2011)	16.0%

SOURCE: U.S. Department of Health and Human Services. *Healthy People 2020 Leading Health Indicators: Progress Update.* Washington, DC: U.S. Department of Health and Human Services; 2014

Information Set (HEDIS) indicates that while some improvements have been made over a 10-year timeframe, many of the preventive health changes have been modest (Table 16-4).

The current metrics on the LHIs and preventive measures indicate that there are large gaps between levels of desired performance and actual practice. To help reduce these gaps, organizational techniques from other industries are being introduced into public health, offering tremendous potential to increase effectiveness and efficiency. Three methods that are known to raise performance will be reviewed next: **quality improvement**, public health accreditation, and performance management.

QUALITY IMPROVEMENT

Quality improvement (QI) techniques are specifically developed to help close gaps between current and desired performances of an organization. The application of QI methods in public health is resulting in measurable improvement in public health services which can eventually translate to enhanced health status of populations. The HHS definition of quality in public health suggests that QI can help achieve the HHS quality goals for public health. In defining quality as the degree to which public health services impact the health of a population, the HHS statement explicitly assumes that quality exists on a continuum from low to high quality.

TABLE 16-4   10-year Trends for Preventive Practices, Selected Measures[12]

Effectiveness of Care Measure: Percentages of Patients Receiving Recommended Intervention	1999	2009
Breast cancer screening	73.4%	71.3%
Cervical cancer screening	71.8%	77.3%
Childhood immunizations – MMR	87.0%	90.6%
Controlling of High Blood Pressure	39.0%	64.1%
Cholesterol Screening	69.0%	85.70%
Comprehensive Diabetes Care – Eye Exams	45.3%	56.5%
Comprehensive Diabetes Care – Monitoring Nephropathy	36.0%	82.9%
Antidepressant Management – Continuation Phase	42.1%	46.2%

SOURCE: The State of Health Care Quality: Reform, The Quality Agenda and Resource Use. The National Committee for Quality Assurance. 2010.

Quality improvement in public health is defined as the application of QI methods and techniques to improve a specific process with a defined beginning and end, using an identified QI model.[13] Five applications have been identified to deploy QI in public health: (1) understand processes and pinpoint critical problems; (2) establish control and reduce variation; (3) determine process capability; (4) design interventions to improve processes and outcomes; and (5) assess service reliability.[14] Defined this way, applying QI in public health presents two opportunities. It increases the level of performance within an organization, and can lead to transformational change to improve desired health outcomes.

Quality Improvement Background

Quality improvement is a prominent management model that supports the short-term growth and long-term success of any organization. Quality improvement involves deployment of process engineering techniques for the analysis, design, and ongoing implementation of public health processes to achieve measurable increases in health department performance and, ultimately, community outcomes. It is an important method urgently needed in public health to enhance public health department effectiveness in improving population health.

Quality improvement has been successfully deployed in many industries for over 90 years. Formal QI methods were first developed in 1924 when Walter Shewhart developed statistical process control techniques and the plan-do-study-act (PDSA) cycle.[15] Following World War II, these techniques were further refined in Japan[16,17,18] but were not largely adopted in the United States until the 1980s when the Six Sigma model was developed by Motorola.[19] General Electric started using Six Sigma as a model to improve quality, and helped QI techniques to proliferate rapidly in the manufacturing industry. Other QI methods also took hold including Lean,[20] The Baldrige Criteria for Performance Excellence,[21] the Deming Approach,[22] and Juran Trilogy.[23]

Quality improvement was introduced to the health care industry in the late 1980s,[22] and is now used extensively in the hospital sector to improve services for patients.[23] Although QI was deployed sporadically in health departments during the mid-1990s, widespread adoption of QI techniques in public health organizations began in 2005 when several states introduced QI methods to their health departments. The last decade has seen rapid expansion of QI into health departments through major support by the Robert Wood Johnson Foundation (RWJF). Currently, 87 percent of local health departments[24] and 96 percent of state health departments[25] have undertaken QI projects within their agencies.

It is now well accepted that QI can be a powerful mechanism to ensure superior performance of public health departments and improve population health. However, unlike other industries, public health has an added layer of complexity; not only are health department employees, and even the departments themselves, accountable for their own performance but they must also provide leadership for the entire public health system. It is anticipated that using the HHS definitions of quality and QI to establish program priorities is likely to improve public health practice. QI is a proactive approach to quality management that features: (1) multidisciplinary teamwork; (2) empowerment so teams can make immediate process changes; (3) an iterative scientific approach to problem solving; and (4) ongoing measurement and monitoring.[26]

Process Design

All public health services are the result of a process. A *process* is a series of steps to produce an outcome. For example, birth and death certificate registrations, a flu vaccination program, and a legislative effort to implement policy to reduce tobacco consumption are all processes. Whenever public health interventions are planned, or programs implemented, the service is a result of a series of steps. Process design refers to the deliberate and intentional development of processes so that they result in the desired outcome. Quality improvement is based on process engineering, and all quality improvement initiatives analyze a process in order to improve performance. Two of the most common tools used to analyze a process are: (a) process maps and (b) cause and effect diagrams. As mentioned above, a *work process* is defined as a series of steps designed to produce an outcome and has three components:

1. It has a beginning point and an end point.
2. It uses inputs (people, equipment, supplies, and facilities) to carry out the process.
3. It produces an output created by the process, which is usually a service.

For example, a client visit to a Women, Infants, and Children (WIC) clinic involves a multiple-step process. The beginning point is when the mother calls for an appointment and the end point is when the client leaves the clinic once the visit is completed. The inputs are dieticians, counselors, receptionists, rooms, equipment, and supplies, while the output is a client (and family) who has been served. The series of steps in a work process are combined to add value to the inputs by changing them or using them to produce a service.

A typical public health department has hundreds, even thousands, of work processes to serve clients and the community. A process improvement team may find it difficult to decide which process to study, and how to draw the boundaries for the process. Creating a process map (also known as a *flow chart*) is a disciplined method to overcome these difficulties as well as to understand and analyze a process. Figure 16-1 illustrates an example of a process map.

Table 16-5 explains the function of each component of a process map. A process map can be created with three different levels of detail: (1) the macro level, which shows key action steps but no decision points; (2) the intermediate level, which shows both action and decision points; and (3) the micro level which shows extensive detail.

Uncovering Problem Areas Using a Process Map

After a process map has been constructed, it can be analyzed for specific problem areas. Many times a process map will uncover a problem in the process that cuts

TABLE 16-5 Components of a Process Map

Component	Function
Oval	Designates the start and finish of the process.
Rectangle/Box	Represents a task or activity. It has one arrow pointing away.
Arrow	Connects various process steps.
Diamond	Designates a decision. It has two arrows pointing away. Note that decisions must have a closed loop. No arrow can end with an activity that does not connect again to the process.

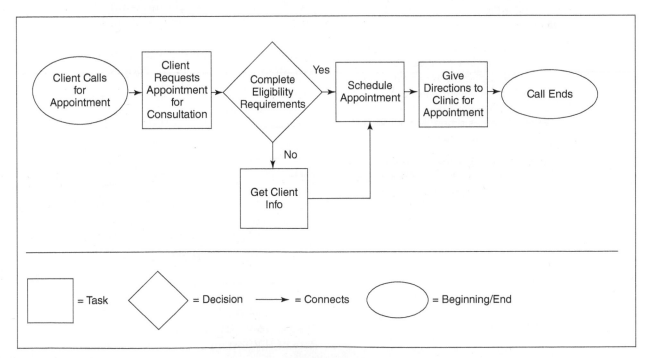

FIGURE 16-1 Basic Process Map for Making an Appointment in Clinic for Women, Infants, and Children

across departments. The process map can also identify where a breakdown may occur or where steps can be eliminated. Table 16-6 lists and defines five types of problems that can be identified by studying a process map.

There are two types of processes: core and support. A *core process* is a process that provides a service to communities or populations, such as a restaurant inspection program. A *support process* is a process that provides key services to enable an organization's core processes to perform. Typical support processes might include the financial department, human resources, and technical support for employees.

Finally, processes are almost always cross-functional, which means they usually go across several different departments in an organization. For example, in the client visit process, several departments can be involved, including the appointment-scheduling department, the

WIC clinic, nutrition counseling, and immunization screening. An organization is only as effective as its processes, and the first step in QI is to define and identify a process to improve, followed by an analysis of the effectiveness and efficiency of the process.

Public health departments are extensively involved in creating governmental policy for their jurisdictions. The process of creating public health policy can be complex, cumbersome, and sometimes requires considerable time periods to be enacted. Process maps have been used effectively in public health to assist in facilitating the process of making public policy, by identifying and rectifying problem areas.

Cause and Effect Diagram

A second important QI technique for process analysis is a cause and effect diagram. A *cause and effect diagram* is a tool used to identify the possible causes of a problem in a process. For example, the cause and effect diagram shown in Figure 16-2 was created because the Infectious Disease Officer was concerned by the low rates of HIV testing at the public health department. A QI team developed a cause and effect diagram to study why clients do not receive HIV testing. They identified four main causes and organized them as headers in the diagram: clients, staff, the test location, and client counseling. There were also subcauses associated with each main cause.

A cause and effect diagram organizes group knowledge about causes of a problem and displays the information graphically. In a cause and effect diagram, the problem is written on the far right, while causes are represented by the diagonal lines connected to the horizontal line which leads to the problem. The cause and effect diagram is also known as a *fishbone diagram* because it resembles a fish (the problem is the "head" of the fish and the causes represent the "bones").

TABLE 16-6   Five Problem Areas Identified by Process Maps

Problem Area	Definition
Disconnect	A disconnect occurs when a handoff from one group to another is poorly managed. For example, the appointment scheduler makes a client appointment on a day the WIC specialist is not in the clinic.
Bottleneck	A bottleneck is a point in a process where volume overwhelms capacity. For example, two clients are scheduled during the same appointment time.
Redundancy	A redundancy is an activity repeated at two points in a process. For example, a client is asked for demographic information at several different times (when the appointment is scheduled, when the client arrives for the visit).
Rework	Rework is when work is fixed or corrected. For example, if the client's demographic information is entered incorrectly or incompletely, extra work is required to retrieve the information at a later time.
Inspection	Inspection is a point in the process where appraisal occurs. This usually is an extra step that can be costly, and also creates potential delay. For example, a cleaned hospital room cannot be occupied until it is inspected by a supervisor.

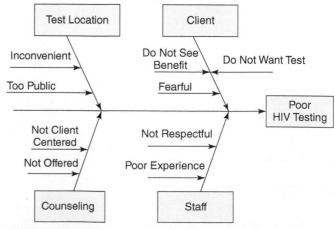

FIGURE 16-2   Cause-Effect Diagram, Analysis of Low Rate of HIV Testing at a Health Department[27]

Courtesy of the Public Health Foundation

Model for Improvement

The Model for Improvement is a common technique used to carry out QI in a public health department and has been used extensively by the Institute for Healthcare Improvement (IHI).[28] Numerous health care organizations and public health departments around the country have adopted the Model for Improvement because it is very comprehensive, yet easy to use.

The Model for Improvement consists of four components:

1. *Set Aim Statement:* An aim addresses the question of what the process improvement team is trying to accomplish.

2. *Establish Measures:* Establishing measures addresses the question of how the team will know that a change is an improvement.

3. *Generate Change Concepts:* Developing changes addresses the question of what changes can be made that will result in improvement.

4. *Conduct Plan, Do, Study, Act (PDSA) Cycle:* The **PDSA cycle** describes how to test a change—by trying it, observing the consequences, and then learning from those consequences. Once a team has set an aim, established measures to indicate whether a change leads to an improvement, and found a promising idea for change, the next step is to test that change in the work setting by conducting a PDSA cycle.

The following discussion will expand on each of the four components of the Model for Improvement.

Set Aim Statement

Improvement begins with setting an aim. A program will not improve without clear and firm intention to do so. Principles of an effective aim statement are:

- State the aim clearly: Achieving agreement on the aim of the project is critical for maintaining progress. Teams make better progress when they have very specific aims.

- Include numerical goals: The aim should be expressed in specific terms. For example, this could be a 50 percent increase in condom use by teenagers, or a 30 percent reduction in sexually transmitted infections (STIs). Using numerical goals is an effective way to communicate expectations. Including a numerical goal clarifies the aim and also suggests a level of support that will be needed from the organization to accomplish the aim. Agreement by the team on the aim of the project is essential so the team is clear about what measures of improvement are feasible and what initial changes it might make for the project.

Establish Measures

The second component of the Model for Improvement is establishing measures. A measure is a metric that provides specific performance levels that are associated directly or indirectly with the aim statement. Establishing the measures is less complicated when the team has accurately articulated its aim statement. Measures need to be identified to indicate whether a change actually leads to improvement.

Generate Change Concepts

Developing changes identifies actionable strategies that will result in improvement. All improvement requires making a change, but not all changes result in improvement. A change concept is a general idea for change that the team believes will result in improvement. It has proven merit and a sound scientific or logical foundation which will stimulate specific ideas for changes that lead to improvement. Using change concepts and combining them creatively can stimulate new ways of thinking about the problem at hand. There are many ways to generate a change concept, including: critical thinking about the current system, creative thinking, watching the process, a hunch, talking with experts who know the process, or a literature review.

Conduct PDSA Cycle

The PDSA cycle is the fourth component of the Model for Improvement. Once a team has set an aim, established measures to indicate whether a change leads to improvement, and found a promising change concept, the fourth step is to test that change in the work setting by conducting a PDSA cycle.

A PDSA cycle describes how to test a change. Its four separate components are:

- Plan: plan the change
- Do: try the change
- Study: observe the consequences
- Act: learn from those consequences

These four components of the PDSA cycle are shown in Figure 16-3. Note that each of the four components of the PDSA cycle has specific questions to be addressed during that phase.

Ideally, public health quality results from comprehensive process design and continuous quality improvement. In reality this is far from the case. Serious quality and efficiency problems in the public health system persist despite the best efforts of public health professionals. While public health personnel are individually committed to quality excellence, organizational processes are often not adequate for ensuring efficiency and effectiveness in a complex system. Quality must be recognized as a system property, which

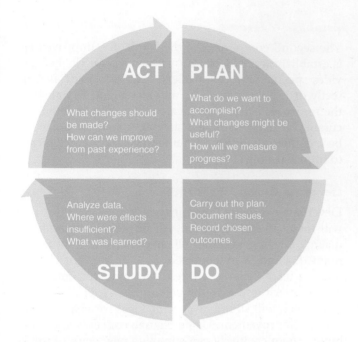

FIGURE 16-3   Components of the PDSA Cycle[29]

Adapted from Kheraj R, Tewani SK, Ketwaroo G, Leffler DA. Quality improvement in gastroenterology clinical practice. *Clinical Gastroenterology and Hepatology.* 2012;10(12):1305–1314.

means that public health processes are deliberately designed to achieve desired outcomes, and process control is in place to detect when system outcomes do not meet expectations. A superior public health service is considered a system, and thus quality is an attribute of the entire structure.

The concept of making quality a system property means ensuring that the system itself is sound, rather than relying solely on individuals to achieve quality. Better quality will not be achieved by imploring public health department staff to work harder or better. In order to improve quality, public health systems need to be redesigned to achieve the desired outcomes.

In summary, QI in public health involves the analysis of a specific process with an identified beginning and end, using a defined QI model with the intent to achieve measurable improvement and efficient output and outcomes. Quality improvement methods and techniques are essential to improving health department results because the quality and performance of the public health system are not where they should be. The high level of preparation for nurses, physicians, dieticians, epidemiologists, and other public health professionals results in a dedicated workforce. However, most quality deficiencies and waste do not occur from lack of professional expertise or individual commitment, but from poorly designed processes.

PUBLIC HEALTH DEPARTMENT ACCREDITATION

Accreditation is the process by which organizations are certified by an external organization to meet specified standards. The largest accreditation body in health care is the Joint Commission, which accredits more than 20,500 organizations and programs (primarily hospitals, home care organizations, nursing homes, medical groups, laboratories, and surgery centers) in the United States. In public health practice, the prominent national accreditation body is the Public Health Accreditation Board (PHAB), which administers the voluntary national public health department accreditation program. Started in 2007, the goal of PHAB is to improve and protect the health of the public by advancing the quality and performance of tribal, state, local, and territorial public health departments.[30]

The PHAB accreditation program has a direct link to the three core functions in public health (assessment, policy development, and assurance), which were identified by the IOM report in 1988. The three core functions were elaborated upon six years later when the 10 Essential Public Health Services were identified.[31] Figure 16-4 shows the 10 Essential Services and how they relate to the three core functions. These essential services provide a foundation for any public health activity and are the basis for both the NPHPS and the PHAB program.

The PHAB scope of accreditation extends to over 3,000 governmental health departments operated by tribes, states, local jurisdictions, and territories (over 500 tribal health departments, 56 state and territorial health departments, and more than 2,500 local health departments). PHAB's vision is of a high-performing governmental public health system that will make the United States a healthier nation.

The purpose of public health accreditation is to: (a) promote high performance and continuous quality improvement; (b) advance public health practices; (c) demonstrate health department accountability to the public and policy makers; and (d) increase the visibility and public awareness of governmental public health.[32] The PHAB system assesses health department performance against a set of standards that are nationally recognized, practice-focused, and evidence-based.

PHAB Domains, Standards, and Measures

The PHAB Accreditation System consists of domains, standards, and measures to assess a range of core public health programs and activities. A *domain* is an area of performance considered necessary to be a

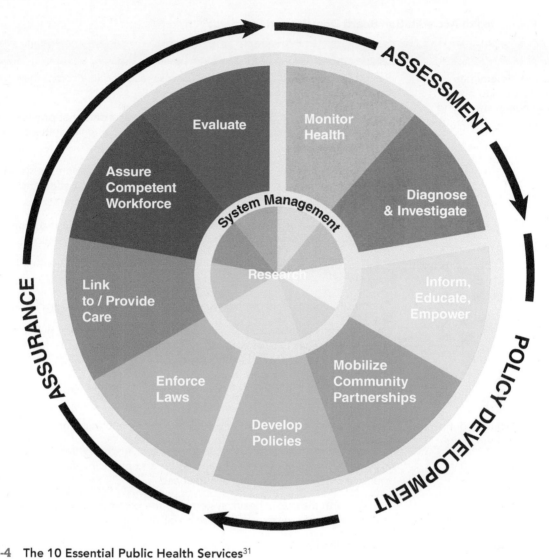

FIGURE 16-4 The 10 Essential Public Health Services[31]

SOURCE: Centers for Disease Control and Prevention. The Public Health System and the 10 Essential Public Health Services. Centers for Disease Control and Prevention Website.

fully functional health department. A *standard* is the required level of achievement that a health department is expected to meet. *Measures* provide a way of evaluating whether a standard is met; the number of measures vary depending on the type of health department (there are 102 tribal measures, 108 state and territorial measures, and 100 local measures). Twelve domains are shown in Table 16-7. The first 10 domains address the 10 Essential Public Health Services, while Domain 11 addresses management and administration, and Domain 12 addresses governance.[33] Table 16-7 also shows that a total of 32 standards are incorporated into the 12 domains.

There are three prerequisites that must be met before a health department can apply for accreditation: completing an organizational strategic plan, a community health assessment, and a community health improvement plan. The PHAB system also incorporates QI as the cornerstone of its accreditation system. Unlike many accreditation systems which focus on auditing programs, the PHAB system focuses on how to continuously enhance quality and promote performance improvement. To ensure that QI is a central component of the PHAB system, a focus on the evaluation of key public health processes and the implementation of a formal quality improvement process has been incorporated into one of the domains. As of September 2015, 80 health departments have been accredited with over 121 million people served by a PHAB-accredited health department. (Information on these departments can be found at http://www.phaboard.org by searching "Accredited Health Departments.")

TABLE 16-7   Public Health Accreditation Board Domains and Standards[33]

Domain	Standard
1. Conduct and disseminate assessments focused on population health status and public health issues facing the community	Participate in or lead a collaborative process resulting in a comprehensive Community Health Assessment.
	Collect and maintain reliable, comparable, and valid data that provide information on conditions of public health importance and on the health status of the population.
	Analyze public health data to identify trends in health problems, environmental public health hazards, and social and economic factors that affect the public's health.
	Provide and use the results of health data analysis to develop recommendations regarding public health policy, processes, programs, or interventions.
2. Investigate health problems and environmental public health hazards to protect the community	Conduct timely investigations of health problems and environmental public health hazards.
	Contain/Mitigate health problems and environmental public health hazards.
	Ensure access to laboratory and epidemiologic/environmental public health expertise in capacity to investigate and contain/mitigate public health problems and environmental public health hazards.
	Maintain a plan with policies and procedures for urgent and nonurgent communications.
3. Inform and educate about public health issues and functions	Provide health education and health promotion policies programs, processes, and interventions to support prevention and wellness.
	Provide information on public health issues and public health functions through multiple methods to a variety of audiences.
4. Engage with the community to identify and address health problems	Engage with the public health system and the community in identifying and addressing health problems through collaborative processes.
	Promote the community's understanding of and support for policies and strategies that will improve the public's health.
5. Develop public health policies and plans	Serve as a primary and expert resource for establishing and maintaining public health policies, practices, and capacity.
	Conduct a comprehensive planning process resulting in a tribal/state/community health improvement plan.
	Develop and implement a health department organizational strategic plan.
	Maintain an all-hazards emergency operations plan.
6. Enforce public health laws	Review existing laws and work with governing entities and elected/appointed officials to update as needed.
	Educate individuals and organizations on the meaning, purpose, and benefit of public health laws and how to comply.
	Conduct and monitor public health enforcement activities and coordinate notification of violations among appropriate agencies.
7. Promote strategies to improve access to health care	Assess health care service capacity and access to health care services.
	Identify and implement strategies to improve access to health care services.

Domain	Standard
8. Maintain a competent public health workforce	Encourage the development of a sufficient number of qualified public health workers.
	Ensure a competent workforce through assessment of staff competencies, the provision of individual training and professional development, and the provision of a supportive work environment.
9. Evaluate and continuously improve processes, programs, and interventions	Use a performance management system to monitor achievement of organizational objectives.
	Develop and implement quality improvement processes integrated into organizational practice, programs, processes, and interventions.
10. Contribute to and apply the evidence base of public health	Identify and use the best available evidence for making informed public health practice decisions.
	Promote understanding and use of the current body of research results, evaluations, and evidence-based practices with appropriate audiences.
11. Maintain administrative and management capacity	Develop and maintain an operational infrastructure to support the performance of public health functions.
	Establish effective financial management systems.
12. Maintain capacity to engage the public health governing entity	Maintain current operational definitions and statements of the public health roles, responsibilities, and authorities.
	Provide information to the governing entity regarded public health and the official responsibilities of the health department and of the governing entity.
	Encourage the governing entity's engagement in the public health department's overall obligations and responsibilities.

SOURCE: Public Health Accreditation Board. Standards & Measures, Version 1.5. Alexandria, VA: PHAB; 2013

PERFORMANCE MANAGEMENT

All governmental health departments have a management structure to develop and achieve the organizational goals. *Management* consists of a set of functions executed within an organizational setting to accomplish the objectives of the enterprise. There are four essential management functions which managers must execute in order to successfully lead an organization: (1) establish strategic plans and operations plans to serve the community; (2) create an organizational structure that establishes authority, responsibility, and accountability; (3) motivate the staff within the health department to perform at consistently high levels; and (4) control the organization by assuring that the plans are achieved as expected. These four processes are listed and defined in Table 16-8.

Performance management (PM) is a coordinated set of activities undertaken to ensure that the goals of a health department are consistently being met in an effective and efficient manner. Viewed this way, performance management is a comprehensive approach

TABLE 16-8   The Four Management Functions

Management Function	Definition
Planning	Defining what needs to be done and methods to accomplish objectives.
Organizing	Establishing a formal structure through which objectives are arranged.
Motivating	Causing people to act in order to achieve objectives.
Controlling	Measure performance against plan to determine if objectives are met.

to manage two critical elements in an organization: the behavior of staff and the results of programs. A performance problem is any gap between desired results and actual results. *Performance improvement* is all activity used to compare desired results with actual results and close the gap between these when it exists. Any discrepancy, where actual is less than desired, constitutes the *performance improvement zone.*

Performance Management Systems

A performance management system is an integrated approach to achieving the goals and objectives of the organization. A performance management system uses performance improvement concepts and quality improvement methods. There are a number of performance management systems including the Turning Point Model, which was developed specifically for public health departments.

The Turning Point Model

Accreditation standards establish expected levels of performance for health departments, but by themselves, these standards will not assure changes in practice. Successful performance improvement hinges on how effectively performance management is implemented in a health department. In 1999, the RWJF partnered with the W.K. Kellogg Foundation to sponsor a national collaborative of public health practitioners to develop a performance management system for health departments. The collaborative defined performance management as follows:

> The practice of actively using performance data to improve the public's health. This practice involves strategic use of performance measures and standards to establish performance targets and goals, to prioritize and allocate resources, to inform managers about needed adjustments or changes in policy or program directions to meet goals, to frame reports on the success in meeting performance goals, and to improve the quality of public health practice.[34]

The Public Health Performance Management System Framework was originally developed in 2002 and underwent a revision in 2012. The Turning Point Performance Management Model is shown in Figure 16-5 and its five components are defined as follows:[35]

▸ *Visible Leadership* is commitment by senior management staff to ensure that the organization's actions adhere to Performance Management practices of quality improvement. This includes considering routine client, community, and stakeholder feedback, and assuring that there are no barriers to understanding performance between leadership and staff.

▸ *Performance Standards* are objective guidelines used to assess an organization's performance (e.g., one epidemiologist on staff per 100,000 people served). Standards may be set based on

- national, state, or scientific guidelines (e.g., National Public Health Performance Standards Program standards or the Public Health Accreditation Board standards);
- benchmarking against similar organizations (e.g., standards available through the National Association of County and City Health Officials); and
- the expectations of leaders or the public (e.g., 100 percent access for clients).

▸ *Performance Measurement* consists of quantitative measures of capacities, processes, and outcomes relevant to the assessment of a performance indicator.

▸ *Reporting of Progress* is how a public health department tracks and reports performance. These data need to be relevant for users, and a robust progress reporting system makes comparisons to national standards. Progress reporting is important to show where gaps may exist within the system. This information should be systematically shared with relevant stakeholders and the public.

▸ *Quality Improvement* is a defined program to implement quality improvement projects in health departments using continuous cycles based on performance standards, measurements, and reports.

The Turning Point Performance Management system is the continuous use of all five components so that they are integrated into the health department operations and programs to provide consistent outcomes. The system constitutes a comprehensive set of accountabilities to monitor the organizational processes and results.

Performance management practices are used four ways: (1) to prioritize and allocate resources; (2) to inform managers about necessary adjustments or changes in policies or programs; (3) to frame reports on success in meeting performance goals; and (4) to improve the quality of public health practice. The three basic levels of performance management for an organization are the strategic, operational, and personnel levels.

1. Strategic performance management: the process which guides the development of a clear mission, vision, and goals to position the organization to serve the community.

2. Operations performance management: all the activities within an organization to achieve objectives (based on clear, measurable steps) to attain these goals.

3. Personnel performance management: the systems to recruit, orient, train, motivate, and evaluate the staff of the organization.

Performance management aligns these three levels so that the mission is clearly understood by all staff. There

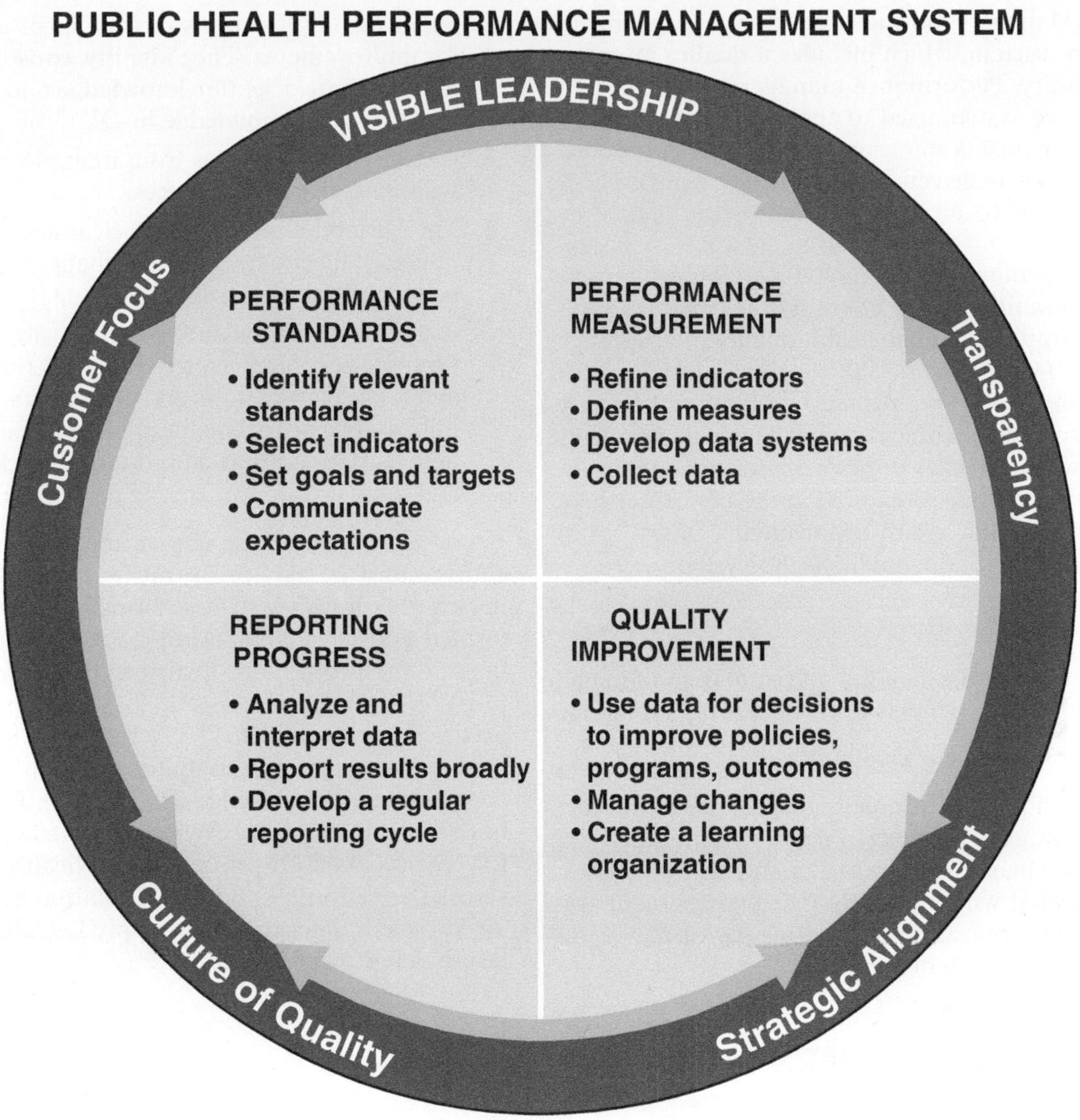

PUBLIC HEALTH PERFORMANCE MANAGEMENT SYSTEM

FIGURE 16-5   The Turning Point Model: A Performance Management System for Public Health[36]
Courtesy of the Public Health Foundation

are five strategies for implementing a performance management system:

1. Work is planned and performance expectations are set. This components applies to all three levels of performance management.

2. Work performance is monitored. Routinely monitoring performance is important to provide positive feedback as well as to intervene early when necessary if standards are not being met.

3. Staff ability to perform is developed and enhanced. Ongoing staff development is important because the work environment is constantly changing and skill sets must continually evolve.

4. Performance is measured and rated. Performance measurement and rating are the basis for formal feedback. Formal and informal feedback are the "breakfast of champions."

5. Top performance is recognized. There are financial and nonfinancial methods to reward top performance. It is difficult to provide financial rewards in a public health department because it is a governmental agency; however, there are numerous nonfinancial means to recognize top performance.

To summarize, traditional management approaches, by themselves, are poorly equipped to help managers create an environment for achieving performance excellence. Managers must also develop a performance management system, which includes a quality improvement capability. Performance management refers to a comprehensive system used to achieve sustained excellence in an organization. A successful performance management system is driven by community health needs and is designed to align closely with the health department vision, mission, and strategic goals. A performance management system includes a comprehensive set of accountabilities, and monitors the organization's processes. Improving public health quality metrics, such as those in *Healthy People 2020* or the nine aims for public health quality established by HHS, will be very difficult to accomplish unless public health departments develop new approaches to performance management. A fundamental change is required in the performance of governmental public health departments, as well as in their interaction with the public health system.

Value Proposition

The value proposition is a key performance management concept and is defined by the following equation:

$$Value = Quality/Cost$$

This relationship links the quality of a service to the cost of a service. Value is maximized for the community and stakeholders when quality increases and cost decreases. When integrated with a performance management system, the value proposition helps drive performance improvement for a health department.

QUALITY IMPROVEMENT COLLABORATIVE

Quality improvement projects can be conducted one at a time, or a number of them can be undertaken simultaneously. A Quality Improvement Collaborative (QIC) consists of numerous teams from one or more organizations cooperating to undertake QI projects using QI methods and techniques to close a performance gap. The QIC is considered one of the most important and well-used approaches by the health system to improve performance.[36,37] A collaborative brings together groups of practitioners from different health departments (or within one health department) to improve one aspect of the quality of their service. It involves teams in a series of meetings to learn best practices from faculty knowledgeable about the content problem as well as from quality improvement experts. A QIC is typically a short-term (3–6 months) undertaking that involves five features[38]:

1. A specified topic for which there is wide variation in performance or gaps between best and current practice.

2. Clinical and QI experts provide ideas and support for improvements. They identify, consolidate, clarify, and share scientific knowledge and best practice as well as knowledge in QI.

3. Interdisciplinary teams from multiple projects are willing to share experiences.

4. The QI model is used to set clear and measurable targets, collect data, and test changes on a small scale to advance learning by doing.

5. A series of structured activities (typically three two-day Learning Session meetings, Actions Periods to test and implement changes and collect data, conference calls, and an active email list) is completed in a given time frame to advance improvement, exchange ideas, and share experiences among participating teams.

The QIC is a powerful way to motivate and support change and is becoming more common in public health.[39] A number of collaboratives have been performed and have yielded impressive results. Examples include the Multi-State Learning Collaborative Series (a RWJF-sponsored series of three collaboratives that occurred between 2005–2011 for 17 states to develop quality improvement capabilities in their public health departments);[40] Public Health Practice: Evaluating the Impact of Quality Improvement (implementation of 32 RWJF-sponsored QI projects by 13 health departments across the nation);[41] and a 2013 kaizen event program for 10 health departments to apply Lean techniques for health department processes.[42]

SUMMARY

Managing performance and strengthening accountability are two prevailing themes confronting public health departments as expectations continue to rise and resources tighten. The increased demand placed on public health departments to perform better and improve health outcomes with less funding cannot be achieved under the design and operation of the current system.[43] Health departments are capable of achieving sustained performance excellence through the delivery of enhanced value to clients, the community, and stakeholders. Performance management systems and public health accreditation provide frameworks to help a public health organization align its resources to improve productivity and effectiveness.

REVIEW QUESTIONS

1. What is the purpose of the National Public Health Performance Standards Program?

2. What is the current state of public health quality in the United States? What methods have been applied to raise quality in health care?

3. How is the PDSA cycle useful in improving quality health care?

4. Explain how the five components of the Turning Point Model work together to improve performance management.

5. Why is a quality improvement collaborative important to improve performance of a health system?

REFERENCES

1. Institute of Medicine. *The Future of Public Health*. Washington, DC: National Academy Press; 1988.

2. Institute of Medicine. *The Future of the Public's Health in the 21st Century*. Washington, DC: National Academy Press; 2002.

3. Bender K, Halverson PK. Quality improvement and accreditation: what might it look like? *Journal of Public Health Management and Practice*. 2010;16(1):79–82.

4. Halverson PK, Nicola RM, Baker EL. Performance measurement and accreditation of public health organizations: a call to action. *J Public Health Manage Pract*. 1998;4(4):5–7.

5. Baker EL, Melton RJ, Stange PV, et al. Health reform and the health of the public. Forging community health partnerships. *JAMA*. 1994;272(16): 1276–1282.

6. U.S. Department of Health and Human Services. *Healthy People 2010: Conference Edition*. Washington, DC: U.S. Dept of Health and Human Services; 2000.

7. National Association of County and City Health Officials. *National Public Health Performance Standards Program: Local Public Health System Performance Assessment Instrument, Version 3*. 2013.

8. Public Health Quality. U.S. Department of Health and Human Services Web Site. http://www.hhs.gov/ash/initiatives/quality/quality/. Accessed October 24, 2014.

9. Frieden TR. Six components necessary for effective public health program implementation. *Am J Public Health*. 2013;e1–e6. doi: 10.2105/AJPH.2013.301608.

10. Healthy People 2020 Leading Health Indicators: Progress Update. Healthy People 2020 Web Site. https://www.healthypeople.gov/2020/leading-health-indicators/Healthy-People-2020-Leading-Health-Indicators%3A-Progress-Update. Published March 2014. Accessed October 24, 2014.

11. Healthcare Effectiveness Data and Information Set (HEDIS) 2013. National Committee for Quality Assurance Web Site. http://www.ncqa.org/ReportCards/HealthPlans/StateofHealthCare Quality.aspx. Accessed October 24, 2014.

12. The State of Health Care Quality: Reform, The Quality Agenda and Resource Use. *The National Committee for Quality Assurance*. 2010.

13. Riley W, Moran J, Corso L, Beitsch L, Bialek R, Cofsky A. Defining quality improvement in public health. *Journal of Public Health Management and Practice*. 2010;16(1):5–7.

14. Parsons H, Riley W. Public health program design and deployment. In: Bialek R, Duffy G, Moran J, eds. *On the Cutting Edge of Quality and Innovation: A Public Health Handbook*. Milwaukee, WI: Quality Press; 2009: 53–60.

15. Taylor MJ, McNicholas C, Nicolay C, Darzi A, Bell D, Reed JE. Systematic review of the application of the plan-do-study-act method to improve quality in healthcare. *BMJ Qual Saf*. 2013;0:1–9.

16. Deming WE. *Out of the Crisis*. Cambridge, MA: MIT; 1991.

17. Juran JM. *Juran on Planning for Quality*. New York: The Free Press; 1988.

18. Ohno T. *Toyota Production System: Beyond Large-Scale Production*. Portland, OR: Productivity Press; 1988.

19. Motorola Lean Six Sigma. Motorola Solutions Web Site. http://www.motorolasolutions.com/US-EN/Training+Home/Lean+Six+Sigma. Accessed October 24, 2014.

20. A Brief History of Lean. Lean Enterprise Institute Web Site. http://www.lean.org/WhatsLean/History.cfm. Accessed October 24, 2014.

21. About the Baldridge Criteria for Performance Excellence. Baldridge Performance Excellence rogram Web Site. http://www.nist.gov/baldrige/publications/bus_about.cfm. Updated December 14, 2013. Accessed October 24, 2014.

22. Berwick DM. Continuous improvement as an ideal in health care. *N Engl J Med*. 1989;320:53–56.

23. Lighter DE, Fair DC. *Quality Management in Health Care: Principles and Methods*. Sudbury, MA: Jones and Bartlett Publishers; 2004.

24. National Association of County and City Health Officials. 2013 National Profile of Local Health Departments. Washington, DC. January 2014.

25. Association of State and Territorial Health Officials. ASTHO Profile of State Public Health Volume 3. 2014. http://www.astho.org/Profile/Volume-Three/. Accessed December 15, 2014.

26. Cretin S, Shortell SM, Keller EB. An evaluation of collaborative interventions to improve chronic illness care: framework and study design. *Eval Rev.* 2004;28:28–51.

27. Moran J. Quality Improvement Methods & Tools. NPHII Grantee Meeting. Public Health Foundation Website. http://www.cdc.gov/stltpublichealth/nphii/nphiimeeting/meetingdocs/qualityimprovement/QIMethods_JMoran_2011.pdf. Published March 30, 2011. Accessed November 4, 2014.

28. Institute for Healthcare Improvement Website. http://www.ihi.org. Accessed November 4, 2014.

29. Kheraj R, Tewani SK, Ketwaroo G, Leffler DA. Quality improvement in gastroenterology clinical practice. *Clinical Gastroenterology and Hepatology.* 2012;10(12):1305–1314.

30. About PHAB. Public Health Accreditation Board Web Site. http://www.phaboard.org/about-phab/. Accessed October 24, 2014.

31. The Public Health System and the 10 Essential Public Health Services. Centers for Disease Control and Prevention Web Site. http://www.cdc.gov/nphpsp/essentialservices.html. Accessed December 15, 2014.

32. Exploring Accreditation Steering Committee. Exploring accreditation: Final recommendations for a voluntary national accreditation program for state and local public health departments. National Association of County and City Health Officials. Winter 2006–2007.

33. Public Health Accreditation Board. Standards & Measures, Version 1.5. Alexandria, VA: PHAB; 2013.

34. Public Health Foundation. *From Silos to Systems: Using Performance Management to Improve Public Health.* Seattle, WA: Turning Point National Program Office at the University of Washington; 2002.

35. About the Performance Management System Framework. Public Health Foundation Web Site. http://www.phf.org/focusareas/performancemanagement/toolkit/Pages/PM_Toolkit_About_the_Performance_Management_Framework.aspx. Accessed October 24, 2014.

36. Mittman BS. Creating the evidence base for quality improvement collaboratives. *Ann Intern Med.* 2004;140:897–901.

37. Lindenauer PK. Effects of quality improvement collaboratives. *BMJ.* 2008;336(7659):1448–1449.

38. Simon LP. Expanding the quality improvement collaborative approach to improving quality of care and services for frail elders and children living in communities of poverty in western and central New York. *Community Health Foundation of Western and Central New York.* 2009.

39. Leape LL, Rogers G, Hanna D, et al. Developing and implementing new safe practices: voluntary adoption through statewide collaborative. *Qual Saf Health Care.* 2006;15:289–295.

40. The Multi-State Learning Collaborative: Lead States in Public Health Quality Improvement. National Network of Public Health Institutes Web Site. http://nnphi.org/CMSuploads/MLC_10-2-2013.pdf. Accessed November 5, 2014.

41. Executive Summary. Public Health Practice: Evaluating the Impact of Quality Improvement. Robert Wood Johnson Foundation Web Site. http://www.rwjf.org/content/dam/farm/reports/program_results_reports/2013/rwjf407971/subassets/rwjf407971_1. Published September 30, 2013. Accessed November 5, 2014.

42. Kaizen. National Network of Public Health Institutes Web Site. http://nnphi.org/program-areas/accreditation-and-performance-improvement/kaizen. Accessed November 5, 2014.

43. Riley WJ, Parsons HM, Duffy GL, Moran JW, Henry B. Realizing transformational change through quality improvement in public health. *Journal of Public Health Management & Practice.* 2010;16(1):72–78.

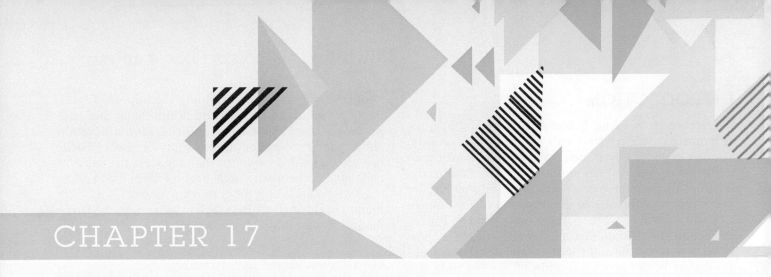

CHAPTER 17

Public Health Services and Systems Research

F. Douglas Scutchfield, MD • Richard C. Ingram, DrPH

LEARNING OBJECTIVES

Upon completion of this chapter, the reader will be able to:

1. Discuss the history of the development of Public Health Services and Systems Research (PHSSR) including the role of the National Public Health Practice Program Office of the Centers for Disease Control and Prevention (CDC).

2. Describe the effect of the Institute of Medicine's 1988 and 2003 reports on the Future of Public Health on PHSSR.

3. Compare and contrast the CDC PHSSR research agenda in 2006 and the PHSSR National Coordinating Center's 2012 research agenda for PHSSR, with a focus on work achieved to address the 2012 research agenda for PHSSR.

4. Describe the role of the Robert Wood Johnson Foundation in enhancing the field of PHSSR.

5. Identify key research areas in public health finance, public health systems organization and structure, public health workforce, and information and technology.

6. Discuss the role of data sources in PHSSR, focusing on the National Association of County and City Health Officials (NACCHO) and Association of State and Territorial Health Officials (ASTHO) Profiles, and the National Longitudinal Survey of Public Health Systems.

7. Discuss the future of PHSSR in the following areas: health care reform, practice-based research in public health, public health accreditation, public health law research, and public health foundational services funding.

KEY TERMS

foundational public health services
practice-based research networks (PBRNs)
public health finance
public health governance
public health services and systems research (PHSSR)
public health system
quality improvement (QI)

INTRODUCTION

Public health is being buffeted by forces that both enhance its potential as well as put it at jeopardy. Efforts to control government spending, combined with a distrust of government and a continued slow recovery from the economic downturn of the late 2000s, are forces that have threatened the provision of governmental public health services.[1,2] At the same time the Patient Protection and Affordable Care Act of 2010 (ACA) provided new resources and specific mandates that encourage public health and prevention.[3–5] For example, the Prevention and Public Health Fund, created and funded by ACA, has provided new resources to governmental public health functions. These events call for a renewed examination of public health programs, activities, and linkages. A potential approach for that effort is the use of science, specifically health services research methodologies, to assist public health practice as it moves into this new era; this discipline is known as public health services and systems research (PHSSR).

Public health services and systems research has been defined as "a field of study that examines the organization, finance, and delivery of public health services in communities, and the impact of these services on public health."[6] It is a multidisciplinary field, and draws on such diverse disciplines as law, geography, and communications, to examine questions related to variations in public health systems characteristics, and the impact of this variation on a number of outcomes, including community health. While PHSSR draws from a spectrum of disciplines, all types of PHSSR have one thing in common: a focus on the public health system, the collection of public and private entities that exist to deliver public health services in communities. Much of PHSSR is focused on providing the public health practice community with an evidence base from which to make informed administrative decisions, by investigating questions related to its three broad areas: finance, system organization and structure, and the public health workforce, and how these impact the delivery of public health services (as opposed to the effectiveness or efficacy of the services themselves). Recognition of PHSSR as a formal research discipline is a fairly recent phenomenon, dating to the early 2000s.

HISTORICAL DEVELOPMENT OF PHSSR

While PHSSR has origins that trace to the early part of the twentieth century, its emergence as a distinct and separate field is fairly recent. It has already distinguished itself by research that has informed practice and policy. PHSSR researchers have produced some of the strongest work to date examining the impact of funding of public health services and health status, and have provided strong evidence supporting efforts to retain and expand funding for public health services.[7] PHSSR has also provided evidence that supports the value of collaboration between public health system members to improve public health programming, practice, and community health status.[8] PHSSR has its roots in the larger discipline of health services research.

Health Services Research

Health services research (HSR) is an area of inquiry that utilizes many disciplines to investigate the impact of variations in financial inputs, health care system and organizational makeup and processes, and the social determinants of health on the quality and cost of care, access to care, and health outcomes.[9] It is distinct from PHSSR in that it is focused on the health *care* system (as opposed to the public health system). Health services research has a relatively long history, and has provided opportunities to undertake research which can and will inform policy in the areas of access, cost, quality, and the health of the population. Recent public policy developments, including the focus on coordinated, efficient, and effective care embodied by aspects of the ACA such as the establishment of the Center for Medicare and Medicaid Innovation, have provided a new and exciting opportunity for health services research to make major contributions to the policy discussions surrounding implementation of health care reform. However, these developments and attendant rapid cycle experimentation in health care delivery have also created new opportunities for the application of health services research techniques to public health, and suggest that PHSSR can play an active and important part in efforts to improve health and health care.

The Emergence of PHSSR as a Research Discipline

While the recognition of PHSSR is a fairly recent phenomenon, attempts to describe the public health system have historical roots that extend to the early twentieth century. From the 1920s to the late 1940s, the American Public Health Association (APHA) fielded a series of surveys that collected data on public health agency capacity and service delivery in the United States.[10] The APHA used these surveys to establish standards for staffing and activities of public health agencies, and published a series of reports detailing the characteristics of public health agencies in the United States. Perhaps the most notable illustration of this effort was the release by the APHA Committee on Municipal Health Department Practice, in 1948, of the so-called "Emerson

Report" that established the six essential services that all health departments should provide.[11] Unfortunately, the Emerson Report marked the apex of research on public health agency capacity for a great deal of the remainder of the twentieth century.

The 1950s till the late 1980s was an era where traditional public health practice had minimal attention as the public health and medical care establishment turned its attention to expanding financial access to medical care. This shift was influenced and accelerated by the passage of Medicare and Medicaid legislation, and the founding and development of the community health centers that began to provide medical services in rural and inner-city underserved communities. While these were important and necessary accomplishments, public health practice suffered as a result and was left without a traditional champion for its efforts. While there were notable exceptions, this period represented a low point in efforts to examine and use research findings to improve public health services provision.

The 1988 IOM Report on the Future of Public Health

This changed with a pivotal event in public health, the publication in 1988 of the Institute of Medicine report, *The Future of Public Health*.[12] This landmark report pointed out that public health was in disarray, suffered from a lack of focus and resources, and was in desperate need of attention if it was to fulfill its potential. The report went on to establish a public health mission statement, "creating conditions in which people can be healthy." The report focused on the governmental public health system at the federal, state, and local level; however, it also pointed out that many organizations and agencies shared this mission, from not-for-profit organizations to academia, and business. It described this broader constellation of actors, who shared this mission in public health, as the *public health system*. It drew the distinction between governmental public health entities and their responsibility, as opposed to the broader public health system, which included these other actors. Focusing on governmental public health, the report described a set of three core functions: assessment, policy development, and assurance.

During the 1990s the Clinton administration, in its efforts to pass a national health plan, prompted the further elaboration of the three core functions into the familiar 10 Essential Public Health Services.[13] Much current public health practice and research are based on these 10 Essential Public Health Services.

The development of a clearly defined mission for public health, and specific activities public health agencies were to provide (the core functions and 10 Essential Public Health Services), led to other critical

developments that supported the growth of PHSSR. A number of those activities were intended to both measure and improve the provision of public health services across the United States. Many of those activities contributed to a reemergence of the critical examination and recommendations about public health practice that had characterized the earlier part of the twentieth century in public health. For example, two major public health professional organizations, the National Association of County and City Health Officials (NACCHO) and the Association of State and Territorial Health Officials (ASTHO), began fielding surveys examining the makeup of local and state public health agencies, in some ways similar to the previously discussed APHA efforts in the early-to-mid-twentieth century. In addition, NACCHO developed tools for local health departments to use to ascertain their capacity to undertake the 10 Essential Public Health Services and assist in community health assessment, such as the Assessment Protocol for Excellence in Public Health (APEX-PH).[14] These early efforts led to more sophisticated and useful tools for public health practice.

Federal Engagement and Leadership in PHSSR

It was also during that period that several federal government efforts occurred in response to the call of the IOM's 1988 report. First, the U.S. Centers for Disease Control and Prevention (CDC) created the Public Health Practice Program Office (PHPPO), designed as a liaison between CDC and state and local health departments to assist them in developing their infrastructure and capacity. Early efforts, supported by CDC, in partnership with the Association of Schools of Public Health (ASPH) focused on measuring performance of the three Core Functions of Public Health by local health departments, and resulted in a set of 20 questions, called the Miller-Turnock 20 (after the researchers who led the teams that developed the instruments).[15] This instrument was designed to measure the performance of local health departments in providing the 10 Essential Public Health Services. The Public Health Practice Program Office also established the National Public Health Performance Standards Program (NPHPSP), designed to assist the local and state public health systems (as opposed to departments) and local governance organizations in assessing their performance of the 10 Essential Public Health Services. The instruments that were developed, in partnership with several national organizations, focused on the measurement of public health systems performance at the state and local levels, as well as the governance structures (e.g., boards of health) supporting public health practice. The use of these instruments allowed researchers, supported by

PHPPO, to examine the performance of public health systems, and related areas such as the determinants and characteristics associated with performance.[16]

The Public Health Practice Program Office also undertook additional efforts to enhance PHSSR; for example, in the early 2000s, they began working with AcademyHealth, an organization of health services researchers, to create a venue that would stimulate, showcase, and help promote PHSSR (known at the time as PHSR, or public health systems research). These efforts led to the creation of AcademyHealth's Public Health Systems Research Interest Group, one of a number of topical interest groups supported by AcademyHealth. Initially, CDC funding supported an interest group meeting, held in conjunction with AcademyHealth's Annual Research Meeting, which provided credibility and visibility in the HSR community for PHSSR. The Interest Group has served PHSSR well and allowed those engaging in PHSSR an opportunity to network, and has given them a venue for research presentations and exchanges. It has also provided additional educational opportunities to assist PHSSR researchers. The Interest Group has also taken on the role of acting as a bridge between the policy and PHSSR communities, facilitating a dialog between research and policy at the national level.

Preparedness for Man-made and Natural Disasters

At the same time PHPPO was working to increase the visibility of PHSSR, unforeseen events were about to unfold that would increase the visibility of public health in the United States, and demonstrate the need for a high-performing public health system. The terrorist attacks on the United States in 2001, along with the anthrax scare that shortly followed, provided a demonstration that the U.S. public health system had been allowed to deteriorate to a degree that hampered its response to acts of mass destruction and bioterrorism. While the anthrax scare prompted some action, and highlighted how ill prepared the U.S. public health system was to respond to bioterrorism, in 2005 the lack of preparedness was again highlighted by a disaster, this time Hurricane Katrina, which ravaged the southern United States, particularly the city of New Orleans, Louisiana. Both episodes demonstrated that public health did not have the resources to respond to natural and man-made disasters, and there was a substantial infusion of new funding provided to public health to address both natural and man-made disaster preparedness.[17,18] As the PHSSR community had gained some credence and visibility, some of this funding was focused on PHSSR, specifically examining the issues of preparedness and how best to allocate resources to meet the threat of disasters.[18]

The Future of the Public's Health in the Twenty-First Century

In the time period between the anthrax scare and Hurricane Katrina, public health had greater visibility, and the IOM again turned its attention to the U.S. public health system. The result, released in 2003, was another report on public health, *The Future of the Public's Health in the 21st Century*.[19] This report was, in some measure, a follow-up to the 1988 IOM report. However, as the 1988 IOM report primarily focused on governmental public health, this report focused primarily on the broader public health system and examined the role that various members of that public health system, from business, to media, to the academy, might play in the mission of public health and their role in working to improve the nation's health. It issued recommendations focused on how other members of the public health system could contribute to the success of public health mission achievement.

The 2003 report also had several recommendations and observations that were key to the continued development of PHSSR. Perhaps one of the most telling comments pointed to the lack of evidence on which to base decisions regarding public health infrastructure, and the delivery of public health services. The report states:

> Research is needed to guide policy decisions that shape public health practice. The committee had hoped to provide specific guidance elaborating on the types and levels of workforce, infrastructure, related resources, and financial investments necessary to ensure the availability of essential public health services to all of the nation's communities. However, such evidence is limited and there is no agenda or support for this type of research, despite the critical need for such data to promote and protect the public's health.[19]

This recommendation was telling and promoted subsequent action in a variety of quarters. The 2003 IOM report also called for the creation of a research agenda that would focus on research to support evidence-based policy making for public health practice. In 2003, the CDC, through PHPPO, led efforts to create that agenda. PHPPO engaged a broad variety of stakeholders, including public health practice organizations, public health researchers, and nonprofit organizations, and other organizations to examine research needs for a broad variety of topics, and to identify a list of research priorities.[20] These priorities focused on four broad areas: public health agency and system structure, public health finance, public health agency and system performance, and quality improvement in public health. While the agenda was broad in scope and ambitious, it lacked depth in the form of specific research questions for each priority. Table 17-1 lists the research priorities developed to guide the early stages of PHSSR and to set priorities for the small body of those engaged in PHSSR.[20]

TABLE 17-1   Research Priorities for the Public Health Systems Research Agenda

1. Determine how public health agency structure affects performance.

2. Define and quantify dimensions of public health systems, including interorganizational relationships (including the role of the agency within the public health system).

3. Explore the relationship between performance and health outcomes (and the chain of impacts that leads from improved performance to improved health outcomes).

4. Define the characteristics of high-performing local, state, and federal public health agencies.

5. Explore the relationship between social determinants of health and system performance.

6. Evaluate the costs of achieving and maintaining acceptable/optimal levels of performance. (This activity includes exploring reasonable models to collect agency financial data.)

7. Explore the relationship between public health infrastructure/performance and the design, implementation, and impact/outcomes of categorical programs (including the use of evidence-based interventions).

8. Conceptualize a framework for high-performing public health systems that includes key elements.

9. Identify, develop, and refine measures of health outcomes that are sensitive to public health systems capacity and performance.

10. Explore models and outcomes of accreditation of public health agencies and/or public health systems as performance improvement methods.

11. Evaluate how shifting policy and financial priorities affect performance of public health systems.

12. Explore what factors and processes facilitate community involvement in using the National Public Health Performance Standards Program in system improvement activities (quality improvement).

13. Evaluate how and to what extent a high-performing public health system is indicative of preparedness.

14. Explore the effectiveness (within the agency and the system) of local and state governance structures.

Adapted from Lenaway et al[20]

Some areas of the agenda received a relatively large amount of attention from the research community. For example, a study examining the feasibility of an accrediting body for public health eventually led to the creation of the Public Health Accreditation Board, a national voluntary nongovernmental body that is responsible for accreditation of local, state, and tribal health departments, and now has created an accreditation-specific research agenda.[21] Other areas have had less attention, in spite of their inclusion on an agenda generated nearly 10 years ago. For example, knowledge of the nature and character of **public health governance** remains, at best, minimal.[22,23] Moreover, many of these research agenda items have reemerged both in a subsequent iteration of the research agenda for PHSSR (see below) and as major items that have prompted substantial PHSSR investment, such as the issue of preparedness.

Engagement of the Robert Wood Johnson Foundation

The early 2000s also saw the initial engagement of the Robert Wood Johnson Foundation (RWJF) in PHSSR, with the hope and anticipation that their efforts would help move the PHSSR field forward and serve as a source of research funding that would be able to drive both practice and policy. The Robert Wood Johnson Foundation has funded a number of activities in the field of PHSSR, including an initial investment that allowed AcademyHealth to continue with its Public Health Systems Research Interest Group. The RWJF added a funding stream for PHSSR through their Health Care Financing and Organization program (the PHSSR arm of which was transferred later to the National Network of Public Health Institutes). The RWJF also began a program, collaboratively with the National Library of Medicine and the University of Kentucky, to develop a site for the listing of databases and PHSSR bibliographic references, which could be used by PHSSR researchers.[24]

The RWJF supported the development of a venue to highlight PHSSR, the Keeneland Conference, an annual conference where individuals who are engaged in PHSSR can present research findings and network with colleagues. The RWJF has also engaged in efforts to create new investigators in the field and provided resources for the funding of pre- and post-doctoral PHSSR awards, as well as mentored scientist research awards, resulting in the development of new investigators who are currently active and have leadership positions in the field of PHSSR.

A NEW PHSSR RESEARCH AGENDA

The lack of progress on key 2006 research agenda items noted earlier (as well as the reorganization of the CDC, leading to the demise of PHPPO) suggested a need for a revised research agenda for PHSSR. In 2010, a consortium of public health researchers, along with staff from RWJF, CDC, and the Altarum Institute, led efforts to create a revised research agenda for PHSSR.[25] This effort was a multistep process, with feedback gathered from multiple stakeholder groups. Systematic reviews of four key areas were commissioned: workforce, quality improvement, organization and structure, and data and methods. These reviews were the basis of a series of stakeholder meetings that yielded a list of key research topics. This list was then vetted with the larger public health research and practice community through a number of venues, and then refined to yield a list of 74 operational research questions. The revised agenda is notable in that, unlike the initial agenda, which contained broader areas of action, it contains specific research questions. Thus, while it may be more proscriptive, it also brings more clarity regarding specific research questions of importance. Table 17-2 contains the broader thematic areas encompassed by the revised research agenda for PHSSR.[25]

TABLE 17-2 Research Agenda for Public Health Services and Systems Research, 2010

The Public Health Workforce

- Enumeration
- Demand, Supply, and Shortages
- Diversity and Disparities
- Recruitment and Retention
- Workforce Competencies
- Educational Methods and Curricula

Public Health System Structure and Performance

- System Boundaries and Size
- Public Health Agency Organization and Governance
- Interorganizational Relationships and Partnerships
- Performance Measurement, Quality Improvement, and Accreditation
- Social Determinants of Health and Health Disparities

Public Health Financing and Economics

- Fiscal Analysis
- Financing Mechanisms
- Costs, Performance, and Outcomes

Public Health Information and Technology

- Capabilities to Assess and Monitor Health Outcomes
- Translation and Dissemination of Research-Tested Public Health Strategies
- Information and Communication Technologies

SOURCE: Consortium from Altarum Institute, Centers for Disease Control and Prevention, Robert Wood Johnson Foundation, National Coordinating Center for Public Health Services and Systems Research

While the revised PHSSR agenda is more comprehensive than its earlier iteration, it is clear when comparing the two that many questions on the original agenda remain. For example, little is still known about the governance of public health agencies, in spite of research that suggests they may play a significant role in the delivery of public health services.[16,23,26–30] Critical questions surrounding the impact of many public health systems characteristics on health outcomes remain. There is a general lack of clarity, for example, on how public health systems may best address health disparities. In spite of the lack of progress on certain key areas, progress has been made in others. For example, there seems to be more clarity regarding the determinants of public health system performance. Basic questions regarding system structure and organization appear to have been addressed, at least superficially.

This revised research agenda and the lack of clarity regarding the impact of the first research agenda led to efforts to track the impact of RWJF-sponsored PHSSR funding to date.[31] Between 2009, when RWJF first began to fund a dedicated PHSSR stream managed by the National Network of Public Health Institutes, through March 2014, RWJF funded 116 PHSSR projects: 8 workforce studies, 56 studies on public health system structure and performance, 34 studies on public health finance and economics, and 18 studies on information and technology. Table 17-3 contains the number of studies funded in specific subareas, from workforce enumeration to translation and dissemination of research.[31]

The examination of RWJF PHSSR projects funded from 2009–2014 also suggests certain areas of PHSSR have garnered the attention of a relatively large number of researchers, while other areas have enjoyed far less attention. As was the case after the first research agenda was developed in 2003, system structure and performance still command the largest share of attention from those engaging in PHSSR. Performance measurement, QI, and accreditation have been relatively well studied, perhaps a result of the launching of a voluntary national accreditation program for public health agencies by the Public Health Accreditation Board. Workforce research, an area of PHSSR that had received relatively little attention after the first agenda, has still spawned very little PHSSR. While data and information deficits were noted in the systematic review commissioned in 2010, there still appear to be relatively few studies that are addressing gaps in data and technology. Finance and economic-related issues have continued to stimulate much research, particularly in the areas of cost, performance, and outcomes. While PHSSR has examined a broad array of topics, current research emphasis is focused on four key, overarching areas: Finance; Structure and Organization; Workforce; and Data, Information, and Technology, described in more detail below.

TABLE 17-3   Content of Robert Wood Johnson Foundation-Sponsored Public Health Services and Systems Research, 2009–2014

Area
Public Health Workforce
Enumeration (1 study)
Diversity/disparities (2 studies)
Recruitment/retention (2 studies)
Workforce competencies (3 studies)
Public Health System Structure and Performance
System boundaries/size (1 study)
Organization/governance (8 studies)
Interorganizational relationships/partnerships (12 studies)
Performance measurement/QI/accreditation (27 studies)
Social determinants of health/health disparities (8 studies)
Public Health Finance and Economics
Fiscal analysis (4 studies)
Finance mechanisms (10 studies)
Costs/performance/outcomes (20 studies)
Information and Technology
Assess/monitor health outcomes (3 studies)
Translate/disseminate research tested strategies (1 study)
Information/communications technology (14 studies)

SOURCE: University of Kentucky, Lexington KY: National Coordinating Center for Public Health Services and Systems Research

Finance in PHSSR

Finance-related PHSSR seeks to provide the public health practice community with an evidence base to allow them to best allocate their resources to meet community health needs, and thus operate in the most efficient manner possible. **Public health finance** research has a long history, dating back to the early 1950s.[32] However, the advent of PHSSR as a field of inquiry saw a concurrent rise in the number of published research studies examining issues related to public health finance. This increased attention to finance was also stimulated by the decreased funding allocated to governmental public health agencies, particularly after the global financial collapse of the late 2000s, and simultaneous calls for increased government accountability. While public health finance research examines a broad array of issues, much focuses on three major domains:[32]

- What is the relationship between public health funding and the delivery of public health services, and public health agency and system performance? What are the costs of various health services provided?

- How do variations in public health funding and public health agency spending impact health outcomes? How does public health spending influence medical care utilization and spending?

- What methodological tools and analytic techniques can be applied to public health finance-related research questions that will allow researchers to answer the questions in the two domains above?

System Organization and Structure in PHSSR

Public Health Services and Systems Research focused on system organization and structure seeks to identify the optimal system and agency makeup that will facilitate the efficient and effective delivery of public health services. While efforts to examine the structure and organization of the U.S. public health system stretch at least as far back as the 1920s, most of the research focused on the organization and structure of the U.S. system dates from the early 2000s onward. The post 9/11 resurgence of interest in the public health system, as well as calls for increased accountability may have contributed to the initial resurgence of interest in preparedness. Similar to finance research, other contemporary events such as continuing economic challenges may have fed interest in this area. Structure and organization-related PHSSR examines a diverse set of issues, but the majority of research studies has focused on four broad questions:[33]

- How are governmental public health agencies and larger public health systems structured and organized?

- How do variations in public health system or agency structure, including partnerships and cross disciplinary and jurisdictional sharing of resources, impact the delivery of public health services?

- What is the relationship between variations in public health system or agency structure and community health outcomes?

- How do activities related to quality improvement, performance measurement, and accreditation impact departmental performance and community health?

The Public Health Workforce

Workforce-related PHSSR seeks to determine the optimal makeup, both in size and composition, of the U.S. public health workforce. Research on the public health workforce dates to at least 1923 when the U.S. Public Health Service (USPHS) attempted to enumerate the public health workforce of the 100 largest U.S. cities.[34] The USPHS not only collected data, but also used the data to recommend staffing levels for public health departments—an early example of attempts to build the evidence base regarding optimal workforce characteristics. Research on the workforce lagged until the early 2000s, with the release of Dr. Kristine Gebbie's seminal report *The Public Health Workforce: Enumeration 2000*, which used a variety of data sources to estimate the size and scope of the U.S. public health workforce.[34] The release of *Enumeration 2000*, along with the advent of PHSSR as a recognized research endeavor, seemed to accelerate the pace of research on the public health workforce. The financial strains of the late 2000s no doubt contributed to this, as public health agencies that faced the prospect of paring down their workforce looked for evidence to guide their decisions about the character of those areas where they might successfully decrease their workforce without damaging their productivity. Workforce-related PHSSR is as diverse as the public health workforce, but much research to date has addressed four overarching questions[35]:

▸ What is the racial and ethnic makeup of the U.S. public health workforce, and how do variations in these characteristics impact the delivery of effective public health services?
▸ What effective recruitment and retention strategies can public health agencies use to maintain an effective workforce, and what challenges will public health agencies face related to separation and retirement of workers?
▸ What educational, training, and credentialing opportunities are necessary to assure a competent public health workforce, and how do variations in these areas impact service delivery?
▸ How satisfied are public health workers with their jobs, and how do variations in pay and promotion impact their performance and service delivery as a whole?

Data, Information, and Technology in PHSSR

Public health, as with any other health-related endeavor, has entered the Information Age. Early surveys from NACCHO asked very simple questions such as, "Does the health department have a computer or a fax machine?" The growth and development of information technology, particularly in the health sector, with the financial incentives for the medical care system to adopt electronic health records (EHRs) and so-called meaningful use to achieve financial rewards or penalties, has resulted in a major new capacity in the health care system. The development of data "warehouses" and routine disease registries as well as interoperability of new information systems have substantial implications

for the health department of the future. The future health department in some cases has been characterized as the health information hub, being a central resource for data collection, analysis, and dissemination.[36] Moreover, the notion of "Big Data to Knowledge" has become a major interest of the National Institutes of Health. Vital statistics and data management, part of the assessment function of the health department, has been a key issue since the 1988 IOM report; however, the area of data and technology has not received the attention in the research community that other areas of PHSSR have received. The major questions related to data and information that have been explored in PHSSR include:

▸ What information and communications technologies, particularly disease registries and data linkage methods, can be used to develop databases for assessment, analysis, and dissemination?
▸ What analytical techniques can best allow the use of information and data to assess health outcomes?
▸ What translation and dissemination strategies have been demonstrated to be successful in public health?

DATA USED TO CONDUCT PHSSR

A key concern in PHSSR is the availability of data to use for research.[24] As with other research endeavors, primary data collection is expensive and requires a substantial investment of time on the part of the research team, thus secondary data analysis is a key method in PHSSR. While the medical care system has claims data that can be used for research, a comparable data source does not exist for PHSSR. Moreover, the accounting systems and varieties of financial data reporting used by various state and local health departments are not uniform with a standard set of definitions, which presents difficulties when trying to compare different health departments in terms of financial or service data. This is also true of programmatic data and definitions as well. However, there is movement in the direction of standardization, such as a uniform chart of accounts that may facilitate financial and economic analysis.[32,37]

The NACCHO and ASTHO Profiles

Much of the data used to conduct PHSSR focused on governmental public health agency finance, structure, and workforce comes from the two major public health practice organizations, ASTHO and NACCHO. ASTHO and NACCHO both collect data on state (ASTHO) and local (NACCHO) public health agencies through their respective *Profile* surveys. NACCHO's *National Profile of Local Public Health Departments* provides data on local public health agency capacity and makeup, including areas such as workforce size and composition, the services delivered by local public health agencies and their partners, and agency financial data such as income and expenditures. NACCHO Profile data are collected using a survey sent to all identified local public health departments, totaling over 2,500 agencies. While NACCHO collected Profile data somewhat sporadically during the 1990s and early 2000s, since 2005 Profile data have been collected in 2–3 year increments.

ASTHO's *Profile of State Public Health* provides data on the characteristics and capacities of state public health agencies. Many questions on the ASTHO Profile are similar to those in NACCHO's survey instrument, and examine the workforce, services provided by the agency, and financial data. ASTHO Profile data are collected using a survey sent to all state and territorial public health agencies. ASTHO has collected Profile data in three-year increments since 2007. Other data on state health agencies were collected by the Public Health Foundation during the 1970s and 1980s,[38] but these data are largely unavailable.

While the ASTHO and NACCHO Profiles are of much utility to researchers, their use does pose some challenges. Neither of the Profiles has undergone reliability testing, providing some uncertainty regarding the quality of the data collected. In addition, questions are sometimes modified, changed, or dropped over the span of multiple surveys, presenting challenges to researchers attempting to use the profiles for longitudinal analysis. In spite of these limitations, the profiles have provided robust datasets for researchers, and can be made even more powerful when their data are combined with other datasets used in PHSSR.

Commonly Used Types/Examples of Data Collected by the Federal Government

The U.S. government maintains a number of datasets of interest to those engaging in PHSSR, particularly related to the financial and demographic characteristics of communities and the larger public health workforce. The recently discontinued Consolidated Federal Funds Report (CFFR) contained data on federal allocations to state and local governments, allowing researchers to track the flow of federal funds into state and local public health systems. The Area Resource File contains county-level data on health care resources, including physician types and demographics, hospital and health care facility size and usage, and community demographic characteristics, economic data, and data related to the environment. The U.S. Census and associated surveys provide a rich source of information on a diverse set of areas from community demographic characteristics

such as racial and ethnic makeup, to employment, home ownership, and disability. The U.S. Bureau of Labor Statistics collects data related to employment, and such data were used in Dr. Gebbie's attempt to enumerate the public health workforce, the first large-scale attempt in the twentieth century.[34]

Data on Performance

Contemporary data on public health system performance is limited. While the CDC supported the collection of two rounds of performance data using versions 1 and 2 of the NPHPSP, as of April 2015, NACCHO and ASTHO manage the Version 3 Score Sheets and Reports (released in summer 2013).[39] Other data on public health systems performance have been collected by researchers using the Miller-Turnock instrument. The instrument was not widely used outside of the Miller-Turnock research teams; however, a modified version of the instrument is used in another rich source of PHSSR data, the National Longitudinal Survey of Public Health Systems (NLSPHS).[40,41]

The National Longitudinal Survey of Public Health Systems

The NLSPHS is the only regularly collected source of longitudinal data on public health system makeup, the effectiveness of public health services delivered, and distribution of effort among public health system partners. The NLSPHS uses a modified version of Miller and Turnock's 20 questions on performance related to the three core functions, but also the delivery of services and the distribution of public health system effort in the activities examined. It is unique in that it provides data on the contribution of effort from specific members of the public health system (e.g., hospitals) to public health services in a community. While the NLSPHS is a rich source of data, it is limited, however, in that it only includes local public health systems that serve over 100,000 people. Three rounds of the NLSPHS have been collected, in 1998, 2006, and 2012.[40]

PRACTICE-BASED RESEARCH IN PUBLIC HEALTH

In addition to heavy investments in PHSSR, RWJF has also invested in a related research enterprise, the use of public health practice-based research networks (PBRNs). Public health PBRNs, initiated with five networks in 2008 and now expanded to cover 28 states with over a thousand state and local health departments included, are comprised of partnerships of state and local public health agency practitioners with researchers, often at major academic institutions. Public health PBRN research answers the call from the public health community for research that is of greater utility to practitioners and can be used to directly and quickly impact their communities.[42,43] The cycle of problem identification in practice, practice-based research to address the question, and the application of the research in practice can be considerably shortened. In addition, the research questions are clearly immediately relevant to public health practice and policy issues. Public health PBRN research has been used to conduct quick-cycle research focused on specific events, such as the 2009 H1N1 flu outbreak in the United States, and also longer-term projects, including identifying which local public health services are most effective in addressing disparities and improving population health. Public health PBRN activities have accelerated, particularly in efforts to address concerns of policy makers regarding the cost of provision of public health services and how best to finance the provision of those services, particularly in a declining funding environment.[42]

THE FUTURE OF PHSSR

Health Care Reform

Efforts to control government spending combined with a distrust of government and a continued slow recovery from an economic downturn have threatened the provision of governmental public health services and had adverse impacts on federal research funding, including support for PHSSR. The ACA has provided new resources and specific mandates that encourage public health and prevention, and as a result there are specific portions of ACA that call for funding of PHSSR; however, that funding has not been forthcoming. The Prevention and Public Health Fund, created and funded by ACA, has provided new resources to governmental public health functions.[44] The requirement that insurance companies provide certain preventive services without a co-pay or deductible has boosted the capacity of the health care system to provide clinical preventive services to a larger population. At the same time, the expansion of health insurance resulting from ACA may impact health departments that have served as a primary care provider of last resort in many communities in the nation—newly covered patients may no longer use safety net providers such as public health agencies for primary care, creating financial and existential crises for those departments. In addition, patients may be unlikely to use public health agencies for the provision of clinical preventive services, such as immunizations. This could result in a net loss of patient-associated revenues for these agencies. This will present challenges to the public health community: while these agencies may now be able to focus on providing more traditional population-based services, they will lose revenues such as Medicaid reimbursements that they previously used to cross-subsidize population services. There will be a need for a renewed examination of public health programs, activities, and linkages, specifically, the role of public health in a changing health care environment that is moving to integrated delivery systems and value-based purchasing, an area PHSSR is well suited to exploring. (Further detail on the impact of ACA on public health practice is provided in Chapter 30.)

Accreditation in Public Health

One of the overarching goals of PHSSR has been to protect the public's health by improving the quality of public health service delivery. **Quality improvement (QI)** activities are formal methods to improve service delivery, and one major QI initiative in public health has been the advent of a voluntary national public health accreditation program guided by the Public Health Accreditation Board (PHAB). PHAB accreditation seeks to foster the development of a culture of continuous quality improvement in state, tribal, and local public health agencies through compliance with a set of standards and measures that reflect best practices in public health.[45,46] However, while accreditation has the potential to improve quality, it also comes with serious costs. These costs include not only accreditation fees, but also the costs associated with the time and workforce needed to engage in accreditation-related activities. PHSSR could play a key role in answering research concerns related to accreditation, including the true costs of accreditation, the impact of accreditation on health department activities and community health, and determining if the benefits of accreditation are commensurate to its costs. It could guide the development of accreditation standards, assuring those standards are based in research that demonstrates that they improve the quality, efficiency, and effectiveness of health department activities.[45,46] In recognition of this, PHAB has developed its own research agenda that attempts to raise many of these questions and provides important direction for PHSSR researchers who are interested in pursuing concerns about public health accreditation.[21]

Public Health Law Research

The field of public health law research has experienced tremendous growth since the early 2000s, in large part due to heavy investment by the RWJF. Policies and laws, such as smoke-free legislation, have shown themselves to be powerful tools in efforts to improve and protect the public's health. In addition, research related to the area of infrastructure law, which determines the character, governance, authority, and responsibility of public health agencies as defined by law, provides a powerful tool to examine the impact of legislation on the ability of public health agencies to perform their duties, and the impact this may have on the public's health. This area of research may provide important insight into factors that impact the quality of services delivered by public health agencies. For example, while some early PHSSR suggests that characteristics of the bodies that govern public health agencies may influence the performance of public health systems, little is known regarding the specific authorities and powers of these bodies. Public health law research has the potential to help answer this and other important questions in PHSSR. Efforts have been developed to assure that there is a dialog between those engaged in PHSSR and public health law research on the questions and issues where there is an overlap in interest on the part of both.[47]

Public Health Foundational Services Funding

The Institute of Medicine, in 2012, completed a study focusing primarily on the financing of public health services. This report added a new paradigm for approaches to examining the public health services that a population would require.[48] Figure 17-1 illustrates that new paradigm.

The IOM report defined the various areas contained in Figure 17-1 as:

▸ **Foundational Capabilities:** Cross-cutting skills needed in state/local health departments everywhere for the health system to work anywhere; essential skills/capacities to support all activities.
▸ **Foundational Areas:** Substantive areas of expertise or program-specific activities in all state/local health departments necessary to protect the community's health.
▸ **Programs/Activities Specific to a Health Department or a Community's Needs:** Additional, critical significance to a specific community's health, supported by Foundational Areas and Capacities; most of a health department's work.
▸ **Foundational Public Health Services**: Comprised of the Foundational Capacities and Areas; a suite of skills, programs/activities that must be available in state/local health departments system-wide.

This new model provides an important point of departure for the consideration of public health services and the requisite funding; it is not a substitute for the 10 Essential Public Health Services, but a new way of looking at the provision of those services. It has also provided a way to examine the approach to costing out the provision of public health services and ascertaining

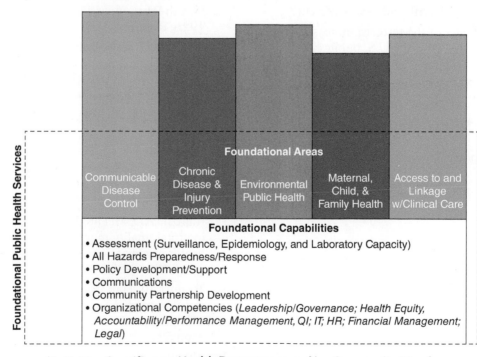

FIGURE 17-1   **Programs/Activities Specific to a Health Department and/or Community Needs**

Adapted from Public Health Leadership Forum[49]

how best to fund the foundational capabilities as opposed to the programs and activities specific to a local health department's response to a community's needs. This work, under the aegis of the RWJF, the Public Health Leadership Forum, and facilitated by RESOLVE, is still in its formative stages, but represents an important potential new development in PHSSR vis-a-vis costs, economics, and financing.[49]

SUMMARY

Health services research has a relatively long history and has provided many answers and much guidance to both practitioners and policy makers regarding access, quality, and costs of medical care. PHSSR is a much newer endeavor, but, given the opportunities provided by ACA, as well as the resurgence of interest in public health services in the United States, those engaged in PHSSR are presented with great opportunities to undertake research which can and will inform policy in the areas of increasing access to care, reducing its cost while simultaneously improving its quality, and ultimately improving and protecting population health. Given this resurgence of interest in population health and public health services, the field of PHSSR is poised to play an active role in efforts to improve health and health care.

REVIEW QUESTIONS

1. In what ways are PHSSR and HSR different?
2. Discuss the impact of the terrorist attacks of September 11, 2001 on the U.S. public health system.
3. Current PHSSR emphasis is focused on which four major themes?
4. Describe the major sources of data used to conduct PHSSR.
5. Describe the potential impact of the ACA on PHSSR.
6. Describe how PHAB accreditation relates to PHSSR.

REFERENCES

1. Erwin PC, Shah GH, Mays GP. Local health departments and the 2008 recession: characteristics of resiliency. *Am J Prev Med.* June 2014;46(6):559–568.
2. Willard R, Shah GH, Leep C, Ku L. Impact of the 2008–2010 economic recession on local health departments. *J Public Health Manag Pract.* March–April 2012;18(2):106–114.
3. Costich JF. Local health departments as essential community providers for health benefits exchange plans. *Am J Public Health.* April 2014;104(4):e12–14.
4. Koo DMDMPH, Felix KMD, Dankwa-Mullan IMDMPH, Miller TD, Waalen JMDMPH. A call for action on primary care and public health integration. *Am J Public Health.* June 2012;102(S3):S307–S309.
5. Calman NS, Hauser D, Chokshi DA. "Lost to follow-up": the public health goals of accountable care. *Arch Int Med.* April 9 2012;172(7):584–586.
6. Mays GP, Halverson PK, Scutchfield FD. Making public health improvement real: the vital role of systems research. *J Public Health Manag Pract.* May–June 2004;10(3):183–185.
7. Mays GP, Smith SA. Evidence links increases in public health spending to declines in preventable deaths. *Health Aff.* August 2011;30(8):1585–1593.
8. Varda DM. Data-driven management strategies in public health collaboratives. *J Public Health Manag Pract.* March–April 2011;17(2):122–132.
9. What is HSR. 2014; http://www.academyhealth.org/About/content.cfm?ItemNumber=831&navItemNumber=514. Accessed October 16, 2014.
10. III. Survey Schedule and Appraisal Form for Certain Typical Activities Common to City Health Work. *Am J Public Health.* January 1926;16(Suppl_1):14–63.
11. Emerson H, Luginbuhl M. *Local health units for the nation.* The Commonwealth Fund; 1945.
12. Institute of Medicine (U.S.). Committee for the Study of the Future of Public Health. *The future of public health.* Washington, DC: National Academy Press; 1988.
13. The Public Health System and the 10 Essential Public Health Services http://www.cdc.gov/nphpsp/essentialservices.html. Accessed August 29, 2014.
14. Kaluzny AD, McLaughlin CP, Simpson K. Applying total quality management concepts to public health organizations. *Public Health Rep.* May–June 1992;107(3):257–264.
15. Turnock BJ, Handler AS, Miller CA. Core function-related local public health practice effectiveness. *J Public Health Manag Pract.* September 1998;4(5):26–32.
16. Bhandari MW, Scutchfield FD, Charnigo R, Riddell MC, Mays GP. New data, same story?

Revisiting studies on the relationship of local public health systems characteristics to public health performance. *J Public Health Manag Pract.* March–April 2010;16(2):110–117.

17. Avery GH, Zabriskie-Timmerman J. The impact of federal bioterrorism funding programs on local health department preparedness activities. *Eval Health Prof.* June 2009;32(2):95–127.

18. Hyde J, Kim B, Martinez LS, Clark M, Hacker K. Better prepared but spread too thin: the impact of emergency preparedness funding on local public health. *Disaster Manag Resp.* October–December 2006;4(4):106–113.

19. Institute of Medicine (U.S.). Committee on Assuring the Health of the Public in the 21st Century. *The future of the public's health in the 21st century.* Washington, DC: National Academies Press; 2003.

20. Lenaway D, Halverson P, Sotnikov S, Tilson H, Corso L, Millington W. Public health systems research: setting a national agenda. *Am J Public Health.* March 2006;96(3):410–413.

21. Riley WJ, Lownik EM, Scutchfield FD, Mays GP, Corso LC, Beitsch LM. Public health department accreditation: setting the research agenda. *Am J Prev Med.* March 2012;42(3):263–271.

22. Wallace H, Tilson H, Carlson VP, Valasek T. Instrumental roles of governance in accreditation: responsibilities of public health governing entities. *J Public Health Manag Pract.* January–February 2014;20(1):61–63.

23. Beckett AB, Scutchfield FD, Pfeifle W, Hill R, Ingram RC. The forgotten instrument: analysis of the national public health performance standards program governance instrument. *J Public Health Manag Pract.* July–August 2008;14(4):E17–22.

24. Scutchfield FD, Lawhorn N, Ingram R, Perez DJ, Brewer R, Bhandari M. Public health systems and services research: dataset development, dissemination, and use. *Public Health Rep.* May–June 2009;124(3):372–377.

25. Consortium from Altarum I, Centers for Disease C, Prevention, Robert Wood Johnson F, National Coordinating Center for Public Health S, Systems R. A national research agenda for public health services and systems. *Am J Prev Med.* May 2012;42(5 Suppl 1):S72–78.

26. Mays GP, Scutchfield FD. Improving public health system performance through multiorganizational partnerships. *Prev Chronic Dis.* November 2010;7(6):A116.

27. Mays GP, McHugh MC, Shim K, et al. Institutional and economic determinants of public health system performance. *Am J Public Health.* March 2006;96(3):523–531.

28. Mays GP, McHugh MC, Shim K, et al. Identifying dimensions of performance in local public health systems: results from the National Public Health Performance Standards Program. *J Public Health Manag Pract.* May–June 2004;10(3):193–203.

29. Scutchfield FD, Bhandari MW, Lawhorn NA, Lamberth CD, Ingram RC. Public health performance. *Am J Prev Med.* March 2009;36(3):266–272.

30. Scutchfield FD, Knight EA, Kelly AV, Bhandari MW, Vasilescu IP. Local public health agency capacity and its relationship to public health system performance. *J Public Health Manag Pract.* May–June 2004;10(3):204–215.

31. *Public health Services and Systems Research Inventory.* University of Kentucky, Lexington KY: National Coordinating Center for Public Health Services and Systems Research 26 March, 2014.

32. Ingram RC, Bernet PM, Costich JF. Public health services and systems research: current state of finance research. *J Public Health Manag Pract.* November 2012;18(6):515–519.

33. Hyde JK, Shortell SM. The structure and organization of local and state public health agencies in the U.S.: a systematic review. *Am J Prev Med.* May 2012;42(5 Suppl 1):S29–41.

34. Gebbie KM, Columbia University. School of Nursing. Center for Health Policy. *The public health work force: enumeration 2000.* Washington, DC: Health Resources and Services Administration, Bureau of Health Professions; 2000.

35. Hilliard TM, Boulton ML. Public health workforce research in review: a 25-year retrospective. *Am J Prev Med.* May 2012;42(5 Suppl 1):S17–28.

36. Keck CW, Scutchfield, F.D., Holsinger, J.W.III. Conclusion: Future of public health *Contemporary public health: principles, practice, and policy.* Lexington, KY.: University Press of Kentucky; 2012:p.251–276.

37. Gans DN, Piland NF, Honore PA. Developing a chart of accounts: historical perspective of the Medical Group Management Association. *J Public Health Manag Pract.* March–April 2007;13(2):130–132.

38. Barry M, Bialek R. Tracking our investments in public health: what have we learned? *J Public Health Manag Pract.* September–October 2004;10(5):383–392.

39. Corso LC, Lenaway D, Beitsch LM, Landrum LB, Deutsch H. The national public health performance

standards: driving quality improvement in public health systems. *J Public Health Manag Pract.* January–February 2010;16(1):19–23.

40. Mays G. *Overview of the National Longitudinal Survey of Public Health Systems.* Lexington, KY: University of Kentucky;2012.

41. Mays GP, Scutchfield FD, Bhandari MW, Smith SA. Understanding the organization of public health delivery systems: an empirical typology. *Milbank Q.* March 2010;88(1):81–111.

42. Mays GP, Hogg RA, Castellanos-Cruz DM, Hoover AG, Fowler LC. Public health research implementation and translation: evidence from practice-based research networks. *Am J Prev Med.* December 2013;45(6):752–762.

43. Mays GP, Hogg RA. Expanding delivery system research in public health settings: lessons from practice-based research networks. *J Public Health Manag Pract.* November 2012;18(6):485–498.

44. Linde-Feucht S, Coulouris N. Integrating primary care and public health: a strategic priority. *Am J Public Health.* June 2012;102 Suppl 3: S310–311.

45. Beitsch LM, Riley W, Bender K. Embedding quality improvement into accreditation: evolving from theory to practice. *J Public Health Manag Pract.* January–February 2014;20(1):57–60.

46. Ingram RC, Bender K, Wilcox R, Kronstadt J. A consensus-based approach to national public health accreditation. *J Public Health Manag Pract.* January–February 2014;20(1):9–13.

47. Burris S, Mays GP, Douglas Scutchfield F, Ibrahim JK. Moving from intersection to integration: public health law research and public health systems and services research. *Milbank Q.* June 2012;90(2):375–408.

48. Institute of Medicine (U.S.). Committee on Public Health Strategies to Improve Health. *For the public's health. Investing in a healthier future.* Washington, DC: National Academies Press; 2012.

49. *Defining and Constituting Foundational "Capabilities" and "Areas" Version 1.* Public Health Leadership Forum; March 2014. Available at http://www.resolv.org/site-healthleadershipforum/files/2014/03/Articulation-of-Foundational-Capabilities-and-Foundational-Areas-v1.pdf

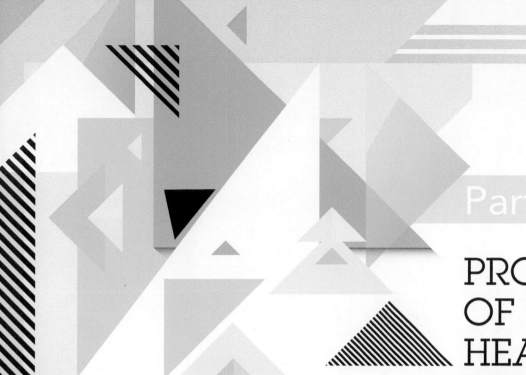

Part Four

PROVISION OF PUBLIC HEALTH SERVICES

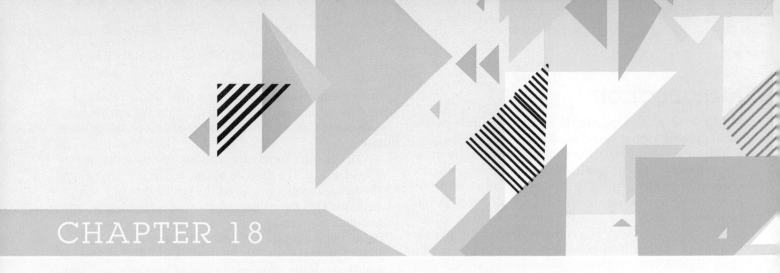

CHAPTER 18

The Public Health Workforce

Matthew L. Boulton, MD, MPH • Edward L. Baker, MD, MPH • Angela J. Beck, PhD, MPH

LEARNING OBJECTIVES

Upon completion of this chapter, the reader will be able to:

1. Identify professions comprising the public health workforce and describe efforts to determine the public health workforce size and composition.

2. Describe the places of employment of the public health workforce, how the workforce is trained, and who is licensed or certified.

3. Describe the efforts underway to ensure and measure the impact of public health workforce development, including leadership development.

4. Describe the essential public health services delivered by the public health workforce.

5. Define leadership and be able to distinguish leadership and management.

6. Understand theories of leadership practice and the related behaviors needed to practice effective leadership.

7. Understand the needs for leadership development at various career stages.

KEY TERMS

certification
competencies
enumeration
leadership
licensure
management
multidisciplinary teams
voluntary health organizations
workforce
workforce capacity

INTRODUCTION

Public health is increasingly at the forefront of the national and global response to new and re-emergent health threats ranging from outbreaks of deadly infectious diseases, to the explosive growth in the obesity epidemic, to disturbing increases in injury and violence, making the need for a highly effective public health system as vital as ever. Perhaps no part of that public health system is as important as the people who work within it as members of the public health workforce. A well-trained and competent workforce is essential to the practice of public health and the successful delivery of essential public health services. The professionals and other workers who comprise the public health workforce share a common awareness of and commitment to improving health through a population focus. These workers are uniquely diverse in terms of the education, skills, and experience they bring to the field, especially relative to other health professions. However, unlike other health professions, the public health workforce has actually become smaller over the last two decades. At the same time the variety of occupations comprising that workforce has diversified and includes new positions such as health informatics specialists, public health geneticists, and emergency preparedness professionals which mostly did not exist just a decade ago. The opportunities for public health worker training and education have also grown dramatically as schools and programs of public health have undergone an unprecedented expansion. This has been accompanied by a rapid development of continuing education and other training, often using distance modalities, offered through national networks of federally funded workforce centers. These efforts are creating an increasingly professionalized workforce that has been reinforced and strengthened through complementary initiatives aimed at development of competency-based education and training, worker certification, and accreditation of public health agencies.

Despite these exciting developments, many contemporary challenges confront attempts to fully characterize the public health workforce—there is still too little known about how many workers it contains, the disciplines they represent, where they deliver services and how effective they are at doing so, their demographic composition, the reasons they enter and leave the workforce, and how they adapt to unstable funding impacting their job security and future career prospects. And, we continue to wrestle with the appropriate benchmarks that define the ideal mix of education, experience, and diversity needed to produce an effective workforce and how that mix contributes to overall workforce capacity. Finally, there is a clear need for more research on the public health workforce to address these many questions and to also ensure that, ultimately, we have the right number of people with the right skills in the right place at the right time to improve and protect the public's health.

The chapter concludes with an extensive discussion of **leadership**. The practice of leadership consists of specific behaviors which lead to the realization of a shared vision through the implementation of core strategies and the application to operational reality of specific tactics. Therefore, the practice of leadership consists of specific behaviors which lead to the realization of a shared vision through the implementation of core strategies and the application to operational reality of specific tactics. A range of theories has developed regarding the skills needed for effective leadership; one of the most compelling for public health practice is servant leadership. As leaders evolve, leadership development needs to change and can be addressed by formal leadership development programs. In public health, leadership is central to addressing the challenges and opportunities needed to improve and protect the public's health.

PUBLIC HEALTH WORKERS

The effective delivery of public health services is dependent upon the availability of a skilled, competent **workforce** (the population employed in a specified occupation). A key challenge for governmental and nongovernmental public health organizations is to employ the appropriate number of workers who possess the requisite skills which can be used where and when they are needed.[1] The public health workforce comprises a highly varied group of professions. The wide diversity of skills, education, and experiential backgrounds that public health workers bring to the field is a strength given the multitude of factors that contribute to population health; however, it also creates challenges in accurately determining the size, composition, job function, and expertise of public health workers, both individually and collectively. The public health workforce has been defined in many ways, with a focus on population health serving as the common element to define a public health worker. According to the Institute of Medicine (IOM), a public health professional is "a person educated in public health or a related discipline who is employed to improve health through a population focus."[2] Given the importance of the public health workforce in promoting and protecting the health of populations, it is key to understand how many workers are currently employed and what skills they possess, as well as where gaps in workforce capacity exist and how to recruit and retain the right types of workers in all public health settings.

WORKPLACE SETTINGS

Public health workers can be found in a wide variety of job settings in both public and private sectors. Some of these settings may not be traditionally characterized as places where public health services are delivered, but services carried out there make important contributions to the public's health nonetheless. Although the settings summarized in this chapter employ substantial numbers of public health workers, not all workers employed in these settings are necessarily part of the public health workforce.

Governmental Public Health

The core public health workforce is employed in governmental settings, including 59 state and territorial public health agencies, nearly 3,000 local health departments (including tribal agencies), and federal agencies that contribute to a public health mission such as the Department of Health and Human Services, Environmental Protection Agency, and Department of Agriculture, among others. Within all three levels of government, public health workers are found in a wide variety of programs that focus on areas such as energy, environmental protection, food safety, health insurance (including Medicaid), immunizations, control of infectious diseases, maternal and child health, mental health, occupational health and safety, substance abuse, rural health, traffic safety, sexually transmitted infections, welfare, and zoning. Many of these programs, originally developed as part of a department or board of health, have since been relocated or combined as policy makers shift preferences for relating programs and people. For example, pesticide control programs now housed in agriculture were once part of health departments, and the function of assuring access to care for the poor encompassed by Medicaid may have been a part of the jurisdiction of a board of health. The IOM described an ideal state health agency that encompasses all of these programs.[3] However, no such agency exists, nor is one likely to appear. Consequently, public health professionals must work collaboratively across program and agency lines and among public and private and voluntary partners.

Nongovernmental Public Health

Public health workers can be found in a range of settings beyond governmental public health agencies. For example, school districts and individual schools (public, private, and parochial) employ many public health nurses to assure the health of school-aged children. They may also have nutrition and environmental health professionals working at a district-wide level to assure the healthfulness and safety of school meal programs. Independent water, sewer, or waste management districts also employ public health professionals to assure that standards for public health protection are met.

In addition, voluntary health organizations (an industry comprising organizations that engage in fund raising for health-related research, health education, and patient services) represent another setting for public health workers. The American Red Cross is a special case of a voluntary agency, given the public health and care-giving role it plays during emergency response in coordination with local, state, and national officials. It also provides extensive public health education in many localities, for example, through sponsorship of HIV/AIDS prevention training. Other voluntary organizations with a strong public health presence include the American Lung Association, the American Cancer Society, the American Heart Association, and the American Diabetes Association. Although each of these employs public health personnel, they also use extensive networks of volunteers, some of whom are also full-time public health workers in other agencies. For their volunteers who are not public health workers, the training given for volunteer tasks results in expanding the public health knowledge within communities. To illustrate, few communities would be as strict in control of indoor tobacco smoke today were it not for the thousands of public health volunteers working through voluntary associations. Local communities also often have nonprofit groups with public health and human services missions who provide important outreach to the population through health education, health advocacy, and other public health efforts.

Hospitals and Healthcare Organizations

Many hospitals and health care organizations (including staff-model and other health maintenance organizations) employ public health professionals. Many of the administrators of personal health care services have earned graduate degrees in administration from programs housed in schools of public health, and may have developed a population focus on their work. Among the most common public health workers in these settings are health educators, outreach workers, and epidemiologists. A large institutional system may have its own sanitarians, environmental engineers, and occupational health staff as well. Further, many localities expect that the clinical portion of public health services, such as immunizations or home-based education and outreach, will be housed with other care services, and not solely in the public health agency, and often are incorporated seamlessly into daily practices such as a pediatrician's ongoing care. Conversely, it should be remembered, however, that just providing a health-related service or activity outside the walls of a hospital does not make it a public health activity. The test for whether something should be considered part of public health is the presence of a focus on a population group or community and on a preventive strategy or a preventable outcome.[4] As public health and health care organizations continue to implement mandates of the Patient Protection and Affordable Care Act of 2010 (ACA),[5] some of the job tasks of public health workers and hospital workers may become more integrated and shared across worker settings.

Occupational Health

For workforce and other strategic considerations, occupational health is a subspecialty of public health practice that may take workers into almost any other field as a part of the organization's infrastructure. These public health professionals include physicians (some board certified in occupational medicine by the American Board of Preventive Medicine), nurses, epidemiologists, and industrial hygienists, and are involved primarily with protection of workers from hazardous working conditions. Some also develop workplace-based health promotion programs or even broader health programs for workers and their families. Workers concerned about their health and safety may also employ public health expertise through unions or professional associations. For example, occupational health advocates on the staff of the American Nurses Association were leading activists in supporting legislation protecting health care workers from occupational exposure to blood-borne pathogens.

WORKER ENUMERATION

Unlike for other health professions such as physicians and nurses, the U.S. government does not employ a system for continuously collecting data to count or characterize the public health workforce. The U.S. Bureau of Labor Statistics (BLS) produces employment and wage estimates annually for over 800 professions.[6] Although public health workers are included in these estimates, most cannot be counted because they are grouped within broader health care professions categories that lack sufficient precision to specifically determine who is a public health worker. As a result, public health professional organizations and public health systems researchers undertake national surveys and studies in an attempt to collect information on different segments of the workforce. Most studies are conducted with state and local health departments because these agencies are easily identifiable, have a clear public health mission, and are often willing to participate in such research activities. Among the most basic of research questions studied is *How many public health workers are employed in*

state and local health departments? Enumeration studies (studies to count the number of workers employed in a defined set of agencies or organizations) have been conducted on the U.S. public health workforce since 1908 to estimate its size. More recent efforts estimated 220 public health workers per 100,000 population in 1980, while a national enumeration study conducted in 2000 yielded a total of approximately 450,000 workers nationally, equivalent to a ratio of 158 public health workers per 100,000 population.[7] These studies used different definitions for "public health worker" and different methods for data collection, making trend comparisons over time difficult. The most recent enumeration study, conducted in 2014, includes workers in local, state, and federal health agencies who are responsible for the delivery of essential public health services, which is a narrower definition than used in previous studies. In this study, approximately 291,000 public health workers in 14 occupational categories were enumerated using survey data collected by multiple organizations (see Table 18-1),[8] equivalent to a rate of 92/100,000 population. Half of the public health workforce worked in local health departments, which is not surprising given that the majority of public health services are provided at the local level; 30 percent worked in state health departments and 20 percent at federal health agencies. Additional detail on the recent trends in governmental workforce data is provided in Chapter 8 (for state health departments) and Chapter 9 (for local health departments). Enumeration studies provide valuable information for assessing the size of the workforce, but usually provide limited information on other characteristics of the workforce, such as demographics, education and training background, and job function because most data are collected from the organization, rather than from individual workers.

Public Health Occupations

The occupational categories listed in Table 18-1 represent the primary professions of public health workers. The occupational diversity of the workforce is apparent. Several disciplines, each with their own skills and training requirements, work in multidisciplinary teams to contribute to the overall delivery of public health services. Administrative and clerical personnel, who may not have a degree in public health but support public health program activities in local, state, and federal health departments, represent almost 20 percent of the workforce. The largest proportions of workers trained in public health service delivery are public health nurses (16 percent), followed by environmental health workers (8 percent), and public health managers (6 percent). Other occupations with fewer workers include laboratory workers, public health physicians, behavioral

TABLE 18-1   Public Health Workforce Occupations and Enumeration Estimates, 2014

Occupation	Job Description	Enumeration Estimates: Governmental Public Health			
		Local	State	Federal	TOTAL
Administrative/ Clerical Personnel	Staff who work in business, finance, auditing, management, and accounting; trained at a professional level in their field of expertise before entry into public health; staff who perform support work in areas of business and financial operations; and staff who perform nontechnical support work in all areas of management and program administration.	35,000	14,559	6,085	55,644
Public Health Nurses	Workers who plan, develop, implement, and evaluate nursing and public health interventions for persons, families, and populations at risk for illness or disability. This includes positions identified at the registered nurse (RN) level, and includes graduates of diploma and associate degree programs with the RN license.	29,191	12,286	5,793	47,270
Environmental Health Worker	Staff who plan, develop, implement, and evaluate standards and systems to improve the quality of the physical environment as it affects health; manage environmental health programs; perform research on environmental health problems; and promote public awareness of the need to prevent and eliminate environmental health hazards.	13,300	4,618	5,920	23,838
Public Health Manager	Health service managers, administrators, and public health directors overseeing the operations of the agency or of a department or division, including the senior agency executive, regardless of education or licensing.	10,100	3,296	4,998	18,394
Laboratory Worker	Staff who plan, design, and implement laboratory procedures to identify and quantify agents in the environment that might be hazardous to human health, biologic agents believed to be involved in the etiology of diseases among animals or humans (e.g., bacteria, viruses, or parasites), or other physical, chemical, and biologic hazards; and laboratory technicians who plan, perform, and evaluate laboratory analyses and procedures not elsewhere classified, including performing routine tests in a medical laboratory for use in disease diagnosis and treatment; preparing vaccines, biologics, and serums for disease prevention; preparing tissue samples for pathologists or taking blood samples; and executing laboratory tests (e.g., urinalysis and blood counts).	2,000	5,699	5,685	13,384
Public Health Physician	Physicians who identify persons or groups at risk for illness or disability and who develop, implement, and evaluate programs or interventions designed to prevent, treat, or ameliorate such risks; might provide direct medical services within the context of such programs, including medical doctor and doctor of osteopathy generalists and specialists, some of whom have training in public health or preventive medicine.	2,100	791	6,700	9,591
Behavioral Health Professional	Workers who provide psychological support and assess, coordinate, and monitor provision of community services for patients or clients. Includes social workers.	4,000	1,839	895	6,734

TABLE 18-1   (Continued)

Occupation	Job Description	Enumeration Estimates: Governmental Public Health			
		Local	State	Federal	TOTAL
Health Educator	Workers who design, organize, implement, communicate, evaluate, and provide advice regarding the effect of educational programs and strategies designed to support and modify health-related behaviors of persons, families, organizations, and communities.	5,100	1,572	43	6,715
Nutritionist	Staff who plan, develop, implement, and evaluate programs or scientific studies to promote and maintain optimum health through improved nutrition; collaborate with programs that have nutrition components; might involve clinical practice as a dietitian.	5,000	1,276	223	6,499
Epidemiologist	Staff who investigate, describe, and analyze the distribution and determinants of disease, disability, and other health outcomes and develop the means for disease prevention and control; investigate, describe, and analyze the efficacy of programs and interventions.	1,800	2,476	—	4,276
Emergency Preparedness Staff	Workers whose regular duties involve preparing for (e.g., developing plans, procedures, and training programs) and managing the public health response to all-hazards events.	2,900	810	—	3,710
Public Health Dental Worker	Staff who plan, develop, implement, and evaluate dental health programs to promote and maintain the public's optimum oral health, including public health dentists who can provide comprehensive dental care and dental hygienists who can provide limited dental services under professional supervision.	2,600	356	443	3,399
Public Health Informatics Specialist	Workers who systematically apply information and computer science and technology to public health practice, research, and learning (e.g., public health information systems specialists or public health informaticists).	2,100	729	—	2,829
Public Information Specialist	Staff who represent public health topics to the media and public, act as a spokesperson for public health agencies, engage in promoting or creating goodwill for public health organizations by writing or selecting favorable publicity material and releasing it through different communications media, or prepare and arrange displays, make speeches, and perform related publicity efforts.	2,100	174	—	2,274
Other or Uncategorized Worker	Public health workers in occupations not listed in the previous categories; workers who cannot be placed in a category due to missing data	30,200	35,960	20,271	86,431
TOTAL		147,491	86,411	57,056	290,988

SOURCE: Beck, A.J. and Boulton, M.L.

health professionals, health educators, nutritionists, epidemiologists, emergency preparedness staff, public health dental workers, public health informatics specialists, and public information specialists. Approximately 30 percent of the workforce in this study was represented by an undesignated occupation or was unassigned to a category due to underreporting of workforce information. This further supports the need for more standardized methodologies for collecting workforce information on a national level.

Public health workers who are often excluded from most public health workforce enumeration studies are community health workers, individuals who conduct outreach for medical personnel or health organizations to implement programs in the community that promote, maintain, and improve individual and community health.[6] Community health workers, sometimes called *lay health workers* or *promotoras*, depending on the community, are a growing segment of the public health workforce; they may be volunteer or paid, are found working in any public health setting, and generally do not have a formal educational background in public health, but are trained to help deliver public health services to the population. The BLS recently began collecting data on this segment of the workforce and estimated that 45,800 community health workers were employed in the United States in 2013, excluding self-employed and volunteer workers for which enumeration estimates are unavailable. The number of employed, paid workers in this discipline is similar to the number of public health nurses enumerated in governmental public health settings. This diverse group of public health workers could soon represent the largest group of public health workers in the United States.

Workforce Taxonomy

One method for improving the quality of data related to enumeration and other workforce characteristics is to develop a common system for classifying workers. A public health workforce taxonomy was developed in 2014 by several public health professional groups and federal agencies providing a framework for worker classification that could lead to a much clearer picture regarding workplace settings, type of employment, job tasks, funding sources for workers, educational background, licensure and certification, and worker demographics.[9] The taxonomy's occupational categories, which include far more than the 14 occupations used in the most recent enumeration study, provide more specificity on the types of disciplines represented in the public health workforce (see Table 18-2). Broadly, public health occupations can be grouped into four main categories: management and leadership; professional and scientific; technical and outreach; and support services. The workforce taxonomy provides a mechanism for standardizing the classification of public health occupations across different workforce surveys, which has been a persistent challenge for workforce researchers, permitting more valid comparisons while also providing a framework for ensuring collection of a set of minimum data elements on all workers in the public health workforce.

TRENDS IN PROFESSIONALIZATION

The field of public health has been aptly described as a "loose confederation of professions" because the breadth of skills and experience needed by public health workers requires highly diverse backgrounds representing many different disciplines. Historically, it was commonplace for workers in health departments, for example, to be primarily trained on the job with no public health degree and little or no formal education or even training in public health. However, that began to change with the IOM's 1988 report, *The Future of Public Health*, which prominently acknowledged the need for significant changes in the training and education of the national public health workforce, including access to more educational offerings. That need was dramatically highlighted and reinforced in the follow-on 2003 IOM report, *Who Will Keep the Public Healthy in the 21st Century?*, which recommended that the CDC and Health Resources and Services Administration (HRSA) "periodically assess the preparedness of the public health workforce, to document the training necessary to meet basic competency expectations and to advise on the funding necessary to provide such training." These ongoing efforts to further develop the skills and competence of the existing public health workforce have increased substantially since 2000, with greater emphasis on certification and licensure of public health workers, and accreditation of governmental public health departments. Although it may have been true at one time that public health workers learned most skills on the job and that any worker in the health department could perform almost any job task in a pinch, even without any training or education in that area, that is rapidly becoming an outmoded perspective and no longer true nor feasible in the modern public health workforce. As several enumeration and other workforce studies have revealed, the public health workforce is becoming increasingly professionalized as workers are charged with carrying out more complex, specialized, and technical tasks that call for an appropriate level of educational and professional background training. This has been driven, in part, by the enormous changes occurring in health information technology with the advent of advanced web-based communicable disease surveillance systems, ever more sophisticated immunization information systems, the development of large and complex health registries, the increasing use of electronic health records, and the need to utilize "big data" to improve health, all of which require high levels of technical and professional expertise. For example, a 2002 national study found that over 40 percent of epidemiologists in state health departments lacked any education or formal training in epidemiology;[10] similarly a state health department reported in 2006 that over 60 percent of their workforce

TABLE 18-2   A Taxonomy for the Public Health Workforce

1.4.   Management and Leadership
  1.4.1.   Public Health Agency Director
  1.4.2.   Health Officer
  1.4.3.   Department or Bureau Director
          (subagency level)
  1.4.4.   Deputy Director
  1.4.5.   Program Director
  1.4.6.   Public Health Manager or Program Manager
  1.4.7.   Other Management and Leadership
          1.4.7.1.   Coordinators
          1.4.7.2.   Administrators
1.5.   Professional and Scientific
  1.5.1.   Behavioral Health Professional
          1.5.1.1.   Behavioral Counselor
  1.5.2.   Emergency Preparedness Worker
  1.5.3.   Environmentalist
          1.5.3.1.   Sanitarian or Inspector
          1.5.3.2.   Engineer
          1.5.3.3.   Technician
  1.5.4.   Epidemiologist
  1.5.5.   Health Educator
  1.5.6.   Information Systems Manager
          1.5.6.1.   Public Health Informatics Specialist
          1.5.6.2.   Other Informatics Specialist
          1.5.6.3.   Information Technology Specialist
  1.5.7.   Laboratory Worker
          1.5.7.1.   Aide or Assistant
          1.5.7.2.   Technician
          1.5.7.3.   Scientist or Medical Technologist
  1.5.8.   Nurse
          1.5.8.1.   Registered Nurse Unspecified
                    1.5.8.1.1.   Public Health or
                               Community Health Nurse
                    1.5.8.1.2.   Other Registered Nurse
                               (Clinical Services)
          1.5.8.2.   Licensed Practical or Vocational
                    Nurse
  1.5.9.   Nutritionist or dietitian

  1.1.1.   Oral Health Professional
          1.1.1.1.   Public Health Dentist
          1.1.1.2.   Other Oral Health Professional
  1.1.2.   Physician
          1.1.2.1.   Public Health or Preventive
                    Medicine Physician
          1.1.2.2.   Other Physician
  1.1.3.   Medical Examiner
  1.1.4.   Physician Assistant
  1.1.5.   Public Information Specialist
  1.1.6.   Social Worker
          1.1.6.1.   Social Services Counselor
  1.1.7.   Statistician
  1.1.8.   Veterinarian
          1.1.8.1.   Public Health Veterinarian
          1.1.8.2.   Other Veterinarian
  1.1.9.   Other Professional and Scientific
  1.1.10. Student Professional and Scientific
1.2.   Technical and Outreach
  1.2.1.   Animal Control Worker
  1.2.2.   Community Health Worker
  1.2.3.   Home Health Worker
  1.2.4.   Other Technical and Outreach
1.3.   Support Services
  1.3.1.   Clerical Personnel
          1.3.1.1.   Administrative Assistant
          1.3.1.2.   Secretary
  1.3.2.   Business Support
          1.3.2.1.   Accountant or Fiscal
          1.3.2.2.   Facilities or Operations
                    1.3.2.2.1.   Custodian
                    1.3.2.2.2.   Other Facilities or
                               Operations Worker
          1.3.2.3.   Grants or Contracts Specialist
          1.3.2.4.   Human Resources Personnel
          1.3.2.5.   Attorney or Legal Counsel
  1.3.3.   Other business support services
1.5   Other

SOURCE: Boulton, M.L., Beck, A.J., Coronado, F., Merrill, J., Friedman, C. et al.

lacked a college degree of any type.[11] However, just a decade later a repeat of the national epidemiology assessment revealed over 60 percent of epidemiologists working in health departments possessed a public health or epidemiology degree and almost 90 percent had received at least some formal training in epidemiology (although this may constitute just a single epidemiology course[12]). The lack of formal training within the workforce resulted in workers who were cross-trained to fulfill many types of duties: a public health nurse may have also performed duties of an epidemiologist, such as outbreak investigation; a health educator may have also assisted with health facility inspection. Although the public health professionals continue to work in **multidisciplinary teams** (work groups composed of

or combining several usually separate fields of expertise) and are cross-trained to some extent, public health disciplines have become much more specialized as the number of accredited schools and programs of public health have increased in the United States (Figure 18-1).

PUBLIC HEALTH EDUCATION

The first U.S. school of public health was founded in 1916 but the process of formally accrediting these schools did not begin until the 1940s; two decades later, the first program of public health (outside of a school of public health) was accredited. The number of schools and programs grew steadily until the 2000s at

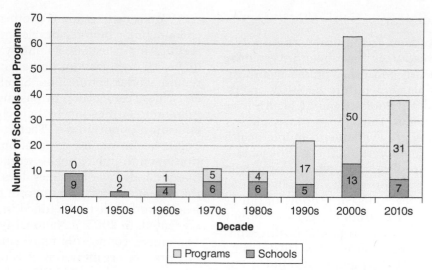

FIGURE 18-1   The Growth of Schools and Programs of Public Health in the United States, 1940s–2010s

which point a dramatic and rapid expansion occurred (see Figure 18-1). The increased availability of public health degree programs at the graduate level and, more recently, at the undergraduate level, in on-campus and distance learning formats has greatly improved the accessibility of public health education. Not all public health graduates choose to work in public health practice; however, it seems reasonable to expect increases in the percentage of public health workers with formal public health education in future years.

The academic core of a public health Master's (MPH) degree program, which is the most common type of public health degree, includes courses in the following five areas: biostatistics, epidemiology, environmental health sciences, health services administration/policy, and social and behavioral sciences, described in Table 18-3. All schools and programs of public health accredited by the Council on Education for Public Health (CEPH), the main national accrediting body, are required to offer courses in these areas; many also offer courses in areas such as global public health, health information/informatics, public health genetics, health disparities, and maternal and child health, among other specialty areas. Some of these areas have more recently been developed into formal degree offerings; in particular global public health, public health preparedness, and health information technology are offered as MPH concentrations through a number of schools and programs of public health.

TABLE 18-3   Knowledge Areas of the Core Academic Components of Accredited Master of Public Health Programs

Biostatistics	Collection, storage, retrieval, analysis, and interpretation of health data; design and analysis of health-related surveys and experiments; and concepts and practice of statistical data analysis
Epidemiology	Distributions and determinants of disease, disabilities and death in human populations; the characteristics and dynamics of human populations; and the natural history of disease and the biologic basis of health
Environmental Health Sciences	Environmental factors including biological, physical, and chemical factors that affect the health of a community
Health Services Administration	Planning, organization, administration, management, evaluation, and policy analysis of health and public health programs
Social and Behavioral Sciences	Concepts and methods of social and behavioral sciences relevant to the identification and solution of public health problems

SOURCE: Council on Education for Public Health

Continuing Education

Beyond educating students for future work in public health, substantial resources have been invested by schools of public health and other public health organizations to train current public health workers. The IOM reported that schools of public health have a responsibility to ensure that appropriate, quality education and training are available to public health professionals, other members of the public health workforce, and health professionals who participate in public health activities.[2] As a result, federally funded training centers were developed at schools of public health across the country to train the existing public health workforce in foundational public health skills. A large national network of Public Health Training Centers (funded by the HRSA) and CDC-funded Preparedness and Response Learning Centers have offered trainings using distance learning and a variety of other modalities to offer instruction which is provided by public health professionals and faculty covering a diverse array of public health topics ranging from short courses related to the five academic core areas of public health, to emergency preparedness and response. These trainings tend to be more applied in nature in order to provide knowledge and skills that the public health worker can integrate into his or her daily job tasks immediately and often provide continuing education credit to meet certification or licensure requirements.

Licensure and Certification

In keeping with trends of greater professionalization and training of the public health workforce, there has been a concurrent increase in the requirement for and monitoring of worker licensure and certification. There are several methods for verifying that workers are adequately trained and capable of performing the duties required by their positions. Some health professionals are required to obtain a state license by passing an examination in order to practice their profession. Examples common among public health workers include M.D. licenses for physicians, R.N. licenses for nurses, R.S. licenses for sanitarians, and R.D. licenses for dietitians. Maintaining licensure generally requires the worker to complete training courses to achieve a minimum number of continuing education credits within specific time intervals and then report those credits periodically to a state licensing board. Licensure may be an effective way to ensure workers continue to hone and maintain their skills; however, only a minority of the overall public health workforce is eligible for licensure, as there is no license for most disciplines within the public health workforce.

Worker certification is another common method for encouraging workforce development. Unlike licensure, certification is usually voluntary, although some public health organizations and agencies may individually require worker certification. Similar to licensure, workers achieve certification by passing an examination and maintain certification by participating in continuing education opportunities. There are many examples of public health worker certification; however, a certification open to public health workers of all educational backgrounds and disciplines does not yet exist. Perhaps the closest example of a uniform certification for public health workers is the Certified in Public Health (CPH) credential. In 2005, a National Board of Public Health Examiners, comprising representatives from academic and practice organizations, was formed to develop and administer a voluntary certification exam for graduates of public health schools and programs. The CPH is intended to distinguish public health workers who have "mastered knowledge and skills relevant to contemporary public health."[13] Eligibility for certification was expanded in 2013 to include public health professionals who have taken core public health courses at an accredited institution and have relevant job experience or other education. The CPH is the field's only certification for which all public health disciplines are eligible.

Other examples of certification in public health are discipline specific. Physicians and nurses may achieve board certification in public health through a combination of completing clinical or preventive medicine residency programs, successfully passing board examinations, and enrolling in other advanced training or fellowship programs. Workers with a degree and/or substantial experience in health education are eligible to sit for a Certified Health Education Specialist (CHES) exam, which is also offered at a Master's level for advanced health educators. Finally, public health laboratory workers are eligible for a variety of generalist and specialist certifications within their field.

WORKFORCE COMPETENCIES

Public health education and training, whether provided by a school of public health or through a training center's online offerings, is increasingly being guided by the development of competencies. Competencies form the cornerstone of efforts by schools and programs of public health, governmental public health agencies, and many public health professional groups to more systematically ensure that public health workers are equipped with the appropriate level of skills and knowledge to competently and effectively carry out their work.

Public health workforce competencies are the foundational knowledge, skills, and abilities necessary for public health professionals to efficiently and effectively deliver the services deemed essential to public health. Competencies themselves should be action-oriented and clearly describable, observable, and measurable. The CDC, IOM, and the Association of Schools and Programs of Public Health (ASPPH) have all strongly endorsed competency development in order to strengthen the public health workforce. Competencies improve the workforce by providing a framework for developing educational and training programs, delineating worker roles and responsibilities, and permitting a means for assessing worker performance and organizational capacity. The first public health workforce competencies were developed in the 1980s; more recently many national public health worker specialty groups including the Council of State and Territorial Epidemiologists (CSTE), the Association of Public Health Laboratorians, the Quad Council of Public Health Nursing Organizations, the

National Commission for Health Education Credentialing, and the CDC, among others, have developed comprehensive worker competencies specific to their profession (see Table 18-4).[14–18] These practitioner and profession-specific competencies are complemented by more general public health competencies such as the Core Competencies for Public Health Professionals developed by the Council on Linkages Between Academia and Public Health Practice—developed for all public health workers[19]—and the more academically oriented public health core competencies for MPH students enrolled in academic degree programs, developed by the ASPPH Education Committee. For educational accreditation, CEPH requires academic programs to clearly identify the competencies expected of their graduates and to indicate how course-specific learning objectives will lead to the acquisition of these competencies.[20] Competencies are further addressed in detail in Appendix B.

A common basis for many of these public health worker competencies is the *10 Essential Services of Public*

TABLE 18-4   Public Health Workforce Competency Sets

Competency Set	Lead Organization	Date	Notes
Bioterrorism and Emergency Readiness: Competencies for All Public Health Workers	Columbia University School of Nursing Center for Health Policy & Centers for Disease Control and Prevention	2002	
Applied Epidemiology Competencies	Council of State and Territorial Epidemiologists	2006	Three tiers: Beginner, Midlevel, and Senior Epidemiologist
Master's Degree in Public Health Core Competency Development Project (v. 2.3)	Association of Schools of Public Health	2006	
Competencies for Public Health Informaticians	Centers for Disease Control and Prevention & University of Washington Center for Public Health Informatics	2009	
Areas of Responsibility, Competencies, and Subcompetencies for Health Education Specialists	National Commission for Health Education Credentialing, Inc.	2010	
Quad Council Competencies for Public Health Nurses	Quad Council of Public Health Nursing Organizations	2011	
Guidelines for Biosafety Laboratory Competency	Centers for Disease Control and Prevention	2011	
Competency Guidelines for Public Health Laboratory Professionals	Centers for Disease Control and Prevention & Association of Public Health Laboratories	2014	
Core Competencies for Public Health Professionals	The Council on Linkages Between Academia and Public Health Practice	2014	(This is the newest version)

Health (ESPH) (Table 18-5), described earlier in this textbook (see, e.g., Chapters 1, 2, and 11). First formulated in 1994 by the Public Health Functions Steering Committee, these 10 key services summarize the major activities of the workforce in carrying out the responsibilities of public health and form the core from which necessary worker knowledge, skills, and abilities are derived. For example, the CSTE Applied Epidemiology Competencies and the six national capacity assessments based on those competencies focus on them largely in the context of carrying out just four ESPH which are perceived to have a significant epidemiological focus: ESPH 1 (Monitoring), 2 (Investigate), 9 (Evaluate), and 10 (Research).

PUBLIC HEALTH WORKFORCE CAPACITY

There have been an increasing number of researchers, practitioners, and policy makers acknowledging the need to identify factors that contribute to **workforce capacity**, or the ability of the public health workforce to perform the necessary tasks to effectively deliver the essential public health services. Deficiencies in organizational capacity have been theorized to negatively impact

TABLE 18-5 The 10 Essential Public Health Services

1. Monitor health status to identify community health problems.
2. Diagnose and investigate health problems and health hazards in the community.
3. Inform, educate, and empower people about health issues.
4. Mobilize community partnerships to identify and solve health problems.
5. Develop policies and plans that support individual and community health efforts.
6. Enforce laws and regulations that protect health and ensure safety.
7. Link people to needed personal health services, and assure the provision of health care when otherwise unavailable.
8. Assure a competent public health and personal health care workforce.
9. Evaluate effectiveness, accessibility, and quality of personal- and population-based health services.
10. Research for new insights and innovative solutions to health problems.

SOURCE: Centers for Disease Control and Prevention

the ability to sustain public health programs and interventions[21-22] and workforce capacity contributes significantly to the overall capacity of an organization to deliver services. Many factors can contribute to workforce capacity. Individual factors such as educational and training background, job experience, and job satisfaction may play a role, as well as organizational factors such as whether the organization supports continuing education for employees. Workforce capacity is an important concept that needs further research to determine how it may be enhanced and to what extent organizational performance may be improved as a result. Consensus among public health systems and services researchers and public health practitioners as to how and what to measure in order to most accurately assess workforce capacity remains elusive although interest in this area continues to grow.

Public Health Department Accreditation

Accreditation is the process by which health department performance is assessed against a set of nationally recognized, practice-focused and evidence-based standards that are continually developed and revised. Ultimately, the goal of the national accreditation program is to improve and protect the health of the public by advancing the quality and performance of tribal, state, local, and territorial health departments while also increasing value and accountability to public health stakeholders. The Public Health Accreditation Board (PHAB), a nonprofit entity charged with developing accreditation standards and measures as well as evaluating health departments' abilities to achieve them, strongly supports development of the nation's governmental public health workforce. In addition to the various standards and measures that detail tasks and responsibilities expected of public health workers, there are also accreditation criteria that focus on ensuring that a sufficient number of workers are staffing health departments, and that those workers are well-qualified. PHAB encourages the development of a competent workforce by requiring health departments to regularly assess staff competencies and address gaps through training opportunities.[23-24] The PHAB standards and measures include a domain focused on maintaining a competent public health workforce. The two standards within this domain require health departments to: encourage the development of a sufficient number of qualified public health workers; and, ensure a competent workforce through assessment of staff competencies, the provision of individual training and professional development, and the provision of a supportive work environment.[24] Accreditation measures such as these promote the development of a well-trained workforce that can effectively deliver public health services in health departments.

WORKFORCE RESEARCH

Research on the public health workforce is typically included under the broader umbrella of public health services and systems research (PHSSR) which is defined as a field of study that examines the organization, finance, and delivery of public health services in communities and the impact of these services on public health.

In the last few years especially, numerous national workgroups have been convened, meetings held; and papers written on public health workforce research needs. Recently, a number of central themes have been developed to guide the public health workforce research agenda[25] and public health workforce has been specifically identified as one of the four main thematic areas of PHSSR in a 2012 journal supplement (as shown in Table 18-6).[26] The progress in the conduct of research on these themes varies and, for example, while the evidence base on public health worker enumeration and competency development have both rapidly advanced, in contrast we have made very little headway in examining issues around (the lack of) workforce diversity and disparities, or in addressing the clear lack of diversity in the current public health workforce, especially in leadership positions. Nonetheless, these themes provide a research roadmap that hopefully will establish a basis for guiding future efforts to develop a competent, sustainable, and diverse public health workforce through evidence-based training, career and leadership development, and strategic workforce planning to improve population health outcomes.

LEADERSHIP

Leadership is the "process of persuasion or example by which an individual influences a group to act toward a common goal."[27] In this definition emphasis is placed on the processes associated with the practice of leadership (rather than the personality of the leader). It then follows that effective leadership is characterized by

TABLE 18-6 Public Health Workforce Research Priority Areas

Worker enumeration
Demand, supply, and shortages
Diversity and disparities
Recruitment and retention
Workforce competencies
Educational methods and curricula

SOURCE: Consortium from Altarum Institute, CDC, the Robert Wood Johnson Foundation, and the National Coordinating Center for Public Health Services and Systems Research

adherence to certain behaviors which can contribute to improved performance by "followers" and to increased organizational effectiveness.

In this section, some of the theoretical research on leadership practice will be reviewed with a particular emphasis on applicability to public health practice. Since an emphasis on practice and improving leadership behaviors flows from that research, a discussion of various programs designed to enhance public health leadership development will be provided. Finally, some guiding principles and best practices will be delineated as a guide for future leader development.

Leadership versus Management

The processes of leadership and management are different. The process of leadership has been distinguished from the process of management by the aphorism: "leadership is doing the right thing, management is doing things right."[28] Perhaps the most useful framework for distinguishing the two processes came from Kotter.[29] In his formulation, management is designed to provide *order and consistency*; leadership is designed to provide *change and movement*. To accomplish these goals, management consists of planning and budgeting, organizing and staffing, and controlling and problem solving. Leadership is about providing direction, aligning people, and motivating and inspiring.[29]

Another approach to distinguishing the practices of management and leadership[30] focused on the role of leaders as providing a compelling *vision* and core *strategies* while management involved translating strategies into *operational reality* using specific *tactics*. In this formulation, a vision should be "something you can see"—a visualizable mental picture that is easily communicated to others. Strategies provide the logic and limited details for how the vision can be achieved. In public health, programs are created to operationalize the strategies and apply concrete tactical solutions to problems.

Theories of Leadership Practice

The commonly used statement that "leaders are born and not made" derives from a trait perspective toward leadership.[27] As a result of this emphasis, early research on leadership practice focused on the personal attributes of effective leaders, leading to the erroneous view that a basic set of unique traits could be delineated and, as a result, aspiring leaders should be assessed with respect to those ideal traits. Selection for leadership positions then utilized an assessment and matching process.

In the mid-twentieth century, this point of view was called into question as an era of leadership development began. Since the trait theory of leadership provides a very static view of what a leader is and should be, systematic development of leadership skills and behaviors was devalued. Once this static view was called into question, the research field expanded to consider a range of theoretical foundations that led into formal approaches to developing leaders.

The Skills Approach

Seminal research[31,32] in the mid- to late-twentieth century created a useful framework for the elucidation of the skills needed for effective leadership. Katz's 1955 paper considered the skills needed at various levels of an organization. At the supervisory level, technical and human skills are needed to a greater degree than conceptual skills. As one moves "up" into a managerial position, all three skill areas take on equal importance. Once an individual reaches a top leadership position, technical skill becomes less important while human and conceptual skills are paramount.

Mumford went further by focusing on the relationship of individual attributes and competencies as they relate to leadership outcomes, such as effective problem solving and enhanced performance.[32] In his formulation, there are four key individual attributes:

- General Cognitive Ability
- Crystallized Cognitive Ability
- Motivation
- Personality

These attributes contribute to specific leadership competencies:

- *Problem-solving skills*—especially when dealing with novel and ill-defined problems
- *Social Judgment skills*—the capacity to understand people and social systems
- *Knowledge*—the accumulation of information needed to apply skills to a particular situation, along with the ability to mentally structure and communicate that knowledge

This skills-based framework has fostered the use of a range of educational approaches designed to enhance creative problem solving, conflict resolution, listening, and teamwork.[27]

The Situational Approach

Building upon the skills approach, research then evolved to consider ways in which leadership styles should be adapted to different situations, particularly as they relate to the developmental level of the follower.[33] This approach takes into account the degree to which leaders should focus energy and attention on tasks versus the development of relationships. For example, in situations where the "follower" is less developed, a directive is called for; whereas, more developed followers can be supported or delegated to. A central challenge of this approach lies in the ability of the leader to correctly assess the developmental level of another person and to adapt his/her style accordingly.

Transformational Leadership

A more popular, recent theory of leadership practice is transformational leadership, which is contrasted with transactional leadership. As described by Burns,[34] transformational leadership taps the motives of followers and establishes an interaction between leaders and followers toward achievement of a common goal. In contrast, transactional leadership relies on the exchange of some type of contingent reward from the leader in order to elicit a behavior on the part of the follower.[35] Transformational leadership is seen as evoking a more enduring level of motivation and a level of performance beyond expectations.

Kouzes and Posner[36] articulated a set of five fundamental practices which provide strategies for practicing transformational leadership:

- Model the Way
- Inspire a Shared Vision
- Challenge the Process
- Enable Others to Act
- Encourage the Heart

This practice-oriented approach emphasizes that certain behaviors can lead to better organizational outcomes and can be learned by the developing leader.

Servant Leadership

Robert Greenleaf in his classic book, *Servant Leadership*,[37] articulated a view of leadership that has resonated for many:

> Servant leadership begins with the natural feeling that one wants to serve, to serve *first*....The best test is: do those served grow as persons and will the least privileged in society benefit.[37]

Servant leadership behaviors can then be described as including listening, showing empathy and awareness, committing to the growth of others, and building community.[38] Within the context of public health practice, the servant leadership philosophy has had particular resonance as a foundation for various approaches to the development of public health leaders.

Leadership Development in Public Health

As theories of leadership evolved and an emphasis on developing leaders increased, organized programs were created to develop public health leaders beginning in 1990.

The National Public Health Leadership Institute

Following the IOM report on *The Future of Public Health*,[3] the CDC, under the leadership of Director

Dr. William Roper, committed to an extensive effort to strengthen the public infrastructure in 1990. Within this context, leadership development was identified as a top priority and the National Public Health Leadership Institute (PHLI) was formed in 1991. The mission of the PHLI was to provide top public health leaders with a high-quality development opportunity in which they were exposed to new perspectives related to the practice of leadership within the public health system. The PHLI program was initially designed and managed by a team of California public health leaders; the program was later managed out of the University of North Carolina.

Over the 20 years of its existence (1991–2011), the Public Health Leadership Institute included nearly 1,000 scholars in top public health leadership positions, including a former U.S. Surgeon General, top CDC and other federal health agency leaders, numerous state and local health directors, the National Association of County and City Health Officials (NACCHO) and Association of State and Territorial Health Officials (ASTHO) presidents, the current Food and Drug Administration commissioner, the CEO of CARE, a senior vice president of a major health foundation, presidents and executive directors of the American Public Health Association, Association of Schools of Public Health, Public Health Foundation, Association of Public Health Laboratories, deans and professors in schools of public health, and leaders in many other major health organizations.[39]

An evaluation[40,41] of the impact of the PHLI program revealed that 81 percent of PHLI graduates developed a better understanding of leadership principles and practices; 73 percent developed new or better leadership skills and behaviors, such as skills in leading collaborations and managing teams; 82 percent developed an enhanced awareness of their own personal leadership behaviors through the use of 360 degree assessment, team interaction, and executive coaching; 55 percent developed a professional knowledge-sharing network focusing on public health leadership practice, which continued for many years after graduation; and 19 percent obtained new or higher level positions as a result of PHLI participation. PHLI graduates also led the creation of new policies and laws guiding the practice of public health such as increasing cigarette taxes, developing a state trauma registry system, and passage of a smoke-free workplace act. Finally, graduates increased funding for public health programs including legislation providing $1.9 million for local public health departments and an increase in funding for school nurses.

Another benefit of the PHLI program was the creation of an alumni network, the Public Health Leadership Society (PHLS), which brought together PHLI alumni and alumni of other similar programs to enhance lifelong learning. An important contribution of the PHLS was the creation of a Public Health Code of Ethics,[42] which is discussed in greater detail in Chapter 5.

The National Public Health Leadership Development Network

In 1994, the National Public Health Leadership Network (led by the Saint Louis University College for Public Health and Social Justice) was formed to share information and to develop collaboration across the growing number of state, regional, and national public health leadership institutes. The network of leadership institutes ultimately expanded through academic and practice collaboration among schools of public health and state public health departments, resulting in the establishment of 12 state-based institutes, 10 regional institutes, 6 national institutes, and 3 international institutes. As a result, 47 states plus the District of Columbia and Puerto Rico had access to a state, regional, or national public health leadership program. These programs graduated over 6,000 public health practitioners from across the world. A full report on these public health leadership programs can be accessed through http://www.heartlandcenters.slu.edu.

Furthermore, the network created a competency set which guided the design and development of public health leadership institutes for over a decade.[43]

The National Leadership Academy for the Public's Health

The National Leadership Academy for the Public's Health (NLAPH) began in 2011 to provide training to four-person multisector teams from across the country to advance their leadership skills and to achieve health equity in their communities. The program, managed by the Public Health Institute in Oakland, California, uses an experiential learning process that includes webinars, a multiday retreat, coaching, peer networking, and an applied population health project.

In its first year, NLAPH was successful in advancing participants' leadership skills, strengthening team functioning, increasing intersectoral collaboration, and helping teams make progress on their community health improvement project. Through 2014, 69 teams from 33 states along with two national teams have participated in the NLAPH program.

Schools of Public Health and Academic Public Health Programs

Some schools of public health and academic public health programs have included courses in the curriculum related to leadership theory and practice. Often, graduate public health students may have access to leadership development experiences through business schools within their own university. Some schools (e.g., University of North Carolina at Chapel Hill, University of Illinois at Chicago, and Harvard) have developed doctoral programs in public health leading to DrPH degrees that focus on leadership practice and provide opportunities to develop leadership skills as part of a formal degree program.

In 2009, the Association of Schools of Public Health developed a set of competencies for DrPH programs which included specific leadership competencies to develop the ability to create and communicate a shared vision for a positive future; inspire trust and motivate others; and use evidence-based strategies to enhance essential public health services. (More information can be found at http://www.aspph.org by searching "DrPH Model.") Graduates of such DrPH programs are expected to acquire the following leadership skills:

▸ Communicate an organization's mission, shared vision, and values to stakeholders.
▸ Develop teams for implementing health initiatives.
▸ Collaborate with diverse groups.
▸ Influence others to achieve high standards of performance and accountability.
▸ Guide organizational decision making and planning based on internal and external environmental research.
▸ Prepare professional plans incorporating lifelong learning, mentoring, and continued career progression strategies.
▸ Create a shared vision.
▸ Develop capacity-building strategies at the individual, organizational, and community level.
▸ Demonstrate a commitment to personal and professional values.

These competencies now provide a basis for curriculum development and course creation in schools of public health and academic public health programs.

Leadership Development Programs Sponsored by National Public Health Organizations

Both ASTHO (http://www.astho.org) and NACCHO (http://www.naccho.org) have sponsored programs designed to enhance leadership skills in directors of state or local health departments. ASTHO has also created a leadership development experience designed for senior deputies. Each of these programs relies on a competency-based format and a cohort model in which peer learning and network development is enhanced. The NACCHO program—the "Survive and Thrive Program"—pairs experienced local health directors

with new health directors in a mentoring relationship. Funding from the Robert Wood Johnson and de Beaumont Foundations has been essential to support these programs.

Leadership Development Needs at Stages of Career Development

As leaders develop, they may evolve through a series of stages in which developmental needs differ.[44] The emerging leader (sometimes referred to as a "rising star") needs to be identified and assisted in developing a personal awareness of their unique talents and abilities. Further, these emerging leaders benefit from exposure to leadership concepts and theories (as noted above) and involvement in a formal mentoring relationship. Emerging leaders should seek out a mentor, rather than hoping one will come along.

At a later stage, often when a young leader enters a full-time job situation, needs evolve as she/he enters the stage of the "early leader." In this stage, technical skills are often central in public health occupations (e.g., epidemiology); however, leadership development must also advance skills in adaptive change. At this stage, formal 360 degree assessments are useful along with participation in formal leadership development programs of the type noted above. Peer networks are also of great value as ways to share lessons learned and promote lifelong learning.

As leaders progress to becoming established leaders, they will continue to benefit from activities noted at earlier developmental stages and should take note of the need for ongoing peer-to-peer interaction with a structured approach to formal executive coaching. Often, established leaders fail to commit to leadership development as they become saddled with increasing responsibilities. Participation in some type of formal development program suited to their needs can offset the tendency to procrastinate with regard to ongoing leadership learning.

Finally, as leaders enter the emeritus stage of their careers, they may be uniquely qualified to serve as coaches and mentors to those at early career stages. In this way, these individuals may pass on the wisdom of experience that goes beyond formal courses or programs in leadership.

PROFILES IN PUBLIC HEALTH LEADERSHIP

Many of the principles and practices noted above are exemplified daily in the work of public health leaders. Two examples (from many hundreds not described here) are useful in providing concrete examples of the practice of public health leadership, as shown below in Exhibit 18-1.

EXHIBIT 18-1   Leadership Profiles

JOHN AUERBACH

As Director of the Massachusetts Commission of Public Health, John Auerbach led efforts to capture and codify the role of public health in the Massachusetts Health Reform effort that has served as a national model for health system change. In an article titled: "Lessons From the Front Line: The Massachusetts Experience of the Role of Public Health in Health Care Reform,"[45] he stated five key principles that enabled public health contributions to landmark health policy change:

1. Get a Seat at the Table
2. Take an Open Minded and Critical Look at What Public Health Does Now
3. Defend the Traditional Public Health Approach When Called For
4. Keep on the Lookout for Opportunities
5. Envision a Better Model and Take Steps to Make It Real

These principles, which were instrumental in leading the Massachusetts Health Reform effort, reflect the leadership attributes described in this section and are broadly applicable to other public health challenges and opportunities.

PAUL KUEHNERT

As Director of the Kane County (Illinois) Health Department, Paul Kuehnert was faced with a daunting challenge during the Great Recession of 2008. Budget cuts prompted an in-depth reassessment of the role of the public health agency that ultimately led to the transfer of personal health services out of the health agency into three federally qualified health centers and a reduction in the agency workforce by 50 percent.[46] This case study exemplifies the practice of front line leadership within a public health agency (in addressing major organizational changes) as well as leadership outside the agency (to navigate major political challenges related to accomplishing unprecedented organizational change).

SUMMARY

The public health workforce comprises a diverse group of health professionals who are uniquely varied in terms of the education, skills, and experience they bring to the job, although all share a common awareness of and commitment to improving health through a population focus. Over the last decade the public health workforce, unlike other health professions, has grown smaller while also increasing in occupational diversity to encompass new fields such as health informatics, public health genetics, and emergency preparedness. The opportunities for public health training and education have never been greater as the number of programs and schools of public health have rapidly expanded along with more options for continuing education. The result is an increasingly professionalized public health workforce that has been further strengthened by enhancements to competency-based trainings, worker certification, and accreditation of public health agencies. Despite these advances, too little is known about the number and type of public health workers and the reasons they enter and leave the workforce.

A key concept related to workforce is that of leadership, defined as the "process of persuasion or example by which an individual influences a group to act toward a common goal." Leadership is essential to the realization of a shared vision, and a number of theories have been developed regarding the skills required for effective leadership, although "servant leadership" is an especially compelling model. Outstanding leadership for the public health workforce will be needed to successfully address the challenges and opportunities to improve and protect the public's health in the twenty-first century.

REVIEW QUESTIONS

1. What are some of the professions that comprise the public health workforce and what do they share in common?

2. What are some of the key trends in public health worker professionalization?

3. What are competencies and why are they valuable? What are some of the public health professions which have developed profession-specific competencies?

4. How does the practice of leadership differ from the practice of management?

5. What are the key features of servant leadership?

6. What do "early leaders" need to enhance their own leadership skill development?

REFERENCES

1. Drehobl P, Stover BH, Koo D. On the road to a stronger public health workforce: visual tools to address complex challenges. *Am J Prev Med.* 2014;47(5S3):S280–S285.

2. Institute of Medicine. *Who will keep the public healthy? Educating public health professionals for the 21st century.* Washington, DC: The National Academies Press; 2003.

3. Institute of Medicine. *The Future of Public Health.* Washington, DC: National Academy Press; 1988.

4. Gebbie K. Community-based health care: an introduction. In: Brennan P, Schneider S, Tornquist E, eds. *Information Networks for Community Health* (pp. 3–14). New York: Springer-Verlag; 1997.

5. Patient Protection and Affordable Care Act, 42 U.S.C. § 18001; 2010.

6. U.S. Bureau of Labor Statistics. Occupational employment statistics: community health workers. http://www.bls.gov/oes/current/oes211094.htm. Published 2013.

7. Merrill J, Btoush R, Gupta M, Gebbie K. A history of public health workforce enumeration. *J Public Health Manag Pract.* 2003;9(6):459–470.

8. Beck AJ, Boulton ML. Enumeration of the governmental public health workforce, 2014. *Am J Prev Med.* 2014;47(5S3):S306–S313.

9. Boulton ML, Beck AJ, Coronado F, et al. Public health workforce taxonomy. *Am J Prev Med.* 2014;47(5S3):S314–S323.

10. CDC. Assessment of epidemiologic capacity in state and territorial health departments—United States, 2004. *MMWR.* 2005;54(18):457–459.

11. Honore PA. Aligning public health workforce competencies with population health improvement goals. *Am J Prev Med.* 2014;47(5S3), S344–S345.

12. Council of State and Territorial Epidemiologists. 2013 National Assessment of Epidemiology Capacity: Findings and Recommendations. Atlanta, GA: CSTE. http://www.cste2.org/2013eca/CSTE EpidemiologyCapacityAssessment2014-final2.pdf. Published 2014.

13. National Board of Public Health Examiners. About NBPHE. http://www.nbphe.org/aboutnbphe.cfm. Published 2014.

14. CDC/Council of State and Territorial Epidemiologists. Competencies for applied epidemiologists in governmental public health agencies. Atlanta, GA: CDC. http://www.cdc.gov/appliedepicompetencies/. Published 2008.

15. CDC/University of Washington School of Public Health and Community Medicine's Center for Public Health Informatics. Competencies for public health informaticians. http://www.cdc.gov/informaticscompetencies/downloads/PHI_Competencies.pdf. Published 2009.

16. Columbia University School of Nursing Center for Health Policy/CDC. Bioterrorism & emergency readiness competencies for all public health workers. New York: Columbia University; 2002.

17. Quad Council of Public Health Nursing Organizations. Quad Council competencies for public health nurses. http://www.phf.org/resourcestools/Pages/Public_Health_Nursing_Competencies.asp. Published 2011.

18. National Commission for Health Education Credentialing, Inc. Areas of responsibility, competencies, and subcompetencies for health education specialists. http://www.nchec.org/_files/_items/nch-mr-tab3-59/docs/areas%20of%20responsibilities%20competencies%20and%20sub-competencies%20for%20the%20health%20education%20specialist%202010.pdf. Published 2010.

19. Council on Linkages Between Academia and Public Health Practice. Core Competencies for public health professionals. http://www.phf.org/resourcestools/pages/core_public_health_competencies.aspx. Published 2010.

20. Council on Education for Public Health Understanding accreditation. http://ceph.org/constituents/understanding-accreditation/. Published 2014.

21. Hawe P, Noort M, King L, Jordens, C. Multiplying health gains: the critical role of capacity building within health promotion programs. *Health Policy.* 1997;39(1): 29–42.

22. Schwartz R, Smith C, Speers MA, et al. (1993). Capacity building and resource needs of state health agencies to implement community-based cardiovascular disease programs. *J Public Health Policy.* 1993;14(4):480–493.

23. Bender KW, Kronstadt JL, Wilcox R, Tilson HH. Public health accreditation addresses issues facing the public health workforce. *Am J Prev Med.* 2014;47(5S3):S346–S351.

24. Public Health Accreditation Board. Standards & Measures v. 1.5. http://www.phaboard.org/wp-content/uploads/SM-Version-1.5-Board-adopted-FINAL-01-24-2014.docx.pdf. Published 2013.

25. Consortium from Altarum Institute, CDC, the Robert Wood Johnson Foundation, and the

National Coordinating Center for Public Health Services and Systems Research. A national research agenda for public health services and systems. *Am J Prev Med.* 2012;42(5S1):S72–S78.

26. Scutchfield FD, Perez DJ, Monroe JA, Howard AF. New public health services and systems research agenda: directions for the next decade. *Am J Prev Med.* 2012;45(5S1):S1–S5.

27. Northouse PG. *Leadership, Theory and Practice, Sixth Edition.* Los Angeles, CA: Sage Publications; 2013.

28. Bennis W, Nanus B. *Leaders: The Strategies for Taking Charge.* New York, NY: Harper & Row; 1985.

29. Kotter J. *A Force for Change: How Leadership Differs from Management.* New York, NY: Free Press; 1990.

30. Baker EL, Orton, SN. Practicing management and leadership: vision, strategy, operations and tactics. *J Public Health Manag Pract.* 2010;16(5):470–471.

31. Katz R. Skills of an effective administrator. *Harvard Bus Rev.* 1955;33(1):33–42.

32. Mumford MD, Zaccaro SJ, Harding FD, et al. Leadership skills for a changing world: Solving complex social problems. *Leadership Quart.* 2000;11(1):11–35.

33. Blanchard K, Zigami P. *Leadership and the One Minute Manager.* New York, NY: William Morrow and Company; 1985.

34. Burns JM. *Leadership.* New York, NY: Harper & Row;1978.

35. Bass BM, Aviolio BJ, Pointon J. The implications of transactional and transformational leadership for individual, team and organizational development. *Research in Organizational Change and Development.* 1990; 231–272.

36. Kouzes J, Posner B. *The Leadership Challenge.* San Francisco, CA: Jossey-Bass; 2002.

37. Greenleaf R. *Servant Leadership.* New York, NY: Paulist Press; 1977.

38. Spears L. *Focus on Leadership- Servant Leadership for the 21st Century.* New York, NY: John Wiley; 2002.

39. Baker EL. Investing in public health leadership. *J Public Health Manag Pract.* 2011;17(3): 291–292.

40. Umble KE, Baker EL, Woltring C. An evaluation of the National Public Health Leadership Institute-1991–2006: part I. Developing individual leaders. *J Public Health Manag Pract.* 2011;17(3):202–213.

41. Umble KE, Baker EL, Diehl SJ, et al. An evaluation of the National Public Health Leadership Institute-1991–2006: part II. Strengthening public health leadership networks, systems and infrastructure. *J Public Health Manag Pract.* 2011;17(3):214–224.

42. Thomas JC, Sage M, Dillenberg J, Guillory VJ. A code of ethics for public health. *Am J Public Health.* 2002;92(7):1057–1059.

43. Wright K, Rowitz L, Merkle A, et al. Competency development in public health leadership. *Am J Public Health.* 2000;90(8):1202–1207.

44. Baker EL. The Evolution of a leader. *J Public Health Manag Pract.* 2011;17(5):475–477.

45. Auerbach J. (2013). Lessons from the front line: the Massachusetts experience of the role of public health in health care reform. *J Public Health Manag Pract.* 2013;19(5):488–491.

46. Kuehnert P, M. K. (2012). Tough Choices in tough times: enhancing public health value in an era of declining resources. *J Public Health Manag Pract.* 2012; 18(2), 115–125.

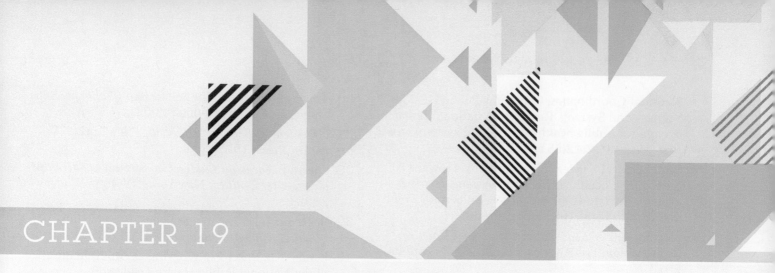

CHAPTER 19

Maternal and Child Health

Carol Hogue, PhD, MPH • Cassandra M. Gibbs Pickens, MPH

LEARNING OBJECTIVES

Upon completion of this chapter, the reader will be able to:

1. Describe the maternal and child health (MCH) impact of 8 of the 10 major public health accomplishments of the twentieth century.

2. Relate these accomplishments to the 10 Essential Public Health Services.

3. Describe the major federal programs that fund MCH services, with respect to their history and current function.

4. Apply this understanding to twenty-first century MCH problems, such as asthma and childhood obesity.

5. Describe the interplay among advocacy, public opinion, public policies, and public health as applied to family planning services and child health and welfare services.

6. Apply this understanding toward framing effective public health advocacy, surveillance, and related programs for the near future.

KEY TERMS

family planning
infant mortality
maternal mortality
Maternal Mortality Review (MMR) Committees
Pregnancy Risk Assessment System (PRAMS)
Women, Infants, and Children (WIC)

INTRODUCTION

The United States ranked 24th in infant mortality among industrialized countries in 2010. To address this persistent and pernicious problem, U.S. Department of Health and Human Services Secretary Kathleen Sebelius formed the Secretary's Advisory Committee on Infant Mortality (SACIM) in 2012, which submitted its recommendations to her in 2013.[1] Their framework for action is based on a core set of public health principles that highlight the unique features of maternal and child health (MCH) as well as underscore the importance of the 10 Essential Public Health Services (EPHSs, first described in Chapter 2): "reflect a life course perspective, engage and empower consumers, reduce inequity and disparities and ameliorate the negative effects of social determinants, advance systems coordination and service integration, protect the existing MCH safety net programs, leverage change through multisector, public and private collaboration," and "define actionable strategies that emphasize prevention and are continually informed by evidence and measurement."[1] While the life course perspective is a relatively new principle, the other principles have inspired public health action for more than a century.

In 1999, the federal Centers for Disease Control and Prevention (CDC) published a series of articles under the general heading "Ten Great Public Health Achievements—United States, 1900–1999."[2] In 2011, CDC scientists updated this list with achievements during the first decade of the twenty-first century.[3]

These achievements reflect major contributors to death and disability that can be effectively prevented. Notably, most achievements address MCH issues. These include ones that were directly targeted at improving MCH (healthier mothers and babies and family planning), those that improved the overall health of women and children (safer and healthier foods), and those that addressed specific childhood diseases and health risks (control of infectious diseases and vaccination, motor-vehicle safety, fluoridation of drinking water, and recognition of tobacco use as a health hazard). A review of the history, current status, and future needs of MCH provides a framework for discussing the scope of these problems and the programs designed to alleviate them. Toward the latter part of the twentieth century, improvements in maternal and infant survival stalled or were reversed. Recent efforts have made some impact, but further improvement in MCH during the twenty-first century will require attention to effective implementation of the 10 EPHSs, especially for vulnerable populations, with particular attention to an examination of the rationale for public health actions and focused research on the remaining major threats to MCH.

TWO GREAT TWENTIETH-CENTURY PUBLIC HEALTH ACHIEVEMENTS

During the twentieth century, two major public health achievements were important to America's health status. The first was a focus on the health of mothers and babies, and the second was family planning.

Healthier Mothers and Babies

Early in the twentieth century, childbirth was extremely dangerous, with more than 800 maternal deaths recorded for every 100,000 live births in the United States. A death is defined as maternal if it occurs during pregnancy or delivery or up to one year after delivery, as a result of complications of the pregnancy or delivery. Sepsis (blood stream infection) related to unsafe delivery practices and illegal abortions (voluntary termination of pregnancy prior to the possibility of survival outside the womb) accounted for 40 percent of the deaths, but most of these could have been prevented if known principles of asepsis (infection control procedures) at the time of the delivery had been uniformly applied. The death rate for infants was even higher, with up to 30 percent of babies in some urban areas dying before their first birthday.[4] Many of these deaths were also preventable but required improvements in living conditions, drinking water safety, nutrition, and pasteurized milk supplies.

Recognizing these critical needs, MCH coalitions advocated for milk pasteurization as well as improved housing, nutrition, sanitation, income, and health care access. Their efforts led to the establishment of the federal Children's Bureau in 1912, which focused attention on the link between poverty and health and advocated for comprehensive welfare services for pregnant women and their infants. In 1921, this approach became law in the Maternity and Infancy Act (also known as the Sheppard-Towner Act). This act prescribed federal matching funds to establish MCH divisions in state health departments, with missions to provide maternity care services, health education, nutrition counseling, and household assistance, especially for underserved populations. However, due to limited political support, the act was not renewed in 1929. During the 1930s, as the Great Depression deepened, Congress passed the Social Security Act of 1935. However, this act separated health care and social welfare into MCH services under Title V and income assistance for indigent families (the forerunner of Aid to Families with Dependent Children [AFDC], which is now Temporary Assistance for Needy Families [TANF]).

These efforts paid off in immediate reductions in infant deaths; from 1915 to 1929, infant mortality (deaths in the first year of life per 1,000 live births) declined by almost one-third. However, it was not until the 1930s that public awareness led to effective action and a dramatic drop in maternal deaths. A 1933 White House Conference report[5] documented the association between poor obstetric practices and maternal deaths. This prompted state medical associations to establish **maternal mortality review (MMR) committees** to assess the preventability of each maternal death. Over the next two decades, these efforts led to obstetrics and delivery guidelines as well as qualifications for physicians delivering in hospitals. At the same time, the proportion of deliveries occurring in hospitals increased from about 50 percent to 90 percent, and **maternal mortality** dropped from approximately 700 to 100 per 100,000 live births. Infant mortality declined another 50 percent during this period. During the last half of the twentieth century, improvement in infant and maternal mortality slowed considerably. Although the twentieth century saw a 93 percent drop in infant mortality, more than two-thirds of that occurred prior to 1950. Factors contributing to ongoing improvement in infant morbidity and mortality in the 1980s and beyond included artificial pulmonary surfactant, which increases lung maturation among premature infants to help prevent respiratory distress syndrome; newborn screening for selected genetic and endocrine disorders, which saves lives and improves the health of several thousand babies each year; and the public health-led "Back to Sleep" movement, which educated the public about safe infant sleep positions and led to a greater than 50 percent drop in SIDS (sudden infant death syndrome) rates during the 1990s.

Only 15 percent of the dramatic drop in maternal mortality during the twentieth century occurred after 1950. Most of the pre-1950 decline may be attributed to improved delivery practices, whereas the last 15 percent was largely owing to improved abortion practices during the 1960s and 1970s. However, pregnancy-related mortality has nearly doubled since 1987, and many state maternal mortality review committees have been reinstated to address this troubling trend. It is estimated that half of the maternal deaths in the United States could be prevented with the uniform application of good obstetrics practices.[6]

Family Planning

Both maternal and child health are affected by fertility levels. Infant health is maximized when pregnancies are spaced two to four years apart. For women, childbirth risks are minimized if pregnancies occur at least two years after menarche. The more children a woman has, the greater her likelihood of experiencing major morbidity or mortality from childbirth. Childbirth risks increase with increasing maternal age, particularly for women in their mid-30s or older. Thus the timing of pregnancies as well as the number of deliveries affects both maternal and child health. Oral contraceptives, which are the most popular form of nonpermanent birth control in the United States, also have noncontraceptive health benefits, including reduced rates of pelvic inflammatory disease, endometrial and ovarian cancer, menstrual cramp discomfort, and more.[7]

Family planning is the deliberate effort by women and couples to determine the number and timing of conceptions that the woman will have. The need for universal access to family planning services was a major public health issue during the twentieth century. At the turn of the century, Margaret Sanger and her colleagues sought to make contraception available to poor women. They challenged the laws and gradually won public acceptance for provision of family planning services to married couples. Some public health departments began offering services in the 1930s, when fertility dropped to nearly replacement (the number of children needed to replace the current generation). Available methods of birth control at that time included the condom, douching, withdrawal, cervical diaphragms, and "rhythm" methods with correct knowledge of ovulation and the fertile period. Abortion was widely practiced, although it was largely illegal and often conducted under dangerous conditions, which contributed substantially to maternal mortality until the late 1960s.

With the return of prosperity following World War II, average family size in the United States increased to a peak of 3.7 children per woman in 1957. Fertility had already begun to decline again before the introduction of modern contraceptives—the first oral contraceptive pill and the first intrauterine device—in the early 1960s. Concern for continued high abortion rates and lack of access to modern contraceptives prompted the Supreme Court in 1965 to nullify all remaining state laws prohibiting contraceptive use by married couples. To improve contraceptive access to poor and underserved individuals, Congress passed the Family Planning Services and Population Research Act in 1970. This created Title X of the Public Health Service Act, with funding targeted at establishing affordable family planning services. By 1980, the way was cleared for contraceptive services to be available to all, irrespective of marital status. By 2010, 8.9 million clients received publicly subsidized contraceptive services through either "publicly funded clinics" (including Title X-funded clinics) or the joint federal-state Medicaid insurance program. However, this was less than half (47 percent) of women in need of these services.[8] The resulting gap in family planning access contributes to the more than fivefold difference in unintended pregnancy rates for poor women compared with wealthier women.[9]

THE 10 ESSENTIAL PUBLIC HEALTH SERVICES FOR THE HEALTH OF WOMEN, INFANTS, AND CHILDREN

So far we have focused only on the two major public health achievements of the twentieth century that contributed most to the remarkable improvements in the health of women and infants. These achievements were social and public health programs that drastically reduced infant and maternal mortality, and improved technology and access to safe family planning practices. Of the other major public health achievements between 1990 and 2010 that were highlighted by the CDC, the following seven had significant impact on reducing morbidity and mortality for children and, to a lesser extent, for mothers:

▹ Safer and healthier foods
▹ Prevention and control of infectious diseases
▹ Vaccination
▹ Motor-vehicle safety
▹ Fluoridation of drinking water
▹ Tobacco control
▹ Reduction in childhood lead poisoning

What is common to all these achievements is that success was accomplished through what have become the 10 EPHSs. Although it is not possible in the scope of this chapter to document how each success transpired or how progress will be maintained, it is possible to illustrate how the 10 EPHSs contribute to this process. Briefly described next are some of the ways that the 10 EPHSs combated the major MCH challenges of the twentieth century as well as how they continue to combat the major MCH challenges of today. These are presented in an order that emphasizes their relevance to past, current, and future MCH impact.

Enforcing Laws and Regulations to Protect Health and Safety (EPHS 6)

Vulnerable infants and young children benefit when evidence-based laws and regulations to protect their health and safety are enforced. Major examples include protection of food and water, protection from vaccine-preventable infectious diseases, protection from motor-vehicle injuries and death, and prevention of dental caries through fluoridation of water supplies.

Food safety legislation has led to drastic decreases in illness and deaths attributable to foodborne diseases, and improved understanding of basic nutritional needs has virtually eliminated nutritional deficiency diseases such as rickets. MCH advocates continue to take the lead in these efforts. Nutritional programs, such as the Special Supplemental Food Program for Women, Infants, and Children (WIC), have reduced iron-deficiency anemia among vulnerable populations. Most recently, neural tube defects associated with folic acid deficiency are decreasing because of food fortification. A major issue yet to be addressed effectively through food safety legislation is childhood and maternal obesity, which are strongly linked to adult chronic diseases.

The sharp decline in deaths attributable to infectious diseases was driven in part by strategic vaccination campaigns and earmarked programs to increase vaccination coverage, particularly for poor children. Since the Vaccination Assistance Act of 1962, federal funds have supported the purchase and administration of a full range of childhood vaccines. Presently, the childhood vaccination schedule averts 42,000 deaths and 20 million illnesses for each birth cohort that is immunized, resulting in an estimated net direct savings of $14 billion.[3] Public school immunization requirements are state-specific and vary "in terms of the school grades covered, the vaccines included...[and] reasons for exemptions (medical reasons, religious reasons, philosophical or personal beliefs)."[10] Required vaccinations may include polio, measles, mumps, rubella, diphtheria, tetanus, and pertussis.[11] Parental refusal of traditional childhood vaccinations due to philosophical or personal beliefs has become more common in recent years, contributing to outbreaks of measles, pertussis, and other serious vaccine-preventable diseases.[10] Public health practitioners must educate parents on the low risks and substantial benefits of childhood vaccination in order to prevent further outbreaks.

One of the greatest scourges among children and youth during the twentieth century was deaths caused by motor-vehicle accidents. However, sustained efforts to increase highway safety contributed to a 90 percent decline in the overall highway death rate throughout the twentieth century. These efforts included state laws mandating car seat use and booster seat use for infants and children, respectively, as well as state laws mandating seat belt use for passengers of all ages (with some exemptions for backseat passengers[12]). Children benefit from enforcement of these laws; car seats decrease the risk of death by up to 71 percent, and booster seats decrease the chance of injury by 45 percent.[13] Encouragingly, motor-vehicle death rates have continued to decline throughout the first decade of the twenty-first century, including a 49 percent drop in pedestrian deaths among children.[3]

Developing Policies and Plans to Achieve Health Goals (EPHS 5)

Pregnant women and children have long been viewed as vulnerable populations for whom health goals require policies that fund direct health care services and supplemental financial assistance. For example, children with special health care needs (CSHCN, "those who have or are at increased risk for a chronic physical, developmental, behavioral, or emotional condition and who also require health and related services of a type or amount beyond that required by children generally"[14]) comprised 15.1 percent of all U.S. children in 2009–2010.[15] Reassuringly, 96 percent of these children had health insurance, and 62 percent reported no difficulties obtaining all the services they needed. However, 22 percent of these children lived in households with financial problems caused by their condition. The federal authorities concluded that "the indicators…paint a picture of a system of services for CSHCN that meets the needs of many children and their families. However, room for improvement still exists, especially in the systems that serve the most vulnerable children."[15]

Early twentieth-century social reformers defined MCH vulnerabilities as due to poverty, and their solutions included eliminating poverty as well as improving public health services. However, the decline in popular support for the Progressive Movement and increased professionalization of health care set the stage for a retrenchment in the 1920s. The Great Depression of the 1930s once again revealed the needs of vulnerable families and children, with public recognition of the government's obligation to protect these citizens. The Social Security Act of 1935—in particular, Title V and income assistance for indigent families—addressed these issues.

As part of the Civil Rights Movement of the 1960s and 1970s, the Progressive approach led to funding of community health centers with a broad mandate to improve public health, provide primary care, and create employment opportunities. Federal funds were distributed to states under mandates for uniform program enactment.

Simultaneously, advocacy groups for specific problems became more influential, giving rise to a checkerboard of programs. These included family planning services, WIC, school lunch programs, Title I educational assistance, and PL 94–142, which guaranteed the right to education for handicapped children. Medicaid (Title XIX), which is jointly funded by state and federal governments and which is the primary government funding mechanism for low-income women's and children's health care, was also enacted in this era. Funding for these public programs reflects a popular view that only certain individuals should receive financial help. Eligibility for assistance varies by state and program, and participation is limited in some states due to insufficient funds. Despite these limitations, numerous evaluations of WIC and other programs have concluded that most are beneficial and cost effective.

Another major shift in public support of MCH services occurred as an outgrowth of the Reagan administration's new federalism in the early 1980s, with an emphasis on saving money and improving efficiency. A smaller amount of federal funds was distributed to the states in the form of block grants with fewer "strings" attached. The MCH block grant consolidated federal funds for seven Title V categorical child health programs into a single program of formula grants. Efficiency improved in some states, but the impact of reduced programming funds and lack of assured equal access to programs within and across states is still undetermined.[16]

In the 1990s, public policies continued to shift away from governmental support for poor families. AFDC was replaced with TANF in 1997. The Personal Responsibility and Work Opportunity Reconciliation Act of 1996 ("welfare reform") established a five-year lifetime limit for cash assistance for most eligible families and required that assistance recipients participate in welfare-to-work programs. States were given more discretion over eligibility and other regulations, resulting in a rapid decrease in the number of families receiving assistance. During the early years of these sweeping changes, both the number of families receiving public assistance and the number of families with children in deep poverty declined. However, the number of families in deep poverty has increased since 2000 and now exceeds the number at the time of TANF's implementation. Concurrently, the number of families receiving TANF benefits has continued to decline.[17] Furthermore, while a principal goal of TANF was to provide employment for single mothers, the program's early successes have been lost. In 2012, 43 percent of families headed by single mothers were in poverty, while only 25 percent of families in poverty were receiving TANF support (compared to 68 percent of families at TANF's outset). Other cash credits and noncash benefits help, but in 2011, there were more than 600,000 families living in abject poverty in the United States.[17]

Although government support for indigent families decreased in the 1990s, access to medical insurance increased for poor and near-poor children through Title XXI of the Social Security Act. Title XXI established the State Children's Health Insurance Program (SCHIP) and extended coverage to children who did not qualify for Medicaid due to family incomes over the eligibility limit. In 2010, Medicaid paid for 45 percent of deliveries,[18] and over 90 percent of children ages 0–18 were covered by health insurance. Of these, 34 percent were enrolled in either Medicaid or SCHIP.[19]

As of 2009, however, 70 percent of the 6.7 million uninsured U.S. children were eligible but not enrolled in Medicaid/SCHIP.[20] The Children's Health Insurance

Program Reauthorization Act of 2009 reauthorized SCHIP and provided funds to enroll additional eligible children, while the Affordable Care Act extended SCHIP funding through 2015.

The Affordable Care Act (ACA), consisting of the Patient Protection and Affordable Care Act and the Health Care and Education Reconciliation Act of 2010, became law in March 2010. The ACA aims to improve health care access, quality, and affordability. It mandates that all individuals, with some exceptions, carry health insurance. Insurance companies can no longer reject individuals due to preexisting conditions (including pregnancy), and premiums for women cannot be higher than those for men. In addition, all plans must provide certain evidence-based preventive services at no cost to the consumer. For women, these services include contraception; screening for sexually transmitted diseases, cervical cancer, and breast cancer; screening for anemia and diabetes during pregnancy; and provision of folic acid supplements, among others.[21] Preventive services for children are numerous and include immunizations as well as assessments of oral health, mental health, behavioral health, and nutrition.[22]

Under the ACA, many individuals are eligible for Medicaid or for financial assistance to help pay for health insurance. The ACA was passed assuming that every state would expand Medicaid to adults making less than 133 percent of the federal poverty level (FPL). Under this scenario, approximately 4.6 million uninsured women aged 19–44 would become eligible for Medicaid.[23] However, as of September 2015, only 31 states and Washington, D.C. chose to expand Medicaid, resulting in an unintended coverage gap. In states that did not expand Medicaid, most adults making less than 100 percent of the FPL are ineligible for both Medicaid and financial assistance.

The ACA's effect on children's insurance coverage is unknown at the time of writing this chapter. Some experts estimate that the number of uninsured children could drop from 7.4 to 4.2 million under the ACA. Nevertheless, the number of uninsured children could increase if SCHIP is not reauthorized or funded in the future.[24] Another issue yet to be resolved is the continuing role of federal funds in support of health care services, such as Title V[25] and Title X.[26]

As the number of U.S. citizens with health insurance increases under the ACA, a competing trend is the large and growing population of undocumented residents who do not qualify for publicly funded services. All babies born in the United States are automatically citizens, which creates fissures in health care access between parents and children. How the public resolves immigration policies in this century remains to be seen.

Linking People to Needed Personal Health Services (EPHS 7)

Because of the history of public funds for vulnerable mothers and children, personal health services for many pregnant women, infants, and children have been and continue to be provided through public health clinics that receive both state and federal funding. Increasingly, states pay private providers for MCH personal health services, primarily through Medicaid and SCHIP. Nonprofit community health centers also provide primary care, health education, and health care–related transportation to medically underserved populations in many areas. Due to expanded funding under the ACA, the role that federally qualified health centers (FQHCs) play in providing primary care to mothers and children is likely to increase. For example, in 2014, a consortium of nongovernmental organizations and FQHCs won the contract for providing Title X services in Georgia, which was previously held by the Georgia Department of Public Health.

The U.S. Constitution reserves authority for health to the states, and each state decides how to organize these services and administer these programs. Some of the key programs are briefly described below.

Title V

Title V (the MCH block grant described above) is the oldest federal-state partnership, dating from the initiation of Social Security in 1935. The aim of Title V is to improve and protect the health and development of the nation's mothers, children, and youth—with emphasis on those with special health care needs and their families—by assuring comprehensive systems of care that meet the population's needs. Title V is administered at the federal level by the Health Resources and Services Administration (HRSA) and at the state level through MCH offices, generally in departments of public health. States match the federal funds on a formula basis and must demonstrate that they will use the funds for objectives within the scope of the Public Health Service's *Healthy People 2020* objectives. The scope of services supported under Title V has evolved over the decades and is currently under scrutiny after enactment of the ACA. The Association of Maternal and Child Health Programs has recommended that Title V priorities be driven by core MCH services that are based on the 10 EPHSs.[25]

WIC

WIC is a federal program administered by the U.S. Department of Agriculture and each state. WIC participation improves pregnancy outcomes and increases the likelihood that infants will receive scheduled vaccinations.[27] Monthly participation exceeds 8.5 million individuals, and eligibility is determined by income and risk of poor nutrition. Eligible pregnant and breastfeeding women and children up to five years of age receive food vouchers, infant formula, nutrition education, and referrals to other MCH services. Breastfeeding has long been recognized to benefit infants and is strongly recommended by both the American Academy of Pediatrics and the American Congress of Obstetricians and Gynecologists. Along with maternal bonding and emotional satisfaction, components of breast milk include maternal antibodies, which reduce infant infections, and oxytocin, which reduces the risk of postpartum complications. Longer-term impacts of exclusive breastfeeding for the first six months include reduced incidence among infants of asthma, ear infections, and diarrhea. For mothers, there may also be reduced risk of developing type 2 diabetes, rheumatoid arthritis, and cardiovascular disease. The *Healthy People 2020* goals for breastfeeding are 81.9 percent for initiation and 60.6 percent for continuation of exclusive breastfeeding to six months. Breastfeeding has been increasing in recent decades and reached 79 percent overall in 2011.[28] However, breastfeeding disparities do exist, and WIC providers are targeting these disparities. Breastfeeding WIC participants receive education and counseling, peer support, and materials such as breast pumps. They also enjoy expanded program eligibility and "enhanced food packages" if they exclusively breastfeed.[29]

Recent WIC program modifications increased participants' access to healthy foods and allowed "states and local WIC agencies more flexibility to meet the . . . cultural needs of WIC participants."[30] WIC benefits depend on the availability of funds, and at times, state funds may run out before the end of the fiscal year.

EPSDT

The Early Periodic Screening, Diagnosis, and Treatment Program (EPSDT) is part of Medicaid. It provides funding for preventive services for children up to age 21 who are enrolled in Medicaid. Established through the Social Security Amendments of 1967 in response to concerns about preventable conditions of military draftees and the poor health status of some children enrolled in Head Start programs, Medicaid requires that state MCH agencies provide case-finding and comprehensive health care through cooperative agreements with state Medicaid agencies. In 1989, Congress broadened comprehensive coverage of health care for children with disabilities, who may qualify for Medicaid even if their families are not otherwise eligible for Medicaid. "In its current form, the EPSDT benefit is uncommonly sweeping, not only in its primary preventive coverage (comprehensive health examinations, assessment of developmental health, and comprehensive vision, dental, and hearing care) but also in the degree to which its terms encompass all medically necessary treatments and services falling within any of Medicaid's dozens of enumerated benefit classes. . . ."[31] For example, EPSDT services include well-child screening, outreach to inform eligible families of this service, and travel assistance as needed. Children in low-income families who do not qualify for Medicaid may be covered by SCHIP or the ACA. The core required services, however, may be more limited than for children covered by EPSDT, particularly those with chronic health conditions for which amelioration can enhance development.[31]

States vary in how they enroll children in Medicaid. Some children who qualify for Supplemental Security Income (SSI) owing to their disability are automatically enrolled in Medicaid, while in other states, they must apply for it separately or do not qualify at all. Some children can get Medicaid coverage even if they do not qualify for SSI. In 2009, almost 34 million children were enrolled in EPSDT, but the percentages enrolled who were eligible to be enrolled varied from 38 percent in Arkansas to 95 percent in Idaho.[32]

Family Planning

The history of family planning was discussed earlier. Currently, family planning services are funded through Title X, Medicaid, Title V, and state funds. Most federal funds for contraceptives are now distributed to the subset of all women in need of them who also qualify for Medicaid. It was estimated that if Medicaid coverage for contraceptive services were expanded to all women in the United States whose incomes were at or below 250 percent of the FPL, there would be 722,600 fewer unintended pregnancies and 291,200 fewer abortions.[33] Title X Family Planning clinics, which include state and local health departments and community health centers, attend to approximately five million individuals annually.[34]

Recent policy developments may result in increased access to contraception in some regions and decreased access in others. Under the ACA, many states expanded Medicaid eligibility criteria, allowing nonpregnant women making up to 133 percent of the FPL to enroll. This will increase the number of women with access to free family planning services. An opposing trend is some states' actions to defund Planned Parenthood by rejecting federal monies for women's health and family planning. This has resulted in the closing of many women's health clinics. Many states also opted not to expand Medicaid.

The ACA's contraceptive mandate requires that all insurance plans cover the cost of FDA-approved prescription contraceptives. However, some employers have successfully challenged this mandate due to moral/religious objections. In the future, it is possible that the federal government may be called upon to cover the cost of contraception in these instances.[35]

Integrated Care: The Medical Home and Accountable Care Organizations

A patient-centered medical home (PCMH) has the potential to improve maternal and child health care quality, affordability, and access. A medical home is "an approach to comprehensive primary care...[It] is a health care setting that facilitates partnerships between individual patients and their personal physicians and, when appropriate, the patient's family."[36] The PCMH is designed to improve care coordination across private, public, and community health care providers and has become a large focus of Medicaid/SCHIP in recent years. Coordination is enhanced through communication between providers and is aided by the use of health information technology.

Although the concept of integrated care in MCH is not new, its importance has grown under the ACA, which provides states with funding and assistance to improve care integration. The ACA has also led to the development of accountable care organizations in Medicare and their counterpart, totally accountable care organizations, in Medicaid. A totally accountable care organization is responsible for all aspects of patient care, including physical, mental, and behavioral health services. Totally accountable care organizations receive bundled payments for each participant, which provides flexibility in how they address health and social needs. This integrated care model has the potential to improve maternal and child health care for the most vulnerable populations.

Monitoring Community Health Status through Surveillance and Surveys (EPHS 1)

Vital statistics (birth and death certificate data) are key to monitoring maternal and infant health. For example, surveillance of birth certificates revealed that an increasing proportion of births were occurring during the "early term" gestations of 37–38 completed weeks.[37] Linkage with infant death certificates further revealed that infants born at these gestations had a much higher risk of death in the first year than infants born at full term (39 completed weeks' gestation).[38] This has inspired "hard stop" quality improvement policies that prohibit elective deliveries before full term, resulting in a concomitant drop in the proportion of early term births.

Several surveillance systems are maintained by the states, with federal sponsorship and funding administered by the CDC. These systems include the Behavioral Risk Factor Surveillance System (BRFSS), the Pregnancy Nutrition Surveillance System (PNSS), the Pregnancy Risk Assessment Monitoring System (PRAMS), and the Pediatric Nutrition Surveillance System (PedNSS). BRFSS and PRAMS are ongoing, population-based surveys, whereas PNSS and PedNSS are program-based systems that use routinely collected data from federally funded public health programs.

Behavioral Risk Factor Surveillance System (BRFSS)

Begun in 1984, BRFSS is the world's largest ongoing telephone health survey system. BRFSS samples adults at random in each state. Participants respond to questions about their general health as well as specific health issues such as asthma and diabetes. They are also asked about access to preventive health care and various health-related practices such as smoking, nutrition, family planning, and more. Information from BRFSS is used to assess the prevalence of smoking, obesity, sedentary behavior, and other behavioral health risks.

Pregnancy Risk Assessment Monitoring System (PRAMS)

PRAMS samples women identified from birth certificates as recently having given birth. Some high-risk pregnancies, such as low birthweight deliveries, are oversampled. In each state, a sample of 1,300 to 3,500 women receive mailed questionnaires each year; if they do not respond, they may be contacted by telephone. As of 2014, 40 states plus New York City were participating in PRAMS.[39] PRAMS provides data not available from other sources about pregnancy intendedness; prenatal care; maternal complications during pregnancy, delivery, and the first few months postpartum; breastfeeding practices; infant health in the early months; and much more. Information from PRAMS has been used to identify women and infants at high risk for health problems (such as domestic violence), to monitor trends in health care (such as access to early prenatal care) and status (such as maternal obesity), and to track progress in achieving national and state public health goals (such as percentage of births that were intended at conception). As an example of how both PRAMS and BRFSS have been used to monitor maternal and infant health status, Huber and colleagues estimated the risk of oral contraceptive failure associated with obesity with data from the 1999 BRFSS and the 2000 PRAMS surveys in South Carolina. They found that, compared to normal-weight women, overweight women (body mass index [BMI] of 25–29.9 kg/m²) and obese women (BMI of ≥30 kg/m²) may have an increased risk of oral contraceptive failure.[40]

The Pregnancy Nutrition Surveillance System (PNSS) and the Pediatric Nutrition Surveillance System (PedNSS)

Unlike BRFSS and PRAMS, which are ongoing, population-based surveys, PNSS and PedNSS use readily available program data from the major federally funded maternal, infant, and child health programs to monitor health status and assess program impact for the population eligible for such services. PNSS uses data from WIC and Title V MCH programs. PNSS data include information on approximately 750,000 low-income, pregnant, and postpartum women. PedNSS data cover more than seven million children from birth to their fifth birthday. In some states, data from the EPSDT Program of Medicaid are combined with WIC and Title V data to provide information on children and adolescents to age 20. With these data, program analysts can track trends in the prevalence of nutritional problems such as anemia, health practices such as breastfeeding, and risk factors such as obesity among the program participants.

Ongoing Surveys

In addition to these ongoing surveillance systems, maternal and child health status may be monitored less frequently but in greater depth through ongoing surveys, such as the National Health and Nutrition Examination Survey (NHANES); the National Survey of Family Growth (NSFG); and the National Survey of Children's Health (NSCH), which will be combined with the National Survey for Children with Special Health Care Needs into an annual survey as of 2016.[41] These surveys have in common a continuous national sampling with periodic release of data for public use.

Diagnosing and Investigating Health Problems and Hazards (EPHS 2)

Investigating and diagnosing health problems and hazards is similar to monitoring community health status through surveillance and surveys, in that it is based on analysis of data. However, surveillance depends on large data sets with uniform data definitions, collected over time, whereas health problem investigation is focused on individual cases, examined with greater specificity. Maternal Mortality Review committees were highly effective during the middle of the twentieth century through application of this methodology, but most committees were disbanded and have only recently been reconstituted in some jurisdictions in response to the alarming doubling of maternal mortality since the late 1980s.

Based on the successful MMR model, HRSA, in conjunction with the American Congress of Obstetricians and Gynecologists and state and local health departments, launched a movement in the 1990s known as Fetal and Infant Mortality Review (FIMR). There are key differences between FIMR and MMR committees that reflect an understanding of the complexities involved in preventing infant mortality. First, health care providers may not be the most important change agents. The major causes of infant deaths are associated with preterm delivery (delivery at <37 completed weeks' gestation) and birth defects, and current knowledge regarding how to prevent these deaths through health care alone is highly limited. Rather, in FIMR, the underlying assumption is that currently preventable fetal and infant deaths are those in which support systems, such as prenatal care programs, are inadequate to meet the demand for services or are of insufficient quality.[42] The FIMR process includes a Community Action Team, whose job is to assure that public programs and services are responsive to the recommended remediation of the Case Review Team. Evaluation of the FIMR process found that better performance of the essential MCH services was associated with the presence of a FIMR program,[43] suggesting that the FIMR process may improve infant outcomes when fully implemented.

Additional examples of diagnosing and investigating health hazards at the local level include epidemiologic investigations of birth defects clusters or pediatric infectious disease outbreaks.

Informing, Educating, and Empowering People Regarding Health Issues (EPHS 3)

Public awareness and advocacy has driven many MCH successes. For example, when infant mortality stopped improving after 1950, public awareness grew that more could be done, especially for high-risk neonates (babies younger than 28 days) whose survival depended on intensive care in state-of-the-art facilities. During the late 1960s and early 1970s, MCH coalitions effectively lobbied to establish regional perinatal centers for high-risk infants. Largely through technological advances and improved health care access, neonatal mortality (neonatal deaths per 1000 live births) dropped 41 percent from 1970 through 1979. Concurrently, concern grew about the continued high proportion of babies born weighing less than 2,500 grams, who are at greatly increased risk of morbidity and mortality when compared to larger babies. In 1989, Congress expanded Medicaid eligibility, arguing that improved access to prenatal care would prevent low birthweight deliveries. However, although more women have entered prenatal care early, the low birthweight rate has not declined.

The information age has transformed health education and information systems. With Internet access now nearly universal, most citizens can access highly accurate information about specific health issues. The recommendations of the HHS Secretary's Advisory Committee on Infant Mortality include designing and implementing new health promotion and social marketing campaigns focused on key preventive interventions, the warning signs of pregnancy and infant complications, and what to do when these signs appear.[1]

The CDC, including the National Center for Health Statistics, NIH, and other governmental-sponsored websites at federal, state, and local levels provide a wealth of data and program information. These are briefly described in Table 19-1.

Numerous nongovernmental organizations maintain websites with easily accessible, relevant information. A few of the key ones are listed in Table 19-2.

TABLE 19-1 Governmental-Sponsored Websites Pertaining to Maternal and Child Health

Title	Website Description	Website
The National Center for Education in Maternal and Child Health's MCH Library	HRSA-sponsored website with resources about MCH for public health professionals and communities	http://www.mchlibrary.info
Title V Information System Snapshots	Annual snapshot of MCH, with data from all Title V recipients	Access https://mchdata.hrsa.gov and click on the link for "Title V Information System." Then click on the link for "State Snaphots."
Healthy People 2020: Maternal, Infant, and Child Health	List of evidence-based programs and clinical recommendations related to MCH	Access http://www.healthypeople .gov and search for "Maternal, Infant, and Child Health."

TABLE 19-2 Nongovernmental-Sponsored Websites Pertaining to Maternal and Child Health

Title	Website Description	Website
CityMatCH: The National Organization of Urban MCH Leaders	Contains detailed information about the National Perinatal Periods of Risk tool, among other topics	http://www.citymatch.org
Kaiser Family Foundation	Nonpartisan information source about women's and children's health and other issues, including data collected and analyzed by the Foundation geared to policy makers, the media, the health care community, and the public	http://www.kff.org
March of Dimes Perinatal Data Center	Provides free access to maternal and infant health-related data gleaned and analyzed from several government agencies and organizations and presented at the national, state, county, and city level, including easy-to-access PowerPoint slides	http://www.marchofdimes .com/peristats
The Alan Guttmacher Institute	Information about sexual and reproductive health in the United States and worldwide, with easy-to-access fact sheets, PowerPoint presentations, and interactive databases at the state level	http://www.guttmacher.org/
Annie E. Casey Foundation: KIDS COUNT	Provides access to the annual KIDS COUNT Data Book, with national- and state-level information on child well-being indicators	Access http://www.aecf.org/ work/ and click on the link for "Kids Count."
National Women's Law Center	Makes the counterpart document for women's health indicators, "Making the Grade on Women's Health," available for ordering	http://hrc.nwlc.org/

Mobilizing Community Partnerships to Solve Problems (EPHS 4)

Coalitions and partnerships are a hallmark of MCH advocacy. The Healthy Mothers/Healthy Babies Coalition has functioned for several decades in all states and serves in many areas as a potent force for public policy review and legislation. One of the most recent coalitions has formed around the need to assure women's health status prior to their pregnancies. Known as Preconception Care,[44] the issue is defined somewhat differently by different members of the partnership. As a known means to improve pregnancy outcome, this effort is supported by child advocacy groups such as the March of Dimes. As a means of improving women's health irrespective of whether they become pregnant, this effort is also supported by women's health advocacy groups. Whether this movement becomes successful will rely, in part, on keeping these somewhat disparate partners together in their advocacy goals.

Assuring a Skilled, Competent Public Health Workforce (EPHS 8)

As part of a larger effort to improve the public health workforce, the CDC and HRSA have focused efforts on increasing the number and competence of MCH epidemiologists, as well as nurses, health technicians, and primary care providers at all levels. Numerous educational programs have been established, including distance learning programs that address the needs of individuals already in the workforce.

MCH educators also emphasize the need of the public health workforce for cultural literacy to address the needs of an increasingly diverse population. Skills in conducting community-based participatory program development are also stressed to assure that services meet the needs of the specific community being served.

Evaluating Effectiveness, Accessibility, and Quality of Health Services (EPHS 9)

Program evaluations are keys to the appropriate use of public resources and can yield valuable information on program effectiveness. Some examples of program evaluations were provided in previous sections of this chapter. In recent years, the focus on evidence-based programming has grown. A 2013 White House brief called for a greater emphasis on evidence-based programming and government accountability, pledging to prioritize funding for programs that "showed a widespread commitment to evidence and innovation."[45] Current MCH programming adheres to this agenda. For instance, 75 percent of funds for HRSA home visiting programs must be allocated to effective program models. These include the Nurse-Family Partnership, which reduces the risk of child abuse/neglect, injuries, and poor cognitive outcomes; and Child FIRST, which reduces the risk of childhood developmental and behavioral problems and possibly childhood maltreatment, among others. Individual states have also enhanced their focus on evidence-based MCH programming. For instance, New York State is currently building an evidence base for MCH programming by funding innovative projects that will be rigorously evaluated.[46]

Another level of evaluation is to consider the impact of policies on the health issues they were designed to address. An example of this type of evaluation is the impact of increasing Medicaid eligibility for prenatal care and deliveries, which was enacted in 1989 as a means to reduce the rates of premature delivery and infant mortality. In a comprehensive review of the published studies of this question, Howell determined that the policy did increase the proportion of pregnant women receiving Medicaid-paid prenatal and delivery services, and some women entered prenatal care earlier than they would have otherwise.[47] However, there is little evidence that this policy change improved birth outcomes, and the solutions to the ongoing problems of premature delivery and birth defects remain elusive. Future policy evaluations should assess the long-term consequences of the ACA on health care affordability, access, and quality.

The ACA aims to shift the focus to quality, rather than quantity, of health services through changes in health care reporting and reimbursement. Moreover, quantity of services will no longer be a proxy for quality of health care. The ACA's emphasis on quality of health services will likely extend to the MCH realm. State Medicaid programs have begun using value-based purchasing and bundled payments, although implementation is not uniform across states.

Under the ACA, hospitals are required to publish patient satisfaction and quality ratings. The ACA's enhanced focus on patient-centered care and quality measurement may improve the standard of health services. Publishing quality and patient satisfaction ratings may be particularly important for maternity and delivery care, in which there are large disparities in quality of care by hospital.[48] However, this information is currently not publicly reported.

Other MCH quality initiatives are also underway. The 2009 SCHIP Reauthorization Act focused on developing criteria to measure quality of pediatric health care, and the Centers for Medicare and Medicaid Services sponsor several MCH-related quality improvement initiatives for Medicaid/SCHIP programs. The Maternal and Infant Health Initiative also focuses on improving the health of Medicaid/SCHIP participants by promoting increased use of postpartum care and reducing the rate of unintended pregnancies.

Researching and Applying Innovative Solutions to Health Problems (EPHS 10)

What solutions to the persistent health disparities in preterm delivery should be explored? This was the topic of a recent Institute of Medicine (IOM) study, *Preterm Birth: Causes, Consequences, and Prevention.*[49] Recommendations for research spanned health care of the pregnant woman and preterm infant as well as epidemiologic investigations of the complex and interrelated potential causes of preterm birth. This should be a key goal for MCH research in the twenty-first century.

Stillbirth (death in the womb of a fetus of at least 20 weeks' gestation), which now accounts for more than one-half of deaths of babies from 20 weeks' gestation through the first year of life, is the topic of a recent large, population-based case-control study sponsored by the Eunice Kennedy Shriver National Institute of Child Health and Human Development. Data derived from this study provided information about the scope and causes of stillbirth and may supply some answers to the cause of preterm delivery in the future.[50]

In addition, a comprehensive study of the impact of environment, stress, genetics, and chronic diseases on human growth and development has long been a high priority of MCH researchers. This ambitious dream will be fulfilled in the form of the National Children's Study, which involves recruiting a random sample of approximately 100,000 women and following them through conception, pregnancy, and delivery and their offspring up to age 21.[51] Study recruitment was originally set to be complete by 2014. However, recruitment was delayed due to logistical challenges, including study design and budgeting difficulties. A 2014 Institute of Medicine/National Research Council report called for improved scientific leadership of the study and additional evaluation of the protocol and data collection methods, among other recommendations.[52] The future of the National Children's Study will depend on the investigators' abilities to address these issues.

Medical care professionals view the management of chronic diseases as "the major challenge for health care professionals who care for infants, children, and young adults and for those who will treat them as they age into adulthood."[53] Public health professionals see a parallel challenge in preventing chronic diseases or postponing their onset. Obesity was classified as a disease in 2013 and is an underlying cause of many chronic illnesses, such as diabetes, that are now appearing at far younger ages than before. Major prevention efforts are underway to reverse the trend toward an ever increasing prevalence of obesity in childhood. Intervention studies designed to increase physical activity and improve nutrition have begun at the individual, family, community, and environmental levels of impact. If the obesity trend is not reversed, it is widely believed that this generation of children will have a lower life expectancy than their parents and grandparents.

A second chronic pediatric illness of increasing importance is asthma, a respiratory disease that causes periodic inflammation and narrowing of small airways. Asthma attacks, which can vary from mild to life-threatening, are triggered by allergens, infections, exercise, weather changes, and irritants such as tobacco smoke. Asthma often requires emergency room visits and interferes with daily activities, such as school attendance. Its prevalence has increased over the past two decades and is highest among children (9.3 percent in 2012[54]). Furthermore, large socioeconomic and racial disparities exist.

Another major child health problem that has only recently begun to receive widespread attention is promoting mental health and caring for those with mental health issues. It is estimated that by the year 2020, childhood neuropsychiatric disorders will become one of the top five causes of morbidity, mortality, and disability among children.[55] Already, mental illness that is severe enough to cause some level of impairment affects about 10 percent of U.S. children, but only about 20 percent of them receive mental health care services. The National Agenda for Action calls for engaging all 10 Essential Public Health Services toward prevention, screening, diagnosis, and adequate treatment.

The ACA has focused attention on the need for public health interventions to be evidence-based. The law established a Patient-Centered Outcomes Research Institute, which funds clinical effectiveness research. Additionally, HRSA encourages local and state health agencies to develop collaborative improvement networks (CoINs) as means to improve quality of services, engage communities in locally relevant programming, and evaluate the impact of programs on improving health throughout the life course. One example is the Collaborative Improvement & Innovation Network to Reduce Infant Mortality.[56] MCH programs are rapidly embracing these initiatives, as illustrated in a special issue of the *Maternal and Child Health Journal* published in February 2014.[57] At the state level, Wisconsin is experimenting with regional funding of MCH programs. Examples of innovative local health department programs include two different approaches (i.e., community organizing and financial empowerment) to reduce disparities in birth outcomes. Enhancements to the Healthy Start Program in one community and pediatric care in another community are translating the life course theory into practice. In another community, homeless pregnant women are being provided improved access to housing. It is likely that these and other local and state initiatives will transform MCH public health practice in the next decades.

SUMMARY

Much of the unprecedented improvement in MCH in the United States occurred during the first half of the twentieth century. Renewed and continued progress will require focus on rigorous application of the life course perspective to the 10 Essential Public Health Services, with particular attention to the elimination of health disparities; recognition of the inextricable connection between moving families out of poverty and improving the health of mothers and children; a focus on improving the impact of programs to solve current problems, such as the obesity epidemic and asthma; and research into the causes of preterm delivery, birth defects, asthma, and other persistent health issues.

REVIEW QUESTIONS

1. How does the principle of the life course perspective apply to the 10 Essential Public Health Services for MCH?

2. What impact on health would you expect because of the fundamental differences in maternal mortality review (MMR) and fetal/infant mortality review (FIMR)?

3. Why is there a difference in eligibility criteria between Medicaid and Medicare? Are these differences likely to remain throughout the twenty-first century? Why or why not?

4. What impact on MCH (positive and/or negative) is likely with the increased public health emphasis on preconception care?

5. How can policy claims be framed to increase political support for improved access to contraceptive services?

REFERENCES

1. Report of the Secretary's Advisory Committee on Infant Mortality (SACIM): Recommendations for Department of Health and Human Services (HHS) Action and Framework for a National Strategy. 2013.

2. Ten great public health achievements—United States, 1900–1999. *MMWR Morb Mortal Wkly Rep.* 1999;48(12):241–243.

3. Ten great public health achievements—United States, 2001–2010. *MMWR Morb Mortal Wkly Rep.* 2011;60(19):619–623.

4. Meckel RA. *Save the babies: American public health reform and the prevention of infant mortality, 1850–1929.* Baltimore, MD: The Johns Hopkins University Press; 1990.

5. Wertz RW, Wertz DC. *Lying-in: A history of childbirth in America.* New Haven, CT: Yale University Press; 1989.

6. Berg CJ, Harper MA, Atkinson SM, et al. Preventability of pregnancy-related deaths: results of a state-wide review. *Obstet Gynecol.* 2005;106(6):1228–1234.

7. Peterson HB, Lee NC. The health effects of oral contraceptives: misperceptions, controversies, and continuing good news. *Clin Obstet Gynecol.* 1989;32(2):339–355.

8. Frost JJ, Zolna MR, Frohwirth L. *Contraceptive Needs and Services, 2010.* New York: Guttmacher Institute; July 2013.

9. Fincr LB, Zolna MR. Shifts in intended and unintended pregnancies in the United States, 2001–2008. *Am J Public Health.* 2014;104 Suppl 1:S43–48.

10. Omer SB, Salmon DA, Orenstein WA, deHart MP, Halsey N. Vaccine refusal, mandatory immunization, and the risks of vaccine-preventable diseases. *N Engl J Med.* 2009;360(19):1981–1988.

11. Centers for Disease Control and Prevention. State Vaccination Requirements. 2011; http://www.cdc.gov/vaccines/imz-managers/laws/state-reqs.html. Accessed October 28, 2014.

12. State Seat Belt Laws. 2014; http://www.ncsl.org/research/health/state-seat-belt-laws.aspx. Accessed October 29, 2014.

13. Centers for Disease Control and Prevention. Child Passenger Safety: Get the Facts. 2014; http://www.cdc.gov/MotorVehicleSafety/Child_Passenger_Safety/CPS-Factsheet.html. Accessed October 29, 2014.

14. McPherson M, Arango P, Fox H, et al. A new definition of children with special health care needs. *Pediatrics.* 1998;102(1 Pt 1):137–140.

15. Maternal and Child Health Bureau, Health Services and Research Administration, US Department of Health and Human Services. The National Survey of Children with Special Health Care Needs Chartbook 2009–2010. Rockville, MD; 2013.

16. Rosenbaum S. The maternal and child health block grant act of 1981: Teaching an old program new tricks. *Clearinghouse Rev.* August/September 1983:400–414.

17. *Chart Book: TANF at 18.* Washington, DC Center on Budget and Policy Priorities;2014.

18. Markus AR, Andres E, West KD, Garro N, Pellegrini C. Medicaid covered births, 2008 through 2010, in the context of the implementation of health reform. *Women's Health Issues.* 2013;23(5):e273–280.

19. Tang SS. Medicaid and Children. 2011; http://www2.aap.org/research/factsheet.pdf. Accessed August 2014.

20. Medicaid Fact Sheets: United States. http://www.aap.org/en-us/Documents/federaladvocacy_medicaidfactsheet_all_states.pdf. Accessed August 2014.

21. Preventive health services for women. https://www.healthcare.gov/preventive-care-benefits/women/. Accessed August 15, 2014.

22. Preventive health services for children. https://www.healthcare.gov/preventive-care-benefits/children/. Accessed August 15, 2014.

23. Kenney G, Zuckerman S, Dubay L, et al. *Opting in to the Medicaid expansion under ACA: Who are the uninsured who could gain health insurance coverage. Timely analysis of immediate health policy issues.* Washington, DC: The Urban Institute;2012.

24. Kenney GM, Buettgens M, Guyer J, Heberlein M. Improving coverage for children under health reform will require maintaining current eligibility standards for Medicaid and CHIP. *Health Aff (Millwood).* 2011;30(12):2371–2381.

25. Association of Maternal & Child Health Programs Board of Directors. Memorandum to Dr. Michael Lu, Associate Administrator, Maternal and Child Health Bureau, Health Resources and Services Administration: "Preliminary Recommendations for the Future of the Title V Maternal and Child Health Services Block Grant." 2013.

26. Sonfield A, Hasstedt K, Gold RB. *Moving Forward: Family Planning in the Era of Health Reform.* New York: Guttmacher Institute;2014.

27. U.S. Department of Agriculture Food and Nutrition Service. The National WIC Evaluation: An Evaluation of the Special Supplemental Food Program for Women, Infants, and Children. Vol. 1: Summary. In: U.S. Department of Agriculture, ed. Alexandria, VA; 1987.

28. Centers for Disease Control and Prevention. Breastfeeding Among U.S. Children Born 2001–2011, CDC National Immunization Survey. 2014; http://www.cdc.gov/breastfeeding/data/NIS_data/index.htm. Accessed October 29, 2014.

29. U.S. Department of Agriculture Food and Nutrition Service. Breastfeeding Promotion and Support in WIC. 2014; http://www.fns.usda.gov/wic/breastfeeding-promotion-and-support-wic. Accessed October 28, 2014.

30. USDA Finalizes Changes to the WIC Program, Expanding Access to Healthy Fruits and Vegetables, Whole Grains, and Low-Fat Dairy for Women, Infants, and Children. US Department of Agriculture Office of Communications 2014.

31. Goldstein MM, Rosenbaum S. From EPSDT to EHBs: the future of pediatric coverage design under government financed health insurance. *Pediatrics.* 2013;131 Suppl 2:S142–148.

32. Medicaid Enrollment and EPSDT Utilization for Children Under 21, FY 2009. In: US Department of Health and Human Services HRaSA, Maternal and Child Health Bureau, ed.

33. Frost JJ, Sonfield A, Bold RB. *Estimating the impact of expanding Medicaid eligibility for family planning services.* New York: Guttmacher Institute; August 2006.

34. Title X Family Planning. http://www.hhs.gov/opa/title-x-family-planning/, 2014.

35. Burwell v. Hobby Lobby Stores, Inc. Vol 573: United States Reports; 2014.

36. American Academy of Family Physicians (AAFP), American Academy of Pediatrics (AAP), American College of Physicians (ACP), (AOA) AOA. Joint Principles of the Patient-Centered Medical Home. Washington, DC: Patient Centered Primary Care Collaborative 2007.

37. Davidoff MJ, Dias T, Damus K, et al. Changes in the gestational age distribution among U.S. singleton births: impact on rates of late preterm birth, 1992 to 2002. *Semin Perinatol.* 2006;30(1):8–15.

38. Martin JA, Hamilton BE, Sutton PD, Ventura SJ, Menacker F, Munson ML. Births: final data for 2002. *Natl Vital Stat Rep.* 2003;52(10):1–113.

39. Centers for Disease Control and Prevention. Participating PRAMS States. 2011; http://www.cdc.gov/prams/states.htm. Accessed August 15, 2014.

40. Brunner Huber LR, Hogue CJ, Stein AD, Drews C, Zieman M. Body mass index and risk for oral contraceptive failure: a case-cohort study in South Carolina. *Ann Epidemiol.* 2006;16(8):637–643.

41. Research & Data. http://mchb.hrsa.gov/researchdata. Accessed September 2014.

42. Hogue CJ. Whither FIMRs? *Matern Child Health J.* 2004;8(4):269–271.

43. Strobino DM, Baldwin KM, Grason H, et al. The relation of FIMR programs and other perinatal systems initiatives with maternal and child health activities in the community. *Matern Child Health J.* 2004;8(4):239–249.

44. Centers for Disease Control and Prevention. Preconception Health and Health Care. 2013; http://www.cdc.gov/preconception/index.html. Accessed August 26, 2013.

45. Burwell SM, Muñoz C, Holdren J, Krueger A. Memorandum to the Heads of Departments and Agencies: "Next Steps in the Evidence and Innovation Agenda." Washington, DC: Executive Office of the President, Office of Management and Budget; 2013.

46. Association of State and Territorial Health Officials. New York Redesigns Maternal and Child Health Programs Arlington, VA; 2013.

47. Howell EM. The impact of the Medicaid expansions for pregnant women: a synthesis of the evidence. *Med Care Res Rev.* 2001;58(1):3–30.

48. Glance LG, Dick AW, Glantz JC, et al. Rates of major obstetrical complications vary almost fivefold among US hospitals. *Health Aff (Millwood).* 2014;33(8):1330–1336.

49. Institute of Medicine Committee on Understanding Premature Birth and Assuring Healthy Outcomes. The National Academies Collection: Reports funded by National Institutes of Health. In: Behrman RE, Butler AS, eds. *Preterm Birth: Causes, Consequences, and Prevention.* Washington (DC): The National Academies Press (US), National Academy of Sciences; 2007.

50. Parker CB, Hogue CJ, Koch MA, et al. Stillbirth Collaborative Research Network: design, methods and recruitment experience. *Paediatr Perinat Epidemiol.* 2011;25(5):425–435.

51. The National Children's Study. 2014; https://www.nationalchildrensstudy.gov/Pages/default.aspx. Accessed October 12, 2014.

52. Institute of Medicine, National Research Council. The National Children's Study 2014: An Assessment. Washington, DC: The National Academies Press; 2014.

53. DeAngelis CD, Zylke JW. Theme issue on chronic diseases in infants, children, and young adults: call for papers. *JAMA.* 2006;296:1789.

54. National Center for Environmental Health, Centers for Disease Control and Prevention. Data and Surveillance: Asthma Surveillance Data. 2014; http://www.cdc.gov/asthma/asthmadata.htm. Accessed August 21, 2014.

55. US Department of Health and Human Services, US Department of Education, US Department of Justice. *Report of the Surgeon General's Conference on Children's Mental Health: A National Action Agenda.* Washington, DC: US Department of Health and Human Services;2000.

56. Collaborative Improvement & Innovation Network to Reduce Infant Mortality. http://mchb.hrsa.gov/infantmortality/coiin/. Accessed October 24, 2014.

57. Maternal and Child Health Journal, Volume 18, Issue 2, February 2014. Special Issue: Advancing MCH Life Course. 2014; http://link.springer.com/journal/10995/18/2/page/1 Accessed October 28, 2014.

58. McFarlane DR, Meier KJ. *The Politics of Fertility Control: Family Planning & Abortion Policies in the American States.* New York: Chatham House Publishers; 2000.

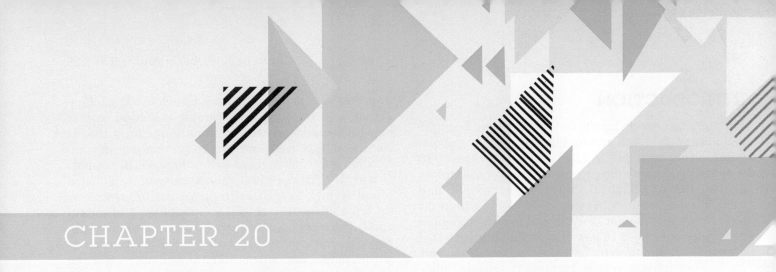

CHAPTER 20

Communicable and Infectious Diseases

Christina A. Mikosz, MD, MPH • Kyle Bernstein, PhD, ScM • Douglas Frye, MD, MPH •
Alan Hinman, MD, MPH

LEARNING OBJECTIVES

Upon completion of this chapter, the reader will be able to:

1. Discuss the methods of transmission of infectious diseases and the role of surveillance in infectious disease epidemiology.

2. List the basic steps in the investigation of a communicable disease outbreak.

3. Discuss the impact of vaccines on rates of vaccine-preventable diseases.

4. Outline the changing epidemiology of HIV/AIDS in the United States and its impact on other sexually transmitted diseases.

5. Highlight the various methods of tuberculosis control employed by local, state, and federal health officials.

6. Compare the differing epidemiology and methods of control of foodborne and waterborne diseases in the United States.

7. Discuss the impact of health-care-associated infections in the United States and the rise of antibiotic resistance.

KEY TERMS

acquired immunodeficiency syndrome (AIDS)
foodborne illness
health-care-associated infections
human immunodeficiency virus (HIV)
immunization
outbreak investigation
sexually transmitted diseases (STDs)
surveillance
tuberculosis (TB)

INTRODUCTION

Throughout history, infectious diseases have been the main causes of death among humans, from major singular events such as the Black Plague and the 1918 "Spanish flu" pandemic, to previously commonplace deaths such as diarrheal illnesses, pneumonia, and tuberculosis, among other causes. It is only within the last century that chronic diseases and injuries have risen to become the major causes of mortality in the United States. The dramatic drop in infectious disease morbidity and mortality is counted among the major public health achievements and is attributable to a number of factors, including measures to improve sanitation and hygiene (e.g., ensuring a clean water supply, sewage disposal, among other examples), wide-scale vaccination programs, and the development of antibiotic drugs.[1] On a global scale, however, infectious diseases are still responsible for millions of deaths each year[2] and nearly two-thirds of deaths in children younger than five years,[3] demonstrating that the threat of infectious diseases continues to persist, and control measures to keep communicable diseases in check are just as necessary now as a century ago.

The field of communicable disease control employs a wide variety of strategies, depending on the disease and population in question, much more than can be adequately covered in a single chapter. Thus, in this chapter we will focus on providing a foundation of general concepts in communicable disease control, starting with an overview of methods of disease transmission, then broadly defining infectious disease surveillance and investigation, and finally demonstrating how these concepts may be put into practice by delving more deeply into a few selected topics, including foodborne and waterborne diseases, immunizations, sexually transmitted infections, HIV/AIDS, tuberculosis (TB), and health-care-associated infections.

TRANSMISSION OF INFECTIOUS DISEASES

Infectious disease transmission can be broadly categorized into four direct and indirect modes. Direct transmission may occur as a result of direct physical contact, such as sexual intercourse, or through the spread of droplet spray (droplet transmission) onto mucous membranes during sneezing, coughing, speaking, or singing.

Indirect transmission may be vehicle-borne, vector-borne, or airborne. Vehicle-borne transmission may occur as a result of contact with contaminated inanimate materials ("fomites") such as toys or eating utensils, or via contaminated water, food, milk, or blood. *Fecal-oral transmission* occurs when infectious particles from feces are ingested by mouth such as via contaminated food or water; an example is a food worker ill with hepatitis A who contaminates food that is consumed by others. Strategies to prevent transmission of blood-borne pathogens, such as hepatitis B, hepatitis C, and HIV/AIDS, include the screening of the donated blood supply, as well as implementation of *universal precautions*, whereby all human blood and certain bodily fluids are considered to be potentially infectious, necessitating universal use of protective gear such as gloves, masks, and gowns when potentially contacting such fluids. Postexposure prophylaxis via vaccination and/or antimicrobial medications may also be strategies to prevent illness in some scenarios. Vector-borne transmission may be mechanical or biological. Mechanical vector-borne transmission includes "simple mechanical carriage by a crawling or flying insect through soiling of its feet or proboscis, or by passage of organisms through its gastrointestinal tract"[4] without further multiplication or development of the organism. With biological vector-borne transmission, some combination of multiplication or development is necessary before an agent can be transmitted to humans. A cornerstone of vector-borne disease control is controlling exposure to the vector, for example, partnering with mosquito abatement programs to reduce mosquito populations and community education about avoiding mosquito bites (e.g., wearing insect repellent and long sleeves and pants) for diseases such as West Nile virus that are transmitted via mosquitoes. In airborne transmission, aerosolized microbials are disseminated through the air and infect others usually via the respiratory tract. Particles may remain suspended for long periods of time, leading to disease transmission even hours after an infected person has left a confined space.

SURVEILLANCE

Surveillance—the ongoing systematic collection, analysis, and interpretation of data about the health of the community—is the foundation of public health practice and an essential element in understanding the epidemiology of infectious diseases. Public health surveillance data are "used to assess public health status, track conditions of public health importance, define public health priorities, evaluate programs, and develop public health research."[5] Data collected through routine health department surveillance can be analyzed for trends and patterns, allowing for the development of targeted policies and interventions to address a population's specific health needs, and ongoing surveillance data can then be used to monitor and evaluate an intervention's effectiveness. Surveillance can be passive—whereby the health department waits to receive a report of a certain disease from a health care provider or laboratory—or active, in which the local health jurisdiction actively solicits reports of a disease.

Certain infectious diseases are *reportable* to state and local health jurisdictions, meaning that by law, health providers and laboratories are required to notify health officials of a case of that disease, in varying time intervals (immediately to several days) depending on the public health urgency of a particular disease. The reportable disease list may vary between health jurisdictions depending on local epidemiology and research interests. In turn, certain infectious diseases are deemed *notifiable* by state health officials on a voluntary basis to the Centers for Disease Control and Prevention (CDC), which aggregates the data on a nationwide scale via the National Notifiable Diseases Surveillance System. In order to ensure uniformity in the disease data being reported across the country, the Council of State and Territorial Epidemiologists defines standard *case definitions* that establish consistent criteria for disease classification. Additional information on surveillance systems is provided in Chapter 12.

OUTBREAK INVESTIGATION

On occasion, close monitoring of incoming surveillance data may suggest that an outbreak is occurring, either of a confirmed disease or possibly a cluster of cases of a clinical syndrome that does not yet have a firm diagnosis. The exact approach for outbreak investigation depends on a number of factors, including the disease or syndrome in question (e.g., an influenza outbreak involves a different approach than an outbreak of norovirus, which causes gastrointestinal illness); the rapidity with which cases are being reported to health officials (e.g., a report of 50 people ill over the past day and another 100 ill today would certainly raise concern, if these numbers were not typical for this particular disease); and the data on hand at the time of reporting (e.g., everyone ill ate at a particular restaurant), among other factors. Public health practitioners at the local and state levels most frequently take the lead in these investigations, but may be assisted by federal partners (e.g., the CDC) depending on the scope and nature of the outbreak. The following is intended to provide a loose framework for a field investigation of an acute outbreak.[4,6,7]

1. *Confirm the existence of an epidemic.* Before declaring that an outbreak is occurring, it is important to determine whether the number of reported cases is above a health jurisdiction's expected baseline, which can vary quite widely depending on the disease and local epidemiology. In some jurisdictions, multiple cases of influenza or norovirus reported in a single week might not be unusual,

but a single case of paralysis due to wild poliovirus occurring in the United States would be considered a potential epidemic because there have been no such cases reported since 1979.[8]

2. *Confirm the diagnosis.* This is ideally done via laboratory testing for at least some cases, provided the remaining cases are clinically compatible with cases in which laboratory confirmation is obtained. Laboratory confirmation should not hold up the investigation of a cluster of illness, if it is clear that an unusual event is occurring.

3. *Establish a case definition and characterize the cases.* A case definition is a workable, flexible set of criteria, initially designed to maximize sensitivity, that may be modified as an investigation progresses and additional data about cases are obtained. A standardized questionnaire used to interview all suspected cases will be helpful to gather other pertinent data for the investigation. For example, if the outbreak involves an acute gastrointestinal illness, collecting data about recently eaten food and drink, restaurants or other food establishments recently visited, onset of symptoms, etc., should reveal commonalities among suspected cases that can focus investigative efforts. Next, characterize cases according to time, place, and person. Characterizing by time typically involves plotting an *epidemic curve* depicting the number of cases by time of onset (by an appropriate time interval). Patterns may begin to emerge: an outbreak attributable to a single, "point-source" exposure typically has an epidemic curve with a single sharp peak centered on the median incubation period following exposure, while "person-to-person" transmission shows a gradual rise in cases, often with a typical incubation period between "generations" of cases, and a gradual decline as the number of still-susceptible persons declines, in the absence of measures to interrupt transmission. Characterization by place can involve constructing a map showing the home or worksite of individual cases to identify any geographic localization. A classic example of place characterization "solving" an outbreak occurred during a large cholera outbreak in London in 1854, when Dr. John Snow plotted the home residences of cholera deaths on a city map; it soon became clear that deaths from cholera clustered around a common water pump that Snow suspected to be supplying contaminated water. Characterization by person involves the obvious—age and gender—but may also entail race/ethnicity, occupation, or other unique variables.

EXHIBIT 20-1 Hypothetical Outbreak Scenario

One Monday morning, the local health department receives an unusual number of phone calls from worried persons who developed vomiting and diarrhea over the weekend—when a typical Monday morning might only involve around five such phone calls, on this day 50 were received. Several persons have already seen their private physicians. Testing for a number of diarrheal illnesses, such as *Escherichia coli*, *Salmonella spp.*, and norovirus is already underway. It appears that an outbreak of an acute gastrointestinal illness is occurring, and local epidemiologists quickly focus on identifying additional cases of vomiting and diarrhea with symptom onset since the previous Friday. A quick series of questions to ill callers elicits the information that while the sick callers spanned a wide range of ages and lived in different nearby towns, nearly all of these persons attended a wedding on Saturday night and developed symptoms around 24 hours after the event. It is hypothesized that given the nature of symptoms, the outbreak was likely related to something the wedding guests ate while attending the wedding, and all wedding guests – healthy and sick – are interviewed about their menu choices. It is discovered that at the wedding, the meal options consisted of steak,

baked chicken, or fish; steamed broccoli; roasted potatoes; rice; and either chocolate cake or pie for dessert. All food was catered by Company X. Data from these cases and controls are statistically analyzed, and it becomes clear that while there is a relatively even distribution of most foods eaten between both healthy and sick patrons, 100 percent of sick attendees ate the baked chicken, compared to only 10 percent of healthy attendees. Suspicion falls on the baked chicken as the exposure of interest. Public health officials inspect the food preparation facilities of Company X and find multiple food safety violations. Meanwhile, some leftover prepared chicken is discovered by inspectors and submitted for laboratory testing, which reveals *Salmonella enteritidis*. At this point in the investigation, laboratory results begin to return from case-patient specimens, several of which have also tested positive for *S. enteritidis*. The leftover chicken is discarded, and Company X is temporarily closed down to address the violations noted on the inspection. As rumors of the outbreak had generated some buzz in the local area, the health department issues a press release describing the outbreak's findings and communicating the message that no further risk is posed to the public from the exposure source.

4. *Formulate and test a hypothesis about the outbreak source.* By now, after careful characterization of the cases, one should be able to formulate a working hypothesis about the culprit exposure that caused the outbreak. Next, the hypothesis can be tested using epidemiologic analytic methods, such as a case-control study, which will involve collecting data on control persons that have similar characteristics as cases but who are healthy (e.g., ate at the same restaurant as a case with gastrointestinal illness but never became sick).

5. *Contain the outbreak.* Once the source of the outbreak is identified, control measures should be implemented to prevent additional exposures or to prevent illness from developing in susceptible persons already exposed (when this is possible, depending on the infectious agent). One example is the widespread vaccination, within a certain time window, of persons without evidence of measles immunity who have been exposed to a measles case; another example is the isolation of an infectious tuberculosis case to prevent further exposure and the rapid identification of contacts to this case to facilitate testing and treatment, if necessary, to prevent secondary transmission. Containing an outbreak often involves other organizations and entities apart from public health officials. For example, the Food and Drug Administration (FDA)

may recommend the recall of an implicated food product in a foodborne illness outbreak.

6. *Prepare and disseminate a report about the outbreak*, which may occur in several forms: a few examples are a formal publication in the scientific literature, a press release, or an administrative memo for public health staff or local stakeholders. This last step is essential to ensure that lessons learned from the investigation can be applied for future planning purposes.

Certain steps in this loose framework may be more prominent in certain investigations as compared to others, and oftentimes multiple steps may occur simultaneously. The hypothetical outbreak described in Exhibit 20-1 "Hypothetical Outbreak Scenario" demonstrates how these steps may be put into practice.

WATERBORNE AND FOODBORNE DISEASES

A variety of parasitic, bacterial, and viral diseases can be transmitted through food and water. Disease results either from infection or from intoxication. Some diseases, such as giardiasis and typhoid fever, result from ingestion of small numbers of microorganisms that subsequently multiply and cause disease, either local or invasive. Others, such as cholera and diarrhea caused by enterotoxigenic *Escherichia coli*, result from ingestion of living bacteria that multiply and produce toxins that act on intestinal mucosa to cause diarrhea. Some conditions such as botulism or *Clostridium perfringens* food poisoning result from ingestion of toxins formed by organisms multiplying in the food before it is eaten. Finally, some fish and shellfish may contain toxins that cause neuromuscular symptoms. Food and water can also carry natural or synthetic toxins (e.g., metals, plant toxins, and insecticides) that may also cause human illness.

These illnesses may vary greatly in symptoms. Some are characterized by mild nausea, vomiting, and diarrhea (e.g., most *Salmonella* infections). Others may be associated with life-threatening profuse diarrhea (cholera), hemorrhagic diarrhea with hemolytic-uremic syndrome (*E. coli* 0157:H7), sepsis (typhoid), infectious hepatitis (hepatitis A), miscarriage (*Listeria monocytogenes*), or cranial nerve and respiratory paralysis (botulism).

Waterborne Diseases

Waterborne illness is less common in the United States due to the protection of our water supply, such as via the routine monitoring of potable water supplies; prevention of cross-connections between water and sewage systems; and mandated inspections of recreational water sources such as pools and water parks, including routine coliform testing of water at beaches, to name a few strategies. However, disease transmission via water does continue to occur. During 2009–2010 the CDC received reports on 33 outbreaks associated with drinking water or other nonrecreational water, causing more than 1,000 persons to become ill.[9] Over half of these outbreaks were due to *Legionella* infection associated with contaminated plumbing systems, although *Campylobacter* caused a greater number of water-associated infections during this time period. If municipal water supplies become contaminated, large numbers of persons may become ill. During a 1965 outbreak of waterborne salmonellosis in Riverside, California, an estimated 16,000 persons became ill.[10] More than 400,000 persons became ill with waterborne cryptosporidiosis in Milwaukee in 1993.[11] Outbreaks have also been associated with recreational water sources, such as public pools and lakes. During 2009–2010, 81 such outbreaks were reported to the CDC, leading to over 1,300 illnesses.[12] Among treated recreational water sources (e.g., pools, spas, water parks), *Cryptosporidium*, a parasite, was the leading cause of illness, while cyanobacterial toxins accounted for the largest proportion of outbreaks attributed to nontreated recreational water (e.g., oceans and lakes).

Foodborne Diseases

Foodborne pathogens are a major cause of morbidity and mortality in the United States, estimated to cause 48 million illnesses yearly, including nearly 500,000 hospitalizations and over 5,000 deaths.[13] Furthermore, only an estimated 9.4 million of these cases are due to known pathogens,[14] suggesting that approximately 80 percent of gastrointestinal illness in the United States is due to an unspecified agent. A specific food source is often never pinpointed as the cause of illness. Additionally, these totals likely underestimate the true burden of foodborne disease as many cases likely go unreported (e.g., an ill patient may never visit his or her physician for evaluation).

Most illnesses do not occur as part of a recognized outbreak,[15] although the study of foodborne illness occurring in a defined outbreak provides interesting insight into the epidemiology of foodborne pathogens in the United States. During 1998–2008, the CDC received reports of over 13,000 food-related outbreaks in the United States, accounting for over 270,000 illnesses, over 9,000 hospitalizations, and 200 deaths. Of the 8,000 of these outbreaks that had a known etiology, 45 percent were each attributed to viruses and bacteria, respectively. The most common viral cause of foodborne illness was norovirus, while *Salmonella* was the most common bacterial species. The food products most commonly associated with foodborne outbreaks in this study period were poultry, fish, and beef, although leafy vegetables were linked most commonly to viral outbreaks.

Prevention of foodborne illness involves all steps in the food chain, from "farm to table." The FDA and U.S. Department of Agriculture primarily share federal oversight for food safety regulations in the United States. Hazards Analysis and Critical Control Points, or HACCP, is a management system that protects our food supply through the systematic analysis and control of potential hazards via the application of seven established principles;[16] adherence to current Good Manufacturing Practices, among other quality measures, is essential for a successful HACCP program. Individual consumers can protect themselves from foodborne illness by adhering to standard food safety recommendations including cleaning hands and food preparation surfaces frequently; avoiding cross-contamination of raw foods; cooking foods to proper temperatures; and promptly refrigerating leftovers to inhibit microbial growth.[17]

IMMUNIZATIONS

Immunization is one of the most important interventions for the control and prevention of infectious diseases. Globally, immunization has resulted in the eradication of smallpox and the near-eradication of poliomyelitis as well as preventing millions of deaths due to other diseases. This section addresses the impact, safety, and effectiveness of vaccines; immunization coverage; immunization schedules; and the immunization infrastructure in the United States.

Vaccines

Vaccines are suspensions of live (usually attenuated) or killed microorganisms (bacteria or viruses) or fractions thereof administered to induce immunity and prevent infectious diseases or their sequelae. Toxoids are modified bacterial toxins (e.g., diphtheria, tetanus) that have been rendered nontoxic but retain the ability to stimulate the formation of antitoxin. They are often included in the general category of vaccines.[18]

Impact of Vaccines

Introduction and widespread use of childhood vaccines have had a dramatic effect on the reported incidence of infectious diseases in the United States. Immunization

has been hailed as one of the 10 great public health achievements of the twentieth century.[19] The United States is currently enjoying historic low levels of disease incidence and historic high levels of vaccine coverage. Tables 20-1 and 20-2 show the typical number of cases reported of childhood vaccine-preventable diseases in the years preceding introduction of vaccines and the number of cases of those diseases reported in 2013. Table 20-1 shows trends for diseases for which vaccines have been available for many years and Table 20-2 shows results for more recently introduced vaccines.[20,21] There has been a reduction in excess of 95 percent in virtually every one of the conditions. Transmission of measles and rubella has been interrupted in the United States, and all cases arise as a result of importation from another country.[22,23]

Table 20-3 shows the 2013 nationwide levels of vaccine coverage in 19- to 35-month-old children.[24] Levels are not uniform throughout the country—for example, state-specific levels of measles vaccination ranged from 86.0 percent (CO, OH, WV) to 96.3 percent (NH). In the past, there has been significant racial variation in coverage rates, with blacks having lower rates than whites. This disparity has narrowed but not yet been eliminated—in 2013, 72.1 percent of white children had received complete series of immunizations compared with 65.0 percent of black children.[24]

TABLE 20-1   Comparison of Twentieth Century Annual Morbidity and Current Morbidity of Vaccine-Preventable Diseases

Disease	Twentieth Century Annual Morbidity	2013 Reported Cases	Percent Decrease
Smallpox	29,005	0	100%
Diphtheria	21,053	0	100%
Measles	530,217	187	>99%
Mumps	162,344	584	>99%
Pertussis	200,752	28,639	86%
Polio (paralytic)	16,316	1	>99%
Rubella	47,745	9	>99%
Congenital Rubella Syndrome	152	1	99%
Tetanus	580	26	96%
Haemophilus influenza	20,000	31*	>99%

Haemophilus influenza type b in children <5 years of age

SOURCE: Roush S.W. and Murphy T.V.

TABLE 20-2   Comparison of Prevaccine Era Estimated Annual Morbidity with Current Estimate of Vaccine-Preventable Diseases

Disease	Prevaccine Era Annual Estimate of Cases	2013 Estimate of Cases	Percent decrease
Hepatitis A	117,333	2,890	98%
Hepatitis B (acute)	66,232	18,800	72%
Pneumococcus (invasive)			
All ages	63,067	33,500	47%
<5 years of age	16,069	1,900	88%
Rotavirus (hospitalizations <3 years of age)	62,500	12,500	80%
Varicella	4,085,120	167,490	96%

SOURCE: Roush S.W. and Murphy T.V.

TABLE 20-3 Vaccination Coverage among Children 19–35 Months of Age, 2012

Vaccine	USA
DTP/DTaP 4+	82.5%
Polio 3+	92.8%
MMR 1+	90.8%
Hib 3+	93.3%
Hep B 3+	89.7%
Varicella 1+	90.2%
PCV 4+	81.9%
Hep A 2+	53.0%
Rotavirus 2+	68.6%

SOURCE: Centers for Disease Control and Prevention

Immunization rates in adults are not as high as those in children. For example, in the 2012–2013 influenza season, only 66.2 percent of adults ≥65 years of age received influenza vaccine, and 59.9 percent had ever received pneumococcal vaccine.[25,26] Both vaccines have been recommended for all persons 65 or older (and for younger persons with certain conditions) for decades.

Immunization Schedules

Recommendations for immunization of children in the United States are developed principally by the Public Health Service's Advisory Committee on Immunization Practices (ACIP) and the American Academy of Pediatrics (AAP) Committee on Infectious Diseases (Red Book Committee). Along with the American Academy of Family Physicians (AAFP), these committees develop harmonized immunization schedules for children and adolescents (Figure 20-1). Immunization of all children

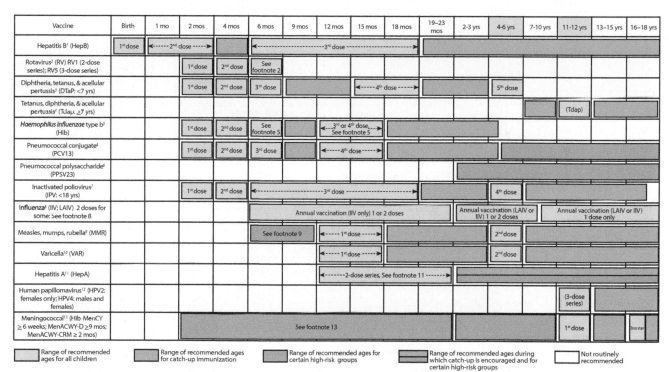

This schedule includes recommendations in effect as of January 1, 2015. Any dose not administered at the recommended age should be administered at a subsequent visit, when indicated and feasible. The use of a combination vaccine generally is preferred over separate injections of its equivalent component vaccines. Vaccination providers should consult the relevant Advisory Committee on Immunization Practices (ACIP) statement for detailed recommendations, available online at http://www.cdc.gov/vaccines/hcp/acip-recs/index.html. Clinically significant adverse events that follow vaccination should be reported to the Vaccine Adverse Event Reporting System (VAERS) online (http://www.vaers.hhs.gov) or by telephone (800-822-7967). Suspected cases of vaccine-preventable diseases should be reported to the state or local health department. Additional information, including precautions and contraindications for vaccination, is available from CDC online (http://www.cdc.gov/vaccines/recs/vac-admin/contraindications.htm) or by telephone (800-CDC-INFO [800-232-4636]).

This schedule is approved by the Advisory Committee on Immunization Practices (http://www.cdc.gov/vaccines/acip), the American Academy of Pediatrics (http://www.aap.org), the American Academy of Family Physicians (http://www.aafp.org), and the American College of Obstetricians and Gynecologists (http://www.acog.org).

NOTE: The above recommendations must be read along with the footnotes of this schedule, available at http://www.cdc.gov/vaccines/schedules/downloads/child/0-18yrs-child-combined-schedule.pdf

FIGURE 20-1 Recommended Immunization Schedule for Persons Aged 0 through 18 Years, United States, 2015

Courtesy of U.S. Department of Health and Human Services, Centers for Disease Control and Prevention

and adolescents in the United States is currently recommended against 16 diseases: diphtheria, hepatitis A, hepatitis B, *Haemophilus influenzu b* (Hib), human papilloma virus, influenza, measles, meningococcal disease, mumps, pertussis, pneumococcal disease, poliomyelitis, rotavirus, rubella, tetanus, and varicella.[18] The CDC produces a valuable textbook on the Epidemiology and Prevention of Vaccine-Preventable Diseases (the Pink Book); it is revised periodically.[27]

Figures 20-2 and 20-3 show 2015 immunization recommendations for adults, who may have special needs for vaccines because of increased risk of illness or death resulting from age, occupation, behavior, or chronic illness.[18] The ACIP recommendations for children, adolescents, and adults are revised annually and are posted on the CDC website. You can review them by going to http://www.cdc.gov and searching "Advisory Committee on Immunization Practices." Recommendations have also been developed for health care workers.[28]

Immunization Infrastructure

Most children in the United States currently receive their immunizations in the private sector, from pediatricians or family physicians. A significant minority receive immunizations in the public sector, typically

from local health departments, 90 percent of which provide child and adult immunization services,[29] although there is considerable variation around the country. Since 1962, the federal government has supported childhood immunization programs through a grant program administered by the CDC (referred to as Section 317). The grants support purchase of vaccine for free administration at local health departments and also support immunization delivery, surveillance, and communication/education. The Patient Protection and Affordable Care Act included provisions to require health plans to cover immunizations recommended by the ACIP with no copayments and also established the Prevention and Public Health Fund, which can supplement Section 317 funds to strengthen surveillance.[30,31]

At 2014 prices, the cost for vaccines alone (irrespective of physician fees) to fully immunize a child from birth to age 18 is more than $1,500 in the public sector.[32] Most insurance plans now cover childhood immunizations. Children who are uninsured, covered by Medicaid, or are Alaska natives/American Indians can receive vaccines free of charge through the Vaccines for Children (VFC) program enacted in 1993.[33] Underinsured children (those whose parents have insurance that does not cover immunizations) may also receive the vaccines free at Federally Qualified Health Centers

VACCINE ▼ AGE GROUP ►	19-21 years	22-26 years	27-49 years	50-59 years	60-64 years	≥ 65 years
Influenza[*,2]	\multicolumn{6}{c}{1 dose annually}
Tetanus, diphtheria, pertussis (Td/Tdap)[*,3]	\multicolumn{6}{c}{Substitute 1-time dose of Tdap for Td booster; then boost with Td every 10 yrs}
Varicella[*,4]	\multicolumn{6}{c}{2 doses}
Human papillomavirus (HPV) Female[*,5]	3 doses					
Human papillomavirus (HPV) Male[*,5]	3 doses					
Zoster[6]					1 dose	
Measles, mumps, rubella (MMR)[*,7]	\multicolumn{4}{c}{1 or 2 doses}		
Pneumococcal 13-valent conjugate (PCV13)[*,8]					1-time dose	
Pneumococcal polysaccharide (PPSV23)[8]	\multicolumn{5}{c}{1 or 2 doses}	1 dose
Meningococcal[*,9]	\multicolumn{6}{c}{1 or more doses}
Hepatitis A[*,10]	\multicolumn{6}{c}{2 doses}
Hepatitis B[*,11]	\multicolumn{6}{c}{3 doses}
Haemophilus influenzae type b (Hib)[*,12]	\multicolumn{6}{c}{1 or 3 doses}

*Covered by the Vaccine Injury Compensation Program

For all persons in this category who meet the age requirements and who lack documentation of vaccination or have no evidence of previous infection; zoster vaccine recommended regardless of prior episode of zoster

Recommended if some other risk factor is present (e.g., on the basis of medical, occupational, lifestyle, or other indication)

No recommendation

Report all clinically significant postvaccination reactions to the Vaccine Adverse Event Reporting System (VAERS). Reporting forms and instructions on filing a VAERS report are available at www.vaers.hhs.gov or by telephone, 800-822-7967.

Information on how to file a Vaccine Injury Compensation Program claim is available at www.hrsa.gov/vaccinecompensation or by telephone, 800-338-2382. To file a claim for vaccine injury, contact the U.S. Court of Federal Claims, 717 Madison Place, N.W., Washington, D.C. 20005; telephone, 202-357-6400.

Additional information about the vaccines in this schedule, extent of available data, and contraindications for vaccination is also available at www.cdc.gov/vaccines or from the CDC-INFO Contact Center at 800-CDC-INFO (800-232-4636) in English and Spanish, 8:00 a.m. - 8:00 p.m. Eastern Time, Monday - Friday, excluding holidays.

Use of trade names and commercial sources is for identification only and does not imply endorsement by the U.S. Department of Health and Human Services.

The recommendations in this schedule were approved by the Centers for Disease Control and Prevention's (CDC) Advisory Committee on Immunization Practices (ACIP), the American Academy of Family Physicians (AAFP), the America College of Physicians (ACP), American College of Obstetricians and Gynecologists (ACOG) and American College of Nurse-Midwives (ACNM).

NOTE: The above recommendations must be read along with the footnotes of this schedule, available at http://www.cdc.gov/vaccines/schedules/downloads/adult/adult-schedule.pdf

FIGURE 20-2   Recommended Adult Immunization Schedule, by Vaccine and Age Group, 2015

Courtesy of U.S. Department of Health and Human Services, Centers for Disease Control and Prevention

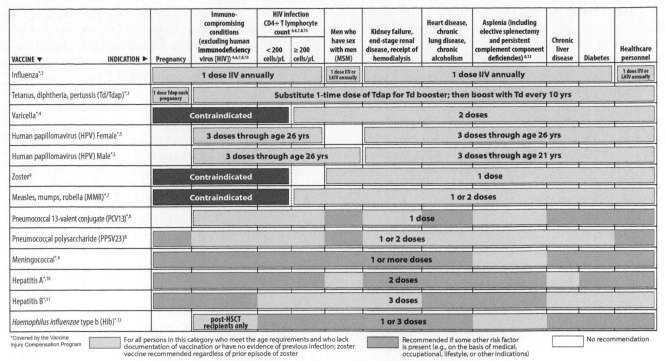

VACCINE ▼ INDICATION ▶	Pregnancy	Immuno-compromising conditions (excluding human immunodeficiency virus [HIV]) 4,6,7,8,13	HIV infection CD4+ T lymphocyte count 4,6,7,8,13 < 200 cells/μL	HIV infection CD4+ T lymphocyte count 4,6,7,8,13 ≥ 200 cells/μL	Men who have sex with men (MSM)	Kidney failure, end-stage renal disease, receipt of hemodialysis	Heart disease, chronic lung disease, chronic alcoholism	Asplenia (including elective splenectomy and persistent complement component deficiencies) 8,12	Chronic liver disease	Diabetes	Healthcare personnel
Influenza*,2	1 dose IIV annually	1 dose IIV annually	1 dose IIV annually	1 dose IIV or LAIV annually	1 dose IIV annually	1 dose IIV annually	1 dose IIV annually	1 dose IIV annually	1 dose IIV annually	1 dose IIV annually	1 dose IIV or LAIV annually
Tetanus, diphtheria, pertussis (Td/Tdap)*,3	1 dose Tdap each pregnancy	Substitute 1-time dose of Tdap for Td booster; then boost with Td every 10 yrs									
Varicella*,4	Contraindicated				2 doses						
Human papillomavirus (HPV) Female*,5	3 doses through age 26 yrs				3 doses through age 26 yrs						
Human papillomavirus (HPV) Male*,5	3 doses through age 26 yrs				3 doses through age 21 yrs						
Zoster6	Contraindicated				1 dose						
Measles, mumps, rubella (MMR)*,7	Contraindicated				1 or 2 doses						
Pneumococcal 13-valent conjugate (PCV13)*,8			1 dose								
Pneumococcal polysaccharide (PPSV23)8			1 or 2 doses								
Meningococcal*,9			1 or more doses								
Hepatitis A*,10			2 doses								
Hepatitis B*,11			3 doses								
Haemophilus influenzae type b (Hib)*,12		post-HSCT recipients only	1 or 3 doses								

*Covered by the Vaccine Injury Compensation Program

For all persons in this category who meet the age requirements and who lack documentation of vaccination or have no evidence of previous infection; zoster vaccine recommended regardless of prior episode of zoster

Recommended if some other risk factor is present (e.g., on the basis of medical, occupational, lifestyle, or other indications)

No recommendation

NOTE: The above recommendations must be read along with the footnotes of this schedule, available at http://www.cdc.gov/vaccines/schedules/hcp/imz/adult-conditions-shell.html

FIGURE 20-3 Vaccines That Might Be Indicated for Adults Based on Medical and Other Indications, 2015

Courtesy of U.S. Department of Health and Human Services, Centers for Disease Control and Prevention

(most Community Health Centers). Approximately one-half of U.S. children are VFC eligible.

Immunization efforts in the United States have been significantly aided by the enactment and enforcement of laws in each state that require immunization before first entry into school. Since 1980, all states have had such laws in place. As a result, approximately 95 percent of children entering school are fully immunized.[34]

Although immunization levels are currently at record high levels and vaccine-preventable disease incidence is at record low levels, there is continuing cause for concern about immunizations in the United States—there are approximately 11,000 children born each day, all requiring immunization; the population is quite mobile (approximately 16 percent of Americans change address in any given year); and the immunization schedule is increasingly complex as new vaccines or additional doses are recommended. All of these factors support the need for automated mechanisms to keep track of children's immunization status and notify parents and providers about needed immunizations.

The National Vaccine Advisory Committee (NVAC) has called for a nationwide network of population-based immunization information systems ("IIS," essentially immunization registries), and the *Healthy People*

2020 objectives call for 95 percent of children to be enrolled in population-based immunization registries by 2020.[35] The Task Force on Community Preventive Services has recommended the use of IIS based on strong evidence of their ability to raise immunization coverage.[36] As of December 31, 2012, 86 percent of children ages 1 through 6 years were enrolled in IIS.[37]

Vaccine Safety and Efficacy

Modern vaccines are safe and effective; however, they are neither perfectly safe nor perfectly effective. Some individuals who receive a vaccine will not be protected against disease, and some will suffer adverse consequences. Adverse events may range from minor inconveniences such as discomfort at the injection site or fever, to serious conditions such as paralysis associated with oral poliovirus vaccine (OPV). The goal is to achieve maximum safety and maximum efficacy. A simple formula exists to determine vaccine efficacy (VE)

$$VE = (ARU - ARV)/ARU \times 100$$

where ARU is the attack rate of disease in unvaccinated individuals, and ARV is the attack rate in vaccinated individuals.[38]

Decisions about use of vaccines are based on the relative balance of risks and benefits. This balance may change over time. For example, recipients of OPV and their close contacts have a risk of developing vaccine-associated paralysis of one (1) in approximately every 2.4 million doses of vaccine distributed. This risk is quite small and was certainly outweighed by the much larger risk of paralysis due to wild polioviruses at the time they were circulating in the United States. However, because wild polioviruses no longer circulate in the United States, and the risk of importation of wild viruses has been greatly reduced by the global effort to eradicate polio, the balance has shifted. Consequently, since 2000 the United States has relied exclusively on inactivated polio vaccine.[39]

It is often difficult to ascertain whether an adverse event that occurs after immunization was caused by the vaccine or was merely temporally related and caused by some totally independent (and often unknown or unidentified) factor. This is particularly a problem during infancy, when a number of conditions may occur simultaneously. In any given instance it may be impossible to determine whether the vaccine was responsible.[18] Particularly when dealing with rare events, it may be necessary to carry out large-scale case-control studies or review comprehensive records of large numbers of infants to ascertain whether those who received a vaccine had a higher incidence of the event than those who did not. The CDC operates a large linked database involving nine large health maintenance organizations. This Vaccine Safety Datalink project includes approximately 3 percent of the U.S. population and has proved to be an invaluable resource in attempting to determine causality.[40]

One result of the extraordinary success of immunization efforts has been the fact that today's young parents (and young physicians) have never seen many of the diseases against which they are being urged to have their children vaccinated. Consequently, they may not be as motivated as were parents and physicians in the past. In the absence of disease, the infrequent known (or alleged) adverse events associated with vaccines assume greater prominence. This imbalance has led some parents, and even some physicians, to question whether use of some (or all) vaccines is still warranted. The rise of the Internet has made it easier for opinions about vaccines to be disseminated, whether based in science or not. This increases the obligation of public health authorities to explain fully the risks and benefits of vaccines. The occasional occurrence of previously unrecognized adverse events actually caused by the vaccine (as with intestinal intussusception and rotavirus vaccine) adds to the complexity of the explanation.[41] Although links between the measles, mumps, and rubella (MMR) vaccine and autism, and thimerosal-containing vaccines and autism have been alleged, repeated studies[42] have shown that there is no causal relationship.* A no-fault National Vaccine Injury Compensation Program has been implemented to provide compensation to children injured by vaccines recommended for universal use.[43]

Accompanying the lack of disease and concomitant relative prominence of known or suspected adverse events has been a rise in parents' unwillingness to have their children vaccinated against any diseases or specific diseases (vaccine hesitancy and vaccine refusal) or to request modified schedules of vaccine administration. This has been reflected in the rising proportion of school entrants whose parents seek "personal belief" exemptions from school immunization requirements as well as by focal outbreaks of vaccine-preventable diseases (e.g., measles and pertussis) that have strained the capacity of local and state health departments to investigate and respond.[44-46]

TUBERCULOSIS (TB)

Tuberculosis (TB) is caused by *Mycobacterium tuberculosis*, a bacterium primarily transmitted through inhalation of airborne droplet nuclei spread by an infectious TB case through coughing or sneezing. Exposure to TB may initially result in an asymptomatic, latent form of infection ("latent TB") that is not transmissible to others but can cause an immune response detectable by standard TB screening tests such as the Mantoux tuberculin skin test (in which a tuberculin purified protein derivative is injected under the skin) or a TB interferon-gamma release assay, a blood test which measures TB immune reactivity. Five to ten percent of immunocompetent persons with latent TB infection ultimately develop active TB disease, in which the TB bacteria are no longer suppressed by the immune system and are now actively multiplying. The highest risk for progression is within the first two years following exposure; however, the risk of progressing to active TB is much higher in immunocompromised persons. While TB disease can present throughout the body, most active infections manifest in the lungs. Classic symptoms associated with active TB are fever, night sweats, weight loss, and cough. Persons with pulmonary TB may also develop cavitary lesions within the lungs and may transmit large numbers of organisms when they cough, speak, sing, or sneeze, exposing others around them who have had

---

*Editor's note: The 1998 article by Wakefield et al (*The Lancet* Volume 351, No. 9103, p637–641, 28 February 1998), which purported to show the association between autism and vaccines, was later retracted (*The Lancet* Volume 375, No. 9713, p445, 6 February 2010), with the statement that "the claims in the original paper that children were 'consecutively referred' and that investigations were 'approved' by the local ethics committee have been proven to be false."

prolonged contact and potentially leading to large contact investigations.

TB is notable for being a slow-growing infection. It may take several weeks for a patient specimen to grow TB bacteria, although the characteristic acid-fast bacilli may be immediately visible by direct staining. Similarly, TB treatment involves a prolonged antibiotic course lasting at least six months, but it is a curable infection if adherence to treatment is high.

Epidemiology of TB in the United States

Globally, TB is a leading cause of death, trailing only HIV/AIDS in deaths due to an infectious agent, with 8.6 million people sick with active TB and 1.3 million dying of TB in 2012, with the vast majority of illness and death occurring in resource-poor settings.[47] In the United States, TB was one of the leading causes of death at the beginning of the twentieth century,[48] but reported mortality from TB declined steadily during the first half of the century, due to improvements in housing that reduced crowding, development of effective antibiotics, and the creation of TB control programs, as well as general improvements in hygiene and sanitation that reduced the rates of many communicable diseases. TB first became nationally notifiable in 1952, and from then until 1985, there was a steady decline in reported incidence, averaging 4–5 percent per year for an overall decline of 74 percent. This marked decline led the CDC and the Advisory Council for the Elimination of

Tuberculosis (ACET) to establish in 1989 a national goal of TB elimination by 2010, defined as a case rate of less than 1 per million people, via a multifaceted approach involving more effective use of existing prevention and control methods; the development and evaluation of new prevention, diagnostic, and treatment technologies; and the rapid transfer of newly developed technologies into clinical and public health practice.[49]

In the late 1980s, however, TB experienced an unfortunate resurgence, driven by a number of factors, including the HIV epidemic; immigration of persons from countries with high prevalence of TB; outbreaks of TB in congregate settings such as hospitals, correctional facilities, and shelters for the homeless; increasing rates of drug-resistant TB; and premature funding reductions to public health programs reducing critical services necessary to control TB. With the implementation of strategies outlined in the ACET plan, since 1993 TB incidence has once again been declining, but the goal of elimination has not yet been met as of 2013, when 30 cases per million people were reported in the United States.

Certain populations are disproportionately affected by TB in the United States.[50] In 2014, the TB incidence rate among foreign-born persons was over 13 times higher than that of U.S.-born persons (see Figure 20-4). Over half of all foreign-born persons with TB originated from five countries: Mexico, the Philippines, Vietnam, India, and China. Four states alone—California, Texas, Florida, and New York—accounted for about half of all TB cases reported in 2013. Furthermore, the TB

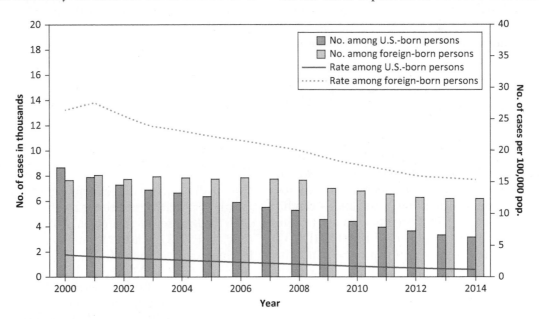

FIGURE 20-4 **Number and Rate* of Newly Diagnosed Tuberculosis (TB) Cases among U.S.-Born and Foreign-Born Persons, by Year Reported—United States, 2000–2014†**

*Per 100,000 population

†Data updated as of February 13, 2015. Data for 2014 are provisional.

DATA SOURCE: Scott et al. Trends in Tuberculosis – United States, 2014 incidence rate for Asians was over 28 times higher than that for whites. Addressing these pockets of higher TB incidence will be a crucial focus if the goal of TB elimination is to be achieved.

TB Prevention and Control

The public health approach to TB prevention and control in the United States has four major components.[51] First is the prompt identification of persons with active TB disease and assurance of treatment completion, to both cure infection and prevent transmission to others. Second, the identification and testing of persons exposed to active TB cases is crucial to prevent the development of secondary cases. Third, public health agencies partner with clinicians to conduct targeted testing among high-risk groups to identify latent TB infection, which can be treated before it progresses to active TB disease. Fourth, identifying settings at high risk for transmission and implementing appropriate infection control strategies can help stem the increasing burden of TB due to recent transmission.

From a public health perspective, TB control can be complicated by a number of factors, including the indolent nature of early infection, which may delay diagnosis and treatment; the prolonged course of multiple antibiotics necessary for successful treatment, raising the risk of suboptimal patient compliance which in turn may give rise to drug-resistant strains; and, due to the airborne nature of transmission, the potential to infect a large number of people through routine activities. TB control programs in the United States thus utilize a number of strategies to combat these barriers and obstacles. One key example is intensive TB case management, which ensures close public health oversight of TB cases throughout treatment by assigning public health staff to follow a TB case throughout the duration of treatment, address barriers to attending medical appointments or other necessary visits via the use of incentives (e.g., grocery coupons) and/or enablers (e.g., subway tokens), and in general serve as a liaison to medical care and social services. In some jurisdictions, medications can be provided free of charge to TB patients who are unable to cover the costs. Directly observed therapy (DOT) is another strategy to ensure treatment compliance, in which public health staff personally administer each dose of medication to a TB patient, either in a clinic, the patient's home or worksite, or some other mutually agreed-upon site. Ideally, DOT could be employed for every TB case to maximize treatment completion rates, but given the resource-intensive nature of this intervention, the CDC has defined priority categories for DOT,[52] including children, homeless persons, and persons with HIV/AIDS, among others.

Given the high public health risk of uncontrolled TB and in the interest of protecting the public's health, public health authorities maintain legal authority that can be exercised in certain situations,[53] namely when the health of the community is felt to be at risk due to the actions of a potentially infectious patient. The exact extent of legal oversight held by public health officials varies by jurisdiction. For instance, in some jurisdictions, a TB patient who is extremely noncompliant with medical evaluation and/or treatment may be served with a health officer directive or court order mandating compliance, and charges may be brought against patients who violate such orders in some jurisdictions. TB patients may be legally detained in isolation (in a hospital, for instance) until deemed noninfectious, or prohibited from going to work or school. The CDC's Division of Global Migration and Quarantine has the legal authority to isolate individuals with infectious TB who are arriving into the United States, and travel may also be blocked for TB patients who are attempting to leave the country.

SEXUALLY TRANSMITTED DISEASES

Sexually transmitted diseases (STDs) represent a range of infections and conditions that are primarily transmitted and acquired through sexual or close intimate contact. These include bacteria (e.g., *Chlamydia trachomatis*, *Neisseria gonorrhoeae*, and *Treponema pallidum*), viruses (e.g., human papilloma virus [HPV] and herpes simplex virus [HSV]), and other pathogens (e.g., *Trichomonas vaginalis*, scabies, and pubic lice or crabs). Additionally, infections whose primary route is nonsexual may also be transmitted sexually or through intimate contact, such as *Shigella*, *Salmonella*, and methicillin-resistant *Staphylococcus aureus* (MRSA).

Epidemiology of STDs in the United States

Chlamydia and gonorrhea represent the two most commonly reported conditions to the CDC.[54] In 2013, 1,401,906 cases of chlamydia, 333,004 cases of gonorrhea, and 17,375 cases of primary and secondary syphilis were reported to the CDC.[55] The corresponding rates were 446.6 per 100,000 population, 106.1 per 100,000, and 5.5 per 100,000, respectively.[56] While other STDs may be monitored locally or nationally, chlamydia, gonorrhea, and syphilis are often the foci of local, state, and federal public health surveillance and intervention. Chlamydia, gonorrhea, and syphilis are effectively cured with simple regimens of antibiotics.[57] Untreated chlamydia and gonorrhea infections in females have been associated with negative reproductive outcomes including pelvic inflammatory disease or salpingitis,[58] which can lead to compromised fertility and ectopic pregnancy. Among males, untreated gonorrhea and chlamydia is less severe, but can result in urethritis, epididymitis, and proctitis.[58] Untreated syphilis is also associated with a number of negative sequelae including congenital syphilis, which can cause severe lifelong deformities and complications, including death.[59] These three bacterial STDs have also been implicated in facilitating the acquisition and transmission of HIV.[60–62] The most recent estimates of the annual costs of all cases of chlamydia, gonorrhea, and syphilis exceeds $700 million.[63]

In the United States, two populations are disproportionately affected by bacterial STDs: adolescents and men who have sex with men (MSM). As shown in Figure 20-5, for both gonorrhea and chlamydia, rates of reported infections among adolescent females (ages 15–24) are significantly higher than rates of reported infections among adult females (ages 25–44). In 2013, the rates of adolescent female chlamydia and gonorrhea were approximately five times as high as those of adult females. Adolescent females are at particularly high risk for STDs due to the greater presence of columnar epithelium on the adolescent cervix[58] which can facilitate STD acquisition. Furthermore, adolescents may move from one monogamous partner to another

quickly, have concurrent (overlapping) sexual partnerships, and be less efficacious in negotiating condom use consistently.[64]

As shown in Figure 20-6, estimated rates of primary and secondary syphilis among MSM were steadily increasing from the 1960s through the late 1970s. The beginning of the U.S. HIV/AIDS epidemic was concurrent with a dramatic decline in primary and secondary syphilis among MSM likely because some MSM were becoming gravely ill with HIV/AIDS and likely not sexually active and many MSM adopted safer sex practices. Beginning in the late 1990s a syphilis resurgence began among MSM, as HIV antiretroviral therapeutic regimens became more efficacious, better tolerated, easier to adhere to, and more widely available, allowing for more sexual activity and increased opportunities for transmission. In 2013, 75 percent of reported primary and secondary syphilis reported in the United States was among MSM.[55] The estimated rate of primary and secondary syphilis among MSM is over 200 times as high as the rate among other males and females, as Figure 20-5 depicts. MSM may be at greater risk for bacterial STDs such as syphilis due to larger and more complicated sexual networks compared to heterosexuals, increased numbers of recent sexual partners, a higher background prevalence

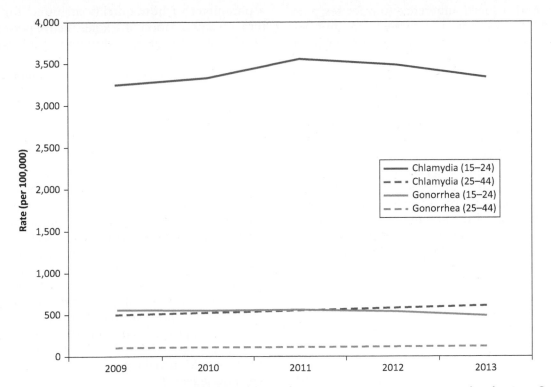

FIGURE 20-5 **Rates (per 100,000) of Reported Chlamydia and Gonorrhea Cases among Females, by Age Group, United States, 2009–2013**

Courtesy of U.S. Department of Health and Human Services, Centers for Disease Control and Prevention

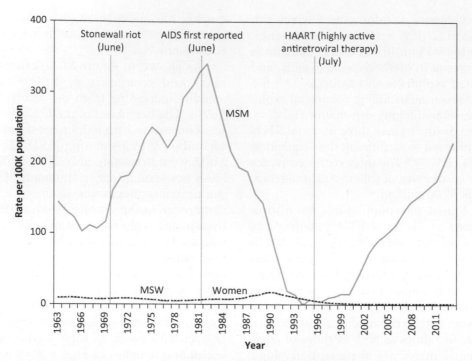

FIGURE 20-6   **Estimated Annual Rate of Primary and Secondary Syphilis among Men Who Have Sex with Men, Men Who Have Sex with Women Only (MSW), and Women. United States, 1963–2013**

DATA SOURCE: Peterman, Su, Bernstein, and Weinstock

of infection, and reduced adherence to safer sex practices as a result of improved HIV treatment and preventive interventions (e.g., preexposure prophylaxis, HIV serosorting).[65–68]

STD Control

Responsibility for the prevention and control of STDs often falls to the local and state health departments. The Anderson and May equation is a useful approach to conceptualizing epidemics of STDs within populations and identifying potential avenues for intervention.[69] Their equation is as follows: $R_0 = \beta cD$. R_0 represents the reproductive rate, or the average number of new infections that occur from one infected person in a population. When $R_0 > 1$, epidemic growth in a population occurs. When $R_0 < 1$, the epidemic is coming under control. In the Anderson and May model, R_0 is influenced by three factors; β, c, and D. β represents the average probability of transmission of the STD in the population; β is influenced not only by the virulence of the pathogen, but also the type of sexual activity (oral versus anal versus vaginal sex), condom use, and population levels of vaccination (for the case of HPV or hepatitis B). In the model, c represents the average rate of sexual contact in the population. This provides

a parameter of how quickly an infection can move through a population of sexually active persons. Finally, D represents the average duration of infection among those who are infected.

The three components of the Anderson and May model can be used to develop intervention priorities to reduce STD morbidity in a population. To halt or slow the spread of an STD in a given population, the R_0 needs to be reduced to a value less than 1. It is worth noting that this can be accomplished by reducing the value of β, c, and D simultaneously or by focusing efforts on one or two of the three parameters. Potential public health interventions that influence the β parameter include increased condom use or vaccination (for certain infections such as HPV or hepatitis B). While educational and social marketing campaigns may help increase condom use, recent data suggest that rates of use are less than optimal to effectively influence the reproductive rate of STD epidemics. Condom use among high school students in the United States in 2013 was approximately 60 percent and has remained unchanged since the 1990s.[70] Among MSM surveyed in 2014, only 25 percent reported always using condoms when having sex.[71]

Even more challenging may be attempts to influence the c component of the reproductive rate equation. The average rate of partner change impacts the potential "velocity" by which an STD moves through a population. Reducing the average number of partners could slow the rate of transmission. However, **c** is often influenced largely by the right tail of the distribution of sexual partners (i.e., those with the largest number of sexual partners). Among high school students, approximately 15 percent reported having had sex with four or more partners in 2013, slightly down from 18.7 percent in 1991.[70] However, among representative samples of adolescents and adults in the United States, the median number of lifetime sexual partners was greater among younger birth cohorts.[72]

From a public health perspective, the **D** parameter may be the most fruitful parameter to influence. The average duration of infection is impacted by a range of factors. Since many STDs are asymptomatic, screening is critical to more expedient diagnosis and treatment. By screening a larger proportion of the at-risk population, the period of infectiousness should be reduced. In the United States, numerous efforts have focused on increasing chlamydia screening. As part of Healthcare Effectiveness Data and Information Set (HEDIS), chlamydia screening is a health care quality indicator, and screening rates among at-risk females has increased.[73] Among those diagnosed with an STD, quick and appropriate treatment also helps reduce the average duration of infection. Ensuring that the sex partners of persons diagnosed with an STD are treated is also a crucial component of reducing **D**. Third-party confidential partner notification involves health department staff interviews of persons newly diagnosed with an STD or HIV and the collection of names and/or contact information of sexual partners who may have been exposed. The health department then contacts these partners (confidentially without disclosing the index patient who named them) and encourages them to be screened. Partner notification programs can help ensure quicker treatment and (in the case of syphilis) offer prophylactic treatment. In the modern age of Internet-based dating, partner notification has incorporated aspects of social media to help facilitate screening and case findings.[74,75] Finally, the national expansion of expedited partner therapy (providing STD treatment or prescriptions for the index patient to hand to his/her partners) may also help reduce **D**.[76]

The CDC supports local and state STD prevention and control activities. In fiscal year 2013, 59 percent of the CDC Division of STD Prevention's budget was allocated to state and local program grants.[77] Local health departments offer primary prevention for STDs through vaccinations for HPV and hepatitis B, as well as the provision of condoms, and secondary prevention

through routine screening for STDs through STD clinics, family planning clinics, HIV testing sites, and other clinical and nonclinical settings. In 2013, 8.9 percent, 14.3 percent, and 24.1 percent of chlamydia, gonorrhea, and primary and secondary syphilis, respectively, were diagnosed in categorical STD clinics.[56] The Patient Protection and Affordable Care Act of 2010 (ACA) will have great impacts on STD prevention and control in the United States. The ACA requires the coverage of services recommended by the U.S. Preventive Services Task Force (USPSTF), such as chlamydia screening for young women, without cost sharing.[78] Furthermore, states expanding Medicaid will increase the number of persons eligible for preventive health care services (including single women) with little or no cost.[78]

HIV/AIDS

Human immunodeficiency virus (HIV) is the agent that invades its human host and reproduces inside host immune system cells (*CD4 T-lymphocytes*) to produce a profound deficiency in host immunity known as **acquired immunodeficiency syndrome (AIDS)**. The syndrome that was soon to be called AIDS was first recognized in 1981 when several large U.S. cities noticed cases of *Pneumocystis* pneumonia and Kaposi's sarcoma in young gay men.[79] HIV itself was first identified by French scientists in 1983 and verified as the cause of AIDS in 1984.[80]

Burden in the United States

In November 2014, the CDC estimated that more than 1.2 million people in the United States were living with HIV (prevalence), including nearly 14 percent who were unaware of their infection.[81] The CDC estimates that about 50,000 Americans have been newly infected with HIV each year since the 1990s (incidence),[82] while new HIV diagnoses reported to the CDC dropped from nearly 57,000 in 2002 to under 42,000 in 2011 in the United States.[83]

In the United States, 880,440 persons were reported to the CDC as living with an HIV diagnosis by the end of 2011, while nearly 48,000 persons were reported as newly diagnosed with HIV in 2012.[84] In Table 20-4, four out of five newly diagnosed HIV cases and three out of four persons living with HIV are male adolescents and adults. By age, the highest rate of new reports is found among persons in their twenties, while those with the highest rate of persons living with HIV are in their forties and fifties. The race/ethnic group with the highest rate of new and prevalent HIV diagnoses in the United States is Black/African American.

TABLE 20-4 Diagnoses of HIV Infection in 2012 and Persons Living with Diagnosed HIV at the End of 2011, by Selected Characteristics—United States

Characteristic	Estimated[a] 2012 Diagnoses		Estimated[a] 2011 Prevalence	
	No.	Rate	No.	Rate
Sex				
Male (Adult or Adolescent)	38,160	29.9	661,072	523.7
Female (Adult or Adolescent)	9,586	7.2	216,756	163.7
Child (<13 years at end of year)	242	0.5	2,612	4.9
Age at Diagnosis (year)				
<13	242	0.5	2,612	4.9
13–14	51	0.6	1,020	12.4
15–19	2,053	9.6	6,701	31.0
20–24	8,187	36.3	31,142	140.6
25–29	7,589	35.5	52,056	244.6
30–34	6,388	30.5	70,415	343.3
35–39	4,939	25.3	86,096	439.4
40–44	5,145	24.5	130,474	620.2
45–49	5,183	23.9	169,080	762.9
50–54	3,800	16.8	143,773	637.1
55–59	2,269	10.9	95,565	471.7
60–64	1,221	6.9	52,497	294.7
≥–65	921	2.1	39,008	94.3
Race/Ethnicity				
American Indian/Alaska Native	228	9.9	2,797	122.2
Asian[b]	959	6.1	10,323	68.0
Black/African American	22,581	58.3	379,985	990.5
Hispanic/Latino[c]	9,816	18.5	172,411	332.3
Native Hawaiian/Other Pacific Islander	79	15.1	813	159.4
White	13,291	6.7	288,760	146.2
Multiple Races	1,036	17.3	25,351	435.2
Total[d]	**47,989**	**15.3**	**880,440**	**282.6**

[a]Estimated numbers resulted from statistical adjustment that accounted for reporting delays, but not for incomplete reporting. Rates are per 100,000 population.
[b]Includes Asian/Pacific Islander legacy cases.
[c]Hispanics/Latinos can be of any race.
[d]Includes persons of unknown race/ethnicity. Because column totals for estimated numbers were calculated independently of the values for the subpopulations, the values in each column may not sum to the column total.

SOURCE: Centers for Disease Control and Prevention

Surveillance

The first five cases of *Pneumocystis* pneumonia among severely immunocompromised homosexual men in Los Angeles, California, were described by the CDC in their June 6, 1981 Morbidity and Mortality Weekly Report.[85] Since then, HIV surveillance has evolved from a one-time report of incident AIDS cases, based on the presence of opportunistic infections (OIs) and other AIDS-defining conditions, to the reporting of laboratory evidence of HIV infection along with markers of immune compromise. Recent changes in prevention and care have led in turn to the longitudinal surveillance of persons living with HIV—requiring serial reported laboratory tests to monitor treatment success and progression of disease—for the entire lifetime of an infected person.

Since 2009, all 50 states, the District of Columbia, and nine U.S. territories have contributed to National HIV Surveillance System (NHSS). NHSS uses a uniform CDC-supplied relational computer database known as "eHARS," Enhanced HIV/AIDS Reporting System, which allows users to collect complete, timely, and high-quality data for HIV and AIDS by collating data from case reports, lab reports, death certificates, birth certificates, and other documents in a document-based data management format. This allows documents to be stored and retained electronically in their original format.[86]

Headed by the CDC's Division of HIV/AIDS Prevention, NHSS is tasked not only to continue traditional surveillance activities—such as monitoring the extent and characteristics of HIV transmission in a complete, timely, and accurate manner—but also to evaluate how states and large local health jurisdictions were achieving National HIV/AIDS Strategy objectives discussed below. Reported serial care provider-ordered laboratory test results are used as evidence for such activities as linkage of newly HIV-diagnosed persons to care in a timely manner (within three months of diagnosis) and retention of HIV-infected persons in care (as evidenced by having at least two medical care visits in the most previous year). In addition, viral suppression—achieved by treatment with a combination of antiretroviral drugs to reduce the amount of virus in the blood to an undetectable level, and which itself has been linked to reduced HIV transmission—is monitored and evaluated on a population basis by NHSS.

Transmission

HIV is spread through contact with the blood, semen, preseminal fluid, vaginal fluids, rectal fluids, or breast milk, from a person infected with HIV.[87] It is most often transmitted through sex with an HIV-infected partner. The highest sexual risk is from "receptive" penile-anal sexual intercourse.[88] The most efficient transmission of HIV is from blood transfusion and tissue transplantation which is now, due to mandatory HIV testing of donors, very rare. Another increasingly uncommon but highly efficient mode of HIV transmission is through *perinatal* exposure—that is, from a (usually untreated) HIV-infected pregnant woman to her fetus/newborn infant during pregnancy, labor and delivery, or breastfeeding. Another common route of transmission is the sharing of needles and syringes contaminated with HIV-tainted blood during the injection of (usually illicit) drugs. Less frequently, HIV may also be transmitted occupationally, for example, through needle stick injury.

For surveillance purposes, the CDC's Division of HIV/AIDS Prevention groups transmission risk into mutually exclusive categories: men who have sex with men (MSM); injection drug use (IDU); MSM/IDU; heterosexual contact; perinatal; and other blood-borne (transfusion, tissue transplantation, hemodialysis, etc.). Table 20-5 presents the breakdown of newly diagnosed HIV and prevalent HIV cases by transmission category for male and female adults and adolescents, as well as for children. For both newly diagnosed HIV and prevalent cases, the predominant mode of transmission in men is male-to-male sexual contact, while for women it is heterosexual contact and, for children, perinatal exposure.[84]

Testing

Identification of HIV infection is usually done by the detection of HIV antibodies in blood (or saliva) and/or of the viral nucleic acid in blood. By 1985, the first licensed test to detect antibodies to HIV was available,[80] but because it would not show a positive result until nearly two months after infection, acute and some recent cases of HIV infection were missed. Subsequent generations of these antibody tests have cut down the window period to detection to 14 days. HIV nucleic acid tests are also available, with the best able to detect HIV in the blood in as little as 9–10 days after infection, making the routine diagnosis of recent and acute HIV infection possible.[89] HIV testing is currently recommended for pregnant women and all adults and adolescents, aged 15–65 years.[90]

Tests are also available to monitor how well a person with HIV is doing in controlling the infection while in care and on treatment. One measures the amount of virus in blood ("viral load"); the other monitors the status of the infected person's immune system ("CD4 count"). Other advances in HIV testing have allowed for rapid testing of antibodies to HIV in saliva as well as blood, making point-of-care testing possible in places and at times not otherwise available. HIV tests can also distinguish the two major types of HIV, the most prevalent in the United States (HIV-1), as well as HIV-2, which is more commonly found in cases presenting from Western Africa. Finally, resistant strains of HIV can be detected using molecular

TABLE 20-5 Diagnoses of HIV Infection in 2012 and Persons Living with Diagnosed HIV at End of 2011, by Transmission Category—United States

Characteristic	Estimated[a] 2012 Diagnoses		Estimated[a] 2011 Prevalence	
	No.	Percent	No.	Percent
Male Adult or Adolescent				
Male-to-male sexual contact	30,695	80.4%	451,656	68.3%
Injection drug use	2,019	5.3%	83,207	12.6%
Male-to-male sexual contact and injection drug use	1,356	3.6%	48,366	7.3%
Heterosexual contact[b]	4,008	10.5%	70,732	10.7%
Perinatal	–	–	3,891	0.6%
Other[c]	81	0.2%	3,220	0.5%
Subtotal	38,160	100%	661,072	100%
Female Adult or Adolescent				
Injection drug use	1,295	13.5%	53,047	24.5%
Heterosexual contact[b]	8,182	85.4%	157,519	72.7%
Perinatal	–	–	4,220	1.9%
Other[c]	109	1.1%	1,969	0.9%
Subtotal	9,586	100%	216,756	100%
Child (<13 years at end of year)				
Perinatal	161	66.5%	2,246	86%
Other[c]	81	33.5%	366	14%
Subtotal	242	100%	2,612	100%
Total	**47,989**		**880,440**	

[a]Estimated numbers resulted from statistical adjustment that accounted for reporting delays, but not for incomplete reporting. Rates are per 100,000 population.

[b]Heterosexual contact with a person known to have, or to be at high risk for, HIV infection.

[c]Includes hemophilia, blood transfusion, and risk factor not reported or not identified.

[d]Includes persons of unknown race/ethnicity. Because column totals for estimated numbers were calculated independently of the values for the subpopulations, the values in each column may not sum to the column total.

SOURCE: Centers for Disease Control and Prevention

genotype tests, which are used to guide the clinician in determining which antiretroviral regimen to use.

Treatment

In 1981, AIDS was an untreatable, overwhelmingly fatal disease, with death often preceded by one or more opportunistic infections (most commonly *Pneumocystis* pneumonia), muscle wasting, and/or HIV-related dementia. Today, once diagnosed, HIV infection is a manageable chronic disease that can be made much less transmissible by successful treatment with the use of highly active antiretroviral therapy, or "HAART," in which three or more drugs of different "classes"—that is, having differing mechanisms of antiretroviral activity—are given in combination.[91] The routine use of HAART in the United States beginning around 1995 resulted in a dramatic decrease in both AIDS-related death and in the progression to severe HIV disease, that is, AIDS (see Figure 20-7).

Since 1990, the federal Health Resources and Services Administration (HRSA) *Ryan White HIV/AIDS*

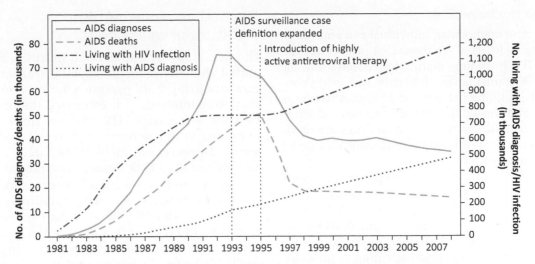

FIGURE 20-7 Estimated Number of AIDS Diagnoses and Deaths and Estimated Number of Persons Living with AIDS Diagnosis* and Living with Diagnosed or Undiagnosed HIV Infection† among Persons Aged >13 Years—United States, 1981–2008

*Yearly AIDS estimates were obtained by statistically adjusting national surveillance data reported through June 2010 for reporting delays, but not for incomplete reporting.

†HIV prevalence estimates were based on national HIV surveillance data reported through June 2010 using extended back-calculation.

Courtesy of Centers for Disease Control and Prevention

Program has funded state and local public health agencies to provide both primary medical care and essential support services for those persons living with HIV unable to afford such care, as well as to support community-planning groups that advise them both on how and where to target these funds and in the development of best practices in HIV care.[92]

Prevention

Although vaccines have been and are being developed, none has proven to be viable for safely and effectively preventing HIV on a large scale. Traditional public health HIV prevention efforts concentrate on both policy-level changes—for example, laws that protect HIV-infected persons from discrimination in the work place and laws that make the sale and replacement of clean needles legally available—and the use of HIV prevention interventions, at the individual and community levels, that have proven efficacy to avert new infections. Examples of the latter include the use of peer navigators to educate and to role-model risk reduction behaviors while also addressing local socioeconomic, cultural, and environmental challenges,[93] and group-level interventions to increase awareness of HIV risk behaviors as well as to support individuals in reducing these risks—such as those focusing on a very high-risk group, young black men who have sex with men.[94] Other topics, such as stigma, homophobia, and racism are often addressed as well. Other prevention modalities promote HIV testing among high-risk groups, as well as increasing availability of condoms and clean needles and syringes for persons who inject drugs.

In 2010, the first-ever *National HIV/AIDS Strategy for the United States* (NHAS) was published by the White House Office of National AIDS Policy with three primary goals: reduce the number of people who become infected with HIV; increase access to care and optimize health outcomes for people living with HIV; and reduce HIV-related health disparities.[95]

According to the CDC, "proven" HIV prevention methods include: HIV testing with prompt linkage to care and antiretroviral treatment to achieve viral suppression; access to condoms; prevention programs for persons infected with HIV, their partners, and persons at high risk for acquiring HIV; substance abuse treatment and access to clean needles/syringes; and screening and treatment of other sexually transmitted infections.[96]

Over 30 years of experience has shown that to successfully reduce HIV transmission a combination of strategies needs to be employed simultaneously,[96,97] including: *educational* (e.g., comprehensive science-based school sexual health education and clinical provider delivered prevention education for HIV-infected patients);[98] *behavioral* (e.g., individual, group, and community-level interventions that are research-proven to provide the tools and support needed to change behavior among high-risk populations);[99] *structural* (e.g., policy and legal changes that empower at-risk communities and expand access to condoms, clean needles, and stable housing);[100] and *biomedical* (e.g., routine prenatal HIV testing,[101] "treatment as prevention,"[102] occupational[103] and nonoccupational postexposure prophylaxis,[104] and preexposure prophylaxis[105]).

Prevention at the Individual Level

The most effective methods an individual can employ to prevent becoming infected are those that protect against exposure to HIV, including: getting tested and knowing a partner's HIV status; having less risky sex; using condoms correctly; limiting the number of sexual partners; getting tested and treated for sexually transmitted infections; not injecting drugs or, if injected drugs are used, using only sterile drug injection equipment and never sharing equipment with others.[106]

State and local public health department activities are instrumental in enabling individuals to protect themselves from HIV: by funding free HIV testing sites through community-based organizations (CBOs); by providing free condoms to CBOs, schools, jails, public fairs, and other venues; and providing counseling and assistance to persons recently diagnosed with STD and/or HIV—not only by identifying and testing their sexual contacts, but also by linking newly diagnosed HIV-infected persons into treatment and helping them to stay in care.[107]

Prevention at the Community Level

State and large local public health agencies, supported by the CDC's Comprehensive Prevention Programs and, often, other state and federal funding sources, are tasked with allocating prevention resources both within the agency and in collaboration with community-planning groups and CBOs to reach those populations at greatest need—through such activities as street outreach, group-level risk reduction, educational efforts, prevention case management, social marketing, lobbying their legislature, as well as capacity building in communities to deliver and evaluate services.[108]

Community-level interventions include targeted social marketing efforts (via billboards, radio, and the Internet) that are culturally relevant and linguistically appropriate, and mobilizing communities to decrease HIV stigma and homophobia (such as by coalitions of faith-based organizations within high-risk populations). Other social structural and environmental changes are meant to aid individual efforts at adopting protective behaviors by changing social norms, laws, and policies. These include: making HIV testing routine for all adults and adolescents; changing sex education curricula in schools both to increase student knowledge of, and tolerance for, alternative sexuality as well as to inform them about behaviors that can reduce the risk for acquiring STDs, including HIV; passing laws that allow for needle exchanges and selling of needles and syringes without a prescription; passing laws that ban discrimination of HIV-infected persons; and increasing housing for homeless and unstably housed persons.[100]

Biomedical Intervention: "Treatment as Prevention"

Citing a study by Marks et al. in 2006,[109] the CDC stated that the majority of HIV transmission was now occurring from persons who were unaware that they were infected.[110] It estimated the proportion of persons living with HIV who are unaware of their status to be 25 percent in 2003[111] and, more recently, 14 percent in 2014.[112] In 2011, the U.S. Preventive Services Task Force recommended that HIV testing be routine for all adolescents and adults in the United States.[90] By then, a preponderance of articles in the scientific literature had shown that early treatment of HIV—at first evidence of infection—was found to be beneficial both in preserving the health of HIV-infected persons as well as in decreasing HIV transmission to others.[35,36,113,114] As a result of these successful biomedical prevention efforts, "treatment as prevention" became one primary focus of the CDC's HIV prevention strategy.[96]

In 1994, it was shown that perinatal (mother-to-newborn infant) transmission of HIV could be successfully reduced from 25 percent to 8 percent through the use of antiretroviral drugs during pregnancy, throughout labor and delivery and, for the newborn, immediately postpartum.[115] Subsequent recommendations for universal prenatal HIV counseling and testing, antiretroviral prophylaxis, scheduled caesarean delivery, and breastfeeding avoidance further reduced perinatal transmission of HIV to less than 2 percent in the United States.[116]

Since 1997, postexposure prophylaxis, or *PEP*, has been recommended for occupational exposure to HIV-infected fluids—most often via needle stick injury. In a 2005 MMWR article, the CDC expanded its recommendation to significant nonoccupational exposures: "For persons seeking care <72 hours after nonoccupational exposure to blood, genital secretions, or other potentially infectious body fluids of a person known to be HIV-infected, when that exposure represents a substantial risk for transmission, a 28-day course of highly active antiretroviral therapy (HAART) is recommended."[104]

Finally, recent studies have also shown that a two-drug FDA-approved antiretroviral combination can reduce HIV transmission in persons at high risk for being infected.[117] According to the CDC, preexposure prophylaxis, or *PrEP*, is recommended as one prevention option for sexually active adult men who have sex with men (MSM), adult heterosexually active men and women who are at substantial risk of HIV acquisition, adult injection drug users at substantial risk of HIV acquisition, and heterosexually active women and men whose partners are known to have HIV infection (i.e., HIV-discordant couples).[105]

HEALTH-CARE-ASSOCIATED INFECTIONS

Health-care-associated infections, or HAIs, have drawn an increasing level of attention due to the threat they pose to patient safety.[118] A recent study examining a large sample of United States acute care hospitals revealed that much work remains to be done to reduce the rates of HAIs: in 2011, 4 percent of inpatients experienced at least one HAI during their hospitalization, leading to an estimated 722,000 HAIs and 75,000 deaths in 2011 alone.[119] Pneumonias and surgical site infections comprised nearly half of these infections, with *Clostridium difficile* illness causing the bulk of health-care-associated gastrointestinal illness.

Collaborative research and surveillance efforts are in place to stem the rise in HAIs in the United States. In 2008, the U.S. Department of Health and Human Services spearheaded an interagency steering committee dedicated to expanding HAI prevention efforts nationwide, leading to the development of a nationwide roadmap to combat HAIs[120] and the Partnership for Patients initiative in 2009. Also, nearly 13,000 U.S. health care facilities contribute yearly data to the CDC's National Healthcare Safety Network, allowing for the timely study and monitoring of HAI rate reduction.

While antibiotic medications have been a large contributor to our success in controlling communicable diseases, their widespread use has given rise to resistant bacterial strains, often associated with HAIs. Vancomycin, an antibiotic routinely used to combat the long-recognized methicillin-resistant *Staphylococcus aureus* (MRSA), has lost effectiveness against some strains of bacteria, including not only some *Enterococcus* species but even some strains of MRSA itself. Resistance to carbapenems, a class of powerful, broad-spectrum antibiotics, is increasingly documented; infections with carbapenem-resistant organisms can be extraordinarily difficult to treat and have caused numerous health-care-associated outbreaks in the United States alone.[121–123] *Antibiotic stewardship* programs in health care facilities and public health agencies are designed to promote the judicious use of appropriate antibiotics to treat infections, to prevent the continued rise of resistant strains.

BIOTERRORISM

The threat of weaponized biological agents intentionally released to cause harm has been a focal point of public health emergency preparedness efforts. The intentional spread of anthrax to Americans through the U.S. postal system in the days following the events of September 11, 2001, highlighted the need to improve public health capacity to identify and respond to such biological threats. The CDC has developed a strategic roadmap for public health stakeholders to assist ongoing preparedness efforts,[124] outlining eight objectives to guide partners in improving preparedness infrastructure.

Biologic agents felt to be of highest threat to national security are designated as Category A, B, or C agents, depending on an agent's ability to spread easily; the severity of illness an agent causes, particularly if fatal; an agent's ability to cause social disruption; and any special preparedness needs for a particular agent. Biologic agents included in Category A, the highest priority category, include anthrax, botulism, tularemia, plague, smallpox, and viral hemorrhagic fevers such as Ebola or Lassa viruses. Category B agents include ricin toxin, Q fever, and agents that may threaten the water supply such as *Cryptosporidium parvum*, among other agents. Emerging agents that may have the potential to be weaponized in the future, such as hantavirus, are grouped into Category C. Further attention is given to bioterrorism in Chapter 26.

SUMMARY

From improved sanitation and clean drinking water, to enhanced surveillance systems and new therapies, to expanded vaccine access and coverage for an increasing number of illnesses, we have come a long way in the control of infectious diseases. However, infectious diseases continue to remain significant causes of morbidity and mortality in the United States, but even more so in low-income countries. In our increasingly global society, introducing an infectious illness into a new environment may be as simple as an airplane flight, only serving to highlight the need for continued vigilance for infectious threats in our public health system.

REVIEW QUESTIONS

1. What are the methods by which infectious diseases are transmitted?
2. What are the major steps of an outbreak investigation?
3. What are some strategies that have supported the widespread availability of vaccines in the United States?
4. How has the HIV/AIDS epidemic in the United States affected rates of other sexually transmitted infections?
5. What are the four main components of TB prevention and control in the United States?
6. Name some strategies used to prevent waterborne and foodborne illnesses.
7. Describe several strategies to study and reduce rates of health-care-associated infections.

REFERENCES

1. Centers for Disease Control and Prevention. Achievements in Public Health, 1900–1999: Control of Infectious Diseases. *MMWR* 48(29):621–629.

2. World Health Organization. Global Health Estimates 2014 Summary Tables. http://www .who.int/entity/healthinfo/global_burden_disease/ GHE_DthGlobal_2000_2012.xls?ua=1. Accessed September 15, 2014.

3. Liu L, Johnson H, Cousens S, et al. Global, regional, and national causes of child mortality: an updated systematic analysis for 2010 with time trends since 2000. *Lancet.* 2012 June 9;379(9832):2151–2161.

4. Heymann D.L. *Control of Communicable Disease Manual.* 19th Edition. Washington, DC: American Public Health Association; 2008.

5. Lee L, Teutsch S, Thacker S, M St Louis. *Principles and Practice of Public Health Surveillance.* New York: Oxford University Press; 2010.

6. Gregg M.B. Chapter 5: Conducting a Field Investigation. In: Gregg M, ed. Field *Epidemiology.* 3rd edition. New York: Oxford University Press; 2008: 81–96

7. Reingold AL. Outbreak Investigations – A Perspective. *Emerg Infect Dis.* 1998 January–March; 4(1):21–27.

8. Strebel PM, Sutter RW, Cochi SL, et al. Epidemiology of poliomyelitis in the United States one decade after the last reported case of indigenous wild virus-associated disease. *Clin Infect Dis.* 1992;14:568–579.

9. Centers for Disease Control and Prevention. Surveillance for waterborne disease outbreaks associated with drinking water and other nonrecreational water - United States, 2009–2010. *MMWR* Morb Mortal Wkly Rep. 2013 September 6;62(35):7147–720.

10. (No authors listed). Collaborative Report: A waterborne epidemic of salmonellosis in Riverside, California, 1965. *Am J Epidemiol.* 1971;93:33.

11. MacKenzie W, Hoxie N, Proctor M, et al. A massive outbreak in Milwaukee of Cryptosporidium infection transmitted through the public water supply. *N Engl J Med.* 1994;331:161–167.

12. Hlavsa MC, Roberts VA, Kahler AM, et al. Recreational Water–Associated Disease Outbreaks — United States, 2009–2010. *MMWR.* 2014 Jan 10;63(1):6–10. Erratum in: *MMWR.* 2014 Jan 31;63(4):82.

13. Scallan E, Griffin PM, Angulo FJ, Tauxe RV, RM Hoekstra. Foodborne Illness Acquired in the United States – Unspecified Agents. *Emerg Infect Dis.* 2011 January;17(1):16–22.

14. Scallan E, Hoekstra RM, Angulo FJ, Tauxe RV, Widdowson MA, Roy SL, Jones JL, Griffin PM. Foodborne Illness Acquired in the United States – Major Pathogens. *Emerg Infect Dis.* 2011 January;17(1):7–15.

15. Gould LH, Walsh KA, Vieira AR, Herman K, Williams IT, Hall AJ et al. Surveillance for foodborne disease outbreaks - United States, 1998–2008. *MMWR Surveill Summ.* 2013 June 28;62(2):1–34.

16. Food and Drug Administration. *HACCP Principles and Applications Guidelines.* Adopted August 14, 1997. At http://www.fda.gov/Food/Guidance Regulation/HACCP/ucm2006801.htm#princ. Accessed December 1, 2014.

17. Keep Food Safe: Check your Steps. At www .foodsafety.gov. Accessed November 20, 2014.

18. Centers for Disease Control and Prevention. General Recommendations on Immunization: Recommendations of the Advisory Committee on Immunization Practices (ACIP). *MMWR* 2011:(RR 60–2):1–61.

19. Centers for Disease Control and Prevention. Ten Great Public Health Achievements – United States, 1900–1999. http://www.cdc.gov/mmwr/PDF/wk/ mm4812.pdf. Accessed December 8, 2014.

20. Roush SW, Murphy TV, Vaccine-Preventable Disease Table Working Group. Historical comparisons of morbidity and mortality for vaccine-preventable diseases in the United States. *JAMA* 2007;298(18):2155–2163.

21. Centers for Disease Control and Prevention. Final 2013 Reports of Nationally Notifiable Infectious Diseases. *MMWR* 2014;63(32):702–715.

22. Katz SL, Hinman AR. Summary and conclusions: measles elimination meeting, 16—17 March 2000. *J Infect Dis* 2004;189(Suppl 1):S43—S47.

23. Centers for Disease Control and Prevention. Elimination of rubella and congenital rubella syndrome – United States, 1969–2004. *MMWR* 2005;54(11):279–282.

24. Centers for Disease Control and Prevention. National, State, and Selected Local Area Vaccination Coverage Among Children Aged 19–35 Months – United States, 2013. *MMWR* 2014;63(34):741–748.

25. Centers for Disease Control and Prevention. Flu vaccination coverage, United States, 2012–2013 influenza season. http://www.cdc.gov/flu/ fluvaxview/coverage-1213 estimates.htm. Accessed September 21, 2014.

26. Centers for Disease Control and Prevention. Non-influenza vaccination coverage among adults – United States, 2012. *MMWR* 2014;63(5):95–102.

27. Centers for Disease Control and Prevention. Epidemiology and Prevention of VaccinePreventable Diseases. http://www.cdc.gov/vaccines/pubs/pinkbook/index.html. Accessed December 8, 2014.

28. Centers for Disease Control and Prevention. Immunization of Health-Care Personnel: Recommendations of the Advisory Committee on Immunization Practices (ACIP). *MMWR* 2011;60(RR07):1–45.

29. National Association of City and County Health Officials. 2013 National Profile of local health departments. http://www.naccho.org/topics/infrastructure/profile/upload/2013–National-Profile-of-Local-Health-Departments-report.pdf. Accessed December 8, 2014.

30. U.S. Department of Health and Human Services. The Affordable Care Act and Immunization. http://www.hhs.gov/healthcare/facts/factsheets/2010/09/The-Affordable-Care-Act-and-Immunization.html. Accessed December 8, 2014.

31. Centers for Disease Control and Prevention. The Prevention and Public Health Fund. http://www.cdc.gov/fmo/topic/Budget%20Information/appropriations_budget_form_pdf/The-Prevention-and-Public-Health-Fund.pdf. Accessed December 8, 2014.

32. Centers for Disease Control and Prevention. CDC Vaccine Price List. http://www.cdc.gov/vaccines/programs/vfc/awardees/vaccine-management/price-list/index.html. Accessed September 2, 2014.

33. Centers for Disease Control and Prevention. Vaccines For Children Program (VFC). http://www.cdc.gov/vaccines/programs/vfc/index.html. Accessed September 21, 2014.

34. Centers for Disease Control and Prevention. Vaccination Coverage Among Children in Kindergarten- United States, 2011–12 School Year. *MMWR* 2012; 61(33):647–652.

35. U.S. Department of Health and Human Services. Healthy People 2020, Immunization and Infectious Diseases. http://www.healthypeople.gov/2020/topicsobjectives2020/objectiveslist.aspx?topicId=23. Accessed September 21, 2014.

36. Task Force on Community Preventive Services. Increasing Appropriate Vaccination: Immunization Information Systems. Available at http://www.thecommunityguide.org/vaccines/imminfosystems.html. Accessed September 21, 2014.

37. Centers for Disease Control and Prevention. Progress in Immunization Information Systems – United States, 2012. *MMWR* 2013;62(49):1005–1008.

38. Orenstein WA, Bernier RH, Dondero TJ, Hinman AR, Marks JS, Bart KJ, Sirotkin B. Field Evaluation of vaccine efficacy. *Bull. WHO* 1986;63:1055–1068.

39. Centers for Disease Control and Prevention. Updated Recommendations of the Advisory Committee on Immunization Practices (ACIP) Regarding Routine Poliovirus Vaccination. *MMWR* 2009;58(30):829–8230.

40. CDC Vaccine Datalink. http://www.cdc.gov/vaccinesafety/Activities/vsd.html. Accessed September 21, 2014.

41. Murphy TV, Gargiullo PM, Massoudi MS, et al. Intussusception among infants given an oral rotavirus vaccine. *New Engl J Med* 2001;344:564–572.

42. Maglione MA, Das L, Raaen L, Smith A, et al. Safety of vaccines used for routine immunization of U.S. children: A systematic review. *Pediatrics.* 20134;134(2):1–15. http://pediatrics.aappublications.org/content/early/2014/06/26/peds.2014–1079.full.pdf. Accessed December 8, 2014.

43. Health Resources and Services Administration. National Vaccine Injury Compensation Program. http://www.hrsa.gov/vaccinecompensation/index.html. Accessed December 8, 2014.

44. Vaccine requirements and exemptions. http://www.vaccineethics.org/issue_briefs/requirements.php. Accessed September 21, 2014.

45. Centers for Disease Control and Prevention. Measles – United States, January 1 – May 23, 2014. *MMWR.* 2014;63(22):496–499.

46. Matthias J, Dusek C, Pritchard PS, Rutledge L, Kinchen P, Lander M. Outbreak of pertussis in a school and religious community averse to health care and vaccinations—Columbia County, Florida, 2013. *MMWR.* 2014;63(30):655.

47. World Health Organization. Global Health Observatory: Tuberculosis. http://www.who.int/gho/tb/en/. Accessed September 10, 2014

48. Centers for Disease Control and Prevention. Leading Causes of Death, 1900–1998. http://www.cdc.gov/nchs/data/dvs/lead1900_98.pdf. Accessed September 10, 2014

49. Centers for Disease Control and Prevention. A strategic plan for the elimination of tuberculosis in the United States. *MMWR.* 1989;38(S-3):1–25.

50. Scott C et al. Trends in Tuberculosis – United States, 2014. *MMWR*. 2014 March 20; 64(10);265–269.

51. Centers for Disease Control and Prevention. Controlling Tuberculosis in the United States. *MMWR*. November 4, 2005. 54(RR12);1–81.

52. American Thoracic Society, CDC, and Infectious Diseases Society of America. Treatment of Tuberculosis. *MMWR*. June 20, 2003 / 52(RR11);1–77.

53. Centers for Disease Control and Prevention. Tuberculosis Control Laws and Policies: A Handbook for Public Health and Legal Practitioners. Published October 1, 2009. Accessed September 11, 2014.

54. Centers for Disease Control and Prevention. Summary of notifiable diseases – United States, 2012. *MMWR*. September 19, 2014 / 61(53);1–121.

55. Centers for Disease Control and Prevention. Sexually Transmitted Disease Surveillance 2013. Atlanta: U.S. Department of Health and Human Services; 2014.

56. Centers for Disease Control and Prevention. Sexually Transmitted Disease Surveillance 2013. Atlanta: U.S. Department of Health and Human Services; 2014.

57. Centers for Disease Control and Prevention. Sexually Transmitted Diseases Treatment Guidelines, 2010. *MMWR*. 2010;59(No. RR-12).

58. Stamm, WE. Chlamydia trachomatis infections in the adult. In. *Sexually Transmitted Diseases*. Holmes, KK, Sparling, PF, Stamm, WE, Piot, P, Wasserheit, JN, Corey, L, Cohen, M, Watts, DH. 4th edition. New York: McGraw-Hill Professional.

59. Shafii T, Radolf JD, Sanchez PJ, Schulz KF, Murphy FK. Congenital Syphilis. In. *Sexually Transmitted Diseases*. Holmes, KK, Sparling PF, Stamm WE, Piot P, Wasserheit JN, Corey L, Cohen M, Watts DH. 4th edition. New York: McGraw-Hill Professional.

60. Bernstein KT, Marcus JL, Nieri G, et al. Rectal gonorrhea and Chlamydia reinfection is associated with increased risk of HIV seroconversion. *J Acquir Immune Defic Syndr*. 2010; 53:537Y543.

61. Craib KJ, Meddings DR, Strathdee SA, et al. Rectal gonorrhea as an independent risk factor for HIV infection in a cohort of homosexual men. *Genitourin Med*. 1995; 71:150Y154.

62. Zetola NM, Bernstein KT, Wong E, et al. Exploring the relationship between sexually transmitted diseases and HIV acquisition by using different study designs. *J Acquir Immune Defic Syndr*. 2009;50:546Y551.

63. Owusu-Edusei K, Chesson HW, Gift TL, Tao G, Mahajan R, Banez MC, Kent CK. The estimated direct medical costs of selected sexually transmitted infections in the United States, 2008. *Sex Trans Dis*. 2013;40(3):197–201.

64. Eaton DK, Kann L, Kinchen S, et al. Youth risk behavior surveillance—United States, 2011. *MMWR Surveillance summaries* (Washington, DC: 2002) 2012;61:1–162.

65. Peterman TA, Su J, Bernstein KT, Weinstock H. Syphilis in the United States: On the rise? *Expert Rev Anti Infect Ther*. 2014 Dec 9:1–8.

66. Snowden JM, Wei C, McFarland W, Raymond HF. Prevalence, correlates and trends in seroadaptive behaviours among men who have sex with men from serial cross-sectional surveillance in San Francisco, 2004–2011. *Sex Transm Infect*.? 2014 Sep;90(6):498–504. DOI: 10.1136/ sextrans-2013–051368. Epub 2014 Mar 31.

67. Paz-Bailey G, Meyers A, Blank S, Brown J, Rubin S, Braxton J, Zaidi A, Schafzin J, Weigl S, Markowitz LE. A case control study of syphilis among men who have sex with men in New York City: association With HIV infection. *Sex Transm Dis*. 2004 Oct;31(10):581–587.

68. Bernstein KT, Stephens SC, Strona FV, Kohn RP, Philip SS. Epidemiologic Characteristics of an Ongoing MSM Syphilis Epidemic, San Francisco. *Sex Transm Dis*. 2013 Jan;40(1):11–17.

69. Anderson, RM. & May, RM. (1991). *Infectious Diseases of Humans*. Oxford: Oxford University Press.

70. Centers for Disease Control and Prevention. Youth Risk Behavior Surveillance-United States, 2013 *MMWR*. 2014;63(SS#4).

71. Kaiser Family Foundation. HIV/AIDS in the Lives of Gay and Bisexual Men in the United States. September 2014

72. Liu G, Hariri S, Bradley H, Gottlieb SL, Leichliter JS, Markowitz LE. Trends and Patterns of Sexual Behaviors Among Adolescents and Adults Aged 14 to 59 Years, United States. *Sex Trans Dis*. January 2015. 42(1):20–26.

73. National Committee for Quality Assurance. The State of Health Care Quality, 2014. October 2014

74. Hightow-Weidman L, Beagle S, Pike E, Kuruc J, Leone P, Mobley V, Foust E, Gay C. "No one's at home and they won't pick up the phone": using the Internet and text messaging to enhance partner services in North Carolina. *Sex Transm Dis*. 2014 Feb;41(2):143–148.

75. Hunter P, Oyervides O, Grande KM, Prater D, Vann V, Reitl I, Biedrzycki PA. Facebook-augmented partner notification in a cluster of syphilis cases in Milwaukee. *Public Health Rep.* 2014 January–February;129 Suppl 1:43–49.

76. Centers for Disease Control and Prevention. Expedited Partner Therapy. Sexually Transmitted Diseases website. http://www.cdc.gov/std/ept/. January 27, 2015. Accessed January 28, 2015.

77. Bolan G. Update from the CDC Division of STD Prevention. National Coalition of STD Directors Annual Meeting, October 28–21,2014. Alexandria, VA.

78. Loosier PS, Malcarney M-B, Slive L, Cramer RC, Burgess B, Hoover KW, Romaguera R. Chlamydia screening for sexually active young women under the Affordable Care Act: New opportunities and lingering barriers. *Sex Trans Dis.* Sept 2014;41(9): 538–544.

79. Centers for Disease Control and Prevention. HIV Surveillance – United States, 1981–2008. *MMWR,* 2011;60:689–693.

80. Gallo RC and Montagnier L. The discovery of HIV as the cause of AIDS. *NEJM.* 2003;349: 2283–2285.

81. Centers for Disease Control and Prevention. *HIV in the United States: At a glance.* Published November 2014.

82. Centers for Disease Control and Prevention. *CDC Fact Sheet: New HIV infections in the United States.* Published December 2012.

83. Satcher-Johnson A, Hall I, Hu X, et al. Trends in HIV infection in the United States, 2002–2011 (Letter). *JAMA.* 2014;312:432–434.

84. Centers for Disease Control and Prevention. *HIV Surveillance Report,* 2012; vol24.

85. Centers for Disease Control and Prevention. *Pneumocystis* pneumonia – Los Angeles. *MMWR.* 1981; 30(21);1–3.

86. Centers for Disease Control and Prevention. *eHARS Technical Reference Guide.* Published July 2014, v4.6.

87. Centers for Disease Control and Prevention. *HIV Transmission.* http://cdc.gov/hiv/basics/transmission.html. Accessed August 26, 2014.

88. Patel P, Borkowf CB, Brooks JT, et al. Estimating per act HIV transmission risk: a systematic review. *AIDS.* 2014;28(10):1509–1519.

89. CSLI. *Criteria for Laboratory Testing and Diagnosis of Human Immunodeficiency Virus Infection; Approved Guideline.* CLSI document M53–A. Wayne, PA: Clinical and laboratory Standards Institute; 2011.

90. United States Preventive Services Task Force. *Final Recommendation Statement: Human Immunodeficiency Virus (HIV) Infection: Screening.* http://www.uspreventiveservicestaskforce.org/Page/Document/Recommendation-StatementFinal/human-immunodeficiency-virus-hiv-infection-screening#consider. Accessed January 7, 2015.

91. National Institutes for Health. *HIV Treatment of HIV Infection.* http://www.niaid.nih.gov/topics/HIVAIDS/Understanding/Treatment/Pages/default.aspx. Accessed January 7, 2015.

92. United State Department of Health and Human Services. About the Ryan White HIV/AIDS Program. HRSA. http://hab.hrsa.gov/abouthab/aboutprogram.html. Accessed January 16, 2015.

93. Ramos RL, Hernandez A, Ferreira-Pinto JB, et al. Designing a capacity-building program to strengthen and expand the role of promotores in HIV prevention. *Health Promotion Practice.* 2006; 7:444–449.

94. Jones KT, Gray P, Whiteside YO, et al. Evaluation of an HIV Prevention Intervention Adapted for Black Men Who Have Sex With Men. *AJPH.* 2008;98:1043–1050.

95. The White House Office of National AIDS Policy. *National HIV/AIDS Strategy for the United States.* Published July 2010.

96. Centers for Disease Control and Prevention. *Proven HIV Prevention Methods.* Published December 2014.

97. Coates TJ, Richter L and Caceras C. Behavioural Strategies to reduce HIV transmission: how to make them work better. *Lancet.* Published online August 6, 2008.

98. AVERT. *Introduction to HIV and AIDS Education.* http://www.avert.org/introduction-hiv-and-aids-education.htm. Accessed September 10, 2014.

99. Centers for Disease Control and Prevention. *Behavioral Interventions.* https://www.effectiveinterventions.org/en/HighImpactPrevention/Interventions.aspx. Danya International. Accessed January 2015.

100. Adimora AA and JD Auerbach. Structural Interventions for HIV Prevention in the United States. *JAIDS,* 2010;55:S132–S135.

101. Nesheim S, Taylor A, Lampe MA, et al. A framework for the elimination of perinatal transmission of HIV in the United States. *Pediatrics.* 2012; 130:738–744.

102. Centers for Disease Control and Prevention. *Background Brief on the Prevention Benefits of IIIV Treatment.* Published January 2013.

103. Cardo DM, Culver DH, Ciescielski CA, et al. A case-control study of HIV seroconversion in health care workers after percutaneous exposure. *NEJM.* 1997;337:1485–1490.

104. Centers for Disease Control and Prevention. Antiretroviral postexposure prophylaxis after sexual, injection-drug use, or other non-occupational exposure to HIV in the United Sates. *MMWR.* 2005; 54(RR2).

105. Centers for Disease Control and Prevention. *Preexposure Prophylaxis for the Prevention of HIV in the United States - 2014: A Clinical Practice Guideline.* USPHS, 2014.

106. National Institutes for Health. HIV Prevention: The Basics of HIV Prevention. *AIDS info.* http://aidsinfo.nih.gov/education-materials/fact-sheets/20/48/the-basics-of-hiv-prevention. Accessed January 9, 2015.

107. Project Inform. *TLC+: Best practices to implement enhanced HIV test, link-to-care, plus treat (TLC-Plus) Strategies in four cities.* Published August 2011.

108. Centers for Disease Control and Prevention. Comprehensive Prevention Programs for Health Departments. http://www.cdc.gov/hiv/prevention/programs/healthdepartments/index.html. Accessed January 21, 2015.

109. Marks G, Crepaz N, Janssen RS. Estimating sexual transmission from persons aware and unaware that they are infected the virus in the USA. *AIDS.* 2006;20:1447–1450.

110. Centers for Disease Control and Prevention. Prevalence of undiagnosed HIV infection among persons aged ≥ 13 year – National HIV Surveillance System, United States, 2005–2008. *MMWR.* 2012;61(suppl):57–64.

111. Centers for Disease Control and Prevention. New Estimates of U.S. HIV Prevalence, 2006. *CDC Fact Sheet,* October 2008.

112. Centers for Disease Control and Prevention. HIV Testing in the United States. *CDC Fact Sheet,* November 2014.

113. Cohen MS, Chen YQ, McCauley M, et al. Prevention of HIV-1 Infection with Early Antiretroviral Therapy. *N Engl J Med.* 2011 August 11; 365(6): 493–505. DOI:10.1056/NEJMoa1105243.

114. Rodger A, Bruun T, Cambiano V, et al. HIV transmission risk through condomless sex if HIV+ partner on suppressive ART: PARTNER study. 21st Conference on Retroviruses and Opportunistic Infections; 2014; March 3–6, 2013, Boston, MA.

115. Connor EM, Sperling RS, Gelber R, et al. Reduction of maternal-infant transmission of human immunodeficiency virus type 1 with zidovudine treatment. *N Engl J Med.* 1994; 331:1173–1180.

116. Whitmore SK, Taylor AW, Espinoza L, et al. Correlates of mother-to-child transmission of HIV in the United States and Puerto Rico. *Pediatrics.* 2012;129(1).

117. Grant RM, Lama JR, Anderson PL. Preexposure Chemoprophylaxis for HIV Prevention in Men Who Have Sex with Men. *N Engl J Med.* 2010; 363:2587–2599.

118. Peleg AY and Hooper DC. Hospital acquired infections due to gram-negative bacteria. *N Engl J Med.* 2010 May 13;362(19):1804–1813.

119. Magill SS, Edwards JR, Bamberg W, Beldavs ZG, Dumyati G, Kainer MA, et al. Multistate Point-Prevalence Survey of Health Care-Associated Infections. *N Engl J Med.* 2014; 370:1198–1208.

120. Department of IIealth and Human Services. National Action Plan to Prevent Health Care-Associated Infections: Road Map to Elimination. Accessible at http://www.health.gov/hai/prevent_hai.asp#hai_plan. Accessed November 17, 2014.

121. Chitnis AS, Caruthers PS, Rao AK, Lamb J, Lurvey R, Beau De Rochars V. Outbreak of carbapenem-resistant enterobacteriaceae at a long-term acute care hospital: sustained reductions in transmission through active surveillance and targeted interventions. *Infect Control Hosp Epidemiol.* 2012 October;33(10):984–992.

122. Epstein L, Hunter JC, Arwady MA, Tsai V, Stein L, Gribogiannis M, et al. New Delhi metallo-β-lactamase-producing carbapenem-resistant Escherichia coli associated with exposure to duodenoscopes. *JAMA.* 2014 October 8;312(14):1447–1455.

123. Centers for Disease Control and Prevention. Notes from the Field: Hospital Outbreak of Carbapenem-Resistant Klebsiella pneumoniae Producing New Delhi Metallo-Beta-Lactamase — Denver, Colorado, 2012. *MMWR.* 2013 Feb 15;62(6):108.

124. Centers for Disease Control and Prevention. A National Strategic Plan for Public Health Preparedness and Response. Issued September 2011. http://www.cdc.gov/phpr/publications/2011/A_Natl_Strategic_Plan_for_Preparedness_20110901A.pdf. Accessed November 19, 2014.

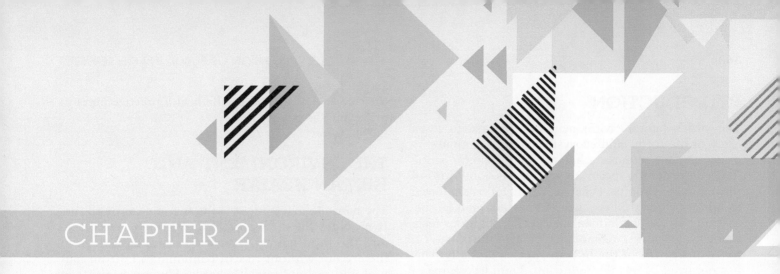

CHAPTER 21

Environmental Public Health

Michael T. Hatcher, DrPH • Siobhan L. Tarver, PhD

DISCLAIMER

LEARNING OBJECTIVES

Upon completion of this chapter, the reader will be able to:

1. Discuss the interplay between human health and the natural environment.

2. Identify critical policy and environmental-related practices that impact sustainability of the natural and man-made environments.

3. Discuss various environmental issues that are global in scope (e.g., acid rain, climate change, ozone, or chemical contaminants) and have widespread impacts on human health.

4. Synthesize current environmental health issues into actionable strategies that public health agencies can take to lessen adverse impacts to human health.

5. Describe public health systems improvements that can be addressed through the use of Environmental Public Health Performance Standards.

KEY TERMS

air pollution
bioaccumulate
climate change
Environmental Public Health Performance Standards (EnvPHPS)
environmental sustainability
essential environmental public health services (EEPHS)
exposure pathways
foodborne illnesses
quality improvement

INTRODUCTION

The earth's natural environment has given rise to a vast array of life forms and ecosystems. The sustainability of ecosystems requires a balance between competing forces in order for species to survive. As conditions of the natural environment change, all life forms are forced to adapt or perish. Few species have adapted as successfully as we, the human species. Through our technological advances, we have manipulated the ecosystem to favor growth of the human species globally. This has occurred largely through control and leveraging of resources in the natural environment, allowing humans to maintain and prosper in spite of fluctuating environmental situations. We as humans try to protect ourselves against adverse natural environmental conditions: temperature extremes, floods and droughts, disease vectors, radiation, earthquakes, volcanic eruptions, tsunamis, and landslides.

The human species has survived to this point in time by creating a relatively healthy and safe environment by:

▶ Adapting biologically through the evolution of the immune system that provides, to some extent, built-in resistance to diseases and sensitivities to allergens and

▶ Developing technologically by modifying both the natural environment and our biological response to threats in the environment.

Extra layers of protection have been added where natural immunity has not evolved or kept pace with environmental change: the development of infrastructures to provide clean drinking water and manage waste; to feed, clothe, and shelter growing populations; and processes and products to care for the sick and prevent the spread of disease. The welfare of populations has been central throughout the evolution in technology with many of the health and safety advances codified in today's practice of public health and its role in monitoring and managing the health protective infrastructures benefiting the human population.

Environmental public health is built on the multidisciplinary approaches of public health and environmental health science. The steps used in public health to protect society from environmental health problems form the basis of environmental health practice. Contemporary environmental health issues faced in public health practice include air quality, climate change, community design and land use, environmental health surveillance, environmental justice, food safety, widespread toxic environmental hazards, vector-borne disease control, water quality and supply, occupational health, and environmental sustainability. In this chapter, we will discuss these contemporary issues and the role environmental public health practice plays in protecting the public.

THE ENVIRONMENT AND HUMAN HEALTH

The natural environment is the foundation of all life. It provides the air we breathe, the water we drink, and the food we eat. These essential resources of life are not without risk of contamination from natural and technological hazards. Human health can be harmed by toxins, toxicants, pathogens, spores, and other environmental threats if safeguards are omitted. In 1962, Rachel Carson's classic and controversial book, *Silent Spring*,[1] introduced the public to the potentially detrimental impacts pesticides have on humans and wildlife. Excerpts from the book were featured in *The New Yorker*, increasing public awareness of the environmental issues, and the need to protect ourselves and the ecosystem, resulting in the birth of environmentalism. Since then, many safeguards have been developed and now are based in contemporary environmental health science and practice. In the sections that follow, there will be a discussion of environmental health risks (associated with water, air, soil, and food) and ways to mitigate health risks through sustainable resource use, environmental public health practice, and changes in managing the built environment.

Water

Safe Water and Environmental Health Practice

Of the earth's entire water supply ($\sim 1.5 \times 10^9$ km^3), only 2.5 percent is fresh (not salty or brackish).[2] Our freshwater needs are limited by its availability. Eighty percent of the globe's freshwater is in glaciers, and therefore is unavailable. The remaining 20 percent of available freshwater is under constant threat of contamination from disease-carrying organisms and toxic chemicals, which could render it unfit for human use. Consequently, public health agencies at all levels of government must be concerned about water supply and water quality. Regulations and guidance for environmental public health practice are provided by federal agencies, specifically the Environmental Protection Agency (EPA), the Centers for Disease Control and Prevention (CDC), and the Food and Drug Administration (FDA). State-level agencies facilitate monitoring and enforcement programs in collaboration with federal agencies. Essential to the success of environmental public health programs are the day-to-day protective actions taken by local environmental health professionals.

Water Needs and Supply

The body of an adult human is about two-thirds water and adults need to consume three or more liters of water at least every few days.[3] Water is needed internally for digestion, circulation of bodily fluids, and elimination of waste products. Aside from human ingestion, water is used for bathing, cooking, cleaning and sanitation, cooling, food production, power generation, and manufacturing. We derive almost all of our fresh water supply from groundwater aquifers (96 percent), and surface water impoundments (4 percent) depending on the regional geology and climate.[3] Water's natural cleansing process is through wetlands and soil filtration, evaporation, dilution (e.g., by rainwater), adsorption (e.g., by carbon or clay in soils), dispersion (e.g., in rivers), and through bioremediation of organisms that consume contaminants.[3] Humans replicate many of these natural processes (e.g., filtration, evaporation, and adsorption) in their water treatment processes. The amount of freshwater available for human consumption makes it a critical resource to protect. As the human population increases in size, water conservation grows in importance, but actions that misuse water are all too common. These actions range from nonessential water usage (e.g., watering lawns and golf courses, filling swimming pools in arid areas) to losing unused water (e.g., dripping faucets, leaking pipes, malfunctioning or overflushed toilets, and broken water mains).

Water Contamination and Health Risks

Allowing water to become contaminated is tantamount to wasting it at the source. Water supplies can be contaminated by its mixing with point sources (identifiable waste stream outlets): wastewater from improperly designed or functioning septic systems, from leaking wastewater conduits, or from manufacturing or waste disposal operations. Contamination also stems from nonpoint sources (runoff from agricultural fields or pavements and atmosphere dispersal of pollutants such as mercury). Existing infrastructure design can also contribute to water contamination. Many municipalities use a Combined Sewage Overflow (CSO) system that combines wastewater derived from residential and commercial drains, including toilets, with storm water drainage from streets and roadways. All of this wastewater is directed to the municipal sewage treatment plants where both sources of wastewater can be treated before being released to the environment. Unfortunately, there are times when this system cannot accommodate all of the sewage and storm water, especially during intense rain storm events. When this happens, the sewage in excess of the capacity of the conduits is discharged, by design, from the CSO system directly to streams without treatment (see Figure 21-1). This results in raw sewage (pathogens and other toxic hazards) being discharged to contaminate surface streams. Once these contaminants reach the water, they disperse via water turbulence and diffusion.

Health risks can arise from water if it contains pathogens (e.g., bacteria, viruses, parasites) or toxic hazards. There are a number of common health problems resulting from the use of contaminated water, especially in low-income countries. Chief among these is diarrhea, a common cause of global death from dehydration, especially among children. Some examples of diseases that can be transmitted by contaminated water include:

- Bacteria: Typhoid fever, Cholera, Dysentery, Salmonellosis, pathogenic *E. coli*. (O157:H7)
- Viruses: Hepatitis A, Poliomyelitis
- Protozoa: Giardiasis, Cryptosporidiosis
- Flukes: Schistosomiasis

Water containing toxic chemicals can also cause health problems. A large number of metals and persistent organic compounds at exposure doses exceeding safe levels during critical fetal developmental windows can cause:

- birth defects (teratogens)
- genetic defects (mutagens)
- cancers (carcinogens)
- nerve damage (neurotoxic)
- organ failure

Common toxic substances in water that cause health problems include moderate to high levels of mercury, arsenic, lead, pesticides, industrial solvents, PCBs, nitrates, and disinfectant byproducts.

Clean Water Regulation

Public water supplies, serving groups of families and whole communities, are monitored and regulated under the scrutiny of the federal and state EPAs. The most frequently monitored contaminants, coliform bacteria, are indicators of contamination of water supplies by sewage.[3] Although most coliform bacteria themselves do not cause disease, sewage contamination may contain other serious disease-causing pathogens as mentioned in the previous section. Private water supplies (wells, cisterns, and springs) may be regulated through construction and health standards permits. In most cases, quality control and continuous monitoring is the responsibility of the owners, increasing the risk of potentially unnoticed contamination unless construction permits also require public health monitoring.

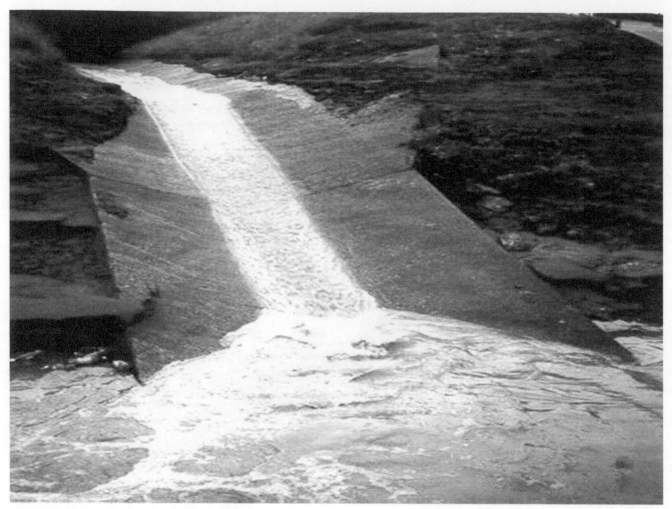

FIGURE 21-1   Combined Sewage Overflow
Courtesy of Sanitation District No. 1 of Northern Kentucky

Regulations developed in the 1970s to implement the Clean Water Act and later the Safe Drinking Water Act, finally put an end to the "right" to pollute water. In the 1980s, standards referred to as Maximum Contaminant Levels, or MCLs, were established for public water supplies.[4] MCLs vary depending on the particular chemical, and if exceeded, require immediate action for reduction (see Figure 21-2).[5] These standards were a big first step to increasing protection and monitoring of drinking water. Truly protective health limits and routine testing to assure compliance may be too costly and technically unfeasible, rendering the price of water too expensive for most communities to maintain. In cases when contamination is suspected, however, the EPA can demand more stringent testing.

Clean Water: Protection Procedures

Public health agencies play a key role in the prevention of contamination in both surface and groundwater supply. All supplies of water for human usage at the surface (natural lakes, surface impoundments, rivers, and wetlands) and even underground water-bearing strata (aquifers) that are shallower than 25 feet can become contaminated. Poorly constructed and maintained water wells are one contributor to groundwater contamination. Private water well rules address the construction and sealing of wells to prevent this contamination. Many public health agencies require permits to install private water supplies. When a permitting process is in place there is opportunity for evaluation of the site conditions prior to installation, inspection of the private water system after construction, testing for bacterial contamination, and, finally, the maintenance of records of test results. Inspection by local health agencies can ensure that improperly constructed or maintained water wells are quickly corrected before aquifers are contaminated. In many instances of contamination, the problem can be

	Contaminant	MCL or TT[1] (mg/L)[2]	Potential Health Effects from Long-Term[3] Exposure above the MCL	Common Sources of Contaminant in Drinking Water	Public Health Goal (mg/L)[2]
OC	Acrylamide	TT[4]	Nervous system or blood problems; increased risk of cancer	Added to water during sewage/wastewater treatment	zero
R	Alpha photon emitters	15 picocuries per liter (pCi/L)	Increased risk of cancer	Erosion of natural deposits of certain minerals that are radioactive and may emit a form of radiation known as alpha radiation	zero
IOC	Arsenic	0.010	Skin damage or problems with circulatory systems, and may have increased risk of getting cancer	Erosion of natural deposits; runoff from orchards; runoff from glass & electronics production wastes	zero
DBP	Bromate	0.010	Increased risk of cancer	Byproduct of drinking water disinfection	zero
D	Chlorine (as Cl)	MRDL=4.0[1]	Eye/nose irritation; stomach discomfort	Water additive used to control microbes	MRDLG=4[1]
M	Cryptosporidium	TT[7]	Short-term exposure: Gastrointestinal illness (e.g., diarrhea, vomiting, cramps)	Human and animal fecal waste	zero
OC	Dioxin (2,3,7,8-TCDD)	0.00000003	Reproductive difficulties; increased risk of cancer	Emissions from waste incineration and other combustion; discharge from chemical factories	zero
IOC	Mercury (inorganic)	0.002	Kidney damage	Erosion of natural deposits; discharge from refineries and factories; runoff from landfills and croplands	0.002
OC	Toluene	1	Nervous system, kidney, or liver problems	Discharge from petroleum factories	1

LEGEND Organic Chemical   Radionuclides   Inorganic Chemical   Disinfection Byproduct   Disinfectant   Microorganism

FIGURE 21-2   EPA National Primary Drinking Water Regulations

SOURCE: U.S. Environmental Protection Agency. EPA National Primary Drinking Water Regulations. Published May 2009.

easily solved by disinfecting the water well and the distribution system.

Surface water protection is a more difficult endeavor. Surface water is easily contaminated through surface spills, airborne contaminants, watershed runoff, and animal or human waste. Public health agencies are often responsible for investigation of surface water contamination when complaints or health concerns are brought to the agency's attention. Agency surveillance programs use their laboratories to test waters that are of public concern and evaluate potential sources for contaminants found.

Protecting water supplies is typically a cooperative venture with public or private water utility suppliers. Surface water makes up most of the fresh water used in the United States, making its protection essential. The U.S. Geological Survey (USGS) provides a report[6] on the *Estimated Use of Water in the U.S.* every five years. In 2010, the fresh water withdrawals from surface waters were estimated at 75.2 percent of total fresh water withdrawals made, with the balance of 24.8 percent being drawn from groundwater wells.[6] Overall 2010 fresh surface water withdrawals were almost 15 percent less than in 2005, and fresh groundwater withdrawals were about 4 percent less than in 2005.[6] Without the surveillance provided by state and local environmental protection programs, it would be impossible for water utilities to manage surface and groundwater supplies and assure the safety of the drinking water. Partnerships between these public and private organizations and branches of government are challenged to collaboratively use the tools of public education, regulation, and sustainable water use practices to minimize water contamination and protect this essential resource.

Air

Clean Air and Environmental Health Practice

Oxygen needed to support human and other life on earth is drawn from the earth's atmosphere. That atmosphere is comprised of nitrogen (78 percent), oxygen (21 percent), argon (0.9 percent), carbon dioxide (0.03 percent), and trace amounts of others gases that often are air contaminants.[7] These gases change in composition, pressure, and temperature from the ground surface upward. Humans must have approximately 20 cubic meters per day of air containing more than 19.5 percent oxygen.[4]

Public health efforts to address airborne pollutants are focused on monitoring and assessing the risks associated with exposure. This work is done at the state and local level in partnership with U.S. EPA. States (e.g., Colorado Department of Public Health and Environment) and local public health agencies issue permits for outdoor burning and approve indoor burning devices, as well as enforce regulations. Some agencies are engaged in emissions control, air quality advisements during times of wild fires, and land use planning to site schools where the air contaminant health risk to children is minimized. Other agencies, such as the New York City Department of Health and Mental Hygiene, are engaged in conducting epidemiological and other studies to determine contaminant sources and population health effects of fine particulate matter and ozone.

Air Pollution and Health Effects

The listing of toxic air pollutants is extensive, with the EPA monitoring 189 pollutants through the National Emission Standards for Hazardous Air Pollutants (NESHAP). (These standards can be accessed at http://www.epa.gov/airtoxics by clicking on the "Rules & Implementation" link and then selecting the "National Emission Standards for Hazardous Air Pollutants Rules" link on the following page.) Among these, the EPA has identified six "criteria pollutants" and developed guidelines known as the National Ambient Air Quality Standards (NAAQS) for setting permissible levels for the protection of public health and welfare. The criteria pollutants are carbon monoxide (CO), nitrogen oxides (NO_x), sulfur dioxide (SO_2), lead (Pb), ground-level ozone (O_3), and particulate matter (PM).[8,9] Environmental and exposure-related health effects for each one are presented below.

First, carbon monoxide is a colorless, odorless gas that contributes to smog formation. At sufficient exposure levels, CO can saturate the lungs and attach to blood hemoglobin, depriving the body of needed oxygen. Insufficient oxygen levels can result in cardiac distress, visual and auditory sensory impairment, and cognitive and neurologic impairment.[10] Nitrogen oxides can irritate and burn the eyes, nose, and throat; cause nausea, coughing, spasms, shortness of breath, tiredness, swelling of tissues in the throat and upper respiratory tract, and a build-up of fluid in the lungs; reduce oxygenation of body tissues; and it can lead to death.[11] Asthmatics are more susceptible to the effects of sulfur dioxide due to its high water solubility. Sulfur dioxide can cause burning of tissue and reduced lung function and edema similar to health effects of nitrogen oxides. Environmentally, rain water can dissolve sulfur and nitrogen oxides in the atmosphere and form acids. This poses a major problem in more industrialized regions near fresh water sources (e.g., Great Lakes Region). When acid rain water impacts surfaces, it can erode building exteriors, and make metallic contaminants in aqueous environments more soluble, placing humans, fish, and animals at increased health risk of absorbing toxic metals.

Chronic exposure to Pb can cause anemia and neurological dysfunction.[12] At high levels of exposure, Pb can severely damage the brain and kidneys in adults or children and ultimately cause death. In pregnant women, high Pb levels may cause miscarriage, and in men, these levels damage the organs responsible for sperm production.[13]

Exposure to ground-level ozone is influenced by where you live and work, and the amount of time you spend outside. Exposure to O_3 can result in higher sensitivity to allergens, aggravated asthma, bronchitis, and emphysema, and increased chances of respiratory illness such as pneumonia or bronchitis.

Particulate matter consists of airborne particles, such as aerosols, dust, soot, smoke, and liquid droplets. Varying in size and composition, some particles are large or dark enough to be seen (e.g., dust, pollen) while others are microscopic, with a diameter of 2.5 microns or less (e.g., combustion pieces, metals). Smaller particles are of greatest exposure concern because they can enter the smallest alveolar sacs of the lungs and in some cases the bloodstream.[14] Being exposed to any kind of particulate matter may cause increased respiratory and cardiovascular problems requiring emergency department visits and hospital stays. It can also cause increased asthma severity, adverse birth outcomes (such as low birth weight), decreased lung growth in children, lung cancer, and mortality.[14]

Clean Air Regulation

The development of clean air laws was slow but gradual as the twentieth century progressed. Events such as the one that occurred on October 26, 1948, in Donora, Pennsylvania, brought air quality issues to the policy forefront. In Donora, industrial gases and dust were emitted from the smokestacks of the local zinc smelter while residents slept, resulting in 20 deaths and 7,000 hospitalizations.[15] With this and other similar events, the U.S. Congress passed the Air Pollution Control Act of 1955, the first in a series of air quality laws in place today. It established the first requirements for conducting research to understand the scope and sources of **air pollution**.

The Clean Air Act (CAA) of 1970[8] was a sweeping set of requirements that are the foundation of today's air quality standards. This act:

▸ Authorized the establishment of NAAQS
▸ Established requirements for state implementation plans to achieve the NAAQS

- ▶ Authorized the establishment of New Source Performance Standards (NSPS) for new and modified stationary sources
- ▶ Authorized the establishment of NESHAP
- ▶ Increased enforcement authority, and
- ▶ Authorized requirements for control of motor-vehicle emissions.

These standards were expanded with the 1990 Amendments to the CAA of 1970. These amendments added new provisions for Acid Deposition Control and a program to phase out the use of chemicals depleting the ozone layer.[9]

Regulation of air pollution across large geographic areas was made possible and authority granted to enforce regulations across city, county, and state jurisdiction lines. The U.S. EPA, state, and some local public health agencies monitor wide geographic areas and track the contaminant sources and direction of plumes; analyze findings; respond to citizen complaints; issue air permits, air pollution alerts, and pollen counts; and monitor air regulation compliance.

Routine regional monitoring of ozone and particulates (less than 2.5 microns, referred to as $PM_{2.5}$) allows actions to be planned to reduce industrial air emissions, including auto exhaust system inspections, public alerts restricting pollution-generating activities such as refueling and grass mowing to certain times of the day, as well as warning the sensitive populations such as the elderly or those with respiratory problems to stay indoors, and limit outdoor activities during smog alerts.

Depletion of stratospheric ozone has been caused by the discharge of chlorofluorocarbons (CFCs) into the atmosphere. CFCs are highly volatile hydrocarbons that are not vaporized into the atmosphere. These compounds typically rise slowly, with the ability to reside in the stratosphere for many years. Here, with the action of a chlorine free radical, the ozone molecule (O_3) reverts back to the normal oxygen molecule (O_2), which does not have UV-radiation absorption characteristics,[3] allowing greater amounts of ultraviolet radiation to reach earth, increasing the chances of skin cancer in humans, fishery depletion, and smog formation.[3] CFCs were manufactured as refrigerants and propellants, and have since been banned or phased out by the Montreal Protocol.

Standards adopted under the CAA and amended in 1990[9] authorized much of the work described above and have proven to be cost effective. Figures 21-3 and 21-4 present the EPA's best estimates, for those health and ecological benefits that can be quantified and converted to dollar values. From these 2020 estimates, the benefits of the CAA programs will total about $2 trillion.[16] This estimate represents the value of avoiding increases in illness and premature death, which would have prevailed without the clean air standards and provisions required

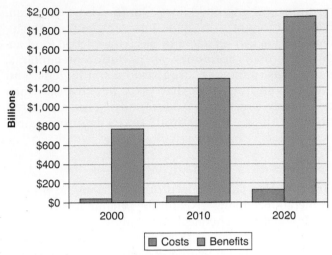

FIGURE 21-3 **Direct Cost and Benefit 2000–2020**

DATA SOURCE: US Environmental Protection Agency. The Benefits and Costs of the Clean Air Act from 1990 to 2020. Washington DC.

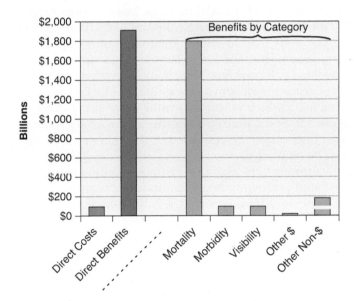

FIGURE 21-4 **2020 Direct Cost and Benefit**

DATA SOURCE: US Environmental Protection Agency. The Benefits and Costs of the Clean Air Act from 1990 to 2020. Washington DC.

by the amendments. By contrast, the detailed cost analysis conducted for this new study indicates that the costs of achieving these health and ecological benefits are likely to be $65 billion in 2020,[16] a fraction of the $2 trillion benefits.

Food

Risks to a Safe Food Supply

Paracelsus (1493–1541), the Father of Toxicology, is credited with the notion that everything is a poison at the proper (or improper) dose. Our food is no exception. Food is thought to provide pure nutrients. Unfortunately, there can be traces of pesticides, feces, food additives, growth hormones, air pollution precipitants, pathogens, parasites, drug residues, allergens, and nutrients in quantities that carry health risks when excessively consumed. Additionally, some plants can produce their own "natural" toxin defense against being eaten.

Food and Risks from Toxicants

Humans also have evolved organ systems to process or metabolize many toxic food contaminants to generally less harmful chemicals by using enzymes to break down toxic substances that are easier for the body to excrete.[17] However, synthetic chemicals manufactured (during the past 70 to 130 years), have structures rare in the natural world. The human body is not equipped with enzymes capable of metabolizing all substances into less toxic chemicals. In some cases, human metabolism can produce a chemical more toxic than the first or the body may be totally incapable of metabolizing some chemicals. For example, toluene, a component of gasoline, can reach and impair the nervous system. The liver contains enzymes that convert toluene into benzoic acid, which is less toxic and more easily excreted from the body. Benzene, another major component of gasoline, cannot be converted in this manner, so it cannot be detoxified.

Although the chemical structure among many natural and synthetic organic compounds is similar, there are subtle differences that inhibit existing enzymes to detoxify some synthetic chemicals.[17] Chlorinated hydrocarbons (e.g., trichloroethylene [TCE] and perchloroethylene [PCE]) for example, are a group of manufactured solvents with carbon-chlorine bonds, which are relatively rare in nature. Chlorinated hydrocarbons have adverse health effects and can bio-concentrate in fatty tissue in the body. Chemically, these compounds are more soluble in the fatty tissue than in water by factors of several hundreds to almost a thousand times more. This means that if you drank water having a PCE concentration of only 0.001 percent, and the PCE were completely absorbed by the fatty tissue, the concentration of PCE in your fatty tissue would be almost 1 percent. Furthermore, if fish that swam in water having a PCE concentration of 0.001 percent are eaten, the PCE would bio-concentrate in the fatty tissue at 1 percent concentrations. As PCE and other fat soluble substances bio-concentrate in fish and other exposed animals, these substances **bioaccumulate** in the food chain and eventually humans are exposed through their diet. Bioaccumulation of these substances is highest in the larger predatory fish and

in animals agriculturally fed contaminated animal byproducts.

Food and Risks from Biologic Agents

Food services and suppliers self-regulate by preventing spoilage in order to protect their inventories. No one will buy foods that look, smell, or taste rotten. Most people can identify spoiled canned foods whose containers are bloated, and detect bad produce or dairy products that show evidence of mold. However, food that looks, smells, and tastes good can still be problematic.

Bacteria, viruses, parasites, and fungi can make food unsafe. Microorganisms may also produce toxins that damage cells. As they grow, the quantity of toxins increases.

FAT TOM is a mnemonic to help us remember conditions conducive for growth of bacteria:

- **F**ood (proteins and carbohydrates),
- **A**cidity (pH of 4.6–7.5),
- **T**emperature (temperature danger zone TDZ = 41°F to 140°F),
- **T**ime (>4 hrs in TDZ),
- **O**xygen (varies), and
- **M**oisture (water activity of 0.85 or higher).

Foodborne illnesses from bacteria include *E. coli* infection, Salmonellosis, Shigellosis, Listeriosis, Gastroenteritis, and Botulism, among others. Bacteria causing these diseases can be found in a variety of foods, both animal and plant derived. *E. coli* bacteria (O157:H7)[18] has been the cause of many serious outbreaks of food poisonings at food establishments. The O157:H7 strain, which produces a powerful toxin, is found in the intestines and bodily waste of people and animals.[18]

Foodborne viral illnesses include hepatitis A, Norwalk virus gastroenteritis, and rotavirus gastroenteritis. They do not reproduce in food although they can be found in food (and water) and on food-contact surfaces.

Foodborne illnesses from parasites include Trichinosis, Giardiasis, and Intestinal Cryptosporidiosis. These parasites are found mostly in animals and fish.

Fungi (molds, yeasts, and mushrooms) may also cause foodborne illnesses either from infection or intoxication.[18]

Foodborne Disease Surveillance and Environmental Health Practice

Public health agencies have a major role in the protection of our food supplies. This role begins with food processing and ends with consumption. It is difficult

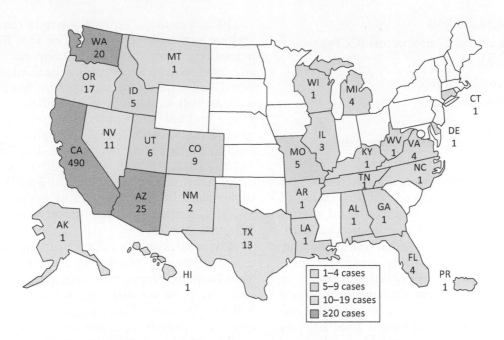

*n = 633 for whom information was reported as of July 24, 2014

A total of 634 individuals infected with the outbreak strains of *Salmonella* Heidelberg have been reported from 29 states and Puerto Rico. Most of the ill persons (77%) have been reported from California. The number of ill persons identified in each state is as follows: Alabama (1), Alaska (1), Arkansas (1), Arizona (25), California (490), Colorado (9), Connecticut (1), Delaware (1), Florida (4), Georgia (1), Hawaii (1), Idaho (5), Illinois (4), Kentucky (1), Louisiana (1), Michigan (4), Missouri (5), Montana (1), Nevada (11), New Mexico (2), North Carolina (1), Oregon (17), Puerto Rico (1), Tennessee (1), Texas (13), Utah (6), Virginia (4), Washington (20), West Virginia (1), and Wisconsin (1).

FIGURE 21-5 **Persons Infected with the Outbreak Strains of *Salmonella Heidelberg*, by State**
SOURCE: U.S. Department of Health & Human Services, Centers for Disease Control and Prevention

to declare that the enforcement of food service (restaurants) and food establishment (groceries) rules decrease the number of foodborne illnesses because their role is prevention and education.

The Centers for Disease Control and Prevention estimates approximately 1 in 6 Americans (or 48 million people) gets sick annually from foodborne diseases, 128,000 are hospitalized, and 3,000 die of foodborne diseases in the United States.[19] Yet, most foodborne illness remains preventable through safe food handling, which is best guaranteed by training food handlers and educating consumers.

Episodes of foodborne illness can be widespread and require a multijurisdictional response. For example, between March 1, 2013 and July 11, 2014, a total of 634 individuals (ages under 1 year to 93 years old) were infected by the multidrug-resistant *Salmonella heidelberg* reported across 29 states and Puerto Rico. Figure 21-5 presents the distribution of those infected. Among 633 persons for whom information was available, 200 were hospitalized and no deaths were reported.[20]

This foodborne outbreak required the collaboration of federal (CDC, FDA), numerous state (California Department of Public Health and Washington State Public Health), and local public health agencies. In this outbreak response, public health investigators used the PulseNet system, a national laboratory diagnostic testing network, to identify outbreak cases through DNA "fingerprints" of the Salmonella bacteria strain. Further, the National Antimicrobial Resistance Monitoring Systems were used in surveillance to detect isolates resistant to various antimicrobial agents (e.g., *Salmonella heidelberg*) in animals and humans.

The federal food safety laws authorize local health departments to inspect according to the potential food hazards associated with each food service or food establishment.

Seven principles applied in the Hazard Analysis and Critical Control Point (HACCP) Program offer a systematic approach to the identification, evaluation, and control of food safety hazards. The seven principles[21] are:

1. Conduct a hazard analysis.
2. Determine the critical control points (CCPs).
3. Establish critical limits.
4. Establish monitoring procedures.
5. Establish corrective actions.
6. Establish verification procedures.
7. Establish recordkeeping and documentation procedures.

HACCP formed the foundation for environmental health practice to analyze chemical, physical, and other biological hazards, and identify critical control points to prevent foodborne illness. Critical control points are examined from time of harvest to the time of consumption in order to apply protective measures at those procedural and operational points in food processing, food preparation, and food service outlets where control measures can be applied. Control is essential to prevent or eliminate food hazards and reduce contamination to acceptable levels. Such inspections involve measuring temperatures of stored foods, investigating the potential for drippings to cross-contaminate foods, searching for the presence of vermin or mold in food preparation or storage areas, and having established hand-washing protocols for food-establishment staff.

WASTE MANAGEMENT: PRINCIPLES AND PROCEDURES

Waste is generated in every aspect of life. It exists in many forms including wastewater or effluent discharge to bodies of water, air emissions, storm water, municipal solid waste, construction and demolition waste, hazardous chemical waste, radioactive waste, and infectious waste. Waste is land filled, incinerated, transported, stored temporarily, processed chemically to be less mobile, toxic, or reduced in volume, physically recycled or reused, injected into deep rock strata, or isolated in repositories (e.g., radioactive waste).

Waste that is not properly managed can cause adverse health effects and create health risks from toxic or infectious waste that enters the environment and is transported through environmental media (air, water, soil, or biota). If exposure pathways are completed (i.e., contaminated media is inhaled, ingested, or absorbed through the skin) and contamination exceeds acceptable risk levels, exposed individuals and/or populations will likely become ill. Those who are elderly, very young, pregnant, sick, or sensitive to environmental contaminates are generally more susceptible to environmental disease and injury.

Proper management of waste is required under various laws and regulations. The U.S. EPA provides federal regulatory oversight in cooperation with state and local environmental public health agencies. Both liquid and solid waste may contain hazardous chemicals as well as pathogens and disease vectors. The design and operation of waste disposal systems must meet EPA standards. These standards are detailed in Title III of the Federal Water Pollution Control Act of 1972 (Pub. L. 92-500), amended by the 1977 Clean Water Act Amendments (Pub. L. 95-217), and further strengthened by the Water Quality Act of 1987 (Pub. L. 100-4). Oversight of waste disposal systems is generally delegated to states.

Disposal systems range from small residential onsite treatment systems to large municipal treatment facilities. Proper treatment and disposal of effluents from these systems are governed by the National Pollutant Discharge Elimination System, which requires issuance of permits for treatment and effluent discharge facilities. Additionally, standards for industrial waste disposed of through municipal sewage systems are set by the National Pretreatment Program so that industrial contaminants are removed prior to reaching the municipal sewage system.

Solid waste standards are addressed under the Resource Conservation and Recovery Act (RCRA). Two issues of importance in solid waste disposal are to assure that solid waste hazards do not leach into aquifers and that off-gassing of decomposing waste is properly managed. Oversight of RCRA is delegated to states and local authorities to monitor. Key strategies to reduce the need for solid waste disposal are (a) decreasing unnecessary packaging to diminish future waste volume and (b) recycling, reuse, and reduction of solid waste mass. Single stream recycling is providing a more efficient means of reclaiming waste and building in opportunities for economic sustainability. Even with this advancement in recycling, major educational efforts to decrease the volume of residential and commercial solid waste are needed.

ENVIRONMENTAL LAWS AND REGULATIONS

In reviewing the environmental protection of air, water, food, and proper handling of waste, the role of environmental law was frequently emphasized. Most laws and regulations address the management of wastes that cause pollution of the environment,[22] while other laws pertain to hazardous materials prior to their becoming wastes. Federal environmental laws have been augmented by state statues and local ordinances.

Together these have been codified into regulations and codes, by regulatory agencies, to guide environmental health practice.

As technology advances so does the need to consider new regulatory protections. Through identification and clarification of environmental contamination, public health agencies can determine situations that require legislative redress and action. To stimulate action, public health agencies can convince politicians to introduce new enabling legislation in order to establish new laws and rules to make enforcement and compliance possible. These laws and rules position public health agencies to inspect and assure compliance by homeowners as well as commercial and industrial corporations. In practice, environmental inspections allow for education to promote compliance, development of documentation to guide compliance and, if necessary, prepare for legal action to force compliance. The practice of environmental public health requires knowledge and capabilities to use regulatory processes to create, implement, and apply legal tools (laws, regulations, code) to protect populations from environmental exposure and harm.

COMMUNITY AND BUILT ENVIRONMENTS

Earlier in this chapter, it was noted that the human species has survived to this point in time by creating a relatively healthy and safe environment. As humans, we have transformed our environment by working together and creating technologies to enrich and safeguard life in communities where we live, work, and play. As with all things, there are lifecycles. Our communities and built environment cope with this process of new to old and the health implications of the built environment lifecycle.

In this section, we will examine our built environment and how homes, industries, and infrastructures in transitions from new to old offer humans both health risks and health protections. We will also examine how community design and land use may enhance or challenge the health of communities and their populations as they interact with their built environments.

Healthy Homes

Shelter has long been recognized as one basic human need. Over time, shelter has transitioned from rock overhangs and caves to the modern single family home and high-rise apartment buildings of the twenty-first century. Homes built in the past and recently built homes can produce health risks to their occupants. Past home building products such as asbestos used in building tiles and insulation products, lead in paint, and general disrepair from poor home maintenance create health risks for the occupants. Newer homes contain manufactured products that can off-gas substances such as formaldehyde and sulfur compounds. Many products in the home are coated with fire retardants made with polybrominated diphenyl ethers (PBDEs) that can degrade and also pose health risks. Other products include carpet backing, electrical cord insulation, vinyl flooring, acoustical ceiling surfaces, and upholstery, all made with phthalates, a "plasticizer," used to increase flexibility and resiliency of materials. New homes also suffer from poor home maintenance and design problems. It is for these and other public health reasons that in 2009 the U.S. Surgeon General issued a healthy homes call to action. This call to action described steps people can take to protect themselves from disease, disability, and injury that may result from health hazards in their houses.[23]

The healthy homes initiative outlined cross-cutting actions and focuses on ways homes support health. The initiative pays attention to how the home is sited, designed, built, renovated, and maintained. The call to action also aligns with the environmental health objectives in *Healthy People 2020* and recognizes that people spend most of their time within home or work structures where they may be exposed to indoor air pollution, inadequate heating and sanitation, structural problems, electrical and fire hazards, and lead-based paint hazards.[24] From this recognition, the national healthy homes initiative is designed to prevent common health hazards in the home and its surroundings, such as:

- Malfunctioning heating and electrical systems producing burns and carbon monoxide poisoning
- Poor lighting and lack of handrails resulting in falls
- Improper storage of firearms, cleaning supplies, and other hazardous substances causing a range of injuries
- Poor home maintenance and surveillance for moisture intrusion or radon gas detection resulting in respiratory illnesses
- Toxic pest control measures which can cause acute poisoning and are suspect in other developmental disabilities and illnesses
- Inadequate supervision of children around stoves, bathtubs, swimming pools, and potentially hazardous household items (medications, cleaning products, and pest control substances) causing injury.

Many factors influence the health and safety of homes, including structure and safety features applied in home design, construction, and maintenance as well as inclusion or omission of safety devices such as smoke detectors. The quality of indoor air and the home water supply are critical to human health as is safe use and storage of potentially hazardous chemicals. Additionally, the environmentally related behaviors of those living in a home and the characteristics of the immediate community surrounding the home can increase or decrease the environmental exposure risks and health outcomes of those who live there.

To effectively improve health through a healthy homes initiative, panels of experts have determined sets of best practices outlined in Table 21-1.[25]

Community Design and Environmental Justice

Healthy homes are building blocks for healthy communities. Through well-planned community design, built environments can provide populations opportunities to be physically active and socially engaged. To create a healthy built environment, planners must examine those factors associated with the ways people behave and interact with one another, the ways communities are organized, and the ways environmental resources are used and sustained. Through this examination, built environments can be designed and organized to provide people healthy options for interacting with one another in all of their daily activities. Health-promoting features of good community design might include considerations for physical activity, resulting in sidewalks, bicycle routes, parks, and sporting facilities. It could also consider sustainability of the built community environment and offer mass transit, protected green spaces, and apply mixed-use development that maintains neighborhood destinations in proximity to homes, schools, work locations, and shopping areas.

Through the work of local, state, and national collaboratives with names such as "Livable Communities," "Healthy Cities," and "Building Healthy Places," the design of built environments is slowly resulting in community changes that promote health. The rule of small wins applies to the many examples of communities taking action to establish well-designed built environments in small and large cities across the nation. Collectively these healthy community initiatives have quietly provided evidence of the health and economic impacts possible. Places such as Falls Park at the Reedy River Falls in Greenville, South Carolina and the Indianapolis Cultural Trail[26] both provide protected places for pedestrians to walk, exercise, gather, and have access to entertainment

TABLE 21-1　Best Healthy Homes Intervention Practices[25]

Panel	Evidence-Based Practice
1. Interior Biological Agents (Toxins)	• Multifaceted tailored asthma interventions • Integrated Pest Management (allergen reduction) • Moisture intrusion elimination
2. Interior Chemical Agents (Toxics)	• Radon air mitigation through active sub-slab depressurization • Integrated Pest Management (pesticide reduction) • Smoking bans • Lead hazard control
3. External Exposures (Drinking water and waste treatment)	• Voluntary drinking and wastewater treatment standards for small systems and private wells • Training for small system personnel • Guidelines for immunocompromised individuals
4. Structural Deficiencies (Injury)	• Installation of working smoke alarms • Isolation 4-sided pool fencing • Preset safe temperature hot water heaters
5. Intersection between Housing and Community	• Rental vouchers (Housing Choice Voucher Program)

SOURCE: National Center for Healthy Housing. Housing Interventions and Health: A Review of the Evidence.

and other services within and bordering these transformed environments.

Over the years, sets of principles have been articulated to guide community planning of healthy built environments. Table 21-2 presents two sets of principles as examples. These principles focus on pedestrian-friendly communities that allow residents to walk to jobs, shops, services, and cultural resources; recognize that healthy places can create enhanced economic value for both the private and public sectors; provide well-defined public places to stimulate social discourse and

TABLE 21-2 Principles for Healthy Environmental Design

Ten Principles for Building Healthy Places[26]	Ten Principles for Livable Communities[27]
1. Put People First	1. Design on a Human Scale
2. Recognize the Economic Value	2. Provide Choices
3. Empower Champions for Health	3. Encourage Mixed-Use Development
4. Energize Shared Spaces	4. Preserve Urban Centers
5. Make Healthy Choices Easy	5. Vary Transportation Options
6. Ensure Equitable Access	6. Build Vibrant Public Spaces
7. Mix It Up	7. Create a Neighborhood Identity
8. Embrace Unique Character	8. Protect Environmental Resources
9. Promote Access to Healthy Food	9. Conserve Landscapes
10. Make It Active	10. Design Matters

SOURCES: Eitler TW, McMahon ET, and Thoerig TC. Ten Principles for Building Healthy Places. Washington, DC: Urban Land Institute; American Institute of Architects. Communities by Design: Ten Principles for Livable Communities.

face-to-face interaction; and design healthy choice opportunities that are safe, accessible, fun, and also easy to make. These and other examples demonstrate that well-designed and maintained built environments can and do impact human health by influencing behaviors, physical activity patterns, social networks, and access to resources.[26,27]

Many considerations go into where homes, roads, waste facilities, parks, transportation facilities, and other services are located in land use and built environment plans. In all decisions regarding land use and built environment plans, it is essential that consideration be given to the potential environmental burden placed on the affected community and its residents. There is ample evidence that minority and low-income populations live in closer proximity to sources of hazardous air pollutants (e.g., Toxic Release Inventory facilities, National Emissions Inventory facilities), hazardous waste facilities, landfills, sewage treatment plants, power plants, major roadways and transportation facilities, and industrial sites.[28] This proximity to environmental hazards is one of several factors associated with poor health outcomes. Poverty, poor health care access, and unhealthy behaviors are also associated; however, research has concluded that these sociodemographic factors cannot fully account for the poorer health in these communities, raising issues of environmental justice. Environmental hazard concentration, coupled with genetic variants (i.e., polymorphisms)[29] and chronic stress,[30] contributes to the differential vulnerability because of the potential to modify the effects of toxicants on human health. Because environmental hazards are central in accounting for poorer health in communities experiencing environmental injustice, it is essential that environmental impacts are not disregarded in land use planning. Such disregard is harmful and unethical and should be guarded against at all time.

Occupational Protection

Built environments should also provide protections for occupational settings that may be impacted by air quality issues, repetitive motion activities, exposure to chemicals, and potential hazards that can cause injury or disease among employees. Control of unhealthy or unsafe conditions includes use of engineering controls, administrative controls, personal protective equipment (PPE) use, and employee training. Engineering controls can include changes in ventilation, lighting, addition of handrails, and noise-absorbing wall or ceiling panels. Administrative controls can include warnings using signs or labels, reduction of time employees spend in hazardous areas, scheduling of training sessions, and health and safety communications (e.g., health and safety plans, spill prevention and control plans, and evacuation plans).

Workers exposed to a health and safety risk should use PPE (e.g., gloves, hardhats, steel-toed boots, and eye and ear protection). They must be fitted and trained to put on, wear, and remove PPE appropriately for the type of health and safety hazard they face (see example in Figure 21-6), be familiar with decontamination procedures, use health and safety monitoring equipment (e.g., contaminant detectors), operate under approved health and safety plans, undergo medical examinations, and be protected under Right-to-Know laws. Managers must undergo their own health and safety training, monitor worker adherence to safety standards, and use administrative and engineering controls to meet Occupational Safety and Health Administration (OSHA) safety and health regulations in the work environment.

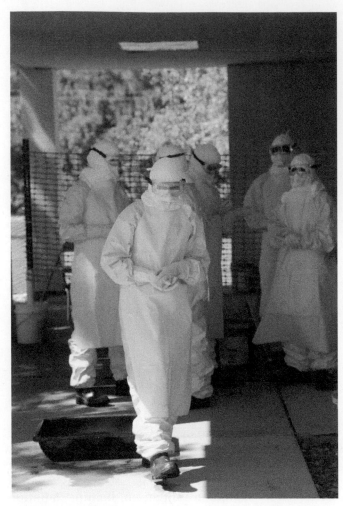

FIGURE 21-6   Personal Protective Equipment for Hazardous Environments
Courtesy of CDC/Nahid Bhadelia, M.D.

ENVIRONMENTAL THREATS AND HEALTH IMPACTS FROM CLIMATE CHANGE

Climate change is an atmospheric phenomenon. It is characterized by extreme shifts in the weather linked often to record high and low temperatures. These shifts include droughts and floods that can impact vast global regions. The root change being observed is a measurable increase in the global temperature.

Data from the National Oceanic and Atmospheric Administration (NOAA) show the globally averaged temperature over land and ocean surfaces in 2014 was, at that time, the highest temperature recorded since 1880,[31] when recordkeeping began. Additionally, the 2014 annually averaged temperature made the 38th consecutive year (since 1977) that the annual global temperature was 0.69°C (1.24°F) above the twentieth century average of 13.9°C (57.0°F).[31]

TABLE 21-3   Top 10 Warmest Years (1880–2014)[31]

Rank 1 = Warmest Periods of Record: 1880–2014	Year	Anomaly °C	Anomaly °F
1	2014	0.69	1.24
2 (tie)*	2010	0.65	1.17
2 (tie)*	2005	0.65	1.17
4	1998	0.63	1.13
5 (tie)*	2013	0.62	1.12
5 (tie)*	2003	0.62	1.12
7	2002	0.61	1.10
8	2006	0.60	1.08
9 (tie)*	2009	0.59	1.06
9 (tie)*	2007	0.59	1.06

*Note: Tie is based on temperature anomaly in °C.

SOURCE: NOAA National Climatic Data Center. State of the Climate: Global Analysis for Annual 2014.

The 10 warmest years since 1880 are listed in Table 21-3, with 9 of the 10 warmest years occurring in the twenty-first century.

A key contributor to the rising global temperature is the emission of greenhouse gases. Naturally occurring gases such as carbon dioxide, methane, water vapor, and nitrous oxide, and synthetic gases such as chlorofluorocarbons (CFCs), hydrofluorocarbons (HFCs) and perfluorocarbons (PFCs), and sulfur hexafluoride (SF6) make up much of the greenhouse gases.[32] Atmospheric concentrations of both the natural and synthetic gases have been rising over the last few centuries coinciding with increased industrial and transportation use of fossil fuels. As the concentration of greenhouse gases increases, less heat escapes the atmosphere resulting in heat build-up.

Climate Change and Potential Health Impacts

Issues of concern from the rising global temperature include more variable weather, heat waves, heavy precipitation events, flooding, sea level rise, droughts, wildfires, air pollution, and more intense hurricanes and other storms. Climate change is a global issue but the effects of climate change will vary across geographic regions and populations.[33–36]

Figure 21-7 presents the CDC's perspective on the impact of climate change on human health, and Table 21-4 presents perspectives on how variable weather events may impact the health of populations at-risk from weather-related events.

The World Health Organization (WHO) has projected global health impacts from climate change for the years between 2030 and 2050, modeling potential impacts under a number of assumptions. The WHO findings compared a future without climate change to one with climate impacts. Projected additional deaths due to climate change for the year 2030 include[36]

▸ 48,000 from diarrheal disease
▸ 60,000 from malaria
▸ 38,000 deaths from heat exposure in elderly people
▸ 95,000 cases of undernutrition among children

Overall WHO estimates approximately 250,000 additional deaths will occur globally each year between 2030 and 2050 due to climate change.[36]

Prevention and Mitigation of Climate Change Impacts

With the challenge of persistent greenhouse gases in the environment, public health and other sectors can use strategies that mitigate and lower greenhouse gas emissions and develop adaptive approaches to lessen potential health effects from climate change. Prevention activities designed to reduce current and future levels of greenhouse gases are largely roles of sectors other than public health; however, the CDC Climate Ready States and Cities Initiative (CRSCI) is working in 16 states and two cities to develop and implement public health adaptation plans for climate change. The focus of CRSCI is to build resilience within these jurisdictions. A five-step process that includes forecasting climate impacts, projecting disease burden, assessing health interventions, developing health adaptation plans, and evaluating health improvement progress will prepare these jurisdictions to be resilient during challenges of climate change. Anticipating impacts of climate change and preparing effectively through processes such as CRSCI will improve adaptive outcomes that better protect population health.[33,37]

Other adaptive measures designed to offset specific environmental risks have been proposed by Frumkin, Sheffield, and others.[34,35] One potential climate risk is coastal flooding from a rise in the sea level. Adaptive behavior to prevent or reduce potential health impacts are the building of seawalls and levees or relocating affected populations. Extreme weather events also present risks of injuries and drowning if populations have not taken steps to prepare emergency plans, establish

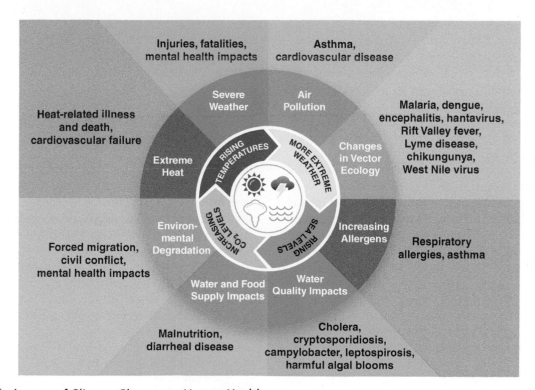

FIGURE 21-7 Impact of Climate Change on Human Health

SOURCE: Centers for Disease Control and Prevention, National Center for Environmental Health. Climate Effects on Health.

TABLE 21-4   Potential Impacts of Climate Change[33–35]

Weather Event	Health and Health-Related Effects	Populations Most Affected
Heat waves	Heat stress, lower birth weight, injuries from transportation infrastructure damage	Extremes of age, athletes, people with respiratory disease
Extreme weather events, (rain, hurricane, tornado, flooding)	Injuries, drowning, and economic disruption	Coastal, low-lying land dwellers, low SES populations
Droughts, floods, increased mean temperature	Vector-food-and-water-borne diseases, and economic disruption	Multiple populations at risk
Sea level rise	Mass population movement, injuries, drowning, water and soil salinization, ecosystem and economic disruption	Coastal populations, low SES populations
Drought, ecosystem migration	Food and water shortages, malnutrition, and economic disruption	Low SES populations, elderly, children
Extreme weather events, drought	Mass population movement, injury, local to international conflict, and economic disruption	General population
Heat with increases in ground-level ozone, wildfires and particulate matter (PM), airborne allergens, and other pollutants	Respiratory disease exacerbations (COPD, asthma, allergic rhinitis, bronchitis); PM associated with preterm births, low birth weight, and infant mortality	Elderly, children, those with respiratory disease
Climate change generally; extreme events	Mental health	Young, displaced, agricultural sector, low SES populations

SOURCES: Centers for Disease Control and Prevention, National Center for Environmental Health. Climate Effects on Health; Sheffield PE, Landrigan PJ. Global climate change and children's health: threats and strategies for prevention. Environ Health Perspect; Frumkin H, Hess J, Luber G, Malilay J, McGeehin M. Framing health matters. Am J Public Health. 2008. 98(3):435–445.

early warning and evacuation systems, and design architectural and engineering protections. Extreme weather cases of drought, flood, and increases in mean temperature, including heat waves are also associated with potential food and water shortages, food-and-waterborne diseases, as well as vector-borne diseases. Adaptive actions that apply technological advances in food production and distribution systems, water conservation, water treatment, watershed management, food and water sanitation, and provision of vector control (accomplished through sustainable farming methods), public education, immunizations, mosquito bed nets, or prophylactic medications are necessary. Adaptive responses for heat waves may include assuring populations have access to air conditioning and fans, public cooling stations, and social support to monitor the well-being of the infirmed and elderly for proper cooling and hydration.

If public health authorities, other governmental agencies, and nonprofit organizations anticipate climate change risks, collective action can be taken to establish policies, warning systems, protective barriers, and support measures to mitigate and adapt to the challenges of climate change and potential population dislocation. Further

environmental public health practice responses to climate change are described below, as they relate to essential environmental public health services (EEPHS).

THE ENVIRONMENTAL PUBLIC HEALTH SYSTEM

In creating environments sufficient to feed, clothe, and shelter a growing human population, humans have developed infrastructure and systems to protect individuals and the communities where they live from environmental harm. The capabilities of environmental public health systems made up of federal, state, and local governmental agencies and nongovernmental partners can be defined by the programs that provide clean drinking water, manage liquid and solid wastes, as well as control air emissions and foodborne disease. Through evolutions in technology, the welfare of populations has been central in development of a strong environmental public health system.

Determining high performance for an environmental public health system has transitioned from assessment of program services to assessment of three core environmental public health functions. The core functions of assessment, policy development, and assurance are measured against optimal model standards associated with 10 Essential Public Health Services.[38,39] In this section, the **Environmental Public Health Performance Standards (EnvPHPS)** are examined in order to optimally describe environmental public health practice and **quality improvement** approaches.

Functional Roles and Practices

Environmental public health has a broad scope of program activities that could be used to describe environmental public health practice; however, defining performance around each potential program activity undertaken would produce a massive number of program performance standards. In the late 1990s, the CDC undertook defining optimal public health system performance standards for the 10 Essential Public Health Services.[38] With the success of the CDC and its national partners in establishing National Public Health Performance Standards (NPHPS), the CDC National Center for Environmental Health (NCEH) undertook refinement of NPHPS and creation of a set of EnvPHPS in early 2002.

The primary goal of the EnvPHPS is to promote continuous improvement of environmental public health practice and foster improvement at the state, tribal, local, territorial, and national levels by building:

▸ Capacity to provide the 10 EEPHS,
▸ Community accountability for EEPHS, and
▸ Consistency of services across the environmental health system.

Generally environmental public health practice is defined by the EEPHS but more specifically by the EnvPHPS associated with each EEPHS.

Environmental Public Health System Response

Frumkin proposes a public health framework that uses the 10 Essential Public Health Services[38] to define the public health role and related actions needed to address climate change. Based on the CDC work to focus the essential public health services on environmental health, the definitions of the 10 essential environmental public health services are presented in Table 21-5.

To demonstrate the utility of the EEPHS, it is used as a framework for environmental public health system actions needed to counter climate change risks. The first of these EEPHS (1) is monitor environmental and health status. For climate change, public health officials can focus their efforts on tracking climate-related diseases and surveillance of indicators of climate change health

TABLE 21-5   10 Essential Environmental Public Health Services[39]

1. Monitor environmental and health status to identify and solve community environmental health problems.

2. Diagnose and investigate environmental health problems and health hazards in the community.

3. Inform, educate, and empower people about environmental health issues.

4. Mobilize community partnerships and actions to identify and solve environmental health problems.

5. Develop policies and plans that support individual and community environmental health efforts.

6. Enforce laws and regulations that protect environmental health and ensure safety.

7. Link people to needed environmental health services and assure the provision of environmental health services when otherwise unavailable.

8. Assure a competent environmental health workforce.

9. Evaluate the effectiveness, accessibility, and quality of personal and population-based environmental health services.

10. Research for new insights and innovative solutions to environmental health problems and issues.

SOURCE: Centers for Disease Control and Prevention, National Center for Environmental Health. Environmental Public Health Performance Standards, (Version 2.0).

risks (e.g., vector range changes, prevalence of infected hosts, water supply conditions, etc.). Associated with monitoring climate-related indicators, public health officials can be diligent in EEPHS 2, diagnosing and investigating climate-related health problems and hazards. In practice, effective surveillance of sentinel environmental conditions such as abundant *Dermacentor* tick populations and the related risk of Rocky Mountain spotted fever can provide an early indication that diagnosis and investigation of potential vector-borne disease outbreaks is needed.

If an extreme climate event is predicted, public health officials employ EEPHS 3: inform and educate those who will likely be impacted so that the population can determine which adaptive action is best for their situation. As an example, there may be a flood warning issued for low-lying areas and some families may wish to leave while others choose to build sandbag embankments to prevent flood damage to their property. EEPHS 4 can guide action to mobilizing community environmental health partnerships and action to identify and solve health problems such as preparing for floods. Undertaking this EEPSH may require public health officials to develop community partnerships with industry to reduce air emissions during times of dangerously poor air quality. A final example is associated with EEPHS 5: developing environmental policies and plans that support individual and community health. In the practice of developing environmental policies and plans, it is essential that public health officials have knowledge of the environmental health situation and understand how to undertake effective interventions in order to recommend appropriate actions within the policy arena and the design of target-specific interventions such as a municipal heat-wave preparedness policy and associated plan.

There are ample indicators that climate change is underway. It is essential that public health officials consider precautionary steps and investigate the environmental health risks and adaptive strategies that may be needed in their jurisdictions to prevent or mitigate the health impacts from climate change. Use of EEPHS as a framework for public health action offers guidance in day-to-day environmental public health practice and should enhance the public health response to environmental and health impacts from climate change.

Quality Improvement in Environmental Public Health Practice

Just as EEPHS elements describe the associated public health practices, the optimal model standards provide measurement indicators for assessing and identifying where performance and quality improvement of EEPHS are needed. To introduce optimal model environmental performance standards, two EEPHS are discussed in relationship to program and/or system-level performance. The *Environmental Public Health Performance Standards (Version 2.0)*[39] provide guidance on use of the EnvPHPS assessment tool. (These standards can be accessed at http://www.cdc.gov by searching for "Environmental Public Health Performance Standards.")

Model standards (MS) set at optimal performance levels for each EEPHS are discussed below. The MS below are modified in that the standards are presented in results-oriented language to describe accomplishment for the following two EEPHS.

▸ EEPHS 2: Diagnose and investigate environmental health problems includes MS 2.1, that optimally requires:
  • A surveillance system that identifies patterns and/or outbreaks of environmentally related health hazards is in place.
  • Epidemiological and environmental health investigation techniques have resulted in collected data that identify environmentally related health threats.

▸ EEPHS 6: Enforce laws and regulations includes MS 6.1, that requires:
  • The impact of state and local laws, regulations, and ordinances on community environmental health are assessed by those in the environmental health system, including those that govern food safety, clean water and air and those that protect environmental health more broadly (e.g., land use, community design, transportation, and agriculture).
  • The scientific merit and best practices in achieving compliance, and the opinions of constituents are reviewed.

Those conducting an EnvPHPS assessment can find resource tools to conduct the assessment and undertake a quality improvement plan. The CDC National Public Health Improvement Initiative provides more information on quality improvement approaches and tools. More information can be found at http://www.cdc.gov by searching under "National Public Health Improvement Initiative."

SUMMARY

Humans have competed for survival advantage within the natural environment through adaptive abilities and technological control of natural resources. Many of the adaptive changes are codified in environmental public health practice. These adaptive actions have provided safe water, air, food (all three are media for exposure pathways for infectious and toxic agents), and shelter to sustain and grow human populations.

If human success is to continue, the overuse of natural resources and contamination of the global environment from technological hazards that harm health and well-being need to be addressed. Humans are now challenged with applying principles of sustainability in maintaining an environment conducive to human health. Critical challenges that lay ahead are:

▸ Developing preventive and adaptive methods to cope with the impacts of global climate change;
▸ Mitigating the legacy environmental toxic pollutants that contaminate our air, water, soil, and food chain;
▸ Improving sanitation and waste treatment processes that are capable of removing infectious pathogens, micro-fibers, nanoparticles, pharmaceuticals, and other toxic substances, including those that mimic endocrine system hormones;
▸ Developing sustainable commercial processes and products that do not harm human health;
▸ Creating living and working environments that are free of hazards and promote health; and

▶ Guarding against acts of environmental disasters and unintended health impacts resulting from the human attempts to control the natural environment and its fluctuations.

Existing environmental sciences, environmentally related laws, and the environmental public health system have evolved and must continue to evolve and adapt to new challenges and threats facing the natural and technological environments that enable humans to prosper.

REVIEW QUESTIONS

1. Identify three critical public health issues projected to occur as a result of climate change.
   a. Discuss the potential human health impacts related to each critical climate change issue.
   b. Describe the mitigating or adaptive environmental public health actions needed to address the climate change issues you identified.
2. Describe the interplay between the natural and built environment and the critical issues of natural environmental sustainability and human health.
   a. In your opinion, what critical policy issues are related to environmental sustainability?
   b. What are the roles of environmental public health professionals addressing the policy issues?
3. Describe why a completed exposure pathway is central to potential health impacts from environmental contaminants.
4. Describe the importance of essential environmental public health services in the practice and quality improvement of the environmental public health system.

REFERENCES

1. Carson, R. *Silent Spring*. Boston, MA: Houghton Mifflin; 1962.
2. Cunningham WP, Cunningham M, Saigo BW. *Environmental Science: A Global Concern*. 8th ed. Boston, MA: McGraw-Hill; 2005.
3. Nadakavukaren A. *Our Global Environment: A Healthy Perspective*. 5th ed. Prospect Heights, IL: Waveland Press, Inc.; 2000.
4. Moore GS. *Living with the Earth: Concepts in Environmental Health Science*. 2nd ed. Boca Raton, FL: Lewis Publishers; 2002.
5. U.S. Environmental Protection Agency. EPA National Primary Drinking Water Regulations. http://water.epa.gov/drink/contaminants/upload/mcl-2.pdf. Published May 2009. Accessed December 29, 2014.
6. Maupin MA, Kenny JF, Hutson SS, Lovelace JK, Barber NL, Linsey KS. Estimated use of water in the United States in 2010: U.S. Geological Survey Circular 1405, 2014. Table 1: Total water withdrawals by source and State, 2010. p9. http://pubs.usgs.gov/circ/1405/pdf/circ1405.pdf. Accessed November 11, 2014.
7. Pani B. *Textbook of Environmental Chemistry*. I. K. International Pvt. Ltd. New Delhi, India; 2007, p2.
8. U.S. Environmental Protection Agency. Clean Air Act of 1970. http://www.epa.gov/air/caa/amendments.html#caa70. Updated August 15, 2013. Accessed October 14, 2014.
9. US Environmental Protection Agency. 1990 Amendments to the Clean Air Act of 1970. http://www.epa.gov/air/caa/amendments.html#caa70. Updated August 15, 2013. Accessed October 14, 2014.
10. U.S. Department of Health and Human Services, Agency for Toxic Substances and Disease Registry. Toxicological Profile for Carbon Monoxide. 2012.
11. U.S. Department of Health and Human Services, Agency for Toxic Substances and Disease Registry. Toxicological Profile for Nitrogen Oxides. 2002.
12. Newman MC. *Fundamentals of Ecotoxicology*. Boca Raton, FL: Lewis; 2002.
13. U.S. Department of Health and Human Services, Agency for Toxic Substances and Disease Registry. Toxicological Profile for Lead. 2007.
14. Centers for Disease Control and Prevention. Air Contaminants: Ozone and Particulate Matter. http://ephtracking.cdc.gov/showAirContaminants.action#pm. Published April 17, 2012. Updated September 16, 2013. Accessed November 1, 2014.
15. Hess D. Historic marker commemorates Donora Smog Tragedy. http://www.donora.fire-dept.net/1948smog.htm. November 3, 1995. Updated 2007. Accessed January 26, 2015.
16. US Environmental Protection Agency. The Benefits and Costs of the Clean Air Act from 1990 to 2020. Washington DC. http://www.epa.gov/air/sect812/prospective2.html. Updated final report April 2011. Accessed December 11, 2014.
17. Rodricks JV. Calculated Risks: The Toxicity and Human Health Risks of Chemicals in our Environment. 2nd ed. Cambridge, New York. Cambridge University Press; 2007. http://dx.doi.org/10.1017/CBO9780511535451. Online Publication August 2009. Accessed January 19, 2015.

18. Centers for Disease Control and Prevention. Diagnosis and Management of Foodborne Illnesses: A Primer for Physicians and Other Health Care Professionals. MMWR: April 16, 2004/53(RR04);1–33. http://www.cdc.gov/mmwr/preview/mmwrhtml/rr5304a1.htm. Accessed December 2, 2014.

19. Centers for Disease Control and Prevention. Estimates of Foodborne Illness in the United States, 2011. http://www.cdc.gov/foodborneburden/2011-foodborne-estimates.html. Published December 15, 2010. Accessed January 12, 2015.

20. Centers for Disease Control and Prevention. Multistate Outbreak of Multidrug-Resistant Salmonella Heidelberg Infections Linked to Foster Farms Brand Chicken http://www.cdc.gov/salmonella/heidelberg-10-13/index.html. Published October 8, 2013. Updated August 1, 2014. Accessed January 12, 2015.

21. U.S. Food and Drug Administration. Hazard Analysis and Critical Control Points: Principles and Application Guidelines. http://www.fda.gov/Food/GuidanceRegulation/HACCP/ucm2006801.htm#princ. Published August 14, 1997. Updated September 19, 2014. Accessed January 12, 2015.

22. Bregman JI, Edell, RD. Environmental Compliance Handbook. Boca Raton, FL: Lewis Publishers; 2002.

23. U.S. Department of Health and Human Services. The Surgeon General's Call to Action To Promote Healthy Homes. US Department of Health and Human Services, Office of the Surgeon General. http://www.surgeongeneral.gov. Published 2009. Accessed January 4, 2015.

24. U.S. Department of Health and Human Services. Office of Disease Prevention and Health Promotion. Healthy People 2020. Washington, DC. https://www.healthypeople.gov/2020/topics-objectives/topic/environmental-health. Updated January 23, 2015. Accessed January 25, 2015.

25. National Center for Healthy Housing. Housing Interventions and Health: A Review of the Evidence. http://www.nchh.org/LinkClick.aspx?fileticket=2lvaEDNBIdU%3d&tabid=229 Published 2009. Accessed December 30, 2014.

26. Eitler TW, McMahon ET, Thoerig TC. Ten Principles for Building Healthy Places. Washington, DC: Urban Land Institute. http://www.uli.org/wp-content/uploads/ULI-Documents/10-Principles-for-Building-Healthy-Places.pdf. Published 2013. Accessed January 17, 2015.

27. American Institute of Architects. Communities by Design: Ten Principles for Livable Communities. http://www.aia.org/about/initiatives/AIAS075369. Accessed January 19, 2015.

28. Maantay J, Chakraborty J, Brender J. Proximity to Environmental Hazards: Environmental Justice and Adverse Health Outcomes. May 12, 2010 Washington, DC: U.S. Environmental Protection Agency. http://www.epa.gov/ncer/events/calendar/2010/mar17/abstracts/brender.pdf. Accessed February 21, 2015.

29. Olden K, White SL. Health-related disparities: influence of environmental factors. Med Clin North Am. 2005. 89(4):721-738. doi: 10.1016/j.mcna.2005.02.001. Published online May 29, 2005. Accessed February 21, 2015.

30. Gee GC, Payne-Sturges DC. Environmental health disparities: a framework integrating psychosocial and environmental concepts. Environ Health Perspect. 112:1645–1653 (2004). doi:10.1289/ehp.7074. http://dx.doi.org/. Published online August 16, 2004. Accessed February 21, 2015.

31. NOAA National Climatic Data Center. State of the Climate: Global Analysis for Annual 2014, http://www.ncdc.noaa.gov/sotc/global/2014/13. Published online December 2014. Accessed January 24, 2015.

32. NOAA National Climatic Data Center. Greenhouse Gases. http://www.ncdc.noaa.gov/monitoring-references/faq/greenhouse-gases.php. Published online December 2014. Accessed January 24, 2015.

33. Centers for Disease Control and Prevention, National Center for Environmental Health. Climate Effects on Health. http://www.cdc.gov/climateandhealth/effects/default.htm. Updated December 22, 2014. Accessed January 24, 2015.

34. Sheffield PE, Landrigan PJ. Global climate change and children's health: threats and strategies for prevention. Environ Health Perspect. 2011. 119(3):291–298. http://dx.doi.org/10.1289/ehp.1002233. Published online October 14, 2010. Accessed January 26, 2015.

35. Frumkin H, Hess J, Luber G, Malilay J, McGeehin M. Framing health matters. Am J Public Health. 2008;98(3):435–445. doi: 10.2105/AJPH.2007.119362. Accessed January 26, 2015.

36. Hales S, Kovats S, Lloyd S, Campbell-Lendrum D. Quantitative risk assessment of the effects of climate change on selected causes of death, 2030s and 2050s. World Health Organization. 2014. http://www.who.int/globalchange/publications/quantitative-risk-assessment/en/. Accessed January 23, 2015.

37. The White House. The Health Impacts of Climate Change on Americans. June 2014. Washington, DC. http://www.whitehouse.gov/sites/default/files/docs/the_health_impacts_of_climate_change_on_americans_final.pdf. Accessed January 24, 2015.

38. Centers for Disease Control and Prevention. National Public Health Performance Standards Program. http://www.cdc.gov/nphpsp/essentialservices.html. Published 1994. Updated May 29, 2014. Accessed January 18, 2015.

39. Centers for Disease Control and Prevention, National Center for Environmental Health. Environmental Public Health Performance Standards, (Version 2.0). http://www.cdc.gov/nceh/ehs/envphps/docs/envphpsv2.pdf. Update May 2014. Accessed January 18, 2015.

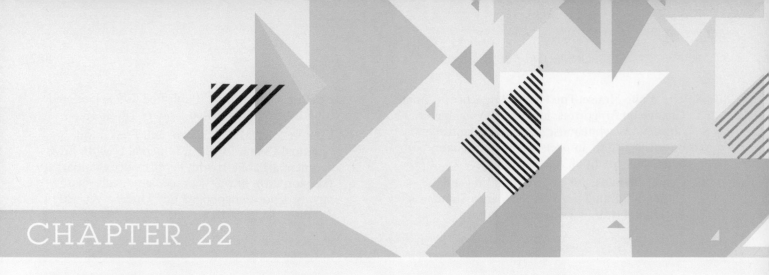

CHAPTER 22

Chronic Disease Prevention and Control

Janet Collins, PhD • Leah Maynard, PhD

LEARNING OBJECTIVES

Upon completion of this chapter, the reader will be able to:

1. Describe the importance of chronic disease prevention as a public health priority.

2. Identify health risk behaviors most highly associated with chronic disease.

3. Identify the types of public health strategies with greatest reach and impact on chronic disease.

4. Identify key settings/locations for public health work to prevent chronic disease.

5. Describe the role of preventive screening and chronic disease management in the control of chronic disease.

KEY TERMS

accessibility
availability
built environment
chronic diseases
chronic disease management
environmental change
nutrition assistance programs
policy, systems, and environmental interventions
socioeconomic factors
systems change

INTRODUCTION

Improving health for the greatest number of Americans requires that chronic disease prevention be a cornerstone of public health.[*][1] **Chronic diseases** such as heart disease, cancer, arthritis, and diabetes are noncommunicable illnesses and are pervasive, prolonged in duration, and rarely completely cured. They are the main cause of poor health, disability, and death in the United States, accounting for approximately 70 percent of deaths.[2] Half of the adults in the United States are living with at least one chronic condition, and a quarter have two or more.[3]

Substantial inequities exist in the burden of chronic disease based on geographic location, race/ethnicity, education, and income. White Americans tend to live longer than black Americans, and life expectancy is much greater in some counties than in others. In fact, the gap in average life expectancy for subpopulations in varying counties can be over 33 years—the difference between dying at 58 years (Native American males in some South Dakota counties) or living to 91 years (Asian females in Bergen County New Jersey).[4] Closing these health disparities is a critical goal for public health professionals.[5]

_____
[*]By "public health" we mean the totality of public health professionals, activities, programs, and policies influencing health behaviors and outcomes at the federal, state, and local levels.

Although the primary focus of public health is on improved health outcomes, the economic consequences of chronic disease are substantial. Chronic illnesses account for the majority of the approximate $2.8 trillion spent on health care each year.[6] By preventing and delaying chronic diseases, people can live longer, healthier, and more productive lives at lower cost.

Given the widespread nature of chronic disease, readers of this text will likely have experienced the effects of cancer, stroke, or diabetes on the lives of a parent, grandparent, aunt, or uncle. Many people have never thought of these diseases as preventable, but public health has a proven track record in preventing and delaying chronic disease. Public health works upstream to maintain health in the first place, in addition to helping people live healthy lives after disease occurs. Working upstream requires preventing a relatively small set of risk factors that contribute to premature mortality, including high blood pressure, tobacco use, obesity, poor nutrition, physical inactivity, and excessive alcohol use.[7,8]

Figure 22-1 is a theoretical model for public health action that compares different public health strategies from smallest impact (top of the pyramid) to largest impact (bottom of the pyramid). Impact is determined by a combination of cost, reach, effectiveness, and sustainability. Most of our focus in this chapter will be on "Changing the Context" to help make a healthy lifestyle

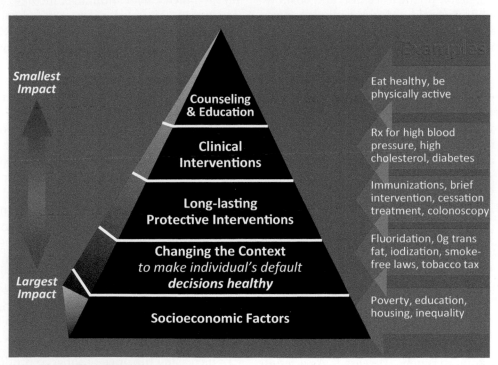

FIGURE 22-1   Factors That Affect Health

SOURCE: U.S. Department of Health and Human Services, Centers for Disease Control and Prevention. Adapted from: Frieden, T. A framework for public heath action: The health impact pyramid. *Am J Public Health*. 2010; April; 100(4): 590–595.

the easier, more affordable, more attractive choice. This "context" encompasses policy, pricing, access, and other aspects of the physical and social environment.

We often refer to strategies to "change the context" as **policy, systems, and environmental interventions**. "Policy" can include formal policies such as laws, executive orders, and regulatory measures, or informal policies such as a company's rules. "Systems" are organizations or institutions such as schools, transportation networks, parks and recreation facilities, and health care providers. Reforming the procedures or principles of these organizations is "**systems change**." One example of a systems change is instituting patient reminders of the need for routine screenings or upcoming visits in health care settings. Finally, "**environmental change**" is an alteration to the physical environment: adding sidewalks or bike paths, building a new street or park, or adding promotional displays for healthier foods in grocery stores or restaurants.

"**Socioeconomic factors**," such as education, housing, poverty, and employment status, have a profound impact on health outcomes. For example, graduating from high school is associated with significantly improved lifelong health outcomes.[9] Public health practitioners are only beginning to understand their role in influencing socioeconomic factors, also called "social determinants of health" (see Chapter 3). These social factors go well beyond the fields of public health and medicine. To be most effective, today's public health professionals work alongside colleagues from the fields of education, agriculture, transportation, labor, political science, and environmental studies to improve health through multiple sectors.

In this chapter our focus is on chronic disease risk factors and the public health strategies associated with risk reduction, rather than on the treatment of chronic diseases. We review evidence-based public health strategies to prevent tobacco use, obesity, poor nutrition, physical inactivity, and excessive alcohol use. While prevention is paramount, we also briefly address the role of public health in controlling chronic diseases through earlier detection and better disease management.

TOBACCO

Tobacco use is the leading cause of preventable death and disease in the United States, resulting in more than 480,000 deaths each year and serious illness for nearly 16 million people.[10] Tobacco use negatively affects nearly every organ in the body, and ongoing research continues to expand our understanding of its harms.[10] Compared to persons who never smoked, smokers are three times more likely to die prematurely, with their lives cut short by approximately 10 years.[11] As a result of smoking, lung cancer went from being a rare disease 150 years ago to being the leading cause of cancer deaths for both men and women by 1987.[12]

Beyond the direct impact of tobacco use, secondhand smoke has a detrimental effect on nonsmokers. Secondhand smoke comes from the burning end of cigarettes and the smoke breathed out by smokers. In infants and children, secondhand smoke increases the severity of asthma attacks, and significantly increases susceptibility to respiratory infections, ear infections, and other health problems. Among adults, secondhand smoke causes coronary heart disease, stroke, and lung cancer. There is no safe level of secondhand smoke exposure.[13]

The history of tobacco prevention and control is one of remarkable progress, deemed one of the greatest public health achievements of the twentieth century.[14] Smoking reached its height in the 1950s and 1960s, when nearly half of American men smoked and women's rates were on the rise.[15] As the result of information about the effects of tobacco on health and a wide range of public policy actions, smoking rates and per capita consumption were cut in half, and exposure to secondhand smoke decreased dramatically by the beginning of the twenty-first century (see Figure 22-2).

Unfortunately, the job of preventing and controlling tobacco use is not finished. In 2013, 18 percent of U.S. adults, 18 years and older, smoked cigarettes during the past month[16] and 21 percent used any tobacco product every day or some days.[17] Among high school students in 2013, 16 percent smoked cigarettes and 22 percent used any tobacco product in the past 30 days.[18] Large disparities in tobacco use exist on the basis of race, ethnicity, education, age, income, and region.[18,19] To support continued progress in reducing tobacco use, President Barack Obama signed the Family Smoking Prevention and Tobacco Control Act into law on June 22, 2009. The Act provides FDA the authority to regulate the manufacture, sale, and marketing of tobacco products, including new standards for nicotine content and other harmful substances in tobacco products.

The 2014 Surgeon General's Report, *The Health Consequences of Smoking—50 Years of Progress: A Report of the Surgeon General*, describes a vision for ending the tobacco epidemic known as the "endgame."[10] The report calls for accelerated efforts to reduce rates of tobacco use by using proven strategies and by considering new strategies such as reducing the nicotine content of cigarettes and increasing restrictions on sales. The Centers for Disease Control and Prevention's (CDC's) *Best Practices for Comprehensive Tobacco Control Programs*, updated in 2014, is an evidence-based guide to help states establish effective tobacco control programs to prevent and reduce tobacco use. Several of the most effective interventions for reducing tobacco use are:

1. increasing the price of tobacco products;
2. establishing and enforcing comprehensive smoke-free laws prohibiting smoking in worksites, restaurants, and bars;

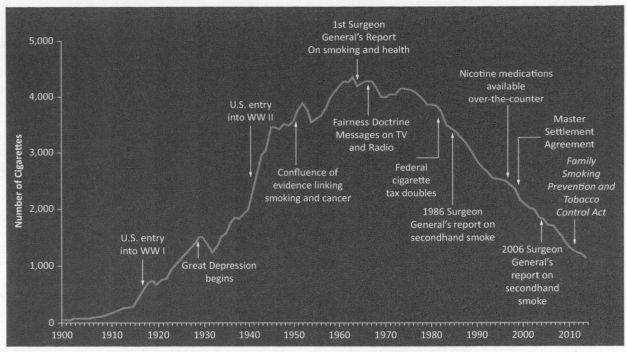

FIGURE 22-2 **Annual Adult Per Capita Cigarette Consumption and Major Smoking and Health Events—United States, 1900–2013**

SOURCES: United States Department of Health and Human Services, The Health Consequences of Smoking—50 Years of Progress: A Report of the Surgeon General. Atlanta, GA, 2014. Adapted from Warner 1985 with permission from Massachusetts Medical Society, ©1985; U.S. Department of Health and Human Services 1989; Creek et al. 1994; U.S. Department of Agriculture 2000; U.S. Census Bureau 2013; U.S. Department of the Treasury 2013.

*Adults ≥18 years of age as reported annually by the Census Bureau.

3. implementing high-impact mass media campaigns; and

4. helping tobacco users quit through health systems change, cessation insurance coverage, and state quitlines.[20]

Tobacco Pricing

Cigarettes and other tobacco products are taxed by federal, state, and local governments, including excise taxes on each pack of cigarettes. Increasing these taxes is one of the most effective ways to reduce smoking and other tobacco use, especially among youth.[21] A 10 percent increase in cigarette prices has been shown to produce a 7 percent decline in youth smoking and a 4 percent decline in total cigarette consumption.[10,22,23] On April 1, 2009, the federal cigarette excise tax increased dramatically from $0.39 to $1.01 per pack. In 2014, state tax rates on a pack of cigarettes ranged from $0.30 to $4.35 with an average of $1.54. Between 2000 and 2014, 47 states and the District of Columbia passed more than 115 state cigarette tax increases.[24]

States can maximize the impact of tobacco taxes by allocating a portion of the revenue to comprehensive

tobacco control programs that prevent smoking initiation and help people to stop using tobacco.[10] Sustained, comprehensive state tobacco control programs funded at CDC-recommended levels accelerate progress toward reducing the health burden and economic impact of tobacco-related diseases in the United States.[20] However, during 2013, despite combined revenue of $25.7 billion from settlement payments and tobacco taxes for all states, only $459.5 million (1.8 percent) was spent on state comprehensive tobacco control programs.[20] Public health professionals can contribute to this area of work by educating local and state legislators and other public officials about the effects of tobacco taxes on health, including the importance of reinvesting a portion of the revenue to support tobacco control efforts.

Smoke-Free Laws

Comprehensive smoke-free laws that prohibit smoking in all indoor areas of worksites, restaurants, and bars are essential to help protect nonsmokers from secondhand smoke in public areas. In addition to protecting nonsmokers, smoke-free laws and policies increase quit rates and reduce tobacco initiation.[10,25]

Like the negative health effects of secondhand smoke, the positive impact of smoke-free policies has been well documented. In parts of North America and Europe, within one year, smoke-free policies resulted in 10 percent declines in the rates of preterm birth and hospital care for asthma attacks.[26] Communities with indoor smoke-free policies have also seen reductions in hospitalizations for heart attack (15 percent), stroke (16 percent), and respiratory disease (24 percent).[27]

Despite the health risks of secondhand smoke, just 49 percent of the U.S. population is protected by state and/or local comprehensive smoke-free laws covering workplaces, restaurants, and bars,[28] and millions of children remain exposed to secondhand smoke in cars and homes. In the United States, 21 million children (35 percent) live in homes where residents or visitors smoke on a regular basis.[29] Efforts are underway to adopt smoke-free policies in private settings such as multiunit housing, as well to promote voluntary smoke-free rules in homes and vehicles.

Considerable work remains for public health professionals to convey the importance and benefits of smoke-free policies, and to help in their design, implementation, and enforcement to ensure maximum effectiveness. Working with the public, including landlords, on protecting children and other nonsmokers from secondhand smoke in apartments and homes is another challenging area in current public health policy and practice.

Cessation Interventions

Cessation interventions are an important element of a comprehensive approach to tobacco control.[20] These interventions ensure that the vast majority of smokers who want to quit (69 percent of all smokers) have access to effective help should they need it.[20,30]

Tobacco dependence treatments, including counseling and medication, are clinically effective and highly cost effective, and health care professionals should routinely recommend them to patients who use tobacco.[10,31] Public health practitioners can work with health care systems and insurers to help ensure that these services are widely available.[31]

Both individual and group counseling are effective, and their effectiveness increases with treatment intensity.[31] Telephone counseling is also effective with diverse populations and has broad reach.[31] Public health departments in all 50 U.S. states, the District of Columbia, Puerto Rico, and Guam operate free quitlines that can be accessed through a 1-800-QUIT-NOW portal. Spanish-language services available from state quitlines can be accessed by calling 1-855-DÉJELO-YA, and the CDC funds a national Asian quitline that provides in-language services to Chinese, Korean, and Vietnamese-speaking callers.

To date, seven FDA-approved cessation medications are available, including five forms of nicotine replacement therapy (the patch, gum, lozenge, nasal spray, and inhaler) and two nonnicotine medications (bupropion and varenicline). The nicotine patch, gum, and lozenge are available over-the-counter; the remaining four medications are available by prescription. Cessation counseling and medications are each effective when used alone, but are even more effective when used in combination.[31]

The 2014 edition of *Best Practices for Comprehensive Tobacco Control Programs* recommends that states take a three-pronged approach to helping tobacco users quit with a focus on policy and systems change.[20] The three components of this approach are: (1) promoting health systems change, (2) expanding insurance coverage and utilization of proven cessation treatments, and (3) supporting state quitline capacity.[20] The goal is to ensure that tobacco screening and cessation interventions are fully integrated into routine clinical practice as a standard of care and that tobacco users who are ready to quit and want help have access to evidence-based treatments.[20]

Mass Media Campaigns

Antitobacco media campaigns are an important strategy to reduce smoking initiation and promote quitting, especially when implemented as part of a comprehensive tobacco control program.[10,32] Effective campaigns involve broad reach, frequent ads, and a sustained presence over time. The most effective ads portray personal testimonials and graphic images illustrating the health effects of smoking and secondhand smoke exposure. Unfortunately, campaigns can be expensive, particularly with the use of paid media. One way to keep costs down is to make use of available, high-quality campaign materials such as those available through the CDC's Media Campaign Research Center.[33]

In March 2012, the CDC launched the first-ever paid national tobacco education campaign—*Tips from Former Smokers (Tips)*. *Tips* encourages people to quit smoking by showing the toll that smoking-related illness takes on smokers and their loved ones. The hard-hitting ads show people living with the real and painful consequences of smoking or exposure to secondhand smoke. During the 12-week campaign, there were more than 200,000 additional calls to 1-800-QUIT-NOW compared to the same period in 2011—a more than 130 percent increase.[34] Additional campaigns were conducted in 2013 and 2014.

Challenges

Tobacco prevention and control continues to be a critical area for public health. While best-practice strategies are clear, major challenges remain. Tobacco is

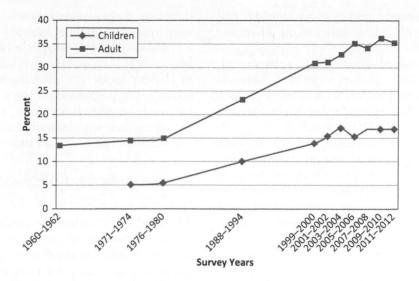

FIGURE 22-3 Obesity Trends among Children and Adults in the United States, 1960–1962 through 2011–2012

SOURCES: CDC/National Center for Health Statistics: National Health Examination Survey 1960–1962 and National Health and Nutrition Examination Surveys for all other year ranges.

a highly addictive, heavily advertised product with a well-resourced industry behind it and an evolving product line. Foremost among the challenges is a tobacco industry that aggressively promotes lethal products, including marketing to youth and young adults.[10] Hookah, flavored cigars, and electronic nicotine delivery systems such as e-cigarettes are particularly attractive to young people. This evolving landscape of tobacco and nicotine products requires timely research on the harmful effects of new and unregulated products. For example, research is underway to help us understand the potential benefits and risks of e-cigarettes on population and individual health, including their potential role in smoking cessation.

OBESITY

Obesity[†] is widespread, affecting 35 percent of adults and 17 percent of children and adolescents in the United States[35] and contributing to nearly 112,000 preventable deaths each year.[36] The prevalence of obesity among adults is higher among non-Hispanic blacks and Hispanics (47.8 percent and 42.5 percent, respectively) than for non-Hispanic whites and non-Hispanic Asians (32.6 percent and 10.8 percent, respectively). When stratified by age, the prevalence of obesity is highest (39.5 percent) among adults who

are 40–59 years.[35] Among children and adolescents, obesity affects 8.4 percent of 2- to 5-year-olds, 17.7 percent of 6- to 11-year-olds, and 20.5 percent of 12- to 19-year-olds. The prevalence of obesity is higher among Hispanic (22.4 percent) and non-Hispanic black youth (20.2 percent) compared to non-Hispanic whites (14.1 percent) and Asians (8.6 percent).[35] Obesity rates for all ages increased dramatically over the past few decades, but recently began to level and stabilize at high rates[35,37–39] (Figure 22-3).

Obesity tracks from childhood into adulthood, with the prediction for adult overweight or obesity being stronger for adolescents than for younger children.[40] Risk of obesity has also been shown to be associated with large birth size (greater than 8.8 lbs.) and overweight during the preschool years,[41,42] with the incidences (new cases) of obesity decreasing with age among children.[41] In the study by Cunningham and colleagues, approximately 50 percent of children who became obese by 8th grade were overweight or obese at entry to kindergarten.[41]

In 2013, the American Medical Association recognized obesity as a disease,[43] but its contribution as a major risk factor for multiple chronic diseases, including coronary heart disease, stroke, type 2 diabetes, some cancers, hypertension, gallbladder disease, osteoarthritis, sleep apnea, complications from pregnancy, and depression has been well documented for years.[44] Obesity can also negatively impact quality of life by reducing an individual's sense of physical, social, and emotional well-being.[45] In terms of psychosocial consequences, a consistent bias, as well as active discrimination, against persons with obesity has been observed in worksite, education, and health care settings.[46] In addition, poor

---

[†]Obesity is defined using body mass index (BMI) measured as weight (in kilograms) relative to height (in square meters). Adults with a BMI of 30 kg/m² or greater, and children and adolescents with a BMI at or greater than their age- and sex-specific 95th percentile, are considered to have obesity.

self-esteem has been shown among some children and adolescents with obesity, especially among Hispanic and non-Hispanic white females.[47,48]

The medical costs of obesity are substantial, amounting to $147 billion dollars annually.[49] Medical spending for adults with obesity is $1,427 more per person per year than medical spending for normal-weight adults, a difference of nearly 42 percent.[49]

The causes of obesity are complex and include genetic, biologic, and environmental components. Population-based public health efforts to prevent obesity focus on changing policy, systems, and the environment to support healthier eating and physical activity. These nutrition and physical activity strategies are described in the following two sections.

NUTRITION

Several of the 10 leading causes of death[2] (e.g., heart disease, cancer, stroke, and diabetes) are associated with nutrition, both directly and indirectly through an association with obesity.[50] The associations of nutrition with morbidity and mortality may differ by disease. For example, excessive sodium intake is a primary risk factor for heart disease and stroke, and consumption of fruits and vegetables reduces the risk of several chronic diseases, such as cancer.[51] In addition, eating fruits and vegetables (which are lower in calories and more nutrient dense) in place of higher calorie foods (such as foods with high amounts of fat and added sugars) can help prevent or reduce obesity.[51]

Healthy diets for persons 2 years of age and older are defined by the *Dietary Guidelines for Americans, 2010*.[51] Healthy diets include fruits, vegetables (especially legumes and those that are dark-green, red, and orange), whole grains (at least half of grains consumed should be whole), fat-free or low-fat milk products (including substitutes such as soy milk), and protein foods (including seafood, lean meats, poultry, eggs, legumes, nuts, and soy). Healthy diets also avoid excessive sodium, added sugars, refined grains, saturated fats, transfats, and cholesterol.[51] For nearly all infants, breast milk is the best source of nutrition and immune protection; thus, encouraging and supporting breastfeeding is a major public health strategy to give children a healthy start in life.[52]

Two primary settings for the implementation of public health nutrition initiatives are: (1) food service facilities where people generally eat away from home, such as restaurants, fast food establishments, schools, worksite cafeterias, and childcare facilities and (2) food retail venues such as grocery stores, convenience stores, and farmers' markets where people buy foods they prepare and eat at home. The key premise of nutrition

initiatives in these settings is to make the healthy options easy, appealing, and affordable.

Below we review public health nutrition strategies to: (1) increase the availability and accessibility of healthy foods, (2) advertise and promote healthier foods, (3) implement nutrition standards in restaurants, cafeterias, concession stands, and vending machines, (4) strengthen supplemental nutrition programs, and (5) encourage and support breastfeeding.

Availability and Accessibility of Healthy Foods

The availability of healthy foods refers to the proximity of food retail or food service venues to residential areas and the presence of healthier foods within these venues. Eating at home can pose a challenge for people who do not live close to supermarkets or grocery stores. Many studies have shown a positive association between the presence of a local grocery store and consumption of fruits and vegetables,[53-58] while others have shown that healthier diets (as measured by various dietary quality indices) were associated with better access to supermarkets.[59,60] In addition to consumption of healthier foods, a lower prevalence of overweight and obesity has also been observed with grocery store proximity.[61-65] Public health initiatives include encouraging grocery stores, farmers markets, and healthier mobile food vendors to locate in underserved areas, and helping convenience stores to carry healthier foods. While the availability of healthy food and beverages is a necessary condition for good nutrition, availability is not enough—accessibility is also important. Accessibility includes availability as well as quality, affordability, variety, and cultural acceptability.[66] For example, if healthier foods are available but are too expensive for the local consumers, then the healthier items are not accessible.

Healthy Food Promotion

Selling healthier foods involves applying the standard components of the marketing mix—product, placement, pricing, and promotion. Sales of healthier foods are affected by variety, quality, taste, and packaging, as well as their location and the effort required to obtain them in grocery stores, cafeteria lines, and other retail and food service venues.[67-69] Coupons, daily specials, differential pricing tactics, in-store displays, item and shelf labeling (including nutritional scoring systems), special menu boards, and table tents are examples of pricing and promotion strategies that can influence the purchase of healthier foods in grocery stores, corner stores, cafeterias, or restaurants.[67-69] These strategies are commonly used to promote overall sales, but could also be used to selectively promote healthy purchases.

Public health practitioners can undertake a number of initiatives to promote healthier foods. These include providing education or technical assistance to store and restaurant owners or managers on marketing strategies; facilitating networking meetings so that owners and managers can learn from each other; helping develop promotional materials; and collecting and disseminating success stories of profitable promotion efforts.

Nutritional Standards

Nutrition standards are explicit principles and nutritional criteria that guide food offerings within an environment to ensure that healthier foods are available. For example, the Child and Adult Care Food Program (CACFP), within the U.S. Department of Agriculture (USDA), established specific nutritional criteria for meals served at facilities such as child care centers, day-care homes (child and adult), afterschool care centers, and emergency centers. These standards must be met for the meals to be reimbursed by the program. To illustrate, adult breakfasts must include one 1-cup serving of nonfat or low-fat milk, one ½-cup serving of fruits or vegetables or 100 percent juice, and one serving of grains or breads made from whole grains or enriched meal or flour.[70]

Nearly 50 percent of food dollars are spent on foods away from home.[71] Foods consumed outside the home typically contain more calories, added sugar, sodium, and fat, and their consumption leads to fewer servings of fruit, vegetables, dairy, and whole grains.[72–74] In addition, the portion sizes at fast food and chain restaurants have increased over time.[75,76] The proportion of calories consumed away from home increased from 17.7 percent in 1977–1978 to 31.6 percent in 2005–2008.[73] People who eat at fast food and chain restaurants generally underestimate the calorie content of the food they eat, particularly high calorie foods.[77] For these reasons, interventions that encourage adoption and implementation of nutrition standards within the food service environment could have a large impact on public health. Public health nutrition programs can work with restaurant owners, chefs, culinary institutes, and food vendors to improve the food and beverage offerings in restaurants and fast food establishments by reducing portion sizes, sodium, calories, and added sugars; eliminating transfats; adding fruits and vegetables; and replacing refined grains with whole grains such as whole wheat or brown rice. Public health practitioners can also encourage restaurant professionals to offer healthier side items as defaults, especially in children's meals: apple slices or carrots rather than fries, for instance, and nonfat or low-fat milk instead of soda.

Beyond restaurants and fast food establishments, institutions such as colleges and universities, hospitals, and other worksites are prime settings to implement nutrition standards. The U.S. Department of Health and Human Services (HHS) and the General Services Administration collaborated to create specific food, nutrition, and sustainability guidelines in their document, *Health and Sustainability Guidelines for Federal Concessions and Vending Operations.*[78] Although this document (commonly referred to as the Food Service Guidelines) was created for use in government-managed facilities, the nutritional criteria are easily applied in other worksite or cafeteria settings.

In 2012, USDA issued new standards for the National School Lunch Program and School Breakfast Program. These standards, which went into effect in the school years 2012–2013 and 2013–2014, respectively, emphasize fruits and vegetables, whole grain foods, nonfat and low-fat milk, and limit calories, saturated fat, and sodium.[79] USDA also developed nutritional standards for competitive foods and beverages sold outside of the school meals programs. These standards, called *Smart Snacks in Schools*, went into effect in the 2014–2015 school year.[80] Public health practitioners can assist schools and other institutions with purchasing of local foods, locating distributors, and training staff on healthier food preparations. In addition, they can ensure current nutrition standards are met and establish requirements that exceed federal standards. Public health practitioners can also serve as a model for other institutions by adopting and implementing the Food Service Guidelines.

Nutrition Assistance Programs

Collaborating with nutrition assistance programs is an effective way for public health practitioners to promote consumption of healthy foods and beverages among low-income individuals and families. There are 49 million Americans who live in food-insecure households[81] defined by having inconsistent access to adequate food.[82] **Nutrition assistance programs** include the Special Supplemental Nutrition Program for Women, Infants, and Children (WIC) and the Supplemental Nutrition Assistance Program (SNAP). SNAP benefits were provided to approximately 47.6 million persons in 2013[83] through designated state agencies that issue Electronic Benefit Transfer (EBT) cards which are similar to debit cards and can be used at any SNAP-authorized retail venue. WIC benefits were provided to approximately 9.2 million consumers in 2010[84] via monthly vouchers, checks, or EBT cards for purchase of approved foods from WIC-authorized retailers. Public health initiatives that focus on nutrition assistance programs include helping the managers of farmers' markets obtain EBT equipment, and promoting incentive programs such as "double bucks" that enable consumers to purchase more fruits and vegetables with their existing benefits.

Food and nutrition assistance is also provided to help supplement the diets of low-income persons in need as part of the Emergency Food Assistance Program. USDA contributes commodity foods to states, and states make the food available to local agencies such as food banks, which then distribute the food to community pantries or soup kitchens that serve the public directly.[85] Public health practitioners can help feeding programs increase the healthfulness of the food they provide and refer persons who are food insecure to appropriate community services.

Breastfeeding

The health benefits of breastfeeding are well documented; breastfeeding is associated with a lowered risk for numerous conditions, including ear infections, nausea and diarrhea, asthma, lower respiratory tract infections, obesity, type 1 and type 2 diabetes, childhood leukemia, sudden infant death syndrome, and inflammatory bowel disease.[52,86] Breastfeeding mothers also have a reduced risk of type 2 diabetes and breast and ovarian cancers.[52,86] In addition, economic savings associated with breastfeeding can be substantial – one study estimated an annual savings of $13 billion in medical and other expenditures if 90 percent of families exclusively breastfed for 6 months.[87] Public health strategies to encourage and support breastfeeding include improving hospital maternity care practices; supporting professional education for nurses, lactation counselors, and other health care professionals; providing peer and professional support for new moms; and helping worksites meet federal law requiring employers to provide break time and a place for hourly paid workers to express breast milk at work.[88]

Challenges

Nutrition is a challenging area of public health. Unlike tobacco control where total abstinence is the clear goal, people must make food choices multiple times each day. These choices are difficult: nutrition information can be confusing or contradictory; there are 15,000 to 60,000 unique food choices available in a typical grocery store;[89] and there is a lack of information about sodium, added sugar, fat, and calories in prepared foods such as restaurant and cafeteria meals. High calorie, low nutrient foods are heavily advertised, easily available, and relatively inexpensive. These challenges are heightened by the pleasure many people experience when they consume salty snacks, candy, cookies, and other sweet foods that are often high in calories.

PHYSICAL ACTIVITY

Although the importance of physical activity to health has been recognized for centuries, physical activity is a fairly recent topic for public health. In 1996, the U.S. Surgeon General released its first *Report on Physical Activity and Health*.[90] This landmark report provided the most thorough review of physical activity and health to date and aimed to create a new physical activity movement in the United States. Twelve years later, HHS released the *2008 Physical Activity Guidelines for Americans*, the first comprehensive set of federal guidelines describing the amount, types, and intensity of physical activity necessary for health.[91] More recently physical activity has been a key recommendation of the *National Prevention Strategy*[92] and the *National Physical Activity Plan*.[93]

An extensive body of research shows a clear relationship between inadequate physical activity and risk of chronic diseases including high blood pressure, heart disease, stroke, colon and breast cancers, type 2 diabetes, obesity, osteoporosis, depression, and premature death.[91] Based on these risks, annual health care expenditures are higher for inactive adults ($1,313 in excess cost) and insufficiently active adults ($576 in excess cost) compared to active adults, with approximately 11 percent of health care expenditures associated with inadequate physical activity.[94]

Current guidelines for aerobic physical activity call for adults to get at least 150 minutes of moderate-intensity or 75 minutes of vigorous-intensity activity or some equivalent combination, per week. In 2012, half (49.6 percent) of U.S. adults met these guidelines while nearly one-third (29.6 percent) of adults engaged in no leisure time physical activity.[95] Guidelines for children call for at least 60 minutes of physical activity each day, most of which should be moderate- or vigorous-intensity aerobic activity. However, only about one-quarter (27.1 percent) of high school students get this amount of activity, with more males (36.6 percent) than females (17.7 percent) meeting the guidelines.[18] While schools can help increase activity levels through daily physical education (PE) classes, such offerings are rare. The percentage of high school students who attend PE classes daily decreased from 41.6 percent in 1991 to 29.4 percent in 2013.[96]

Public health strategies to increase physical activity often focus on increasing access and opportunities for physical activity in key locations such as childcare, preschool and school settings, and worksites.[97,98] Other strategies are designed to make neighborhoods and communities safer, more attractive, and easier places to walk, bike, and play. Three major areas of intervention— school programs, social support, and built-environment supports—are reviewed here.

School Programs

On most days, children spend 6–7 hours a day at school, making the school environment an excellent location to assure adequate physical activity. Giving students opportunities to be active throughout the school day improves their concentration during class time.[99,100] Higher activity levels among students are also associated with better academic performance.[99,101] Physical activity is not only an important lifelong behavior, but it contributes to the primary role of schools to increase learning.[102]

Public health practitioners can help schools identify opportunities to increase physical activity before, during, and after the school day. All schools should ensure that students receive PE daily, totaling at least 150 minutes per week for elementary school students and 225 minutes per week for middle and high school students.[103] Quality PE programs increase physical activity levels, help develop lifelong fitness and motor skills, and build students' appreciation and enjoyment of various sports and fitness activities.[104] PE classes can be augmented with recess and before- and after-school options such as open gyms, running and walking clubs, and informal sports. Schools can promote Safe Routes to School or similar programs that ensure students can walk and bicycle to school safely. Some schools have established joint use agreements that allow students, families, and the broader community to use school facilities such as playgrounds, fields, and running tracks after school, on weekends, and during the summer.

Social Support

Social support interventions focus on increasing physical activity through social networks that provide supportive relationships for walking, running, hiking, biking, or playing sports. Social support can come in the form of a buddy system that establishes a consistent schedule for activity, group activities such as aerobic classes or hiking clubs, or campaigns that involve residents in meeting a workplace or community-wide physical activity goal. Family members can provide social support by including the entire family in shared activities. Social support provides motivation to be active and can make the activity more enjoyable.[98]

Built Environment

Being physically active often depends on the availability of safe, convenient, and attractive places such as parks, recreation areas, sidewalks, and trails where people can walk, bike, run, and play. Improved pedestrian and cycling infrastructure such as sidewalks and bike lanes make walking and cycling easier, safer, and more appealing.[105,106] Street-scale design, zoning reforms, and land use practices can increase mixed-use development, parks and green space, safety, walkability, community cohesion, and reductions in crime and stress. People walk more in neighborhoods that are safe and aesthetically pleasing. They also walk more when they are close to public transportation, stores, jobs, and schools.[107]

Some **built environment** interventions can be as simple as improved street lighting. Others require long-term partnerships with policy makers and urban planners to make physical activity a priority in the design of streets and communities. Building or repairing playgrounds and sidewalks, redeveloping underutilized land, and building multiuse paths on abandoned rail lines all increase the attractiveness of an area for business and home ownership while promoting and supporting physical activity.

Challenges

Many societal factors run counter to the promotion of physical activity including sedentary jobs; distances to schools, jobs, and stores that require use of a car; more time spent with TV, smartphones, computers, and video games; and concerns about neighborhood safety. Solutions to these challenges will require engaging groups beyond public health: community and transportation planners, law enforcement, leaders in business and education, and community-based organizations that play important roles in supporting safe and active communities. Greater attention to this area of public health—including expanding the research base and building public health infrastructure at the local, state, and national levels—will be vital to confronting our country's lack of sufficient physical activity.

ALCOHOL

Excessive alcohol use is responsible for an average of 88,000 deaths each year and shortens the lives of those who die by an average of 30 years.[108] These deaths are due to health effects from drinking too much over time, such as breast cancer, liver disease, and heart disease, as well as health effects from consuming a large amount of alcohol in a short period of time, such as injuries from car crashes and drowning, interpersonal violence, and alcohol poisoning. In addition, excessive alcohol consumption cost the United States $223.5 billion in 2006—about $1.90 per drink. These costs included losses in workplace productivity (72 percent of the total cost) and health care expenses (11 percent of total).[109]

Excessive alcohol use includes binge drinking, heavy drinking, and any drinking by pregnant women or people under the minimum legal drinking age of 21 years.[110] Binge drinking is defined by the National Institute on Alcohol Abuse and Alcoholism as a pattern of drinking that brings blood alcohol concentration levels to 0.08 g/dL. This typically occurs after four drinks for women and five drinks for men—in about two hours.[111] Heavy drinking is defined as 15 or more drinks per week for men and 8 or more drinks per week for women; and any drinking by pregnant women or people under the minimum legal drinking age of 21 years.[110] Binge drinking is the most common form of excessive drinking in the United States, and is responsible for over half the deaths, two-thirds of the years of potential life lost, and three-quarters of the economic costs due to excessive alcohol use.[112] Thirty-eight million U.S. adults report binge drinking an average of four times per month, and consume an average of about eight drinks per binge occasion.[112]

Addressing excessive drinking at a population-level depends primarily on changes to the alcohol environment at the neighborhood and community level. Persons who are addicted to alcohol may require more clinically focused drug-treatment interventions than are reviewed here. However, nine in 10 excessive drinkers are not alcohol dependent or addicted to alcohol.[113] Therefore, public health strategies that involve policy, systems, and environmental change are likely to have the greatest impact on excessive drinking and at the lowest societal cost. Below we review recommendations on the prevention of excessive drinking from the Community Preventive Services Task Force—an independent, nonfederal body of public health and prevention experts, and the U.S. Preventive Services Task Force, who have systematically reviewed the scientific evidence on reducing excessive alcohol use. To date, the primary strategies to reduce excessive alcohol consumption are increasing price, reducing alcohol availability, and providing electronic screening and brief intervention. Other strategies to reduce motor-vehicle-related injuries include 0.08 percent blood alcohol concentration laws, publicized sobriety checkpoint programs, mass media campaigns to reduce alcohol-impaired driving, and ignition interlocks.[114]

Alcohol Pricing

Increasing the price of alcohol is consistently related to reductions in excessive alcohol consumption and related harms, including fewer motor-vehicle crashes and fatalities; less alcohol-impaired driving; reduced mortality from liver cirrhosis; and reduced all-cause mortality.[115] Alcohol prices can be increased through wholesale, excise, *ad valorem*, or sales taxes. Taxes can be levied at the federal, state, or local levels on beer, wine, or distilled spirits, and are intended to reduce alcohol-related harms, raise revenue, or both.

Increases in federal excise tax rates have been rare, happening only once for beer and wine since 1951

(on January 1, 1991) and only twice for distilled spirits (on October 1, 1985, and January 1, 1991). Inflation-adjusted tax rates have declined significantly over the years. For example, after adjusting for inflation, the federal excise tax on beer has fallen from $2.39 a gallon in 1951 to $0.58 a gallon in 2009, a 75 percent decline.[116] State taxes vary widely, from $1.50 to $14.27 per gallon of distilled spirits and from $0.02 to $1.15 per gallon of beer.[117] Increasing alcohol taxes at the state or federal levels provides additional revenue, while reducing the occurrence and costs of alcohol-related harms.

As in the area of tobacco control, public health professionals can educate local and state legislators and other public officials on the effects of alcohol taxes on public health.

Availability of Alcohol

There are several evidence-based strategies available to public health practitioners to limit or reduce access to alcohol, including (1) regulating the concentration or density of retail alcohol outlets in a particular geographic location, (2) limiting days and hours when alcohol is sold, (3) enforcing laws prohibiting sales to minors, (4) maintaining governmental control of the retail sales of alcohol (i.e., not privatizing alcohol sales), and (5) establishing commercial host liability, which holds retailers liable for harms resulting from the illegal sale of alcohol to persons who are drunk or under age 21.[118]

Alcohol outlet density refers to the number of retail alcohol outlets in a defined geographic area that sell alcohol such as bars, restaurants, grocery stores, and liquor stores. Research has established a positive association between alcohol outlet density and excessive alcohol consumption and related harms.[119] Alcohol outlet density can be controlled through zoning restrictions and limiting the number of business licenses available for locations that sell alcohol. However, states vary widely in the amount of control they allow local governments to have over the issuance of new alcohol licenses.

Screening and Brief Intervention

Screening and brief intervention (SBI) consists of a short conversation between a health professional and patient to determine typical drinking patterns and to provide feedback about risks and behavior change strategies for those who screen positive for excessive drinking. Electronic screening and brief intervention (e-SBI) is a variant of face-to-face SBI and involves the use of computers, telephones, or mobile devices as part of the assessment and/or counseling process.

Studies have shown that e-SBI not only reduces the frequency of binge drinking episodes, it also decreases the number of drinks consumed per binge drinking episode by about 25 percent.[115,120] Although SBI is a more individualized intervention, it can complement policy strategies, such as increasing alcohol taxes, by focusing resources on excessive drinkers who are at high risk for negative health outcomes. However, a recent study found that only 1 in 6 U.S. adults report ever being asked by a health professional about alcohol consumption, emphasizing the need for systems-level approaches to increase the utilization of SBI, such as e-SBI.[121]

Challenges

Despite significant benefits to public health, there are many practical challenges to the prevention of excessive alcohol use. First is the role of the alcohol industry in promoting and advertising its products. Second is how deeply embedded alcohol use is from a cultural perspective, along with social norms that often encourage binge drinking. Other challenges include a constantly expanding array of alcoholic products such as "alcopops" (flavored malt beverages with varying alcohol content) and powdered alcohol. These new products may be particularly appealing to underage youth, thus increasing the risk of alcohol use among those younger than 21 years of age. Compounding these challenges is the fact that there is not a public health workforce devoted to addressing excessive alcohol use at the state or local levels as there is for tobacco.

CHRONIC DISEASE CONTROL THROUGH SCREENING AND DISEASE MANAGEMENT

So far this chapter has covered preventing and delaying chronic disease by reducing key risk factors. Maintaining health in the first place is the highest priority of public health. However, public health also has a role to play in detecting chronic disease early and helping those who live with chronic illness to manage their disease.

Screening and Early Detection

Some chronic diseases, such as some forms of cancer, have much better outcomes when detected early. Public health practitioners work to increase the availability and use of evidence-based exams such as mammography, colonoscopy, pap tests, and screenings for high blood pressure and high cholesterol. As one example, the CDC's Breast and Cervical Cancer Early Detection Program screens low-income women in all 50 states and the District of Columbia. Similarly, the CDC's Colorectal Cancer Screening Program works to increase screening rates for colonoscopy. About one-third of adults ages

50–75 have not been tested for colorectal cancer as recommended.[122] These numbers can be increased through the use of patient reminders, patient navigators, small media, and provider assessment and feedback. Through the Patient Protection and Affordable Care Act, more Americans have access to health coverage and preventive services such as colorectal cancer screening tests. Many screening tests are available at no additional cost based on recommendations by the U.S. Preventive Services Task Force. Part of the role of public health is to help ensure that patients make use of these life-saving services.

Chronic Disease Management

Public health also has a role in working with the nearly one-half of adults in the United States who live with one or more chronic diseases. This role includes chronic disease management as well as the reduction of risk factors such as poor nutrition and physical inactivity for all people including those living with chronic illness. The strategies discussed above are relevant to this population. In addition, more intensive behavioral interventions such as individual counseling and small group interventions can be helpful. For example, the Diabetes Prevention Program has been shown to prevent or delay the development of diabetes among persons with prediabetes.[123]

Medical care is a critical feature of maintaining optimal health for persons living with chronic disease. For example, treatment for high blood pressure can be the difference between having a heart attack or stroke, or preventing one. Similarly, appropriate monitoring and control of blood sugar levels among persons with diabetes can prevent blindness or amputation.[124] Care of persons living with chronic illness resides at the intersection of clinical medicine and public health. Clinical medicine provides patient care on an individual-by-individual basis. Public health helps ensure that the entire population of persons living with chronic disease receives appropriate care. This can include helping connect patients to care and helping ensure the widespread application of evidence-based preventive care such as the control of high blood pressure.

One of the best-known models for improving patient care is the Chronic Care Model.[125–127] The Chronic Care Model incorporates six elements in the care continuum that include the community, the health system, self-management support, delivery system design, decision support, and clinical information systems. By engaging informed patients who are active in their own care and connecting health care and community support, the Chronic Care Model transforms a reactive health care system into one that works to keep its patients as healthy as possible through planning, proven strategies, and good management.

SUMMARY

Chronic diseases such as cancer, heart disease, and diabetes greatly reduce quality of life and are the leading causes of death in the United States. Chronic diseases result in enormous health care costs for families and society and they compromise productivity during the prime of life. Many chronic diseases can be prevented or delayed through lifestyle behaviors that promote and protect health. Public health helps to maintain health by intervening on the major risk factors for chronic disease: tobacco use, obesity, poor nutrition, physical inactivity, and excessive alcohol consumption.

Public health has achieved many successes in the area of chronic disease. For example, death rates for heart disease and stroke dropped by one-third between 1998 and 2008.[128] Approximately half of this progress can be attributed to new medicines and advances in clinical care and half to the substantial declines in tobacco use over the same time.[129] Public health has contributed to numerous other successes including increased breastfeeding; a halt in increasing obesity rates; increases in leisure time physical activity; and prevention of type 2 diabetes among high-risk individuals. Public health has contributed to the reduction of some long-standing disparities—eliminating disparities in breast cancer screening rates, for instance.[130] The contribution of public health to chronic disease outcomes is encouraging, but so much more remains to be done. Chronic disease public health is one of the most exciting and important areas of work in public health today. As goes chronic disease prevention, so go the health and health care costs of the nation.

REVIEW QUESTIONS

1. What is chronic disease and why is it important to public health?
2. What are the major behavioral risk factors for chronic disease?
3. How can policy play a role in chronic disease prevention?
4. How does the environment play a role in chronic disease prevention?
5. What roles does public health play in chronic disease prevention and chronic disease control?

ACKNOWLEDGMENTS

We would like to thank Seth Gannon for his valuable insights and editorial assistance, and CDC experts Stephen Babb, Heidi Blanck, Bob Brewer, Susan Carlson, Joan Dorn, Janet Fulton, Deborah Galuska, Brian King, Carol MacGowan, Jessica Mesnick, Terry Pechacek, Ken Rose, Kelley Scanlon, and Jennifer Seymour who reviewed and contributed content in the areas of tobacco, obesity, nutrition, physical activity, and alcohol. We also thank Haley Zwecker for her assistance in helping prepare the manuscript.

DISCLAIMER

The findings and conclusions in this report are those of the authors and do not necessarily represent the official position of the Centers for Disease Control and Prevention.

REFERENCES

1. Frieden TR. Asleep at the switch: local public health and chronic disease. *Am J Public Health.* 2004;94(12):2059–2061.
2. Murphy SL, Xu JQ, Kochanek KD. *Deaths: Final Data for 2010.* U.S. Department of Health and Human Services, Centers for Disease Control and Prevention, National Center for Health Statistics, National Vital Statistics System;2013.
3. Ward BW, Schiller JS, Goodman RA. Multiple chronic conditions among US adults: A 2012 Update. *Preventing Chronic Disease.* 2014;11:E62.
4. Murray CJL, Kulkarni SC, Michaud C, et al. Eight Americas: investigating mortality disparities across races, counties, and race-counties in the United States. *PLoS Med.* 2006;3(12):e545.
5. Centers for Disease Control and Prevention. CDC Health Disparities and Inequalities Report—United States, 2013. *Morbidity and Mortality Weekly Report.* 2013;62(Suppl 3):1–186.
6. Agency for Healthcare Research and Quality. Total Expenses and Percent Distribution for Selected Conditions by Source of Payment: United States, 2011. *Medical Expenditure Panel Survey Household Component Data* 2013. Accessed July, 2014.
7. Bauer UE, Briss PA, Goodman RA, Bowman BA. Prevention of chronic disease in the 21st century: elimination of the leading preventable causes of premature death and disability in the USA. *The Lancet* July 5, 2014;384(9937):45–52.
8. Goodarz D, Ding EL, Mozaffarian D, et al. The preventable causes of death in the United States: Comparative risk assessment of dietary, lifestyle, and metabolic risk factors. *PLOS Medicine.* 2009.
9. Freudenberg N, Ruglis J. Reframing school dropout as a public health issue. *Preventing Chronic Disease.* 2007;4(4).

10. United States Department of Health and Human Services. *The Health Consequences of Smoking: 50 Years of Progress: A Report of the Surgeon General.* Atlanta, GA: U.S. Department of Health and Human Services, Centers for Disease Control and Prevention, National Center for Chronic Disease Prevention and Health Promotion, Office on Smoking and Health;2014.

11. Jha P, Ramasundarahettige C, Landsman V, et al. 21st-century hazards of smoking and benefits of cessation in the United States. *The New England Journal of Medicine.* January 24, 2013;368(4):341–350.

12. Witschi H. Profiles in toxicology: a short history of lung cancer. *Toxicological sciences.* 2001;64:4–6.

13. United States Office on Smoking and Health. *The Health Consequences of Involuntary Exposure to Tobacco Smoke: A Report of the Surgeon General.* Atlanta, GA: Centers for Disease Control and Prevention;2006.

14. Centers for Disease Control and Prevention. Ten great public health achievements—United States, 2001–2010. *Morbidity and Mortality Weekly Report.* 2011;60(19):619–623.

15. Giovino G. Epidemiology of tobacco use in the United States. *Tobacco Control.* 2002;21(48):7326–7340.

16. Jamal A, Agaku IT, O'Connor E, King BA, Kenemer JB, Neff L. Current cigarette smoking among adults—United States, 2005–2013. *Morbidity and Mortality Weekly Report (MMWR).* 2014;63(47):1108–1112.

17. Agaku IT, King BA, Husten CG, et al. Tobacco product use among adults—United States, 2012–2013. *Morbidity and Mortality Weekly Report (MMWR).* 2014;63(25):542–547.

18. Kann L, Kinchen S, Shanklin S, et al. Youth risk behavior surveillance—United States, 2013. *Morbidity and Mortality Weekly Report.* 2014;63(SS04):1–168.

19. Blackwell DL, Lucas JW, Clarke TC. *Summary Health Statistics for U.S. Adults: National Health Interview Survey, 2012.* National Center for Health Statistics, Vital and Health Statistics;2014.

20. Centers for Disease Control and Prevention. *Best Practices for Comprehensive Tobacco Control Programs—2014* Atlanta, GA: U.S. Department of Health and Human Services, Centers for Disease Control and Prevention, National Center for Chronic Disease Prevention and Health Promotion, Office on Smoking and Health;2014.

21. Chaloupka FJ, Yurekli A, Fong GT. Tobacco taxes as a tobacco control strategy. *Tobacco Control.* 2012;21:172–180.

22. Guide to Community Preventive Services. Reducing tobacco use and secondhand smoke exposure: interventions to increase the unit price for tobacco products. http://www.thecommunityguide.org/tobacco/internet.html. Accessed August 13, 2014.

23. United States Department of Health and Human Services. *Preventing Tobacco Use Among Youth and Young Adults: A Report of the Surgeon General.* Atlanta, GA: U.S. Department of Health and Human Services, Centers for Disease Control and Prevention, National Center for Chronic Disease Prevention and Health Promotion, Office on Smoking and Health;2012.

24. Campaign for Tobacco-Free Kids. Cigarette tax increases by state per year 2000–2014. 2014; http://www.tobaccofreekids.org/research/factsheets/pdf/0275.pdf. Accessed August 27, 2014.

25. Guide to Community Preventive Services. Reducing tobacco use and secondhand smoke exposure: Smoke-free policies. http://www.thecommunityguide.org/tobacco/smokefree policies.html. Accessed, October 8, 2014.

26. Been JV, Nurmatov UB, Cox B, Nawrot TS, van Schayck CP, Sheikh A. Effect of smoke-free legislation on perinatal and child health: a systematic review and meta-analysis. *The Lancet.* May 3, 2014;383(9928):1549–1560.

27. Tan CE, Glantz SA. Association between smoke-free legislation and hospitalizations for cardiac, cerebrovascular, and respiratory diseases: a meta-analysis. *Circulation.* October 30, 2012;126(18):2177–2183.

28. American Nonsmokers' Rights Foundation. Summary of 100% smokefree state laws and population protected by 100% U.S. smokefree laws. 2014; http://www.no-smoke.org/pdf/SummaryUSPopList.pdf. Accessed December 8, 2014.

29. Schuster MA, Franke T, Pham CB. Smoking patterns of household members and visitors in homes with children in the United States. *Arch Pediatr Adolesc Med.* November 2002;156(11):1094–1100.

30. Malarcher A, Dube S, Shaw L, Babb S, Kaufmann R. Quitting smoking among adults—United States, 2001–2010. *Morbidity and Mortality Weekly Report (MMWR).* 2011;60(44):1513–1519.

31. Fiore MC, Jaen CR, Baker TB, et al. Treating Tobacco Use and Dependence: 2008 Update:—Clinical Practice Guideline. Rockville, Maryland: U.S. Department of Health and Human Services, Public Health Service; 2008. http://www.ahrq.gov/professionals/clinicians-providers/guidelines-recommendations/tobacco/clinicians/update/index.html.

32. Durkin S, Brennan E, Wakefield M. Mass media campaigns to promote smoking cessation among adults: an integrative review. *Tobacco Control.* March 2012;21(2):127–138.

33. Centers for Disease Control and Prevention. Smoking & Tobacco Use: Media Campaign Resource Center (MCRC). http://www.cdc.gov/tobacco/media_campaigns/index.htm. Accessed December 8, 2014.

34. Augustson E, Bright MA, Babb S, et al. Increases in quitline calls and smoking cessation website visitors during a national tobacco education campaign—March 19-June 10, 2012. *Morbidity and Mortality Weekly Report.* 2012;61(34):667–670.

35. Ogden CL, Carroll MD, Kit BK, Flegal KM. Prevalence of childhood and adult obesity in the united states, 2011–2012. *JAMA.* 2014;311(8):806–814.

36. Flegal KM, Graubard BI, Williamson DF, Gail MH. Excess deaths associated with underweight, overweight, and obesity. *The Journal of the American Medical Association.* April 20, 2005;293(15):1861–1867.

37. Fryar CD, Carroll MD, Ogden CL. *Prevalence of overweight, obesity, and extreme obesity among adults: United States, trends 1960–1962 through 2011-2012.* Centers for Disease Control and Prevention/Division of Health and Nutrition Examination Surveys;2014.

38. Ogden CL, Carroll MD, Flegal KM. Epidemiologic trends in overweight and obesity. *Endocrinol Metab Clin N Am.* 2003;32:741–760.

39. Ogden CL, Carroll MD, Kit BK, Flegal KM. Prevalence of obesity and trends in body mass index among US children and adolescents, 1999–2012. *Journal of the American Medical Association.* 2012;307(5):483–490.

40. Guo SS, Roche AF, Chumlea WC, Gardner JD, Siervogel RM. The predictive value of childhood body mass index values for overweight at age 35 y. *American Journal of Clinical Nutrition.* 1994;59:810–819.

41. Cunningham SA, Kramer MR, Venkat Narayan KM. Incidence of childhood obesity in the United States. *The New England Journal of Medicine.* 2014;370(5):403–411.

42. Yu ZB, Han SP, Zhu GZ, et al. Birth weight and subsequent risk of obesity: a systematic review and meta-analysis. *Obesity Reviews.* 2011;12(7):525–542.

43. American Medical Association. AMA Adopts New Policies on Second Day of Voting at Annual Meeting. AMA News Room: American Medical Association; 2013.

44. National Heart Lung and Blood Institute and The National Institute of Diabetes and Digestive and Kidney Diseases. *Clinical Guidelines on the Identification, Evaluation, and Treatment of Overweight and Obesity in Adults: The Evidence Report.* National Institutes of Health;1998.

45. Kushner RF, Foster GD. Obesity and quality of life. *Nutrition.* 2000;16:947–952.

46. Puhl R, Brownell KD. Bias, discrimination, and obesity. *Obesity Research.* 2001;9(12):788–805.

47. French SA, Story M, Perry CL. Self-esteem and obesity in children and adolescents: a literature review. *Obesity Research.* 1995;3(5):479–490.

48. Strauss RS. Childhood obesity and self-esteem. *Pediatrics.* January 1, 2000;105(1):e15.

49. Finkelstein EA, Trogdon JG, Cohen JW, Dietz W. Annual medical spending attributable to obesity: payer-and-service-specific estimates. *Health Affairs.* July 27, 2009;28(5):w822–w831.

50. Dietary Guidelines Advisory Committee. *Report of the Dietary Guidelines Advisory Committee on the Dietary Guidelines for Americans, 2012.* 2010.

51. United States Department of Agriculture and United States Department of Health and Human Services. *Dietary Guidelines for Americans, 2010.* Washington, DC; December 2010

52. United States Department of Health and Human Services. *The Surgeon General's Call to Action to Support Breastfeeding.* Washington, DC: U.S. Department of Health and Human Services, Office of the Surgeon General;2011.

53. Bell J, Mora G, Hagan E, Rubin V, Karpyn A. *Access to healthy food and why it matters: A review of the research.* Policy Link and The Food Trust 2013.

54. Morland K, Wing S, Diez Roux A. The contextual effect of the local food environment on residents' diets: the atherosclerosis risk in communities study. *Am J Public Health.* November 2002;92(11):1761–1767.

55. Michimi A, Wimberly MC. Associations of supermarket accessibility with obesity and fruit and vegetable consumption in the conterminous United States. *International Journal of Health Geographics.* 2010;9:49.

56. Robinson PL, Dominguez F, Teklehaimanot S, Lee M, Brown A, Goodchild M. Does distance decay modelling of supermarket accessibility predict fruit and vegetable intake by individuals in a large metropolitan area? *J Health Care Poor Underserved.* February 2013;24(1 Suppl):172–185.

57. Bodor JN, Rose D, Farley TA, Swalm C, Scott SK. Neighbourhood fruit and vegetable availability and consumption: the role of small food stores in an urban environment. *Public Health Nutrition.* April 2008;11(4):413–420.

58. Powell LM, Han E, Chaloupka FJ. Economic contextual factors, food consumption, and obesity among U.S. adolescents. *Journal of Nutrition.* 2010;140:1175–1180.

59. Laraia BA, Siega-Riz AM, Kaufman JS, Jones SJ. Proximity of supermarkets is positively associated with diet quality index for pregnancy. *Preventive Medicine.* 2004;39:869–875.

60. Moore LV, Diez Roux AV, Nettleton JA, Jacobs Jr DR. Associations of the local food environment with diet quality—comparison of assessments based on surveys and geographic information systems: The Multi-ethnic Study of Atherosclerosis. *American Journal of Epidemiology.* 2008;167(8):917–924.

61. Inagami S, Cohen DA, Finch BK, Asch SM. You are where you shop: grocery store locations, weight, and neighborhoods. *American Journal of Preventive Medicine.* July 2006;31(1):10–17.

62. Larson NI, Story MT, Nelson MC. Neighborhood environments: disparities in access to healthy foods in the U.S. *American Journal of Preventive Medicine.* January 2009;36(1):74–81.e10.

63. Morland K, Diez Roux AV, Wing S. Supermarkets, other food stores, and obesity: the atherosclerosis risk in communities study. *American Journal of Preventive Medicine.* 4// 2006;30(4):333–339.

64. Bodor JN, Rice J, Farley T, Swalm C, Rose D. The association between obesity and urban food environments. *Journal of Urban Health.* 2010/09/01 2010;87(5):771–781.

65. Powell LM, Auld MC, Chaloupka FJ, O'Malley PM, Johnston LD. Associations between access to food stores and adolescent body mass index. *American Journal of Preventive Medicine.* 2007;33(4 Suppl):S301–S307.

66. Centers for Disease Control and Prevention. *Healthier Food Retail: An Action Guide for Public Health Practitioners.* Atlanta, GA;2014.

67. Glanz K, Bader MD, Iyer S. Retail grocery store marketing strategies and obesity: an integrative review. *American Journal of Preventive Medicine.* May 2012;42(5):503–512.

68. Glanz K, Hoelscher D. Increasing fruit and vegetable intake by changing environments, policy and pricing: restaurant-based research, strategies, and recommendations. *American Journal of Preventive Medicine.* September 2004;39 Suppl 2:S88–93.

69. Robert Wood Johnson Foundation, The Food Trust. *Harnessing the Power of Supermarkets to help reverse childhood obesity.* 2011.

70. United States Department of Agriculture. Child and Adult Care Food Program (CACFP): Meals and Snacks. Accessed October 10, 2014.

71. United States Department of Agriculture. Food Expenditures. http:/www.ers.usda.gov/datafiles/Food_Expenditures/table10.xls. Accessed August 18, 2014.

72. Bowman SA, Vinyard BT. Fast food consumption of U.S. adults: impact on energy and nutrient intakes and overweight status. *Journal of the American College of Nutrition.* April 1, 2004;23(2):163–168.

73. Lin B-H, Guthrie JF. *Nutritional Quality of Food Prepared at Home and Away from Home, 1977–2008.* U.S. Department of Agriculture, Economic Research Service;2012.

74. Todd JE, Mancino L, Lin B-H. *The Impact of Food Away from Home on Adult Diet Quality.* 2010.

75. Young LR, Nestle M. The contribution of expanding portion sizes to the US obesity epidemic. *American Journal of Public Health.* February 2002;92(2):246–249.

76. Young LR, Nestle M. Expanding portion sizes in the US marketplace: implications for nutrition counseling. *Journal of the American Dietetic Association.* February 2003;103(2):231–234.

77. Burton S, Creyer EH, Kees J, Huggins K. Attacking the Obesity Epidemic: The Potential Health Benefits of Providing Nutrition Information in Restaurants. *American Journal of Public Health.* September 1, 2006;96(9):1669–1675.

78. United States Department of Health and Human Services and General Services Administration. Health and Sustainability Guidelines for Federal Concessions and Vending Operations. http://www.cdc.gov/chronicdisease/pdf/guidelines_for_federal_concessions_and_vending_operations.pdf.

79. United States Department of Agriculture/Food and Nutrition Service. Nutrition Standards in the National School Lunch and School Breakfast Programs; Final Rule. *Federal Register.* 2012;77(17).

80. United States Department of Agriculture Food and Nutrition Service. School Meals: Smart Snacks in Schools. http:/www.fns.usda.gov/school-meals/smart-snacks-school. Accessed August 18, 2014.

81. Coleman-Jensen A, Mark N, Singh A. *Household Food Security in the United States in 2012.* United States Department of Agriculture, Economic Research Service;2013.

82. United States Department of Agriculture/ Economic Research Service. Food Security in the U.S. http://www.ers.usda.gov/topics/ food-nutrition-assistance/food-security-in-the-us/ key-statistics-graphics.aspx#insecure. Accessed August 27, 2014.

83. United States Department of Agriculture/Food and Nutrition Service. Supplemental Nutrition Assistance Program (SNAP). http://www.fns.usda .gov/pd/supplemental-nutrition-assistance- program-snap. Accessed August 26, 2014.

84. United States Department of Agriculture/Food and Nutrition Service. WIC Program. http://www.fns .usda.gov/pd/wic-program. Accessed August 26, 2014.

85. United States Department of Agriculture. The Emergency Food Assistance Program. *Food and Nutrition Service Nutrition Program Fact Sheet.* 2014.

86. Ip S, Chung M, Raman G, et al. *Breastfeeding and Maternal and Infant Health Outcomes in Developed Countries. Evidence Report/Technology Assessment No. 153.* Agency for Healthcare Research and Quality;2007.

87. Bartick M, Reinhold A. The burden of suboptimal breastfeeding in the United States: a pediatric cost analysis. *Pediatrics.* April 5, 2010.

88. Centers for Disease Control and Prevention. *Strategies to Prevent Obesity and Other Chronic Diseases: The CDC Guide to Strategies to Support Breastfeeding Mothers and Babies.* Atlanta: U.S. Department of Health and Human Services;2013.

89. Food Marketing Institute. Supermarket Facts: Industry Overview 2013. 2013. Accessed October 9, 2014.

90. United States Department of Health and Human Services. *Physical Activity and Health: A Report of the Surgeon General.* Atlanta, GA: U.S. Department of Health and Human Services, Centers for Disease Control and Prevention, National Center for Chronic Disease Prevention and Health Promotion;1996.

91. United States Department of Health and Human Services. *2008 Physical Activity Guidelines for Americans.* Washington, DC: U.S. Department of Health and Human Services.

92. National Prevention Council. *National Prevention Strategy.* Washington, DC: U.S. Department of Health and Human Services, Office of the Surgeon General;2011.

93. National Physical Activity Plan. http://www .physicalactivityplan.org/NationalPhysical ActivityPlan.pdf. Accessed August 27, 2014.

94. Carlson SA, Fulton JE, Pratt M, Yang Z, Adams EK. Inadequate physical activity and health care expenditures in the United States. *Progress in Cardiovascular Diseases.* Volume 57, Issue 4, January–February 2015, Pages 315–323.

95. National Center for Health Statistics. *Health, United States, 2013: With Special Feature on Prescription Drugs.* Hyattsville, MD;2014.

96. Centers for Disease Control and Prevention. Youth Online: High School YRBS. http://nccd .cdc.gov/youthonline/App/Default.aspx. Accessed August 27, 2014.

97. Guide to Community Preventive Services. Increasing Physical Activity. October 9, 2014.

98. Task Force on Community Preventive Services. Recommendations to increase physical activity in communities. *American Journal of Preventive Medicine.* 2002;22(4S):67–72.

99. Fedewa AL, Ahn S. The effects of physical activity and physical fitness on children's achievement and cognitive outcomes: a meta- analysis. *Research Quarterly for Exercise & Sport* 2011;82(3):521–535.

100. Sibley B, Etnier J. The relationship between physical activity and cognition in children: a meta-analysis. *Pediatric Exercise Science* 2003;15:243–256.

101. Centers for Disease Control and Prevention. *The Association Between School-based Phys- ical Activity, Including Physical Education, and Academic Performance.* Atlanta, GA: U.S. Department of Health and Human Services;2010.

102. Institute of Medicine. *Educating the Student Body: Taking Physical Activity and Physical Education to School.* Washington, DC: The National Academies Press;2013.

103. National Association of Sport and Physical Edu- cation. *Moving into the Future: National Standards for Physical Education* Reston, VA: National Asso- ciation for Sport and Physical Education; 2004.

104. Centers for Disease Control and Prevention. *A Guide for Developing Comprehensive School Physical Activity Programs.* Atlanta, GA: U.S. Department of Health and Human Services;2013.

105. Pratt RH, Evans IV JE, Turner SM, Jeng CY, Nabors D. TCRP Report 95: Traveler Response to Transportation System Changes: Chapter 16—Pedestrian and Bicycle Facilities. Washington, DC: Transit Cooperative Research Program; 2012.

106. Heath GW, Brownson RC, Kruger J, et al. The effectiveness of urban design and land use and transport policies and practices to increase physical activity: a systematic review. *Journal of Physical Activity and Health.* 2006;3(Suppl 1):S55–S76.

107. Ewing R, Cervero R. Travel and the built environment: a meta-analysis. *Journal of the American Planning Association.* 2010;76(3):265–294.

108. Stahre M, Roeber J, Kanny D, Brewer RD, Zhang X. Contribution of excessive alcohol consumption to deaths and years of potential life lost in the United States. *Preventing Chronic Disease.* 2014;11:E109.

109. Bouchery EE, Harwood HJ, Sacks JJ, Simon CJ, Brewer RD. Economic costs of excessive alcohol consumption in the U.S., 2006. *American Journal of Preventive Medicine.* 2011;41(5):516–524.

110. Centers for Disease Control and Prevention. Alcohol and Public Health. http://www.cdc.gov/alcohol/faqs.htm#bingeDrinking. Accessed October 9, 2014.

111. National Institute on Alcohol Abuse and Alcoholism. Drinking Levels Defined. http://www.niaaa.nih.gov/alcohol-health/overview-alcohol-consumption/moderate-binge-drinking. Accessed October 9, 2014.

112. Kanny D, Liu Y, Brewer RD. Vital signs: binge drinking prevalence, frequency, and intensity among adults—United States, 2010. *Morbidity and Mortality Weekly Report.* 2012;61(01):14–19.

113. Esser MB, Hedden SL, Kanny D, Brewer RD, Gfroerer JC, Naimi TS. Prevalence of alcohol dependence among US adult drinkers, 2009–2011. *Preventing Chronic Disease.* 2014;11(140329).

114. Guide to Community Preventive Services. Motor Vehicle-Related Injury Prevention: Reducing Alcohol-Impaired Driving. http://www.thecommunityguide.org/mvoi/AID/index.html. Accessed October 9, 2014.

115. Elder RW, Lawrence B, Ferguson A, et al. The effectiveness of tax policy interventions for reducing excessive alcohol consumption and related harms. *American Journal of Preventive Medicine.* February, 2010;38(2):217–229.

116. Marr C, Brunet G. Reversing the Erosion in Alcohol Taxes Could Help Pay for Health Care Reform. 2009. http://www.cbpp.org/files/5-27-09health.pdf. Accessed October 9, 2014.

117. Federation of Tax Administrators. State tax rates on distilled spirits (January 1, 2014). 2014; http://www.taxadmin.org/fta/rate/liquor.pdf. Accessed August 27, 2014.

118. Guide to Community Preventive Services. Preventing Excessive Alcohol Consumption. http://www.thecommunityguide.org/alcohol/index.html. Accessed October 10, 2014.

119. Campbell CA, Hahn RA, Elder R, Task Force on Community Preventive Services. The effectiveness of limiting alcohol outlet density as a means of reducing excessive alcohol consumption and alcohol-related harms. *American Journal of Preventive Medicine.* 2009;37(6):556–569.

120. Jonas DE, Garbutt JC, Brown JM, et al. *Screening, Behavioral Counseling, and Referral in Primary Care to Reduce Alcohol Misuse.* Rockville, MD: Agency for Healthcare Research and Quality;2012.

121. McKnight-Eily LR, Liu Y, Brewer RD, et al. Vital signs: communication between health professionals and their patients about alcohol use—44 states and the District of Columbia, 2011. *Morbidity and Mortality Weekly Report.* 2014;63(1):16–22.

122. Klabunde CN, Joseph DA, King JB, White A, Plescia M. Vital signs: colorectal cancer screening test use—United States, 2012. *Morbidity and Mortality Weekly Report.* 2013;62(44):881–888.

123. Diabetes Prevention Program Research Group. Reduction in the incidence of type 2 diabetes with lifestyle intervention or Metformin. *New England Journal of Medicine.* 2002;346(6):393–403.

124. National Diabetes Information Clearinghouse. DCCT and EDIC: The Diabetes Control and Complications Trial and Follow-up Study. October 10, 2014.

125. Coleman K, Austin BT, Brach C, Wagner EH. Evidence on the Chronic Care Model in the new millennium. *Health Affairs.* 2009;28(1):75–85.

126. Bodenheimer T, Wagner EH, Grumbach K. Improving primary care for patients with chronic illness: The Chronic Care Model, part 2. *Journal of the American Medical Association.* 2002;288(15):1909–1914.

127. Wagner EH, Austin BT, Davis C, Hindmarsh M, Schaefer J, Bonomi A. Improving chronic illness care: translating evidence into action. *Health Affairs.* 2001;20(6):64–78.

128. Cooper R, Cutler J, Desvigne-Nickens P, et al. Trends and disparities in coronary heart disease, stroke, and other cardiovascular diseases in the United States: findings of the national conference on cardiovascular disease prevention. *Circulation.* 2000;102:3137–3147.

129. Ford ES, Ajani UA, Croft JB, et al. Explaining the decrease in U.S. deaths from coronary disease, 1980–2000. *New England Journal of Medicine.* 2007;356:2388–2398.

130. Klabunde CN, Brown M, Ballard-Barbash R, et al. Cancer screening—United States, 2010. *Morbidity and Mortality Weekly Report.* 2012;61(3):41–45.

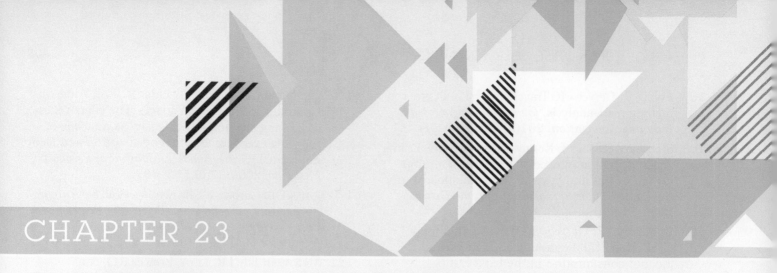

CHAPTER 23

Oral Health in Public Health Practice

Caswell A. Evans, DDS, MPH • Maria C. Dolce, PhD, RN • Tracy E. Garland, MUP • Anita D. Glicken, MSW • Judith Haber, PhD, MA, BSN • Susan Hyde, DDS, MPH, PhD • George W. Taylor, DMD, MPH, DrPH • Darien J. Weatherspoon, DDS, MPH

LEARNING OBJECTIVES

Upon completion of the chapter, the reader will be able to:

1. Describe the burden of oral disease and its public health impact.

2. Identify elements of oral health in the practice of public health.

3. Recognize interprofessional education, training, and practice initiatives regarding oral health.

4. Describe the ways in which incorporating oral health services can reduce the public health burden of diabetes.

5. Demonstrate roles that public health practitioners can play to integrate oral health into primary care and public health practice.

KEY TERMS

community water fluoridation
dental caries
dental sealants
early childhood decay
edentulism
interprofessional education (IPE)
oral health workforce
periodontal diseases

INTRODUCTION

The significance of the oral-pharyngeal complex, and consequently the significance of oral health, is often overlooked and underappreciated.[1] What we eat and drink, all verbal communication, as well as nonverbal communication and expression, depend upon the function of the mouth and upon our oral health. Our vision of ourselves, how we are seen by others, our capacity to smile upon the world around us, and often our employment and subsequent promotion are influenced by our oral appearance. The oral-pharyngeal complex is a distinguishing feature of human existence and the physical structure is present throughout our life span. In that context, one's oral health status and related issues exist and change throughout the life span.[2]

The mouth is a portal as well as a barrier to infection. The oral cavity is susceptible to genetic disorders, acquired diseases and conditions, and to disruption by trauma. Dental caries (cavities) is the most common chronic disease among children, more common than asthma, and oral-pharyngeal cancers are the sixth most common malignancies among adults.[1,3] Oral infections can exacerbate and are associated with general health disorders and conditions. For example, periodontal disease is associated with poor glycemic control among diabetic patients. Strong associations between oral health status and respiratory and cardiovascular disease have also been demonstrated.

Oral health and issues of oral health status are ubiquitous among humans. Dental care—services provided by a dentist or hygienist or other provider—can make significant contributions to improving the oral health of individuals; however, millions of people lack the means to access dental care. A recent Institute of Medicine (IOM) report noted that in 2008 4.6 million children in the United States did not receive dental care due to lack of family financial resources, and that in 2011 there were over 33 million unserved people living in dental health professional shortage areas.[4] That report went on to note that lack of access to oral health care is a fundamental determinant of "profound and persistent" oral health disparities. These disparities are disproportionate and are most evident among racial and ethnic minorities, rural and low-income populations, and those with special needs.

Other than dentists and other members of the dental care team, few others in the health care workforce complete even a rudimentary assessment of the oral cavity. If a tongue blade is used to examine the throat, the assessment typically does not include the oral cavity. However, pediatricians,[5] nurses,[6] and physician assistants[6] are beginning to pay more attention to the oral health status of the populations they serve. Even so, significant opportunities are still lost to identify cavities in children as well cancerous lesions in older adults, among other observations that might entail a referral for care by a dentist or other form of intervention.

This chapter will discuss the importance of "putting the mouth back in the body" in relation to population health. The chapter will provide a brief overview of the burden that oral diseases represent in the U.S. population, a synopsis of public health interventions to decrease the burden through disease prevention and control measures, and the traditional dental care workforce. From there the chapter focuses on the efforts to ensure that public health and primary care professionals understand and are prepared to address oral health and its relation to overall health. Examples of interprofessional education (IPE) and collaboration including physicians, nurse practitioners, physician assistants, pharmacists, and public health practitioners working together to address oral health as a population health issue, will be described. Models will illustrate how education and practice strategies are being used to develop interprofessional (IP) oral health competencies and build IP and collaborative workforce capacity. Finally, the chapter will demonstrate how IP collaboration regarding the associations between oral disease and diabetes can benefit people and populations affected by diabetes.

Traditionally, education of health professionals has occurred in silos. Professional practice silos have been documented to have a negative impact on the quality and safety of patient care.[7] Moreover, the silos minimize the likelihood that health or health problems will be conceptualized as population health issues. As such, it is not hard to understand how a major public health problem such as oral health and its relation to overall health has been largely omitted in the education of other health professionals such as physicians, nurses, physician assistants, and pharmacists.

Healthy People 2020 identified oral health as one of the 10 Leading Health Indicators.[8] In its 10th report to the Secretary of the Department of Health and Human Services and Congress, the Health Resources and Services Administration's (HRSA) Advisory Committee on Training in Primary Care Medicine and Dentistry made recommendations regarding promotion of IP training through the curricula of Title VII training grants.[9] Additionally, a recent IOM report [10] documents the need to build an IP workforce capable of effectively addressing oral health as a population health issue. The report—*Core Competencies for Integrated Collaborative Practice*[7]—coupled with the recent HRSA Report,[6] *Integrating Oral Health and Primary Care Practice*, have provided momentum for primary care educators and clinicians to reach across their academic and practice silos in order to integrate IP oral health core competencies in their curricula and "best practices." An IP and population perspective on oral health is a paradigm shift.

BURDEN OF ORAL DISEASE IN THE UNITED STATES

Dental Caries

Dental caries (sometimes referred to as dental decay or tooth decay) is a bacterial infection that results from the interaction between bacterial microorganisms, diet substrate, and a susceptible host. As this disease progresses it leads to the demineralization and breakdown of tooth structure.[11]

Dental caries is a highly prevalent, chronic disease. Approximately 92 percent of adults in the United States have experienced dental caries in their permanent teeth.[12] Additionally, in 2007–2010, 15.6 percent of children ages 6–19 years had untreated dental decay, while the prevalence of untreated decay was 23.7 percent in adults ages 20–64 (2005–2008).[13] Like many other chronic diseases, the burden of untreated dental caries is not equally distributed in the population, as rates are substantially higher in minorities and individuals living in poverty.[14] Figure 23-1 highlights these disparities in minorities and low-income individuals.

The consequences of untreated dental caries can be detrimental to both the affected individual and society at large. When left untreated in children, caries can negatively impact their quality of life [15] and their development in the classroom by causing pain, missed school days, and impaired academic performance.[16] Additionally, adults miss over 164 million hours of work annually because of dental problems.[17]

The cost of treating dental pain also places a large financial burden on the health care system. Dental caries have been shown to be the leading cause of dental-related Emergency Department (ED) visits.[18] In 2009 there were over 830,000 visits to the ED in the United States for preventable dental conditions, resulting in enormous health care costs to states, which are ultimately passed on to taxpayers.[19] From 2008 to 2010, the mean cost of dental-related ED treatment was approximately $760 per visit, and the total ED charges across the entire United States during the same time period were estimated to be $2.7 billion for the 4 million visits for dental care in hospital EDs.[18] Considerable hospital resources are required to treat these dental conditions in the ED.[20]

In children 6 years of age or younger, dental caries (or teeth missing or filled due to caries) that affect the primary teeth are referred to as Early Childhood Caries (ECC).[21] ECC is also commonly referred to as early childhood decay or baby bottle tooth decay. The primary maxillary incisors are the most commonly affected teeth, and inappropriate feeding practices with baby bottles containing sugar contents (such as juice or milk) are often implicated in the etiology of ECC.[21] Although the prevalence of caries has decreased for most age groups in the United States over time, in large part due to the availability of a variety of fluoride sources,[22] of great concern was an increase in the prevalence of dental caries seen in 2- to 5-year-old children between the 1988–1994 (24 percent) and 1999–2004 (28 percent) time periods.[23] As with caries in adults,

Characteristic	Untreated dental caries				Dental restoration			
	Age in years							
	Total	5–19	20–64	65 and over	Total	5–19	20–64	65 and over
Total	21.5	16.6	23.7	19.9	75.5	45.9	84.3	88.5
Race and ethnicity								
Non-Hispanic white[1]	17.8	13.3	19.3	17.8	80.1	46.2	88.8	91.6
Non-Hispanic black	[2]34.2	[2]22.6	[2]39.7	[2]35.8	[2]62.6	[2]40.4	[2]73.1	[2]63.7
Mexican American	[2]31.1	[2]22.4	[2]35.2	[2]36.4	[2]61.8	50.1	[2]67.4	[2]69.3
Poverty level								
Below 100%	[2]35.8	[2]25.4	[2]41.9	[2]41.3	[2]62.7	48.6	[2]71.5	[2]63.3
100% to less than 200%	[2]30.5	[2]19.3	[2]37.7	[2]22.5	[2]68.8	46.3	[2]75.1	[2]85.6
200% or higher[1]	15.5	12.1	16.6	15.3	80.2	44.5	89.0	92.6
Sex								
Male	[2]24.6	17.6	[2]27.2	[2]25.1	[2]72.1	44.8	[2]80.5	[2]86.3
Female[1]	18.6	15.5	20.2	15.6	78.7	47.0	88.0	90.4

[1]Reference group.
[2]$p < 0.05$.

FIGURE 23-1   **Prevalence of Untreated Dental Caries and Existing Dental Restorations in Teeth, by Sex, Race and Ethnicity, and Poverty Level: United States, 2005–2008**
SOURCE: CDC/NCHS, National Health and Nutrition Examination Survey, 2005–2008.

minority and low-income children are disproportionately affected.[24] High caries rates are especially worrisome in children because severe ECC usually requires treatment under general anesthesia which not only adds to the cost of treatment, but also has the potential for complications.[20,21] Establishing a dental home for children by age 1 year where appropriate diet, behavior, preventive, and treatment strategies can be developed is a way to prevent and control ECC.[25]

Periodontal Diseases

Periodontal diseases are a group of diseases usually caused by bacterial plaque that affect the periodontal tissues in the oral cavity, with the two largest disease categories being gingivitis and periodontitis.[26,27] Periodontitis is distinguished from gingivitis in that it involves inflammation that has progressed past the localized gums around teeth and into deeper periodontal tissues resulting in connective tissue attachment and bone loss.[26,27] As periodontitis progresses to more advanced stages it can ultimately lead to tooth loss, which greatly impacts tooth function and the quality of life.[28]

Gingivitis is usually caused by local plaque retention around the teeth, and is often related to poor oral hygiene.[26,27] The prevalence of gingivitis in children is approximately 60 percent, and close to 50 percent of adults have gingivitis.[29,30] A recent U.S. survey estimated that 47 percent of adults age 30 or older (or 64 million adults) have some form of periodontitis.[31] The prevalence of periodontitis increases with age, and is higher in males, minority groups, and individuals of lower socioeconomic status.[31] In terms of severity, it has been estimated that 8 percent of the adult population displays a mild form of periodontitis, 30 percent a moderate form, and 8 percent severe periodontitis.[31] While gingivitis is usually associated with localized plaque build-up, additional risk factors exist for periodontitis including smoking, uncontrolled diabetes, and potentially genetic factors.[26,27] Similar to dental caries, disparities are observed with periodontal diseases, with minority and low-income individuals showing greater levels of disease than their counterparts.[32]

Oral Cavity and Pharyngeal Cancers

Oral cavity and pharyngeal cancers (sometimes referred to generally as **oral cancers**) are identified by the International Classification of Diseases, 10th edition codes: C00-C14. In 2014, there were approximately 42,000 new cases and 8,000 deaths attributed to these cancers.[33] The current incidence rate for oral cancers is 11 cases per 100,000 people and the mortality rate is 2.5 deaths per 100,000.[34] Oral cancers represent 2.5 percent of all new cancer cases, and 1.4 percent of all cancer deaths.[34]

Oral cancers have distinct etiologic factors and epidemiologic trends based on their anatomic locations.[35] Tobacco and alcohol use are well-established risk factors for cancers of the oral cavity.[36] The incidence for oral cavity cancers has decreased over time in the United States, and this decline is thought to be related to the declines in smoking and alcohol use in the population.[35] In contrast to oral cavity cancers, oropharyngeal cancers have shown an increase in incidence over time.[35] The human papillomavirus (HPV) is strongly associated with oropharyngeal cancers, and the increasing incidence overtime may be due to changing sexual behaviors in the population.[35] The current five-year relative survival rate for oral cancer is approximately 62 percent; however, African Americans have considerably lower survival than their white counterparts.[34,37]

Survival is greatly improved when oral cancers are detected at earlier stages,[34] thus it is imperative that health care providers have a strong understanding of the risk factors for oral cancers, and educate their patients about these risk factors. Additionally, health care providers should ensure that they perform regular oral cancer examinations on their patients so that any potential cancer can be detected at an early stage, where the chances for survival increase.[34]

Tooth Loss

In most cases, tooth loss represents the end stage of oral disease. Edentulism is the term used to describe complete tooth loss. Tooth loss is associated with a lower quality of life, due to the functional limitations and pain that presents as tooth loss increases.[38] The prevalence of edentulism (complete tooth loss) continues to decline in the United States, with lower rates seen in younger age cohorts.[39] Current U.S. estimates show that the overall prevalence of edentulism in the population is 4.9 percent, with a prevalence of 13.7 percent in people age 65–74, and a prevalence of 24 percent in people over age 75.[39] Individuals with lower socioeconomic status experience a higher prevalence of edentulism which is likely related to their lower access to dental care.[39] Although the prevalence of edentulism is expected to continue to decline, the rate of this decline is expected to slow in the future.[39]

ORAL HEALTH CARE IN PUBLIC HEALTH PRACTICE

Public health services and interventions to prevent oral diseases and protect and promote oral health practice are also important. This section will briefly review various modalities of oral health prevention and treatment in public health practice.

Community Water Fluoridation

In the early 1900s, Dr. Fredrick McKay made a discovery that would ultimately help contribute to a dramatic decrease in dental caries prevalence in the United States over time. He noted that many of his patients had staining on their teeth, from which he coined the phrase "Colorado brown stain" (later termed fluorosis).[40] Interestingly, he also noticed that there was a lower caries experience in these patients.[40] Further studies by Dr. H. Trendley Dean, the first dentist at the National Institutes of Health, tested the hypothesis that consumption of fluoride-containing water was associated with reduced caries levels.[40] Dean's research ultimately helped lead to the adoption of fluoridating drinking water to an optimum level as a measure for preventing dental caries without increasing the risk for fluorosis.[41]

The fluoridation of drinking water has been recognized as one of the ten greatest public health achievements in the twentieth century.[42] **Community Water Fluoridation** (CWF) is the controlled addition of fluoride to the water supply.[43] Since 1962, the U.S. Public Health Service has recommended fluoride levels between 0.7-1.2 mg/L based on geographic temperature as a way to get the benefits of caries prevention without the adverse risks associated with overexposure to fluoride.[44] In April 2015, the recommendation was updated to a single level of 0.7mg/L. In 2012, a total of 210,655,401 people in the United States had access to fluoridated water, which equated to 61.7 percent of the population, and 74.6 percent of people on community water systems had access to fluoridated water.[45]

Low levels of fluoride act to prevent dental caries primarily by topical mechanisms after tooth eruption has occurred, by enhancing the remineralization of teeth, by inhibiting the demineralization of teeth, and inhibiting specific bacterial enzymes.[46] The Community Preventive Service Tasks Force recommends CWF based on its demonstrated effectiveness in reducing dental caries in the population.[43] A systematic review used by the task force concluded that the best available evidence showed that fluoridation of drinking waters is effective in reducing caries prevalence.[47] In addition to being effective in preventing dental caries, fluoridation has been shown to provide cost savings to communities [48] and has not been demonstrated to have any unwanted health effects at the levels recommended.[43] The fluoridation of drinking water is a powerful public health modality because of the large number of people that can benefit from it in communities, including underserved groups who may have trouble accessing regular dental care.[49] Community fluoridation, however, has not been without its detractors (even from its earliest days), as innumerable websites attest; however, the major public health and oral health scientific and professional organizations—from the CDC, to the American Dental Association—continue to support CWF.

Dental Sealants and School-Based Dental Sealant Delivery Programs

Dental sealants are plastic, resin-based materials applied to the biting surfaces of back teeth that prevent the formation or progression of dental caries by providing a physical barrier to diet substrate used by cariogenic bacteria.[50] The effectiveness of sealants in preventing dental caries in children and adolescents has been well documented and the effectiveness is related to the long-term retention of the sealant.[50–52] Studies have shown that after placement of sealants, reduction of caries incidence in children and adolescents ranges from 86 percent at one year to 78.6 percent at two years, and 58.6 percent at four years.[50–52] The general thought is that a well-placed and retained sealant is synonymous with a caries-free tooth.[53,54] There has been consistent evidence that sealants placed on first and second permanent molars are associated with reduced restorative dental care for children and adolescents.[50]

Although sealants have been shown to be highly effective, many low-income and minority children do not have access to the benefits of dental sealants, and thus have a lower prevalence of sealants than their counterparts.[55] Children attending schools in lower socioeconomic areas have a higher prevalence of caries, greater untreated dental needs, and lower access to care than children attending schools in higher socioeconomic areas.[56] Therefore, school-based sealant programs (SBSPs) used to target high-risk schools (with children at high risk for caries) can be an effective way of reducing oral health inequities by increasing sealant prevalence and reducing dental caries in these high-risk populations.[56,57] Sealants have also been shown to be cost effective, especially for individuals who have low access to dental care.[56–59]

Other Oral Health Care Delivery Models in Public Health Practice

In addition to community water fluoridation and school-based sealant programs, other oral health care delivery models exist to provide care to special populations. Two examples of such models include hospital-based dental care and dental care provided in Federally Qualified Health Centers (FQHCs). Dental providers who work in hospitals have the advantage of being able to access additional resources than what are normally found in a private practice office, such as general anesthesia equipment.[60] Having access to general anesthesia and other hospital resources allows hospitals to be an appropriate setting for treating children with severe decay; performing certain oral surgery procedures; performing cleft-palate procedures; or providing dental care for patients with serious medical conditions.[60] In addition to having the capability to provide these dental services, hospitals serve as an important training site for many dental general practice residency programs, and therefore, produce future practitioners who will be able to treat patients requiring dental treatment in hospital settings.[60] FQHCs are health clinics that are partially funded by the federal government and serve as a safety net for millions of people who lack regular access to health care.[61] In addition to providing primary care services to low-income and disadvantaged populations, these clinics provide dental care to approximately 4 million patients annually and serve an important role in increasing access to care and reducing oral health inequities in the United States.[61,62] The majority of dental services provided at FQHCs are diagnostic, preventive, restorative, and surgical procedures.[61] The capacity for these clinics to treat underserved populations is expected to increase once the Patient Protection and Affordable Care Act is fully implemented.[63] The U.S. Armed Forces, the U.S. Department of Veterans Affairs, and the U.S. Public Health Service (including Indian Health Service) also provide dental services for people who are eligible for such care.

ORAL HEALTH CARE WORKFORCE

The oral health workforce has historically been concentrated in private practice settings where dentists lead teams comprised of dental hygienists, dental assistants, laboratory technicians, and office personnel. These independent practices are located in various urban, suburban, and rural settings. The last American Dental Association (ADA) dentist distribution survey estimated that there were 186,084 active dentists in the United States in 2009.[64] In 1997, 91.1 percent of practicing dentists were in private practice and the vast majority of these were in solo practices;[65] however, currently less than 75 percent of practicing dentists are in private practice as increasing numbers are opting for employed positions in large group practices, practices operated by corporations, FQHCs, and other public sector service sites.[64-67]

There are other significant changes in the composition of the oral health workforce. Driven largely by concerns about access to care and disparities regarding the oral health status of various populations, some innovative approaches to the provision of dental care have been initiated. Among the Alaska Native Tribal Health corporations, the education, training and practice of dental health aide therapists has produced a cadre of oral health care providers who address the dental needs of native Alaskan people, particularly in remote areas of the state.[68] In 2009, a change in the dental practice act in Minnesota permitted the training and practice of

dental therapists in that state [68] and in 2014 the state of Maine took action to allow the education and practice of dental therapists.[69] In Alaska, candidates for training and practice as dental health aide therapists are high school graduates, but are not required to have a prior background in health services. The two educational programs in Minnesota offer options for students who are college graduates who may, or may not, have a background in health services as well as opportunities for dental hygienists seeking additional training and skill development. The dental therapist education and training program in Maine is for dental hygienists only.

In 2006, responding to the need to improve access to preventive and restorative care among underserved populations, the ADA sponsored training programs for Community Dental Health Coordinators (CDHCs). Working in underserved rural, urban, and Native American communities, CDHCs are trained to increase oral health literacy in the communities they serve and bring more people into the oral health system.[70]

While 46 percent of state health agencies provided direct oral health treatment services in 2012,[71] only approximately 24 percent of local health departments provide oral health services.[72] Local health departments are an important resource for individuals who have limited access to care. The limited oral health services provided through state and local health agencies underlines the need for continued oral health care workforce development.

ORAL HEALTH AND COLLABORATIVE PUBLIC HEALTH PRACTICE

Current Trends

Two major trends are currently working their way through the health system. One relates to the need to increase the capacity of health professionals prepared to work effectively as members of a team with interests of patients as the central focus. Demand for increased effectiveness of teamwork in health care practice arose as a result of concerns about patient safety and care quality.[73] This translated into a demand for increased opportunities for health professional students to learn with, from, and about each other as a standardized part of their education. The 2011 report of the Interprofessional Education Collaborative on Core Competencies for Interprofessional Collaborative Practice provided clear guidance regarding competencies that all members of a health care team need to share.[7] Academic program accreditation standards pertaining to IP education (IPE) have further prompted this movement. The intent is to imprint health professional students with a team ethic as part of their education experience so that they enter practice with the expectation and competency to work effectively together. Health professionals working as a team represent interprofessional practice (IPP); this form of teamwork is also referred to as Interprofessional Collaborative Practice (IPCP).

The second trend relates to reform of the payment and delivery structures for health care. This trend entails the following facets: whole person care; proactive prevention; early detection; care coordination with primary care as the hub for collaboration; patient engagement in managing their own health; and, delivery of quality care that is "the right care, at the right time, in the right way for the right person and having the best possible result."[74] The goal of this trend is to achieve the "triple aim" of health reform: improving the experience of care (including the quality of care), improving the health of populations, and reducing per capita health care costs.[75] The two trends combine to provide a platform for considering how improvements in oral health, given its relationship to overall health, can provide an important contribution to achieving the "triple aim" through IPCP.

National Interprofessional Initiative on Oral Health (NIIOH)

In 2008, three foundations (DentaQuest Foundation, Washington Dental Service Foundation, and Connecticut Health Foundation) saw the possibility of harnessing the energy of the movement toward IPE and collaborative practice to establish a new standard of care for the oral health of patients and populations. The new standard would be: Every patient has access to oral health services and appropriate referrals. At the core of this vision and new standard of care was the goal that primary care clinicians could become skilled at and comfortable with addressing the oral health needs of their patients and interacting effectively with dentists. The funders thought that, with changes in the education, practice, and financing of health care, it would be possible to reach populations in which oral diseases were most prevalent—populations underserved by the oral health care delivery system as currently configured.

In 2009, the shared vision of this funding collaboration led to the development of the National Interprofessional Initiative on Oral Health (NIIOH). The NIIOH Theory of Change (Figure 23-2) is that patients would benefit and experience improved oral health if their primary care providers addressed their oral health needs, including referrals. Further, primary care providers would be more likely to enter practice ready and willing to address the oral health needs of their patients, as a component of overall health needs, if they had the opportunity to acquire core oral health clinical competencies during their education and training. The REACH Healthcare Foundation has recently joined in supporting the NIIOH initiative.

The focus of the NIIOH has been to align oral health in primary care education and practice with larger health care industry trends. The vision of the NIIOH is that primary care clinicians and dentists would share oral

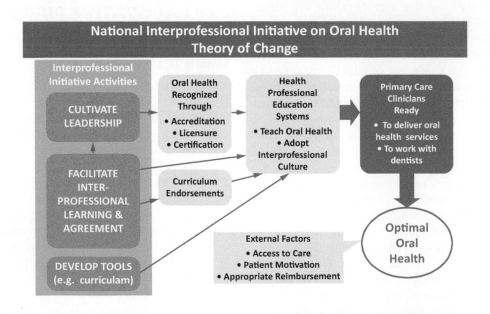

FIGURE 23-2   NIIOH Theory of Change
Courtesy of National Interprofessional Initiative on Oral Health

health core clinical competencies as depicted in Figure 23-3. The NIIOH recruited individuals from primary care who are influential in their professions and considered expert in how to affect change. In addition, they could be counted on to support activities aimed at bringing oral health into the domain of their professions. These activities include faculty development workshops for educators; IPE events which use oral health as a clinical focus; service-learning events for faculty and students; and, convening meetings of leaders from education and practice, including representatives from accrediting and certifying bodies. The NIIOH has encouraged articles for publication in a broad array of professional journals to bring additional attention to this effort.[76,77]

The NIIOH has also sponsored a series of annual Symposia on Oral Health and Primary Care to acknowledge the accomplishments of these leaders, to facilitate cross-pollination among the professions, and to provide a window into the IP oral health agenda for those who are new to, or curious about, this initiative and how it is being advanced. These events are designed to enable relationship development and generative thinking. The yearly symposia have been a vehicle for maintaining and growing momentum and have attracted a mix of professions, from both the education and practice sectors, as well as funders.

Oral Health in Primary Care Practice

Led by HRSA, the federal government's recent report on Integration of Oral Health and Primary Care Practice (IOHPCP)[6] made a major contribution to advancing the

IP movement in oral health. The report presents the case for expanding the oral health workforce in order to reach those not served by the current health and oral health care systems by clearly identifying the role of primary care providers to address the oral health needs of their patients within their scope of practice. It recommends five domains of IP oral health core clinical competencies that should be integrated into primary care practice in order to promote access to oral health and patient-centered provision of care: risk assessment, oral health evaluation, preventive interventions, communication and education, and IPCP. The definition of "Interprofessional Oral Health Core Clinical Competencies" in the HRSA Report was a milestone event providing clarity to the field. The report urged that IP oral health "best practices" can, and should, be provided in primary care.

In addition to HRSA's work, state-specific efforts to engage primary care clinicians in oral health are underway in many states including North Carolina's "Into the Mouths of Babes,"[78] Colorado's "Cavity Free at Three,"[79] and Washington's "Access to Baby and Child Dentistry" programs.[80] Profession-specific work on children's oral health issues has been well organized and funded by the American Academy of Pediatrics since the release of the 2000 Surgeon General's Report on Oral Health.[1] In addition, community-based organizations in multiple states across the country were funded by the DentaQuest Foundation to mobilize a broad array of constituents to develop innovative systems and policy changes to increase access to oral health services and enhance IP regarding oral health as part of an initiative called Oral Health 2020.[81]

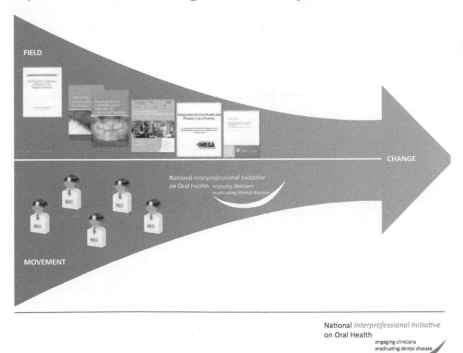

FIGURE 23-3 The Vision of the National Interprofessional Initiative on Oral Health: Aligning the Oral Health Core Clinical Competencies

Courtesy of National Interprofessional Initiative on Oral Health

Core leadership for the IP oral health agenda within the health professions also came from Family Medicine. Beginning in 2008, the Society of Teachers of Family Medicine (STFM) Group on Oral Health, which included representatives from dentistry and pediatrics, initiated the creation of the *Smiles for Life* curriculum.[82] The modular curriculum is intended to meet the oral health education needs of primary care educators, students in the health professions, and practitioners. The main vision was to develop a curriculum that would enable family medicine residents to learn enough about oral health to enable them to address the oral health needs of their patients across the lifespan.

The work of the STFM Group on Oral Health has led to the active engagement of other health professional groups in a concentrated effort to put oral health into primary care education and practice nationwide. The *Smiles for Life* Steering Committee now includes representatives of family medicine, dentistry, nursing, pediatrics, and physician assistants.

NEW MODELS OF EDUCATION: LINKING ORAL HEALTH WITH OVERALL HEALTH

The Oral Health Nursing Education and Practice Experience

There are 2.8 million nurses in the United States, and until a few years ago, oral health and its linkages to overall health was not a prominent focus of the nursing profession.[83] However, a unique organizational partnership of the New York University Colleges of Nursing and Dentistry has provided an innovative platform for developing an IP clinical education model, the *Oral Health Nursing Education and Practice (OHNEP)* program.[84] Developed by the College of Nursing, the OHNEP program is designed to advance a national nursing oral health agenda by promoting linkages between oral health and primary care. This is accomplished through faculty development, curriculum integration, and establishment of "best practices" in the clinical settings for registered nurses and advanced practice nurses, including nurse practitioners and nurse-midwives. The overarching goal of the OHNEP initiative is to develop an infrastructure for the nursing profession to build IP oral health workforce capacity. This goal includes having a nursing workforce competent to address oral health and its relation to overall health as an IP population health issue (Figure 23-4).[85]

The specific aims of OHNEP are to: (1) engage national nursing stakeholders representing licensure, accreditation, certification, education, practice, and policy in advancing an action plan and recommendations that support oral health nursing education, practice, and policy changes; (2) implement a strategy for integrating oral health into undergraduate and graduate nursing curricula; and (3) implement a strategy for integrating oral health "best practices" in registered nurse and advanced practice nurse clinical practice settings.[84] Working toward achievement of these aims, the program has developed a replicable clinical education model that demonstrates how population-focused oral health knowledge and clinical competencies can be woven into the curriculum and clinical practice experiences of nurse practitioners and nurse-midwives. Accomplishing this

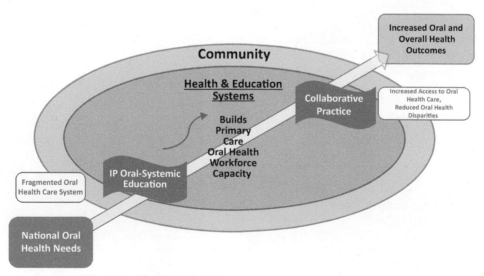

FIGURE 23-4   Interprofessional Oral Health Care Model

Adapted from World Health Organization (WHO) (2010). Framework for Action on Interprofessional Education & Collaborative Practice. Geneva: World Health Organization

objective would also create alignment with the Core Competencies for Interprofessional Collaborative Practice[7] and the HRSA Interprofessional Oral Health Core Competencies.[6]

Engaging internal, external, local, and national stakeholders to create a shared vision has been a critical element of advancing the OHNEP agenda. In efforts to raise awareness among nurses about oral health as a population health issue, two invitational nursing oral health summits have been conducted. The summits were aimed at increasing organizational commitment to promote nursing's role in improving oral health and expanding access to care in the context of IP collaboration. The meetings were attended by leaders from over 35 national nursing and professional organizations responsible for policy related to licensure, accreditation, certification, education, and practice.[84]

The HRSA interprofessional oral health core competencies report, *Integration of Oral Health and Primary Care Practice*,[6] provided the inspiration to create an innovative approach to integrating oral health in nursing clinical encounters by transforming the traditional HEENT (Head, Eye, Ear, Nose, and Throat) component of the health history and physical exam to the HEENOT (adding "O" for oral) approach. By using the HEENOT approach, oral health cannot be excluded from consideration of the overall health status of patients.[76]

OHNEP has used workshops, simulations, virtual cases, webinars, and blended learning modules as innovative strategies for faculty development programs, reaching over 5,000 nursing and IP faculty, preceptors, and clinicians.

Physician Assistants

For almost 50 years, certified physician assistants (PAs) have been integral members of the health care team. With 187 PA education programs in 49 states, there are currently more than 100,000 PAs in the United States. The Bureau of Labor Statistics has projected that by 2022 demand for PAs will increase 38 percent, making PAs one of the fastest growing health professions in the country.[86] Educated in the medical model and working with physician supervision, PAs diagnose and treat patients across all specialties, with approximately one-third of them working in primary care.

Physician Assistants can educate patients about good eating habits, maintaining good oral hygiene, and the risks associated with alcohol and tobacco use. As part of their physical examination, PAs can conduct a caries risk assessment and check the mouth for swollen or bleeding gums, untreated tooth decay, infections, and signs of trauma or soft tissue lesions, particularly those that might suggest oral cancer. They can explain the importance of oral health care to their patients as part of an overall strategy to prevent illness and facilitate referral to a dentist for patients who lack a dental home.

The Physician Assistant Leadership Summit in Oral Health became the vehicle for activating PA's focus on oral health. Supported by the NIIOH, the first summit was convened in August 2010. The purpose of the summit was to provide a forum for sharing new knowledge and information about the oral-systemic connection, oral disease prevention and health promotion, as well as the role of the primary care provider in oral health services. As of 2014, into its fifth year, the Summit's network of partners has grown to include physician groups, pharmacists, nurses, dentists, and public health practitioners, among others. Other entities such as the Primary Care Progress initiative, the Patient-Centered Primary Care Collaborative, representatives from HRSA, and the National Center for Interprofessional Practice and Education, have joined PAs at the summit and are pushing change across the health care system by broadening IP collaboration on oral health.

The Bouvé Experience

Bouvé College of Health Sciences at Northeastern University is the largest health sciences college in metropolitan Boston, Massachusetts, with approximately 4,000 undergraduate and graduate students within its three schools of Health Professions, Nursing, and Pharmacy. Its major academic programs include health science, nursing, pharmacy, physical therapy, physician assistant studies, speech-language pathology/audiology, and public health. The goal at Bouvé College is to enrich students from across the health professions with an IPE experience to enable their future professional collaboration with a shared commitment to improve the health of individuals, families, communities, and populations. The academic programs in public health integrate interdisciplinary education and experiential learning to prepare graduates with the competencies to promote and protect the health of populations and urban communities.

Bouvé College is at the vanguard of preparing a health care workforce equipped with core competencies for IPCP. The overarching goal of its *Innovations in Interprofessional Oral Health Care: Technology, Instruction, Practice, Service* program[87] is to strengthen the primary health care system by infusing a collaborative practice-ready[85] health professions workforce, including public health practitioners, with the team-based competencies to integrate oral health and primary care practice. The specific aims of the program are to integrate oral health across interdisciplinary health sciences curricula, and to promote the integration of oral health in primary care and community-based settings.

DIABETES: A MODEL FOR PUBLIC HEALTH AND INTEGRATED PRACTICE REGARDING ORAL HEALTH AND DISEASE CONTROL

Diabetes: A Brief Review

Diabetes is group of metabolic diseases characterized by their common feature, hyperglycemia due to defects in insulin secretion, insulin action, or both. This chronic hyperglycemia leads to the long-term damage, dysfunction, and failure of a number of organs, including the eyes, kidneys, heart, and blood vessels. Long-term complications of diabetes, resulting from organ involvement, coupled with the markedly increased incidence and prevalence of diabetes, due mostly to type 2 diabetes rates, create a large burden of disease.

Classification of diabetes mellitus currently includes four categories: type 1, type 2, gestational, and diabetes caused by other factors. Type 1, type 2, and gestational diabetes comprise the vast majority of cases of diabetes.[88,89]

Diabetes and Public Health

Approximately 29.1 million or 9.3 percent of the U.S. population have diabetes and 27.8 percent of people with diabetes are undiagnosed.[90] The burden of diabetes is measured by the associated morbidity, mortality, and costs. The substantial economic costs of diabetes for the individual and community are due to overall diminished quality of life, including indirect costs resulting from disability, work loss and premature death, and the direct costs of providing health care for affected persons.[89,90]

From a public health perspective, the importance of diabetes is based on several factors beyond the overall burden of the disease, including the ongoing increase in the incidence and prevalence of diabetes; high proportion of undiagnosed diabetics; disproportionate rates of diabetes experienced by vulnerable populations, including racial and ethnic minority groups;[91,92] and, evidence demonstrating that type 2 diabetes can be prevented or delayed, either through lifestyle intervention or with medicines.[89] Another well-known factor contributing to the public health importance of diabetes is the strong association between the markedly increasing rates of obesity and type 2 diabetes over recent decades.

The Relationship between Diabetes and Oral Health

Oral health is important to people with diabetes in several ways. The association between periodontal disease and diabetes has the most extensive evidence in the literature and perhaps represents the greatest overall oral health impact.[93–96] Periodontal disease, one of the two most common types of oral diseases, occurs in two major forms, gingivitis and chronic periodontitis, and is a common chronic condition, as is type 2 diabetes. A large body of evidence in the scientific literature supports the role of diabetes in increasing the risk for the occurrence, progression, and severity of chronic periodontal disease.[93,96] An emerging body of evidence also supports the association of chronic periodontal disease with increased risk for poorer glycemic control, the development of complications of diabetes, and possibly the development of type 2 diabetes.[95,96] The local chronic inflammatory response of chronic periodontal disease results in highly vascular, inflamed, and ulcerated periodontal tissues that create a ready portal of entry for bacteria from the dental plaque biofilm as well as several of the same inflammatory mediators that have been linked to insulin resistance and the chronic systemic inflammatory burden caused by the adipose tissue in obesity. Hence, the inflamed periodontal tissue behaves as a potential endocrine-like source for increased chronic systemic inflammatory challenge.[94] This forms the biologic basis for emerging evidence linking chronic periodontitis with persisting hyperglycemia, poorer glycemic control, and other adverse outcomes of diabetes.

In considering the relationship between diabetes and oral health it is also important to recognize the emerging body of evidence regarding the association of gestational diabetes mellitus (GDM) with poorer periodontal health.[97–105] Several studies published since 2006 concluded that women with GDM have significantly greater odds of poorer periodontal health than women who have not had GDM.[97–105]

Identification of dental patients with dysglycemia (i.e., prediabetes or diabetes) is gaining increased recognition as a meaningful way in which the clinical dental practice setting can contribute to reducing the burden of diabetes. Almost 28 percent of people with diabetes are not diagnosed, and the vast majority of the 79 million U.S. adults (i.e., 37 percent of adults ages 20 years or older) with prediabetes do not know they have a condition of increased risk for type 2 diabetes.[106] Since over 60 percent of U.S. adults have seen a dental provider in the preceding year[107] and large numbers of individuals seek routine and preventive dental care more often than routine and preventive medical care,[108–110] the dental care setting has potential for being an important health care setting to identify patients with undiagnosed dysglycemia and to refer them to medical care providers for further evaluation. The importance of screening for both diabetes and prediabetes is that prediabetes can be a risk factor for diabetes and can place individuals at risk for diabetes complications before overt diabetes is diagnosed.[111]

There are several aspects about the role of oral health and dental care regarding diabetes that the public health practitioner and administrator should consider in implementing the core public health functions and providing the essential public health services. First, scientific evidence supports a bidirectional relationship between oral health problems—specifically chronic periodontitis—and diabetes.[93,94] That is, diabetes increases the risk for the occurrence, progression, and severity of chronic periodontitis, and tooth loss and chronic periodontal disease can contribute to poorer glycemic control, the development of diabetes complications, and possibly the development of type 2 diabetes. There is also an important body of emerging evidence that supports the role of routine, nonsurgical periodontal therapy in improving glycemic control.[112] The role of periodontal therapy in contributing to reducing the burden of diabetes complications through its impact on improving glycemic control is promising, although not yet explicitly supported by empirical evidence.

Another important oral health-diabetes relationship of importance to public health practice in the realm of maternal and child health is the adverse effect of gestational diabetes (GDM) on periodontal health in pregnant women.[97–105] Closely related is the erroneous yet widely held concern by health care providers that routine dental care is unsafe for pregnant women. There is now credible evidence that provision of essential dental care, including routine periodontal treatment, is safe and prudent for pregnant women.[113]

Serving as a model for integrating oral health into patient-centered care, collaboration and networking among health team members, with the participation or leadership of public health practitioners, offers an approach to improve diabetes management, prevent disease progression, improve health outcomes and quality of life, and lower health care costs.[114]

A number of resources are available to public health practitioners related to public health considerations in addressing diabetes and oral health and their bidirectional relationship. These resources also emphasize the value of IPCP in addressing diabetes as a public health issue. Examples are provided in Table 23-1:

TABLE 23-1   Resources for Addressing Diabetes and Oral Health

Resource	Description	URL
National Diabetes Education Program	The Centers for Disease Control and Prevention, National Diabetes Education Program developed a toolkit, "Working Together to Manage Diabetes: a Toolkit for Pharmacy, Podiatry, Optometry, and Dentistry (PPOD)." This PPOD toolkit describes to PPOD practitioners how they can work collaboratively with each other, as well as with all other members of the health care team, such as primary health care providers, physician assistants, nurse educators, and community health workers to promote better outcomes in people with diabetes. The toolkit includes a guide-book, medications supplement, presentation slides, information for patients, and promotional tools.	Access http://www.cdc.gov/diabetes and search "Working together to manage diabetes"
Smiles for Life	A National Oral Health Curriculum developed by the Society of Teachers of Family Medicine Group on Oral Health. This resource includes a section on obesity and diabetes in its module on oral and systemic disease.	http://www.smilesforlifeoralhealth.org
Wisconsin Diabetes Mellitus Essential Care Guidelines 2012; Section 9: Oral Care	These guidelines were prepared by the Wisconsin Diabetes Prevention and Control Program. The guidelines were designed to be used by primary care providers, other health care professional health systems (e.g., managed care organizations, other insurers, clinics purchasers, etc.), and a companion piece for consumers interested in learning about essential diabetes care. Section 9 focuses on Oral Care.	Access http://www.dhs.wisconsin.gov/publications and search for "Diabetes mellitus essential care guidelines"
International Diabetes Foundation (IDF), Clinical Guidelines Task Force International Diabetes Federation: Guideline on Oral Health for People with Diabetes	In 2007 and 2008 experts in diabetes care and dental care, representing the International Diabetes Federation and the World Dental Federation, collaborated under the lead of the IDF Task Force on Clinical Guidelines to address whether the evidence base in this area allowed formal recommendations on oral health and diabetes care to be made.	Access http://www.idf.org and search for "Oral health for people with diabetes"

SUMMARY

What is the practice of public health in the context of improving oral health? First, the practice of public health embodies the core competencies for collaboration and IPP[7] to improve the population's oral health. Public health practitioners interfacing with other health professionals are expected to (a) demonstrate mutual respect and shared values to improve oral health equity; (b) share roles and responsibilities for addressing oral health promotion and oral disease prevention; (c) demonstrate effective communication practices to improve the oral health of populations; and (d) apply effective teamwork strategies to support quality patient- and population-centered oral health care. Second, the practice of public health embraces interdependence between primary care and public health in "fulfilling society's interest in assuring conditions in which people can be healthy."[115] Collaborative public health practitioners recognize that by working together with primary care workers, both will achieve greater collective impact on improving the oral health of individuals, communities, and populations.[85] Third, public health practitioners understand the inextricable connection between oral health and overall health and well-being for individuals and populations. Oral diseases and many chronic diseases share common risk factors. Public health practitioners and primary health care workers are uniquely positioned to contribute discipline-specific strategies and interventions to address important population health issues, including poor oral health, unhealthy diet and poor nutrition, tobacco and excessive alcohol use, poor water supply, and unsafe behaviors, among others.[116]

REVIEW QUESTIONS

1. What are the connections between oral health and general health?

2. What are three public health interventions relative to oral health?

3. What are three interprofessional collaborations focused on improving the public's oral health status?

4. What is the association between diabetes and oral health?

REFERENCES

1. U.S. Department of Health and Human Services, National Institute of Dental and Craniofacial Research, National Institutes of Health. Oral health in America: A report of the Surgeon General. *Rockville MD: National Institute of Dental and Craniofacial Research.* 2000.

2. Jablonski R, Mertz E, Featherstone JD, Fulmer T. Maintaining oral health across the life span. *The Nurse Practitioner.* 15 June 2014;39(6):39–48.

3. Warnakulasuriya S. Global epidemiology of oral and oropharyngeal cancer. *Oral Oncology.* April–May 2009;45(4–5):309–316.

4. Institute of Medicine. Improving Access to Oral Health Care for Vulnerable and Underserved Populations. *Washington DC: National Academies Press.* 2011.

5. Lewis CW, Boulter S, Keels MA, et al. Oral health and pediatricians: results of a national survey. *Academic Pediatrics.* November–December 2009;9(6):457–461.

6. U.S. Department of Health and Human Services. Integration of Oral Health and Primary Care Practice. *Rockville MD: U.S. Department of Health and Human Services, Health Resources and Services Administration.* 2014.

7. Interprofessional Education Collaborative Expert Panel. Core competencies for interprofessional collaborative practice: Report of an expert panel. *Washington DC: Interprofessional Education Collaborative.* 2011.

8. U.S. Department of Health and Human Services, Office of the Surgeon General, National Prevention Council. National Prevention Strategy. *Washington DC: National Prevention Council.* 2011.

9. U.S. Department of Health and Human Services, Health Resources and Services Administration. Interprofessional Education. Advisory Committee on Training in Primary Care Medicine and Dentistry, 10th annual report. July 2013. p.27.

10. Institute of Medicine. Primary Care and Public Health: Exploring Integration to Improve Population Health. Washington (DC). National Academies Press. 2012.

11. Usha C, R S. Dental caries—A complete changeover (Part I). *Journal of Conservative Dentistry: JCD.* April 2009;12(2):46–54.

12. National Institute of Dental and Craniofacial Research. Dental Caries (Tooth Decay) in Adults (Age 20 to 64). http://www.nidcr.nih.gov/DataStatistics/FindDataByTopic/DentalCaries/DentalCariesAdults20to64.htm. Accessed October 2014.

13. Centers for Disease Control and Prevention. Untreated dental caries, by selected characteristics: United States, selected years 1971–1974 through 2007–2010. http://www.cdc.gov/nchs/hus/contents2013.htm#071. Accessed October 2014.

14. Dye BA, Li X, Beltran-Aguilar ED. Selected oral health indicators in the United States, 2005–2008. *NCHS data brief.* May 2012(96):1–8.

15. Ramos-Jorge J, Pordeus IA, Ramos-Jorge ML, Marques LS, Paiva SM. Impact of untreated dental caries on quality of life of preschool children: different stages and activity. *Community Dentistry and Oral Epidemiology.* August 2014;42(4):311–322.

16. Jackson SL, Vann WF, Jr., Kotch JB, Pahel BT, Lee JY. Impact of poor oral health on children's school attendance and performance. *Am J Public Health.* October 2011;101(10):1900–1906.

17. Centers for Disease Control and Prevention, Division of Oral Health. Oral Health for Adults. December 2006. http://www.cdc.gov/oralhealth/publications/factsheets/adult_oral_health/adults.htm. Accessed October 2014.

18. Allareddy V, Rampa S, Lee MK, Allareddy V, Nalliah RP. Hospital-based emergency department visits involving dental conditions: profile and predictors of poor outcomes and resource utilization. *Journal of the American Dental Association.* April 2014;145(4):331–337.

19. The Pew Center on the States. A Costly Dental Destination: Hospital Care Means States Pay Dearly. February 2012.

20. Allareddy V, Nalliah RP, Haque M, Johnson H, Rampa SB, Lee MK. Hospital-based Emergency Department Visits with Dental Conditions among Children in the United States: Nationwide Epidemiological Data. *Pediatric Dentistry.* 2014;36(5):393–399.

21. Colak H, Dulgergil CT, Dalli M, Hamidi MM. Early childhood caries update: A review of causes, diagnoses, and treatments. *Journal of Natural Science, Biology, and Medicine.* January 2013;4(1):29–38.

22. Carey CM. Focus on fluorides: update on the use of fluoride for the prevention of dental caries. *The Journal of Evidence-based Dental Practice.* June 2014;14 Suppl:95–102.

23. Dye BA, Tan S, Smith V, et al. Trends in oral health status: United States, 1988–1994 and 1999–2004. *Vital and health statistics. Series 11, Data from the national health survey.* April 2007(248):1–92.

24. Guarnizo-Herreno CC, Wehby GL. Explaining racial/ethnic disparities in children's dental health: a decomposition analysis. *Am J Public Health.* May 2012;102(5):859–866.

25. Ng MW, Chase I. Early childhood caries: risk-based disease prevention and management. *Dental Clinics of North America.* January 2013;57(1):1–16.

26. Pihlstrom BL. Periodontal risk assessment, diagnosis and treatment planning. *Periodontology 2000.* 2001;25:37–58.

27. Pihlstrom BL, Michalowicz BS, Johnson NW. Periodontal diseases. *Lancet.* November 19, 2005;366(9499):1809–1820.

28. Martin JA, Page RC, Kaye EK, Hamed MT, Loeb CF. Periodontitis severity plus risk as a tooth loss predictor. *Journal of Periodontology.* February 2009;80(2):202–209.

29. Albandar JM, Kingman A. Gingival recession, gingival bleeding, and dental calculus in adults 30 years of age and older in the United States, 1988–1994. *Journal of Periodontology.* January 1999;70(1):30–43.

30. Bhat M. Periodontal health of 14-17-year-old US schoolchildren. *Journal of Public Health Dentistry.* Winter 1991;51(1):5–11.

31. Eke PI, Dye BA, Wei L, Thornton-Evans GO, Genco RJ. Prevalence of periodontitis in adults in the United States: 2009 and 2010. *Journal of Dental Research.* October 2012;91(10):914–920.

32. Borrell LN, Crawford ND. Socioeconomic position indicators and periodontitis: examining the evidence. *Periodontology 2000.* February 2012;58(1):69–83.

33. American Cancer Society. Cancer Facts & Figures 2014. http://www.cancer.org/acs/groups/content/@research/documents/webcontent/acspc-042151.pdf. Accessed October 2014.

34. Surveillance, Epidemiology, and End Results Program. SEER Stat Facts Sheet- oral cavity and pharynx cancer. http://seer.cancer.gov/statfacts/html/oralcav.html. Accessed October 2014.

35. Chaturvedi AK, Engels EA, Anderson WF, Gillison ML. Incidence trends for human papillomavirus-related and -unrelated oral squamous cell carcinomas in the United States. *Journal of Clinical Oncology.* February 1 2008;26(4):612–619.

36. Radoi L, Luce D. A review of risk factors for oral cavity cancer: the importance of a standardized case definition. *Community Dentistry and Oral Epidemiology.* April 2013;41(2):97–109, e178–191.

37. Saba NF, Goodman M, Ward K, et al. Gender and ethnic disparities in incidence and survival of squamous cell carcinoma of the oral tongue, base of tongue, and tonsils: a surveillance, epidemiology and end results program-based analysis. *Oncology.* 2011;81(1):12–20.

38. Visscher CM, Lobbezoo F, Schuller AA. Dental status and oral health-related quality of life. A population-based study. *Journal of Oral Rehabilitation.* June 2014;41(6):416–422.

39. Slade GD, Akinkugbe AA, Sanders AE. Projections of U.S. Edentulism prevalence following 5 decades of decline. *Journal of Dental Research*. October 2014;93(10):959–965.

40. Burt B, Eklund S. Dentistry, dental practice, and the community. 6th edition. St. Louis: Elsevier Saunders; 2005. Chapter 24. p.307–11.

41. Burt B, Eklund S. Dentistry, dental practice, and the community. 6th edition. St. Louis: Elsevier Saunders; 2005. Chapter 22. p.288–292.

42. Centers for Disease Control and Prevention (CDC). Ten great public health achievements—United States, 1900–1999. *Morbidity and Mortality Weekly Report*. April 2, 1999 48(12):241–3.

43. Community Preventive Services Task Force. The Community Guide- Preventing dental caries: community water fluoridation. [Accessed October 2014]. http://www.the communityguide.org/oral/fluoridation.html.

44. Federal Register. Proposed HHS recommendation for fluoride concentration in drinking water for prevention of dental caries. [Accessed October 2014]. https://www.federalregister.gov/articles/2011/01/13/2011-637/proposed-hhs-recommendation-for-fluoride-concentration-in-drinking-water-for-prevention-of-dental.

45. Centers for Disease Control and Prevention. 2012 water fluoridation statistics. [Accessed October 2014]. http://www.cdc.gov/fluoridation/statistics/2012stats.htm.

46. Featherstone JD. Prevention and reversal of dental caries: role of low level fluoride. *Community Dentistry and Oral Epidemiology*. February 1999;27(1):31–40.

47. McDonough M, Whiting P, Bradley M, Cooper J, Sutton A, Chestnutt I, et al. A Systematic Review of Public Water Fluoridation. National Health Service Centre for Reviews and Dissemination. York(UK): University of York; 2000. [Accessed October 2014]. URL: http://www.nhs.uk/Conditions/Fluoride/Documents/crdreport18.pdf.

48. Griffin SO, Jones K, Tomar SL. An economic evaluation of community water fluoridation. *Journal of Public Health Dentistry*. Spring 2001;61(2):78–86.

49. Burt B, Eklund S. Dentistry, dental practice, and the community. 6th edition. St. Louis: Elsevier Saunders; 2005. Chapter 25. p.333–334.

50. Beauchamp J, Caufield PW, Crall JJ, et al. Evidence-based clinical recommendations for the use of pit-and-fissure sealants: a report of the American Dental Association Council on Scientific Affairs. *Journal of the American Dental Association*. March 2008;139(3):257–268.

51. Ahovuo-Saloranta A, Forss H, Walsh T, et al. Sealants for preventing dental decay in the permanent teeth. *The Cochrane database of systematic reviews*. 2013;3:Cd001830.

52. Llodra JC, Bravo M, Delgado-Rodriguez M, Baca P, Galvez R. Factors influencing the effectiveness of sealants--a meta-analysis. *Community Dentistry and Oral Epidemiology*. October 1993;21(5):261–268.

53. Burt B, Eklund S. Dentistry, dental practice, and the community. 6th edition. St. Louis: Elsevier Saunders; 2005. Chapter 27. p.333–334.

54. Dental sealants. ADA Council on Access, Prevention and Interprofessional Relations; ADA Council on Scientific Affairs. *Journal of the American Dental Association*. April 1997;128(4):485–488.

55. Impact of targeted, school-based dental sealant programs in reducing racial and economic disparities in sealant prevalence among schoolchildren–Ohio, 1998–1999. *Morbidity and Mortality Weekly Report*. August 31, 2001;50(34):736–738.

56. Siegal MD, Detty AM. Targeting school-based dental sealant programs: who is at "higher risk"? *Journal of Public Health Dentistry*. Spring 2010;70(2):140–147.

57. Gooch BF, Griffin SO, Gray SK, et al. Preventing dental caries through school-based sealant programs: updated recommendations and reviews of evidence. *Journal of the American Dental Association (1939)*. November 2009;140(11):1356–1365.

58. Bhuridej P, Damiano PC, Kuthy RA, et al. Natural history of treatment outcomes of permanent first molars: a study of sealant effectiveness. *Journal of the American Dental Association*. September 2005;136(9):1265–1272.

59. Bhuridej P, Kuthy RA, Flach SD, et al. Four-year cost-utility analyses of sealed and nonsealed first permanent molars in Iowa Medicaid-enrolled children. *Journal of Public Health Dentistry*. Fall 2007;67(4):191–198.

60. Burt B, Eklund S. Dentistry, dental practice, and the community. 6th edition. St. Louis: Elsevier Saunders; 2005. Chapter 6. p.70–71.

61. Bailit HL, Devitto J, Myne-Joslin R, Beazoglou T, McGowan T. Federally qualified health center dental clinics: financial information. *Journal of Public Health Dentistry*. Summer 2013;73(3):224–229.

62. Bureau of Primary Health Care. Primary care: the health center program: 2011 national data. Rockville (MD): Health Resources and Services Administration; 2011. [Accessed October 2014]. http://bphc.hrsa.gov/uds/datacenter.aspx?year.

63. Edelstein BL, Samad F, Mullin L, Booth M. Oral health provisions in U.S. health care reform. *Journal of the American Dental Association.* December 2010;141(12):1471–1479.

64. American Dental Association, Health Policy Institute, Distribution of Dentists in the United States by Region and State, 2009. Chicago: American Dental Association; 2011.

65. American Dental Association Survey Center. 1997 Survey of dental practice. Characteristics of dentists in private practice and their patients. 1998.

66. Garcia RI. The restructuring of dental practice: Dentists as employees or owners. *Journal of the American Dental Association.* October 2014;145(10):1008–1010.

67. Guay A WM, Starkel R, Vujicic M. A proposed classification of dental group practices. American Dental Association Health Policy Institute Research Brief. February 2014.

68. Friedman JW, Mathu-Muju KR. Dental therapists: improving access to oral health care for underserved children. *Am J Public Health.* June 2014;104(6):1005–1009.

69. The Pew Charitable Trusts. Pew commends Maine for authorizing dental hygiene therapists. April 2014. http://www.pewtrusts.org/en/about/news-room/press-releases/2014/04/29/pew-commends-maine-for-authorizing-dental-hygiene-therapists. Accessed November 2014.

70. American Dental Association. Breaking down barriers to oral health for all Americans: The Community Dental Health Coordinator. October 2012. http://www.ada.org/~/media/ADA/Public%20Programs/Files/barriers-paper-cdhc.ashx. Accessed November 2014.

71. Association of State and Territorial Health Officials. ASTHO Profile of State Public Health, Volume Three. http://www.astho.org/Profile/Volume-Three/. Accessed November 2014.

72. National Association of County and City Health Officials. 2013 National Profile of Local Health Departments. http://www.naccho.org/topics/infrastructure/profile/upload/2013-National-Profile-of-Local-Health-Departments-report.pdf. Accessed November 2014.

73. Institute of Medicine Committee on Quality of Health Care in America. Crossing the Quality Chasm: A New Health System for the 21st Century. Washington (DC). 2001

74. Peek CJ and National Integration Academy Council. Lexicon for Behavioral Health and Primary Care Integration: Concepts and Definitions Developed by Expert Consensus. AHRQ Publication No. 13-IP001-EF. Rocville, MD: Agency for Healthcare Research and Quality. 2013. http://integrationacademy.ahrq.gov/sites/default/files/Lexicon.pdf. Accessed August 2014.

75. Berwick DM, Nolan TW, Whittington J. The triple aim: care, health, and cost. *Health Affairs.* May–June 2008;27(3):759–769.

76. HEENOT article. Judith Haber. Manuscript submitted for publication. 2014.

77. Oral Health in Pregnancy. Erin Hartnett. Manuscript submitted for publication. 2014.

78. North Carolina Department of Health and Human Services. Into the Mouths of Babes/Connecting the Dots. http://ncdhhs.gov/dph/oralhealth/partners/imb.htm. Accessed August 2014.

79. Caring for Colorado Foundation. Cavity Free at Three. http://www.caringforcolorado.org/post/special-initiatives/cavity-free-three. Accessed August 2014.

80. Washington Dental Service Foundation. Access to Baby and Child Dentistry. http://abcd-dental.org. Accessed August 2014.

81. DentaQuest Foundation. Oral Health 2020. http://dentaquestfoundation.org/oh2020. Accessed August 2014.

82. Smiles for Life. A national oral health curriculum. http://www.smilesforlifeoralhealth.org/. Accessed August 2014.

83. Clemmens DA, Kerr AR. Improving oral health in women: nurses' call to action. *MCN. The American Journal of Maternal Child Nursing.* January–February 2008;33(1):10–14; quiz 15–16.

84. Dolce MC, Haber J, Shelley D. Oral health nursing education and practice program. *Nursing Research and Practice.* 2012;2012:149673.

85. World Health Organization. Framework for Action on Interprofessional Education and Collaborative Practice. 2010.

86. Bureau of Labor Statistics, U.S. Department of Labor. Occupational Outlook Handbook, 2014 15 Edition: Physician Assistants. 2014. http://www.bls.gov/ooh/healthcare/physician-assistants.htm. Accessed July 2014.

87. Dolce MC, Aghazadeh-Sanai N, Mohammed S, Fulmer TT. Integrating Oral Health into the Interdisciplinary Health Sciences Curriculum. *Dental Clinics of North America.* October 2014;58(4):829–843.

88. American Diabetes Association. Diagnosis and classification of diabetes mellitus. *Diabetes Care.* 2014;37 Suppl 1:S81–90. Epub December 21, 2013/12/21.

89. Curtis JM, Knowler WC. Classification, epidemiology, diagnosis, and risk factors of diabetes. In: Lamster IB, editor. Diabetes mellitus and oral health: an interprofessional approach First ed. Ames, Iowa: John Wiley & Sons, Inc.; 2014. p. 27–44.

90. Centers for Disease Control and Prevention. National diabetes statistics report: estimates of diabetes and its burden in the United States, 2014. 2014; http://origin.glb.cdc.gov/diabetes/pubs/statsreport14.htm.

91. Agency for Healthcare Research and Quality. Diabetes Disparities Among Racial and Ethnic Minorities Fact Sheet. http://archive.ahrq.gov/research/findings/factsheets/diabetes/diabdisp/diabdisp.html. Accessed September 2014.

92. Centers for Disease Control and Prevention. Diabetes Public Health Resource. http://www.cdc.gov/diabetes/. Accessed September 2014.

93. Taylor GW, Graves DT, Lamster IB. Periodontal disease as a complication of diabetes mellitus. In: Lamster IB, editor. Diabetes mellitus and oral health: an interdisciplinary approach. First ed. Ames, Iowa: John Wiley & Sons, Inc.; 2014. p. 121–41.

94. Taylor GW, Borgnakke WS, Graves DT. Association between Periodontal Diseases and Diabetes Mellitus. In: Genco RJ, Williams RC, editors. Periodontal Disease and Overall Health: A Clinician's Guide. Yardley, Pennsylvania: Professional Audience Communications, Inc.; 2010. p. 331.

95. Borgnakke WS, Ylostalo PV, Taylor GW, Genco RJ. Effect of periodontal disease on diabetes: systematic review of epidemiologic observational evidence. *Journal of Periodontology.* April 2013; 84(4 Suppl):S135–152.

96. Lalla E, Papapanou PN. Diabetes mellitus and periodontitis: a tale of two common interrelated diseases. *Nature Reviews. Endocrinology.* December 2011;7(12):738–748.

97. National Maternal Child Oral Health Resource Center. Oral Health Care During Pregnancy: A National Consensus Statement: Summary of an Expert Workgroup Meeting: National Maternal and Child Oral Health Resource Center, Georgetown University; 2012.

98. Chokwiriyachit A, Dasanayake AP, Suwannarong W, et al. Periodontitis and gestational diabetes mellitus in non-smoking females. *Journal of Periodontology.* July 2013;84(7):857–862.

99. Esteves Lima RP, Miranda Cota LO, Costa FO. Association between periodontitis and gestational diabetes mellitus: a case-control study. *Journal of Periodontology.* September 2013;84(9):1257–1265.

100. Kumar J, Samelson R. Oral health care during pregnancy recommendations for oral health professionals. *The New York State Dental Journal.* November 2009;75(6):29–33.

101. Michalowicz BS, DiAngelis AJ, Novak MJ, et al. Examining the safety of dental treatment in pregnant women. *Journal of the American Dental Association.* June 2008;139(6):685–695.

102. Novak KF, Taylor GW, Dawson DR, Ferguson JE, 2nd, Novak MJ. Periodontitis and gestational diabetes mellitus: exploring the link in NHANES III. *Journal of Public Health Dentistry.* Summer 2006;66(3):163–168.

103. Steinberg BJ, Hilton IV, Iida H, Samelson R. Oral health and dental care during pregnancy. *Dental Clinics of North America.* April 2013;57(2):195–210.

104. Xiong X, Buekens P, Vastardis S, Pridjian G. Periodontal disease and gestational diabetes mellitus. *American Journal of Obstetrics and Gynecology.* October 2006;195(4):1086–1089.

105. Xiong X, Elkind-Hirsch KE, Vastardis S, Delarosa RL, Pridjian G, Buekens P. Periodontal disease is associated with gestational diabetes mellitus: a case-control study. *Journal of Periodontology.* November 2009;80(11):1742–1749.

106. Saremi A, Nelson RG, Tulloch-Reid M, et al. Periodontal disease and mortality in type 2 diabetes. *Diabetes Care.* January 2005;28(1): 27–32.

107. Shultis WA, Weil EJ, Looker HC, et al. Effect of periodontitis on overt nephropathy and end-stage renal disease in type 2 diabetes. *Diabetes Care.* February 2007;30(2):306–311.

108. Beltran-Aguilar ED, Barker LK, Canto MT, et al. Surveillance for dental caries, dental sealants, tooth retention, edentulism, and enamel fluorosis--United States, 1988–1994 and 1999–2002. *Morbidity and Mortality Weekly Report. Surveillance summaries (Washington, DC: 2002).* August 26, 2005;54(3):1–43.

109. Thorstensson H, Kuylenstierna J, Hugoson A. Medical status and complications in relation to periodontal disease experience in insulin-dependent diabetics. *Journal of Clinical Periodontology.* March 1996;23(3 Pt 1): 194–202.

110. Volzke H, Schwahn C, Dorr M, et al. Gender differences in the relation between number of teeth and systolic blood pressure. *Journal of Hypertension.* July 2006;24(7):1257–1263.

111. Starr JM, Hall R. Predictors and correlates of edentulism in healthy older people. *Current Opinion in Clinical Nutrition and Metabolic Care.* January 2010;13(1):19–23.

112. Simpson TC, Needleman I, Wild SH, Moles DR, Mills EJ. Treatment of periodontal disease for glycaemic control in people with diabetes. *The Cochrane database of systematic reviews.* 2010(5):Cd004714.

113. Nunn ME. Essential dental treatment (EDT) in pregnant women during the second trimester is not associated with an increased risk of serious adverse pregnancy outcomes or medical events.

The Journal of Evidence-based Dental Practice. June 2009;9(2):91–92.

114. Hellquist K, Bradley R, Grambart S, Kapustin J, Loch J. Collaborative practice benefits patients: An examination of interprofessional approaches to diabetes care. Health and Interprofessional Practice. Health and Interprofessional Practice [Internet]. 2012; 1(2):eP1017. http://dx.doi.org/10.7772/2159–1253.1017.

115. Petersen PE, Kwan S. Equity, social determinants and public health programmes--the case of oral health. *Community Dentistry and Oral Epidemiology.* December 2011;39(6):481–487.

116. Institute of Medicine. *The Future of Public Health.* Washington, DC: National Academies Press. 1998.

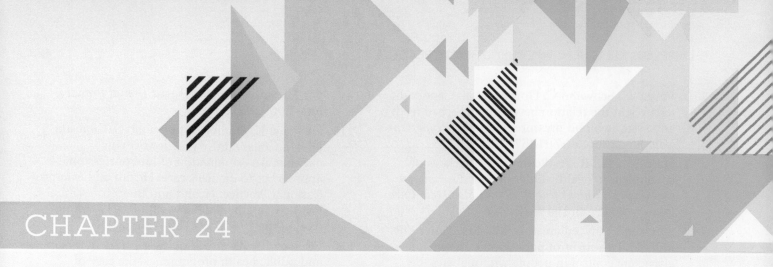

CHAPTER 24

Primary Care and Public Health

Mina Silberberg, PhD • Brian C. Castrucci, MA • Kevin A. Pearce, MD, MPH • Samuel C. Matheny, MD, MPH •
Denise Koo, MD, MPH • J. Lloyd Michener, MD

LEARNING OBJECTIVES

Upon completion of this chapter, the reader will be able to:

1. Explain the concept of primary care and its relevance for and relationship to public health.

2. Explain how primary care has evolved in the United States, including the history of attempts to integrate the activities of public health agencies and primary care providers.

3. Describe the benefits of primary care for cost and quality of care, access to care, and health outcomes.

4. Assess current opportunities and challenges for the primary care sector and the forces that will shape it in the immediate future.

5. Explain "integration" of primary care and public health, provide examples, and describe the potential benefits.

6. Discuss developments and trends that provide new incentives and opportunities for integration.

7. Explain potential challenges and pitfalls of integration, and describe the principles behind effective integration.

KEY TERMS

Area Health Education Centers (AHECs)
Community-Oriented Primary Care (COPC)
family medicine
Federally Qualified Health Centers (FQHCs)
Health Professional Shortage Areas (HPSAs)
integration
population health
primary health care
synergy

INTRODUCTION

Why discuss primary care in a textbook on public health practice? In this chapter, we argue that primary care and public health professionals are natural partners; moreover, the challenges and opportunities attendant upon health and health care in the United States today favor their collaboration. The primary care and public health sectors both strive to improve the health of the public; meet people's basic and essential health care needs, including preventive care; connect people to integrated, accessible, high-quality health services; partner with—and empower—people to improve their well-being; and understand and address the ways in which families and communities shape health. While they share these goals, many of the strengths of the primary care and public health sectors are complementary. Most notably, while primary care providers have access to patients and the opportunity to address their individualized health care needs, public health departments reach out to the population at-large. The services offered by primary care providers and public health agencies and the ways in which they interact with the public are also complementary, as are the data available to inform their work. Arguably, as data use for health care delivery evolves and as the health care marketplace fuels competition based on outcomes and accountability, primary care providers are likely to become increasingly population-oriented, thus strengthening commonalities with the public health sector and interest in their complementary strengths.

Historically in the United States, there have been tensions as well as commonalities and complementarities between public health and the medical sector, including primary care. In this chapter we explore those commonalities, complementarities, and tensions, and argue that integration of the work of primary care and public health—if done right—can reduce tensions and move us from the benefits of "siloed" complementarity to the even greater benefits of synergy. While there has been a history of attempts at integrating public health and primary care, we explain why now is a particularly opportune time to pursue this strategy for improving the health of the nation.

One assumption underlying this chapter is that there are different ways that primary care can be organized and delivered and different ways of conceptualizing and operationalizing the relationship between primary care and public health. The chapter focuses on primary care and its relationship to public health as they are configured in the United States; however, some comparisons are made to other countries, and some of the concepts addressed are applicable outside of this country.

PRIMARY CARE

What Is Primary Care?

Primary care is not a new concept, but its definition and our understanding of its role in the health care system have changed somewhat over the past 50 years. In 1978, the International Conference on Primary Health Care, meeting in Alma-Ata in the former Soviet Union, issued a declaration envisioning primary care as the center of the health care system. The declaration stated that "primary health care is . . . the first level of contact of individuals, the family, and community with the national health system, bringing health care as close as possible to where people live and work, and constitutes the first element of a continuing health care process." This definition was incorporated into the World Health Assembly Global Strategy of Health Care for All by the Year 2000.[1] The Declaration of Alma-Ata also affirmed a relationship between primary care and the social determinants of health such as poverty, education, and the economy, stating that "primary health care . . . involves, in addition to the health sector, all related sectors and aspects of national and community development."[2]

In 1996, the Institute of Medicine (IOM) highlighted the coordinating and facilitating functions of primary care within the health care system, while still indicating a connection to the social aspects of health. The IOM defined primary care as "the provision of integrated, accessible health care services by clinicians who are accountable for addressing a large majority of personal health care needs, developing a sustained partnership with patients, and practicing in the context of family and community."[3] In 2008, in the report *Primary Care: Now More Than Ever*, Dr. Margaret Chan, Director-General of the World Health Organization (WHO), reaffirmed the foundational role of primary care in the health care system and the central role of primary care in addressing the broader determinants of health. Noting current social and political demands for health equity, Dr. Chan described primary care as more than just a sector of medicine, referring to an "ambitious vision of primary health care as a set of values and principles for guiding the development of health systems."[4]

Primary care is usually, but not always, the portal of entry through which individuals obtain medical services.[5] Individual health care services routinely delivered through primary care include diagnosis and treatment of both acute and chronic illnesses, health promotion, disease prevention, health maintenance, counseling, and patient education. Other key responsibilities of primary care providers include coordination of individuals' health care services, advocacy for individuals as they navigate the health care system, and promotion of safe, high quality, and cost-effective care.

Some observers distinguish between primary medical care and primary health care, with primary health care incorporating both primary medical care and the focus on the health of populations typically associated with public health. Primary health care involves teams that go beyond traditional medical providers to include, for example, community health nurses.[6] Vuori states that primary health care can be understood in four ways: as a set of activities, as a level of care, as a strategy of organizing health care, or as a philosophy of care.[7]

The Importance of Primary Care

There is significant evidence that individuals, populations, and countries with adequate access to primary care realize a number of health and economic benefits. At the county, state, national, *and* international levels, there is evidence that primary care (sometimes in contrast to specialty care) decreases long-term morbidity and mortality, reduces cost and overuse of health care resources, and reduces health disparities. Having a primary care physician as a usual source of care is associated with better health outcomes than receiving care only from specialists. It is also a stronger predictor of good health outcomes than insurance status.[8–13]

Primary Care Providers

During the first part of the twentieth century, the majority of medical care in the United States was provided by physicians functioning as general practitioners to those who could afford it, or by the public wards of larger city hospitals to some who could not. Modern medicine had coalesced around the ideals of biomedicine and open market competition, and by the end of World War II, specialization in medicine had accelerated greatly. There was little in the way of national health policy, and with all physicians competing against one another, general practice was becoming a "residual field." The American patient grew accustomed to direct access to specialists, without need for referral from the primary care physician. In contrast, in Great Britain, it was understood that general practitioners were the first point of contact for the patient, making specialty referrals when needed and providing continuity of care before, during, and after specialty care was received. This professional division of labor was cemented with the creation of Britain's National Health Service at the end of World War II.[14]

By the 1950s, the status of the general practitioner in the United States, and the numbers of medical students entering general practice, had reached an all-time low. Concern about adequate provision of first-line care had reached high levels among the American public

and within the health professions. In 1966, two reports by the American Medical Association called for the development of a new discipline to meet the needs of primary care in the United States.[15,16] In 1969, family medicine became the twentieth medical specialty, designed specifically to meet the need for primary care. The rapid expansion of family medicine training halted what had been a decline in the number of generalist physicians, and by 2014, there were approximately 477 family medicine residency programs educating over 10,000 physicians.[17] In the second half of the twentieth century, other specialties such as internal medicine and pediatrics, which train both generalists and subspecialists, began creating special tracks for training primary care physicians within their programs. Today, the term "primary care physicians" includes all of those trained in family medicine and generalists from internal medicine and pediatrics.

Primary care physicians include Doctors of Osteopathy (DOs) as well as Medical Doctors (MDs). DO and MD training is substantially similar, although osteopathic medicine emphasizes the musculoskeletal system and manipulative therapy.[18] Examinations for DO and MD licensure are different, but both DOs and MDs are fully licensed physicians. Steady progress is being made to create a single graduate medical education system for these two professions. Historically, DOs have been particularly committed to primary care; in 2011, almost one-quarter of osteopathic residents were in family medicine alone. DO training slots have increased steadily over the last decade.[19]

Physicians are not the only primary care providers in the U.S. health care system. Over the past few decades, the training of physician assistants (PAs) and advanced practice nurses—including nurse practitioners (NPs), many of whom work in primary care—has grown rapidly. There are approximately 192,000 NPs[20] and 95,000 PAs[21] currently in clinical practice; in 2010, approximately 56,000 NPs and 30,000 PAs were practicing primary care.[22] These clinicians enhance the primary care workforce in two ways. In many practices, they serve as members of primary care teams, focusing, for example on well visits, patient education, or less complex patients. However, a growing number of states now allow PAs and NPs to function as independent practitioners, diagnosing and treating patients and prescribing medications without physician supervision.

In addition to physicians, NPs, and PAs, primary care clinics depend on the efforts of a large variety of service providers and support staff. Staffing varies from office to office, but employees of primary care offices are likely to include nurses, medical assistants, call center staff/receptionists, and increasingly, social workers, nutritionists, health educators, and community health workers.

Challenges in Primary Care

Availability of, Access to, and Utilization of Care

According to a 2012 report on the findings of the National Health Interview Survey, 79 percent of civilian, noninstitutionalized adult Americans reported having a usual source of care in the form of a physician, Health Maintenance Organization, health center, or health clinic.[23] With one-in-five Americans without a usual source of medical services, it is clear that a large segment of the population is not experiencing the continuity that is a key component of primary care. Moreover, having a usual source of care does not necessarily mean having—and certainly does not mean utilizing—a usual provider, let alone a primary care provider. As will be described in more detail later, the passage of the federal Patient Protection and Affordable Care Act (ACA) in 2010 is shrinking the ranks of the uninsured; however, it is clear that insurance coverage alone will not address the many barriers to accessing and utilizing primary care.

The inadequate supply of primary care providers is one such barrier. Experts recommend that primary care and specialty providers be equally represented in a health care system,[13] and in many developed nations, this balance is achieved, along with proportional distribution of providers among the population. This is not the case in the United States, which has both a high ratio of subspecialty to primary care physicians, and geographic maldistribution.

In 2012, there were 46.1 primary care physicians and 65.5 specialists available per 100,000 U.S. population—essentially the same picture seen over the previous decade.[24] The Bureau of Health Professions at the federal Health Resources and Services Administration (HRSA) projects a shortfall of approximately 20,400 physicians by 2020,[25] while the Association of American Medical Colleges estimates this need to be closer to 45,000.[26] In either scenario, the need is great. It is a matter of ongoing debate whether PAs and NPs can fill the need for primary care providers, either as independent practitioners or members of physician-led teams. Their overall numbers are growing, and more and more states are allowing them to practice independently, expanding their potential role in meeting the need for primary care.[27,28] However, recent data show just under one-half of practicing NPs and fewer than one-third of practicing PAs are working in primary care; for a number of years, there has been a downward trend in the percentages of recent graduates in these professions choosing primary care, although there are indications that that trend may be turning around.[28]

Overall provider numbers offer an incomplete picture of primary care supply. They hide the significant geographic maldistribution of medical providers in the United States, which results in an overabundance of health care services in most metropolitan and suburban areas, and provider shortages in many inner-city and rural areas. The geographic distribution of primary care physicians is much closer to the distribution of the general population than that of subspecialists, with primary care physicians constituting the main bulwark against catastrophic physician shortages in rural and underserved areas in the United States; nonetheless, many areas in the United States have a shortage of primary providers. (There is also variation in distribution even among primary care providers. Family physicians are more likely than other primary care providers to work in high-need areas.[29])

There are several ways to identify physician shortages for an area or population. One of the most commonly used is the U.S. government's Health Professional Shortage Areas (HPSAs) designation. Primary care HPSAs are defined as having fewer than one full-time-equivalent (FTE) primary care physician for each 3,500 residents (with some variation under circumstances, such as poverty or language, that increase barriers to medical care).[30] Currently, there are approximately 6,100 designated primary care HPSAs in the United States; meeting those shortages would require an estimated 8,200 primary care physicians to be added to HPSAs.[30]

Another prominent method of identifying shortages of primary care services is the geographic area-based Medically Underserved Areas or the population-specific Medically Underserved Populations, which identifies subpopulations within an area who experience significant barriers to care. Criteria for these designations incorporate poverty levels, percentage of the population over age 65, infant mortality rates, and providers per 1,000 population. Dozens of federal programs designed to improve health care in underserved areas depend on these two methods to determine program eligibility and funding.[31]

In addition to supply barriers, there are financial barriers to utilization of primary care. In 2013, 13 percent of Americans (17 percent of the nonelderly) were uninsured.[32,33] While the ACA mandates that all legal residents of the United States have insurance, many states have chosen not to participate in the ACA's expanded Medicaid program. A number of the ACA's provisions are being contested and worked out in the court system, and we do not know what enforcement of ACA mandates will look like. (See Chapter 30 for more detail on the ACA.)

The high cost of medical care has made it prohibitive for many uninsured people to purchase care on their own (often referred to as "out of pocket").[33] Even for many of those *with* insurance, copayments and deductibles are a barrier to utilizing care. Deductibles for employer-sponsored insurance in the United States rose

47 percent in only five years from 2009 to 2014,[34] and out-of-pocket costs for insulin can now exceed $1,000/bottle.[35] Yet, in 2013, 14.5 percent of the U.S. population lived below the Federal Poverty Level;[36] among the uninsured, 27 percent were below the poverty line, and approximately 90 percent lived below 400 percent of the poverty level, exacerbating the impact of high medical costs on access to care.[33] Moreover, the millions of undocumented immigrants in the United States are ineligible for Medicaid or ACA subsidies.

Access to care is also affected by a number of non-financial factors that are not directly remedied by the ACA. Transportation is consistently cited as one of the top barriers to accessing medical care.[37] For many immigrants, language continues to be a barrier,[38] and, despite a number of policy efforts in this area, cultural insensitivity on the part of providers can keep people from accessing care as well. Another significant barrier for the working American is not being able to get to a clinic during work hours.[39]

Over the past half-century, a number of programs have been instituted to address inadequate access to primary care through public insurance, educational and economic incentives to practice in underserved areas, training of safety net providers, and other mechanisms. Medicaid was created in 1965, providing reimbursement for medical services to specific categories of poor and near-poor individuals, expanding access to care. The federal government mandates that state Medicaid programs cover certain services, including a number of items that are particularly important for primary care, such as physician and NP services, specific screening and treatment services for children, and services of safety-net providers. The program has been modified in a number of ways since its inception, with experimentation taking place in different states. Many providers are unwilling to accept Medicaid, and some changes in state Medicaid programs have tried to increase access to care through the provision of "per member per month" capitation fees to the PCP. The State Children's Health Insurance Program (SCHIP) was launched in 1997 to provide coverage for low-to-moderate income children who were ineligible for Medicaid. As of the writing of this chapter, almost 68 million individuals were enrolled in Medicaid/SCHIP.[40]

An important federal incentive for physicians providing care in urban and rural areas lacking an adequate supply of primary care providers was the establishment of Medicare bonus payments in 1989. This measure, and designations at the state and federal levels improving reimbursement via Medicare and Medicaid, have added to the financial incentive to practice in communities with primary care shortages and participate in programs that enhance the care for underserved populations.[31] In 1965, community health centers

(CHCs) were created as part of the "war on poverty."[41] Today, these centers are part of the Federally Qualified Health Centers (FQHCs) program funded under Section 330 of the Public Health Service Act to meet the needs of medically underserved and low-income populations. In addition to CHCs, FQHCs include Migrant Health Centers, Homeless Health Centers, and Public Housing Health Centers. These centers are local, nonprofit, community owned, and located in areas designated by HRSA as medically underserved or including medically underserved populations. In 2013, FQHCs served over 21 million individuals,[42] providing affordable comprehensive primary and preventive care services, and, in many cases, onsite dental, pharmaceutical, mental health, and/or substance abuse services. Services are provided without regard for patients' ability to pay, and fees are based on a proportional sliding scale that depends on patients' family size and income.[43] The overwhelming majority of physicians working in FQHCs are trained in primary care.

Other government programs and initiatives, such as the Rural Health Clinic Program, so-called FQHC "look-alikes," state-funded health centers, and local health department primary care clinics, together with private nonprofit clinics, have also enhanced primary care services and the safety net for underserved populations. There is evidence that these "community health clinics" perform as well as private physicians or health maintenance organizations in the delivery of preventive services to lower income populations.[44] (For more information, see Table 24-1.)

The National Health Service Corps (NHSC) is the main health professional deployment program instituted by the federal government to help balance geographical access to primary care. Since its inception in 1970, more than 45,000 health professionals (physicians, PAs, NPs, and dental and mental health providers) have participated in this program, receiving either scholarships or loan repayment assistance.[45] In exchange, providers commit to a defined period of practice in underserved areas. Evidence indicates that NHSC participants are more likely than non-NHSC providers to locate in underserved communities, often staying in or near the location of their service commitment.[46] Because of the success of the NHSC, most states have developed their own loan repayment and scholarship programs. Another program allows graduates of foreign medical schools to obtain a waiver of the J-1 visa's required two-year return to their home country, provided that they deliver health care services for three years in primary care or mental health shortage areas.

The federal and state governments' role in supporting medical education has been leveraged at times to support an increase in the supply of primary care. Medicare is required to pay for Graduate Medical

TABLE 24-1   Facts on Federally Qualified Health Centers and "Look-Alikes," Their Patients, and Their Impact*

Health Centers (2013):[42]	Measures
People served	22.7 million
Facilities	9,518
Staff	162,000
Physician assistants, nurse practitioners, and certified nurse midwives	8,481
Patients Served (2013):[42]	
≤200% of Federal Poverty Level	93%
≤ 100% of Federal Poverty Level	73%
Uninsured	32%
Medicaid/SCHIP	40%
Racial or ethnic minorities	~66%
Hispanic/Latino	35%
African American	25%
<18 years of age	32%
>64 years of age	7%
Homeless individuals	1,151,425
Impact:[43]	
Access	Uninsured who use a CHC are more likely to have a usual source of care. Uninsured living near CHC are more likely to have a general medical visit.
Prevention	Uninsured living near CHC are less likely to have unmet medical needs, visit ERs or be hospitalized.
Cost-effectiveness	Health centers' lower cost of care produces *$24 billion in annual health system savings.*
Quality of care	Studies have found that the quality of care provided at health centers is *equal to or greater* than the quality of care provided elsewhere; 99% of patients are satisfied with their care.
Health disparities	Do not exist, even when controlling sociodemographics.
Chronic care	Meets or exceeds national standards, improved outcomes, lower cost.
Birth outcomes	10% lower infant mortality compared to non-CHC communities. Lower rates of low birth-weight babies.
Community economic impact	In 2012, health centers generated over $23 billion in economic activity for their local communities and provided over 212,000 jobs largely in economically disadvantaged neighborhoods.

*Federally Qualified Health Centers (FQHCs) include Community Health Centers, Migrant Health Centers, Health Care for the Homeless, Public Housing Primary Care, and other Health Care Centers Funded Under Section 330 of the Public Health Service Act. Look-Alikes operate and provide services consistent with all requirements that apply to Health Center Program grantees, but do not receive funding under Section 330. FQHCs represent the vast majority of the sites and serve over 95 percent of the patients described in this table.

SOURCES: HRSA. Health Center Data. 2013; http://bphc.hrsa.gov/healthcenterdatastatistics; NACHC. America's Health Centers October 2014.

Education (GME), and state governments provide direct funding to medical schools and indirect support of GME though Medicaid payments. Since the 1970s, the federal government and states have adopted new funding models to expand primary care education; however, GME funding strategies change over time, and Medicare GME payments do not cover all the costs of GME, nor all residents, nor training in all settings.

A novel approach to addressing the maldistribution of physicians has been the creation of rural community-based family medicine residency programs. A related strategy has been the creation of comprehensive selection and training programs—and even sometimes new medical schools—with a clear mission to produce rural primary care physicians. These "pipelines" begin at the high school level, extend through formal medical training, and encompass recruitment, placement, and retention of residency-trained physicians in areas of need. The evidence demonstrates that physicians from a rural background and physicians engaged in rural medicine during their training are more likely to practice in rural areas upon graduation.[47] Graduates of Jefferson Medical College's Physician Shortage Area Program account for 21 percent of family physicians practicing in rural Pennsylvania who graduated from one of the state's seven medical schools, but represent only 1 percent of graduates from those schools.[48]

HRSA's Area Health Education Centers (AHECs), created in 1971, also enhance training of health care providers to work in underserved areas by recruiting and training minority students and students of lower socioeconomic status for health careers; placing health professions students in community-based clinical practice settings, particularly in primary care, and promoting continuing education resources for health professionals in underserved areas.[49] Almost every state now has AHEC programs, as does the District of Columbia, with almost 12,000 training sites nationally.[50] As a final example of government policies to improve access to primary care, the Office of Rural Health Policy (ORHP) in the U.S. Department of Health and Human Services was established by Congress in 1988 through an amendment to the Public Health Service Act, establishing a network of rural health research centers and supporting the development and dissemination of telemedicine for rural areas.

These many efforts to increase access to primary care, while significant, are unlikely to prevent shortages. Due to population growth, insurance expansion, and the aging of the population, demand for primary care is growing together with—and likely faster than—supply.[51] Increasingly, it is recognized that primary care must embrace the team model,[52] but it is not clear that practice redesign alone is the answer. What is clear is

that without significant redesign of primary care delivery and/or a substantial increase in the supply of providers, we are facing a significant shortage of primary care in the United States.

Quality of Care and Impact on Health

As described earlier in this chapter, we now have a great deal of evidence demonstrating primary care's positive impact on the health of individuals and populations. At the same time, there are limits to what medical care in general has been able to achieve in improving health status. Some of these limits can potentially be overcome. The IOM report, *The Quality Chasm: A New Health System for the 21st Century*, brought national attention to inconsistencies and deficits in the quality of U.S. health care, including wasteful and even harmful overuse of services, high rates of medical error, system fragmentation, duplication of care, and barriers to timely access to care.[53] Moreover, a significant body of literature—including another IOM report, *Unequal Treatment: Confronting Racial and Ethnic Disparities in Healthcare*—indicates that institutionalized and personal bias in health care delivery contribute to systematic variation in the treatment of different socioeconomic and racial groups.[54] Another mutable factor is the insufficiency of current research platforms and institutional structures (e.g., linkages between clinicians and researchers) to support the "translation" of medical evidence into real-world practice, or to inform priorities for research.[55]

The organization and financing of our health care system incentivizes overuse of some services (e.g., those procedures for which reimbursement is ample) and underuse of others (e.g., many preventive services) and generates fragmentation in the delivery of health care services.[53] Our current system of health care financing, organization, and delivery also makes it impossible for the primary care provider to fulfill all her responsibilities. Research shows that "the 15-minute physician visit can no longer accomplish what society expects." [52] For example, one study indicates that adhering to the practice guidelines for only 10 chronic illnesses requires more time than primary care physicians have available for patient care overall.[56] How then is the primary care provider to diagnose and treat chronic and acute illnesses, provide well-care, counsel and educate the patent, coordinate his other health services, advocate for him in the health care system, keep up on changing medical knowledge, and participate in maintenance—let alone improvement—of practice quality?

Primary care providers are also challenged by the limits of what medical care alone can do to improve health. The Health Impact Pyramid, described by Centers for Disease Control and Prevention (CDC) Director Dr. Thomas Frieden, shows the relative importance of five different approaches to improving health

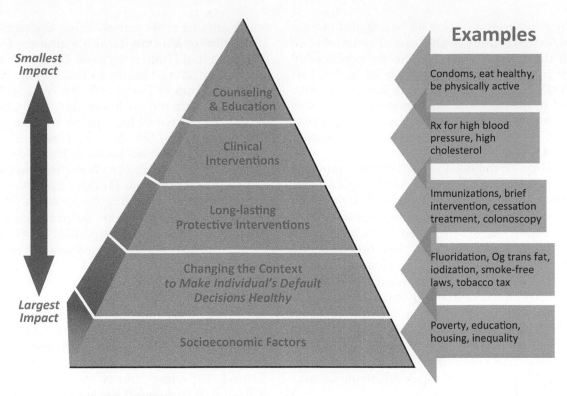

Examples

Condoms, eat healthy, be physically active

Rx for high blood pressure, high cholesterol

Immunizations, brief intervention, cessation treatment, colonoscopy

Fluoridation, Og trans fat, iodization, smoke-free laws, tobacco tax

Poverty, education, housing, inequality

Smallest Impact

Counseling & Education

Clinical Interventions

Long-lasting Protective Interventions

Changing the Context *to Make Individual's Default Decisions Healthy*

Largest Impact

Socioeconomic Factors

FIGURE 24-1 Factors that Affect Health

SOURCE: U.S. Department of Health and Human Services, Centers for Disease Control and Prevention. Adapted from: Frieden, TR. A framework for public health action. *American Journal of Public Health.* 2010;100(4):590–595.

(see Figure 24-1). As illustrated by its placement at the broad base of the pyramid, changing socioeconomic conditions, such as income, education, and housing, will have the largest effect on population health. Clinical care and health education and counseling have the least widespread impact on population health. Despite the importance of medical care, the capacity of medical providers to improve the health of their patients is limited by lack of a strong public health infrastructure and adverse socioeconomic, economic, and cultural contexts.

Over the past few decades, there has been growing attention to improving the quality of medical practice. Commonly used approaches include the development of practice guidelines or practice parameters for specific conditions, measurement of adherence to these guidelines and patient health outcomes, and promotion of "continuous quality improvement"—"an approach to quality management that . . . emphasizes organization and systems, focuses on 'process', . . . recognizes both internal and external 'customers', and promotes the need for objective data to analyze and improve processes."[57] Government agencies such as HRSA and the Agency for Healthcare Research and Quality (AHRQ) have supported evidence-based practice and measurement of care quality, and, through the Physician Quality Reporting

System, providers are given an economic incentive to report data on quality metrics to the Centers for Medicare and Medicaid. Private payers have also contributed to these efforts, most notably through the development of the National Committee for Quality Assurance and its widely utilized Healthcare Effectiveness Data and Information Set (HEDIS) measures assessing care processes and outcomes. Continuous quality improvement is promoted by clinicians' access to evidence-based practice guidance, and is being improved through the development of prompt, systematic, and critical reviews of new research that are fed into electronic medical literature databases that are extensively cross-referenced. Major efforts are under way to meet the human and technological challenges inherent to bringing high-quality information to the point of medical care. Notable examples are the Cochrane Project devoted to putting the results of clinical trials into usable evidence bases,[58] support of medical informatics, evidence-based practice centers and technological assessments by AHRQ,[59] and the Family Physicians Inquiries Network, funded by the American Academy of Family Physicians.[60]

Practice-based research networks (PBRNs), which have been operating in the United States, Canada, and Europe for over 30 years, aim to improving the evidence-base for clinical care and its translation into practice by promoting research on health and disease in the context of routine health care. The number of PBRNs in the United States has grown significantly since their inception, increasing from 28 in 1994 to 111 in 2003. While few in number compared with other types of medical "research laboratories," PBRNs have garnered support from the federal government through HRSA, AHRQ, and most recently the National Institutes of Health (NIH).[61]

Recognition of the need to actively facilitate and promote the translation of research into evidence-based medical practice also led to the NIH's nearly $500 million Clinical and Translational Science Awards program, supporting the development of infrastructure for translational activity at more than 60 Academic Health Centers nationwide.[62] This includes a new focus in the medical world on "implementation science" (studying factors facilitating and impeding effective dissemination and implementation of evidence-based practices), PBRNs, and "community engagement" to support research and health improvement efforts that meet important community needs and have the community support required for implementation and sustainability.

The "triple aim"—improving the quality of care and the patient experience while reducing costs—was first defined by Donald Berwick and colleagues in 2008,[63] and has become a watchword in practice improvement. The federal Center for Medicare and Medicaid Innovations is funding experimentation in new models of care with a focus on the triple aim. This recognition has spawned whole new industries that are devoted to advancing health information systems to allow providers to use clinical data (e.g., test results, biometric measurements) and administrative and encounter data (e.g., provider claims for payment, hospital length of stay) for CQI that, it is hoped, will help achieve the triple aim.

There is also great interest in improved designs for health care delivery systems. The patient-centered medical home (PCMH) is currently the premier design for primary care delivery. It promotes comprehensive, patient-centered, coordinated, accessible, high-quality and cost-effective medical care in a setting that serves as the patient's "medical home" through a physician who serves as first point of contact and understands all of the patient's health needs. The PCMH is designed to be accountable to patients and the community. This model is now being promoted by the federal government, health care payers, and professional associations, and is a prominent feature of the ACA.

National attention to disparities in health and health care has grown over the last few decades. In 1985, the U.S. Department of Health and Human Services issued the "Report on the State of Black and Minority Health," also known as the Heckler report,[64]

which, among other things, led to the creation of the U.S. Office of Minority Health within the Department of Health and Human Services. Many states followed suit, establishing similar offices. In the late 1990s and early years of the twenty-first century, Dr. David Satcher continued to bring national attention to health disparities in his role as U.S. Surgeon General and Assistant Secretary for Health. The National Institutes of Health added an Office of Minority Programs in 1990, which eventually became the Institute of Minority Health and Health Disparities. The most recent iteration of *Healthy People* has a greater focus on health disparities than do previous versions.[65] Attention to the issue of disparities has been substantially propelled by the work of researchers, advocacy groups, and others.

The Affordable Care Act

The most important development in health care of the past decade was the passage in 2010 of the ACA. While Chapter 30 will provide much greater detail on the ACA, it is important to emphasize here the features that relate directly to primary care. The law is designed to expand access to care in a number of ways, including broadening Medicaid eligibility, creating health marketplaces to facilitate informed purchase of health care plans in the individual and small group markets, providing subsidies to the cost of health insurance for low-income individuals, mandating that most Americans have health insurance and that larger businesses provide health insurance or pay into the public system, and prohibiting exclusion from health insurance on the basis of preexisting conditions or gender.

In addition to addressing access to care, the ACA also aims to improve quality of care and to change the incentives around health care utilization and expenditures. Key features of the ACA that touch on challenges facing primary care include: a requirement that most health plans cover recommended preventive medical care without out-of-pocket expenses for patients and that Medicare provide certain preventive services for free; mandates and supports for expanded use of health information technology; expansion of CHCs; new infrastructure to monitor health disparities and create a diverse, "culturally competent" health care workforce; and Medicare programs that reimburse providers on the basis of adherence to quality metrics rather than "fee-for service", and promote the creation of Accountable Care Organizations (networks of providers and health care systems providing coordinated care and sharing cost savings for a defined population). Because the ACA has not yet been fully implemented and many of the changes it promotes will take time, its ultimate impact on quality of care, like access, has yet to be seen.

INTEGRATION OF PRIMARY CARE AND PUBLIC HEALTH

Of primary interest for this chapter is the call for the medical community to enter the field of population health, defined as "the health outcomes of a group of individuals, including the distribution of such outcomes within the group."[66] Given the importance of the social and environmental determinants of health, it is argued, population health improvement must be collaborative, bringing together the sectors (housing, education, job development, medical care, etc.) that have the resources, skills, and expertise to address all the levels of the Health Impact Pyramid. Many observers see one of the foundational collaborations for population health to be that between the primary care and public health sectors. An IOM report, issued in 2012, called for the "integration" of public health and primary care, i.e., "the linkage of programs and activities to promote overall efficiency and effectiveness and achieve gains in population health."[67]

Commonalities and Tensions between Primary Care and Public Health

Historically, the public health and primary care sectors in the United States have operated with relatively little coordination, let alone true partnership. A recent study of state-level public health agency personnel working on chronic disease found that most reported working with health care providers; however, these collaborations were much more likely to be around provision of individual client services than to be system-wide. Moreover, most such collaborations are with community health centers as opposed to other types of clinical sites. Only a small number of respondents even reported having been involved with support or development of patient-centered medical homes. Finally, most collaboration takes place around a limited set of activities, including smoking cessation, cancer screening, and promotion of cardiovascular health.[68]

Arguably, the sharp distinction in the United States between public health and medicine is an artifact of history. The most important turning points in that history include the Flexner report and the formalization of medical education, mirrored by the Welch-Rose Report and its emphasis on research in public health; the growing dominance of the hospital, with its focus on acute tertiary care, as the locus of medical practice; and the increasing power of medical practitioners across multiple aspects of society.[69]

This history of division obscures the fact that medical providers and public health practitioners have a common aim of promoting and maintaining health. This is particularly true for the primary care and public health sectors, which share many of the same goals and paradigms, including:

▸ improving the health of the public
▸ meeting people's basic and essential health care needs
▸ serving as a gateway for people to connect to the services they need, and bringing those services closer to the people who need them
▸ promoting use of integrated, accessible, high-quality health services
▸ practicing within the context of family and community
▸ partnering with and empowering people to take care of their own health
▸ emphasizing prevention, and
▸ recognizing that health is multifaceted and determined by multiple factors

Paradoxically, the common concerns of medicine and public health have often contributed to conflict between the two sectors. For example, early in the twentieth century, some physicians believed that public health efforts to prevent illness were unnecessary given the seemingly limitless growth in biomedical knowledge, and, furthermore, that it would undercut physicians' livelihood. Conversely, public health officials and educators have fiercely guarded their independence from medicine, pointing to the greater power and prestige of the medical field as a threat to the survival of public health and its approaches should the two sectors become too close.[69]

Some unique concerns arise from the overlapping relationship between primary care, in particular, and public health. For example, many public health departments become the primary care "provider of last resort" for underserved and disadvantaged populations. Eleven percent of local health departments provide comprehensive primary care services, with others providing components.[70] There is debate within the public health and medical communities around the benefits of having public health departments meet the medical care needs of the indigent and the risks that meeting these needs will lead public health to shift resources and attention away from their essential role in improving the health of populations. Moreover, public health departments working in primary care are subject to changes in the private primary care market. For example, in the 1990s, when a number of state Medicaid programs moved to managed care, many patients receiving primary care at health departments in those states migrated to private physicians, truncating the Medicaid funding stream into the health departments.[71]

Tensions arise between the primary care and public health sectors because of their differences, as well as the ways in which they overlap. Medicine is deeply rooted in what has been called the "biomedical paradigm," focused on individual patients, the study of specific diseases, the biological origins of disease, and procedural, surgical, and pharmacological remedies.[69] Public health activities, in contrast, are concerned with populations, prevention, social determinants of health and disease such as education and living conditions, and health education, communications, and policy change. Although both approaches are necessary for improving health, at times it seems as if they are in competition, with medicine afforded more resources and greater prestige than public health. Public health practitioners have often felt the need to "accommodate" to the biomedical model, with collaborations between public health and medicine sometimes leading to an emphasis on the biological origins of disease at the expense of social, behavioral, and environmental epidemiology.[69]

There are a number of key language differences between medicine and public health that reflect and reinforce larger paradigmatic differences. For example, in public health, "population health" refers to the health of a defined community—generally a geographic community (e.g., residents of a county)—for whom they are responsible. For many primary care practitioners, "population health" refers to the health of their patient population.

Public health professionals most often think of prevention as primary prevention delivered on a mass basis (e.g., through fluoridation of water) or individually (e.g., through vaccination) or as secondary prevention, for example through large-scale screening to detect cervical and breast cancer. In contrast, primary care practitioners generally deliver preventive care individually and are generally more likely to address secondary and tertiary prevention than primary prevention.

Because the public health sector is committed to the health of the public, and primary care providers to the health of the individual, differences can also arise in their approaches to medical information and confidentiality, as well as resource allocation. These differences create tensions precisely because the public health and primary care sectors may have overlapping responsibilities in regard to a single patient. (Chapter 5 includes further exploration of the differences between medical and public health ethics.)

The Call for Integration

Despite, and in part, because of the tensions between them, there have been many calls for greater integration of the public health and primary care sectors. In the early twentieth century, attempts were made by the Commissioner of Health of New York to bring public health and medical care closer together.[72] Similar attempts followed in Britain in 1920, but not until 1921 was an actual model devised and constructed along these lines by Dr. John Grant in China. The Karks followed in 1940 with the development in rural South Africa of **Community Oriented Primary Care (COPC)**, defined by Nutting as "a variation of the primary care model in which major health problems of a defined population are identified and addressed through modifications in both primary care services and other appropriate community health programs."[73] (This model is discussed in further detail in Exhibit 24-1.) With the advent of the National Health Service in Great Britain, increasing strides that were made to coordinate the Medicine in the Community initiative merged public health and primary care; in

EXHIBIT 24-1   Community-Oriented Primary Care (COPC)

Community-Oriented Primary Care (COPC) is the best-known conceptual model of the integration of primary care and public health approaches. The COPC process, in its simplest form, consists of the following four stages: (1) identification and definition of the community, (2) identification of community health problems, (3) development of some intervention in the health care program, and (4) evaluation of the effectiveness of the program. This approach is designed to define communities, and through the use of various forms of data, identify areas of special concern to a specific community or practice. The intervention may have various forms, but frequently, it is designed to facilitate the delivery of care or provide a measure of preventive services in an attempt to improve the overall health status of the community. One of the other important features of community-oriented primary care is that representatives of the community itself should be involved with prioritizing the areas of emphasis in this model.

This model has been attempted for a number of years in community health centers, the Indian Health Service, family medicine residency programs, and in individual and group practices. Some reported projects have included programs to reduce rural neonatal mortality rates,[77] initiatives to reduce teenage substance abuse,[78] and statewide interventions for prevention of cardiovascular disease.[79]

There have been some concerns about the COPC model. It has been difficult, up to the present time, to accurately obtain community-level information on health and to develop the resources to integrate this information into that of a specific practice. COPC programs require time, and in a fee-for-service model, time allocations for community-based approaches have not been readily compensated. Critics have also expressed concern that evaluations of program effectiveness have been inadequate.[80] However, data are becoming easier to access and many expect the fee-for-service model to be eclipsed by alternative financial approaches in the near future. Some observers are calling for the integration of COPC into the patient-centered medical home model to move the latter to a true focus on population health.[81]

EXHIBIT 24-2   The Cuban National Health System

The Cuban National Health System may be the best example in the world of the population health benefits realized when medicine and public health are melded into a single system based on maximizing health through population-level interventions and universal access—free of charge—to prevention-oriented primary care provided at the community level. Even in the low-resource environment that is Cuba, its health status rivals that of the United States. Cuba has become a leader among nations responding to the consensus goals of the Alma-Ata International Conference on Primary Health Care and has achieved most of the United Nations' Millennium Development Goals (e.g., the Cuban infant mortality rate in 2010 was 4.7 deaths per 1,000 live births compared to 6.1 for the United States). (Gorry 2013)

Approximately 11,000 family physician and nurse teams live within and serve defined populations of up to 1,500 people in every corner of the country, implementing a strategy of integrated, community-oriented care emphasizing prevention, health promotion, public participation, and patient responsibility. Every citizen is individually registered into a Continuous Assessment and Risk Evaluation (CARE) process carried out through interviews at both office and home visits that allows individuals to be characterized into one of four groups—well, at-risk, ill, or disabled—allowing those most in need of services to be prioritized. Aggregate data from this process are used to formulate an annual community health analysis that requires identifying the socio-psychological, economic, historical, geographic, cultural, and environmental characteristics having an impact on the health of the population for the purpose of developing remedial actions—a focus on the social determinants of health. Gorry 2013, Keck 2012

Approximately 450 community polyclinics, essentially multispecialty group practices, are the next link in an integrated system of primary care. Each polyclinic provides supervision, support and specialist consultation for 40 to 60 surrounding family physician and nurse offices (20,000 to 60,000 patients). Services provided include laboratory, X-ray, social work, rehabilitation, and dentistry. Also included at the primary care level are over 300 maternity homes for high risk pregnancies and over 200 senior day care centers. Patients requiring hospital care have access to over 200 municipal, specialty and research institutions across the country with care and hospital follow-up care coordinated by their local polyclinic and family physician and nurse team. (Gorry 2013, Keck 2012)

Cuba's National Statistics Division utilizes robust disease surveillance techniques to provide early warning and response to population health threats, strategic analysis of epidemiological data from all levels to develop and prioritize intervention strategies, and evaluation of health outcomes to determine the success of interventions. This informs the continual search for answers to the system's central policy question, "What can be done now, given our limited resources, to further improve health status?" (Keck 2012)

Understanding how the Cuban system melds public health and medical care may be difficult for U.S. health professionals to understand. When we think of "integration," we think of collaboration among two siloed disciplines. In Cuba, those silos do not exist. Cubans and many others call the Cuban National Health System a "public health system." In that context, teaching one to use condoms is a public health service and cardiac surgery is a public health service. It is the Ministry of Public Health that is in charge of the curriculum for medical schools, nursing schools, dental schools, medical technician training programs, etc., and the national school of public health. It is also the ministry that is in charge of family physician and nurse offices, polyclinics, hospitals, research institutes, disease surveillance, data analysis and policy development. It all deserves the word "system." It is true that there are more than two dozen medical schools, 34 nursing schools and 6 dental schools in the country and only one school of public health. Only one school of public health is needed to train the epidemiologists, biostatisticians, managers and policy analysts, because every other health professions school has a strong public health element in its curriculum—exactly, by the way, what the AAMC, ACPM, APTR and others say we should do here in the United States. Even transplant surgeons talk about the importance of their integrated approach and have as much respect for primary care and prevention as they do for their specialty. The words "Public Health" in Cuba refer to anything related to the health of the public. There are no local public health departments in Cuba so the thought that "public health workers" would work in one context and "clinical workers" would operate in another is completely and refreshingly foreign.

C. William Keck, MD, MPH
Gorry C. Primary care forward: Raising the profile of Cuba's nursing profession. *MEDICC Review.* 2013;15(2):5–9.

Keck CW, Reed GA. The curious case of Cuba, *Amer. J. Pub. Health*, 2012; 102(8): e1–e10.

the 1990s, the initiative was altered to emphasize family medicine access. Physicians in Cuba have both personal and public health responsibilities for the communities they serve (see Exhibit 24-2).[74] Training in Community Medicine as a discipline began at the University of Kentucky in the 1960s, and the concept of merging preventive and primary care medicine became central to the newly developed Community Health Centers of that time.[75] In

1997, the New York Academy of Medicine issued a call for greater collaboration between public health and medicine that included case studies of successful partnerships.[76] Today, the call for integration is being issued again.

Integration of public health and primary care, its proponents argue, allows for synchronized campaigns, common messages, and the allocation of work to the sectors to which it is best suited.[67] Rather than seeing public health and medicine as competitive sectors, observers argue, it is better to think of them as bringing different essential resources and approaches to the same goal. If public health practitioners were to adopt the "medical model" or medical providers were to offer only population health services, we would lose half of our arsenal for promoting health. Collaboration between the public health and medical sectors, particularly primary care, allows not just for deployment of their complementary resources, but synergistic and strategic deployment of these resources.[67,69] In particular:

1. Public health activities often reach hard-to-serve populations such as homeless veterans and migrant families, and employ staff to connect those in need with services. Through partnerships, public health workers can guide vulnerable individuals to a primary care medical home *and* support them with their care plans as case managers and health educators.

2. Managing one's health is a daily challenge. Providers can impart medical information and motivate individuals to care for their health, but can only do so much to support their patients once they leave the clinic. Public health practitioners can deploy targeted communications and education campaigns to promote patient participation in lifestyle-based approaches to health improvement outside of the clinic. By working together, primary care and public health sectors can refer individuals to each other's services, reinforce common messages, and make sure that available resources meet population needs, for example, ensuring that parks and recreation offerings meet the needs of the full spectrum of residents.

3. For health care providers, optimizing diagnosis of disease requires marshalling all available information, including that provided by the public health sector. Knowing, for example, that a certain disease is increasingly prevalent will make the provider more attentive to symptoms of that disease in her patients, facilitating appropriate screening and differential diagnosis.

4. Primary care practices and public health agencies have complementary strengths in regards to data collection and analysis. Clinical data are updated on an almost-daily basis, while there is often a significant time lag between the initiation of public health data collection (think, for example of population-based surveys) and data dissemination. Clinical data also provide the best information available on chronic diseases. While syndromic surveillance and laboratory reporting can facilitate quick identification of acute, infectious disease outbreaks, such systems do not currently exist for chronic diseases. Moreover, clinical data include ZIP codes, allowing for the analysis of data at the county, municipal, and even neighborhood level; public health data are sometimes not available at the appropriate level of geographic aggregation for community health work. On the other hand, clinical data exclude those who do not access health care, and are fragmented across different practices and different systems. Public health data are designed to capture an entire geographic community and often include not only clinical data, but also data on exposures and health behaviors. Public health data also can identify relevant community characteristics, such as restaurants that have failed inspections, locations of alcohol outlets, and locations of unsafe pools. In addition, public health professionals have among their ranks many individuals trained in the development, analysis, and use of population data. The Health Insurance Portability and Accountability Act (HIPAA) Privacy Rule permits providers to share personally identifiable health information with public health authorities for public health purposes. Combining the data-related resources of public health and primary care allows primary care clinics to better understand their patients' social profiles, provides public health with the ability to aggregate timely clinical data to assess community health needs and trends, and creates a platform for the two sectors to work together on data-driven population health improvement initiatives.

5. Primary care and public health have different strengths for addressing the social determinants of health; working together, they can coordinate their efforts. For example, primary care providers might see an uptick in disease among their patients, but are likely to lack the time, information, and analytical resources to conduct the data analysis necessary for substantiating the perceived trend or investigating its underlying causes. If they bring what they have observed to the attention of a public health department, the latter will generally have the capacity to carry out the necessary epidemiological investigations to identify the determinants of the observed trend, including social determinants. They also generally have strong relationships with other governmental and community agencies that are concerned about these social determinants. Through their convening role, programs and policies, research function, and access to other policy makers, public health agencies can inform policy and regulatory responses to population health

problems, as they have done with child booster seat laws, clean indoor air ordinances, and zoning restrictions on bars and alcohol outlets. These policies can be shaped by the input of primary care providers, and advocacy from primary care can also be a factor in the passage and effective implementation of policy.

6. Historically, research on the causes and patterns of population health has been a strength of academic public health, providing a crucial evidence base for primary care. Through collaboration, primary care and public health practitioners can enhance the quality and relevance of research by pooling their analytic skills, their data, their knowledge of biomedicine and the socioecological determinants of health, and their understanding of the health-related issues that are currently most salient to clinical practice and the community. Moreover, public health departments serve as an outlet for the dissemination of new health care knowledge, particularly for diagnosis and treatment of infectious disease.

7. Infrastructure is needed to support primary care physicians as public health sentinels. Computerized medical records and other practice data, the Internet, and e-mail have enhanced the potential efficiency of intersectoral communication creating new capabilities for detection and communication during an emerging epidemic. During an epidemic or natural disaster, primary care services also provide education, screen and triage patient concerns and symptoms, and treat affected individuals. Public health agencies play a crucial role in mediating the demands placed on primary care at these times. Recent concerns with disaster preparedness after Hurricane Katrina, bioterrorism, and potential epidemics or pandemics of influenza show the importance of a responsive public health and primary care workforce collaborating in preparation for, and during, these crises to develop and allocate needed resources.

8. Public health departments' role in convening, facilitating, and mobilizing multidisciplinary, multistakeholder community initiatives makes this sector an invaluable partner in all multisectoral collaborations.

The potential impact of integration on population health is illustrated by the dramatic reduction in cigarette consumption in the late twentieth century. The percentage of American adults who smoke declined over 30 years from approximately 45 percent in 1962 to 25 percent. It is impossible to disentangle the relative contribution to this decline of public health campaigns, physician education of patients, changing social norms, increased cigarette taxes, regulation of smoking, and pharmacotherapies. It is most likely the compounded and synergistic effects of these and other factors—a combination of public health and medical efforts—that fuelled this sea change in health behavior.[69]

Two case studies are presented here to further illustrate integration between the public health and primary care sectors. While these cases are fictitious, they present

CASE 1: TREATMENT AND CONTROL OF INFECTIOUS DISEASES

John S. was a 48-year-old street vendor who shared a cramped apartment with his mother, sister, and his sister's four children. He had a girlfriend who lived at a different address. After a cough persisted for over two months, John S. visited a doctor who, suspecting active pulmonary tuberculosis (TB), consulted with the local health department (LHD) for the most-up-to-date advice on the diagnosis and management of the disease. After an appropriate diagnostic evaluation, with laboratory confirmation, John's doctor started him on treatment and established a care plan to monitor his status, in collaboration with the LHD.

Tom W. was a 38-year-old bisexual physical therapist with a recent diagnosis of HIV infection that had not yet progressed to AIDS. In addition to initiating treatment, his doctor also offered to notify Tom's sexual partners. Concerned that word would spread if his partners were notified about his condition, Tom declined.

In both these cases, the law required that the laboratories providing positive test results and the diagnosing providers report the patient's condition to the LHD. In both cases, the health department followed up with the patients and individuals at risk of disease because of their contact with these patients. For John, the health department identified persons who lived in close contact with him (his mother, sister, and sister's children) or spent significant amount of time with him in closed air space (his girlfriend) or otherwise might have been exposed (the health care workers at his primary care office), and offered them tuberculin skin testing, a clinical evaluation, and prophylactic treatment for those testing positive. The health department's disease investigation specialist, specifically trained to deal with the sensitive issue of a sexually transmitted disease, followed up with Tom and diplomatically elicited the list of his sexual partners, reassuring Tom that he would protect his confidentiality (not revealing the source) when he approached these contacts.

This example of collaboration between primary care and public health demonstrates the support that each provides the other and the benefits of that collaboration for the individual patients initially involved and the broader public.

CASE 2: ADDRESSING OBESITY

Dr. Jones is a pediatrician working in an urban community in the South, who has become concerned about the growing prevalence of obesity among his patients. Dr. Jones cannot recall attending a lecture or case presentation on pediatric obesity during his training in the 1980s. Today, obesity is common and has even been classified as a disease—although there are no clear treatment protocols. Dr. Jones and his patients' families worry that obesity will lead to chronic conditions such as type 2 diabetes. Dr. Jones talks to his patients and their families about obesity, but is frequently met with denial, assertions of blame, and frustration about the likelihood of change. He has extended his practice to include a nutritionist, social worker, and exercise specialist, but the demand exceeds his capacity. Moreover, many patients have refused to meet with his extended team.

Mr. Dolan is director of the local health department, and was recently asked to speak about obesity at a city council meeting. The survey-based data Mr. Dolan presented showed only a small increase in prevalence. Mr. Dolan knows the increase in pediatric obesity is probably greater among the poor sectors of the community than among those with more wealth, so the overall county obesity rate obfuscates the obesity problem among the poor. During the city council meeting, and a later press conference, Mr. Dolan was criticized for having no data reflecting the reality seen by the community and for the fact that his data are almost two years old. Members of the business community, frustrated with rising health care costs

and loss of productivity due to obesity, have suggested that they might relocate. Jones and Dolan have come together to reduce childhood obesity. Dr. Jones convinced other pediatricians to provide the health department with their patients' de-identified data on height, weight, residence (at the census tract-level), race/ethnicity, and age. Health department epidemiologists analyzed these data to produce maps identifying "hot spots" where obesity rates are greatest. Health department staff added the location of low-cost resources for physical activity. These maps were shared with clinicians, community groups, faith-based organizations, and the business community.

With that accomplishment under their belts, the partnership expanded to include a local professor who worked with the pediatricians to ensure that information on obesity rates and community resources would be seamlessly integrated into each practice's electronic medical record. Mr. Dolan engaged the media and Dr. Jones made himself available for interviews. Public health department staff held town hall meetings with community residents to develop strategies to combat obesity. Mr. Dolan convened other city governmental leaders—the school superintendent, the police commissioner, representatives from local public health and child welfare—to discuss a multi-sector approach to the problem. Six months later, Mr. Dolan proposed local policies and regulations aimed at combatting obesity. Providers involved in the partnership rallied their colleagues to advocate for these changes, contributing to their passage.

features of known collaborations. The first example illustrates a long-standing (although not always fully realized) type of partnership between the two sectors addressing infectious disease. The second example demonstrates the collaboration envisioned in current calls for integration, with primary care and public health working together to effect change in chronic disease at the population level.

Despite the history of failed or semisuccessful attempts to bring public health and primary care closer together, many observers think that now is an opportune time for widespread system-level integration of public health and primary care as a way to improve population health. New innovations in integrated health information systems, such as interfaced electronic health records systems or electronic health networks, could provide the population data repository to inform and evaluate integrated community-level preventive and disease interventions. Moreover, state and federal interests in quality care measures provide the policy emphasis to one day realize large-scale community health data sets that can be used to drive joint public health and primary care interventions for populations of people.

The epidemic of chronic disease also poses challenges to both the public health and primary care sectors in their traditional forms. Our traditional model of health care delivery was designed to respond to acute illnesses with drugs or procedures. However, there is no treatment, pill, or vaccine to address the lack of fresh fruits and vegetables to support a healthy diet, limited options for physical activity, exposures to environmental toxins, or the disproportionate distribution of alcohol and tobacco advertising and outlets. Chronic diseases are not currently included among "reportable diseases" for public health surveillance in part because they lack the urgency of an infectious disease outbreak, but also because of the complexity and the number of data sources needed to monitor them. While some chronic diseases can be tracked through laboratory data, others—such as hypertension—cannot. Lack of access to chronic disease data restricts the role public health agencies play in confronting this epidemic. At the same time, primary care cannot adequately support patients with chronic disease in the daily routines and lifestyle changes necessary to manage these diseases.

Both public health and primary care practitioners will need to dramatically change their ways of working and/ or work together (and with other sectors) to meet the challenge of chronic disease.

Finally new models of care, such as Accountable Care Organizations and the PCMH, require primary care providers to incorporate population health thinking and strategies into their practice: the ACA incentivizes providers to partner with other sectors to improve population health and reduce health care utilization. For all these reasons, influential organizations such as the IOM, the National Association of County and City Health Officials, and the Association of State and Territorial Health Officials are calling on both health departments and clinicians to expand beyond their traditional strategies and siloed work to address the unacceptable state of health and health care in the United States by leveraging their respective strengths.

Meeting the Challenge of Integration

If it is true that we are poised to see an unprecedented growth in integrated population health initiatives, it is also true that these initiatives will face many of the same challenges to effective integration confronted in previous years: differences in language and world views, competition for scarce resources and "turf," an unwillingness or inability to do the hard time-consuming work integration requires, and failure to adequately evaluate this work and identify best practices.

The IOM (2012) has delineated five principles for meeting the challenges of integrating public health and primary care:[67]

▸ a shared goal among partners of population health improvement;
▸ community engagement to define and address population health needs;
▸ aligned leadership across partners to reduce fragmentation, clarify roles, create accountability, align incentives with goals, and manage change;
▸ a focus on sustainability of efforts; and
▸ sharing and collaborative use of data and analysis.

Other entities are also offering practical guidance, empirical research, and resources to support integration. This endeavor will grow along with integration itself. A simple but profound reality, however, underlies much of this guidance and research: the recognition that collaboration has both great potential and great challenges— that, despite their common goals, public health and primary care professionals are often divided by competing interests, opposing worldviews, and differing, urgent demands on their time. Effective collaboration requires not only abstract mutual respect and a theoretical commitment to working together, but a willingness to engage in the difficult work of understanding each other and hammering out concrete new ways to work together on a daily basis.

While recognition of this reality should guide integration of primary care and public health, major changes in the financing of primary care and public health services will also be required for success. At present, alignment of financial incentives across the primary care and public health sectors are the exception. More commonly, malalignment of financial incentives causes counterproductive competition for resources, and policy changes lead to disruptions that usurp productive long-term planning. Strong and enduring linkages of funding to evidence-based processes and partnerships that improve population-level health-related outcomes will be needed for successful integration of primary care and public health.

SUMMARY

In many ways, the primary care and public health systems are natural partners. The two sectors share goals of improving integration of and access to health care services, meeting people's basic and essential health care needs, partnering with—and empowering—people to improve their well-being, and understanding and addressing the ways in which families and communities shape health. Many of the strengths of primary care and public health are complementary. While primary care providers have access to their patients and the opportunity to address their individualized health care needs, public health activities reach out to an entire population, including those who do not utilize health care, and can do so on an ongoing basis, addressing multiple determinants of health. The data available to primary care and public health professionals to inform their work are also complementary; primary care data are available in real-time and rich in individual-level medical information, while public health data are population-based and inclusive of environmental factors.

Historically, there have been tensions, as well as commonalities and complementarities between the public health and medical sectors, including primary care. Many observers argue that "integration" of the work of primary care and public health—if done right—can reduce tensions and move us from complementarity in the efforts of these two sectors to the greater benefits of synergy. While there has been a history of unsuccessful or semisuccessful attempts at integrating public health and primary care in the United States, it has been argued that current circumstances provide unusual incentives and opportunities for integration. Effective integration will require development and dissemination of evidence-based best practices and principles and alignment of financial incentives.

REVIEW QUESTIONS

1. What is the importance of primary care for health care delivery? What is its role in promoting population health?

2. What are the key challenges facing the primary care sector in the United States? Name three ways in which policy makers and institutions are attempting to address these.

3. What is "integration" of public health and primary care?

4. Why do some observers consider integration an important vehicle for population health improvement, particularly now?

5. What key concerns (challenges, pitfalls, and principles of practice) should practitioners of integration keep in mind as they do their work?

REFERENCES

1. *Global Strategy for Health for All by the Year 2000* New York: United Nations General Assembly;1981.

2. *Declaration of Alma-Ata International Conference on Primary Health Care.* Alma Ata, USSR September 1978.

3. IOM. *Primary Care: America's Health in a New Era.* Washington D.C.1996.

4. WHO. *The World Health Report 2008: Primary Health Care (Now More Than Ever).* 2008.

5. WHO. 2004; http://www.euro.who.int/en/health-topics/Health-systems/primary-health-care/main-terminology. Accessed December 21, 2014.

6. Ashton J. Public health and primary care: Towards a common agenda. *Public Health.* 1990(104):387–398.

7. Vuori H. Primary health care in Europe—problems and solutions. *Community Medicine.* September 1984;6(3):221–231.

8. Phillips RJ, Starfield B. Why does a US primary care physician workforce crisis matter? *American Family Physician.* October 15, 2003;68(8):1494–1500.

9. Shi L, Macinko J, Starfield B, Politzer R, Xu J. Primary care, race, and mortality in US states. *SocSci Med.* July 2005;61(1):65–75.

10. Starfield B, Shi L, Grover A, Macinko J. The effects of specialist supply on populations' health: assessing the evidence. *Health Affairs.* 2005; January–June(Suppl Web Exclusives):W5-97-W95-107.

11. Starfield B, Shi L, Macinko J. Contribution of primary care to health systems and health. *Milbank Quarterly.* 2005;83(3):457–502.

12. Leiyu S, Starfield B. Primary care, income inequality, and self-rated health in the United States: a mixed-level analysis. *International Journal of Health Services.* 2000(30):541–555.

13. Shi L. The impact of primary care: a focused review. *Scientifica.* 2012:22 pages.

14. Stevens R. The Americanization of family medicine: contradictions, challenges, and change, 1969–2000. *Family Medicine.* 2001;33(4):232–243.

15. Millis J. *The Graduate Education of Physicians: Report of the Citizens' Commission on Graduate Medical Education.* Chicago: American Medical Assocation;1996.

16. Willard_Committee. *Meeting the Challenge of Family Practice: The Report of the Ad Hoc Committee on Education for Family Practice of the Council on Medical Education.* Chicago: American Medical Association;1966.

17. AAFP. American Academy of Family Physicians Annual Residency Census Survey. 2014; http://www.aafp.org/about/the-aafp/family-medicine-facts/table-18.html.

18. AOA. What is a DO? 2014; http://www.osteopathic.org/osteopathic-health/about-dos/what-is-a-do/Pages/default.aspx. Accessed December 4, 2014.

19. Future Osteopathic Physicians Committed to Primary Care Training [press release]. May 7, 2012.

20. AANP. NP Fact Sheet. 2014; http://www.aanp.org/all-about-nps/np-fact-sheet. Accessed December 21, 2014.

21. NCPAA. 2013 Statistical Profile of Certified Physician Assistants. 2013; http://www.nccpa.net/Upload/PDFs/2013StatisticalProfileofCertifiedPhysicianAssistants-AnAnnualReportoftheNCCPA.pdf. Accessed December 21, 2014.

22. AHRQ. The Number of Nurse Practitioners and Physician Assistants Practicing Primary Care in the United States. *Primary Care Workforce Facts and Stats* 2011; http://www.ahrq.gov/research/findings/factsheets/primary/pcwork2/index.html. Accessed December 21, 2014.

23. Blackwell D, Lucas J, Clarke T. *Summary Health Statistics for U.S. Adults: National Health Interview Survey, 2012.* National Center for Health Statistics;2012.

24. Hing E, Hsiao C. *State variability in supply of office-based primary care providers: United States,*

2012. Hyattsville, MD: National Center for Health Statistics;2014.

25. USHDHHS. *Projecting the Supply and Demand for Primary Care Practitioners Through 2020.* Rockville, MD: U.S. Department of Health and Human Services, Health Resources and Services Administration, National Center for Health Workforce Analysis;2013.

26. AAMC. Physician Shortages to Worsen Without Increases in Residency Training. 2010; https://www.aamc.org/download/153160/data/physician_shortages_to_worsen_without_increases_in_residency_tr.pdf.

27. Dunker A, Krofah E, Isasi F. *The Role of Physician Assistants in Health Care Delivery.* Washington DC: National Governors Association Center for Best Practices; September 22, 2014.

28. USDHHS. *Highlights From the 2012 National Sample Survey of Nurse Practitioners. Rockville, Maryland: U.S. Department of Health and Human Services, 2014.* Rockville, MD: U.S. Department of Health and Human Services, Health Resources and Services Administration, National Center for Health Workforce Analysis;2014.

29. AAFP. The Value and Scope of Primary Care. http://www.aafp.org/medical-school-residency/choosing-fm/value-scope.html. Accessed December 21, 2014.

30. HRSA. Shortage Designation: Health Professional Shortage Areas & Medically Underserved Areas/Populations. http://www.hrsa.gov/shortage/. Accessed December 21, 2014.

31. *Physician Distribution and Health Care Challenges in Rural and Inner-City Areas.* Washington DC: US Department of Health and Human Services;1998.

32. KFF. Health Insurance Coverage of the Total Population. 2014; http://kff.org/other/state-indicator/total-population/. Accessed November 24, 2014.

33. KFF. Key Facts about the Uninsured Population. 2014; http://kff.org/uninsured/fact-sheet/key-facts-about-the-uninsured-population/. Accessed November 24, 2014.

34. KFF. Employer-Sponsored Family Health Premiums Rise 3 Percent in 2014. 2014; http://kff.org/health-costs/press-release/employer-sponsored-family-health-premiums-rise-3-percent-in-2014/. Accessed November 24, 2014.

35. Silverman E. Sticking point: the price of an old insulin skyrockets [Wall Street Journal Blog]. 2014; http://blogs.wsj.com/pharmalot/2014/09/11/ sticking-point-the-price-of-an-old-insulin-skyrockets/. Accessed December 21, 2014.

36. US_Census_Bureau. Poverty. 2014; https://www.census.gov/hhes/www/poverty/about/overview/. Accessed December 21, 2014.

37. Syed ST, Gerber BS, Sharp LK. Traveling towards disease: transportation barriers to health care access. *Journal of community health.* 2013;38(5):976–993.

38. Flores G. Language barriers to health care in the United States. *New England Journal of Medicine.* 2006;355(3):229–231.

39. Kullgren J, McLaughlin C, Mitra N, Armstrong K. Nonfinancial barriers and access to care for US adults. *Health Serv Res.* February 2012;47(1 Pt. 2): 462–485.

40. CMS. *Medicaid & CHIP: August 2014 Monthly Applications, Eligibility Determinations and Enrollment Report.* October 17, 2014.

41. HRSA. About Health Centers. http://bphc.hrsa.gov/success/criticalconnections.htm. Accessed November 16, 2006.

42. HRSA. Health Center Data. 2013; http://bphc.hrsa.gov/healthcenterdatastatistics/. Accessed December 1, 2014.

43. NACHC. *America's Health Centers.* October 2014.

44. O'Malley A, Mandelblatt J. Delivery of preventive services for low income persons over age 50: a comparison of community health clinics to private doctors' offices. *J Community Health.* 2003;28(3):185–197.

45. NHSC. About the NHSC. http://nhsc.hrsa.gov/corpsexperience/aboutus/index.html. Accessed November 24, 2014.

46. Holmes G. Does the National Health Service Corps improve physician supply in underserved locations? *Eastern Economic Journal.* 2004;30(4):563–581.

47. Garrison-Jakel J. Patching the rural workforce pipeline—why don't we do more? *Journal of Rural Health.* 2011;27(2):239–240.

48. Physician Shortage Area Program 2014; http://www.jefferson.edu/university/jmc/psap.html. Accessed November, 2014.

49. HRSA. Area Health Education Centers. http://bhpr.hrsa.gov/grants/areahealtheducationcenters/. Accessed December 21, 2014.

50. NAO. *2013 Annual Report.* National Area Health Education Centers Organization;2013.

51. Petterson S, Liaw W, Phillips Jr RL, Rabin D, Meyers D, Bazemore A. Projecting US primary

care physician workforce ceeds: 2010–2025. *Annals of Family Medicine.* November/December 2012;10(6):503–509.

52. Bodenheimer T, Laing BY. The teamlet model of primary care. *The Annals of Family Medicine.* 2007;5(5):457–461.

53. IOM. *Crossing the quality chasm: a new health system for the 21st century.* Washington DC: Committee on Quality of Health Care in America, Institute of Medicine;2001.

54. Smedley B, Stith A, Nelson A. *Unequal Treatment: Confronting Racial and Ethnic Disparities in Health Care.* Washington DC: Committee on Understanding and Eliminating Racial and Ethnic Disparities in Health Care;2002.

55. Zerhouni E. Translational and clinical science — time for a new vision. *N Engl J Med.* October 13 2005(353):1621–1623.

56. Østbye T, Yarnall KS, Krause KM, Pollak KI, Gradison M, Michener JL. Is there time for management of patients with chronic diseases in primary care? *The Annals of Family Medicine.* 2005;3(3):209–214.

57. Graham N. *Quality in Health Care: Theory, Application and Evolution.* Gaithersburg, MD: Aspen Publishers; 1995.

58. http://www.cochrane.org/. Accessed December 21, 2014.

59. AHRQ. Clinicians and Providers. http://www.ahrq.gov/professionals/clinicians-providers/index.html. Accessed December 21, 2014.

60. FPIN. 2014; http://www.fpin.org/. Accessed December 21, 2014.

61. Green L, Hickner J. A short history of primary care practice-based research networks: from concept to essential research laboratories. *Journal of the American Board of Family Medicine.* January–February 2006;19(1):1–10.

62. Clinical and Translational Science Awards: Foundations for Accelerated Discovery and Efficient Translation Progress Report 2009–2011. U.S. Department of Health and Human Services.

63. Berwick D, Nolan T, Whittington J. The triple aim: care, health, and cost. *Health Affairs.* 2008;27(3):759–769.

64. Heckler M. *Report of the Secretary's Task Force on Black and Minority Health.* Washington DC: US Department of Health and Human Services;1985–1986.

65. USDHHS. Healthy People 2020—Disparities. 2014; http://www.healthypeople.gov/2020/about/foundation-health-measures/Disparities. Accessed December 21, 2014.

66. Kindig D, Stoddart G. What is population health? *Am J Public Health.* March 2003;93(3):380–383.

67. IOM. *Primary Care and Public Health: Exploring Integration to Improve Population Health.* Washington DC;2012.

68. Elliott L, McBride TD, Allen P, et al. Health care system collaboration to address chronic diseases: a nationwide snapshot from state public health practitioners. *Preventing Chronic Disease.* 2014;11.

69. Brandt A, Gardner M. Antagonism and accommodation: interpreting the relationship between public health and medicine in the United States during the 20th century. *Am J Public Health.* May 2000;90(5):707–714.

70. NACHHO. *2013 National Profile of Local Health Departments.* The National Connection for Local Public Health;2014.

71. Wall S. Transformations in public health systems. *Health Affairs.* 1998;17(3):64–80.

72. Jones M. *Protecting Public Health in New York City: 200 Years of Leadership.* New York: New York City Department of Health and Mental Hygiene;2005.

73. Nutting P. Community-oriented primary care: an integrated model for practice, research, and education. *Am J Prev Med.* 1986(2):140–147.

74. Cooper R, Kennelly J, Orduñez-Garcia P. Health in Cuba. *International Journal of Epidemiology.* 2006;35(4):817–824.

75. Kark S. Community-oriented primary health care: a review. *COPaCETIC.* 1998;5(1):1–6.

76. Lasker RD. Medicine and public health: the power of collaboration. 1998.

77. Marquardt D. Improvement in rural neonatal mortality: A case study of medical community intervention. *Fam Med.* 1993;23:269–274.

78. Frame P. Is community-oriented primary care a viable concept in actual practice? An affirmative view. *J Fam Pract.* 1989;28:203–208.

79. Mittelmark M, Luepker R, Grimm RJ, Kottke T, Blackburn H. The Role of Physicians in a Community-Wide Program for Prevention of Cardiovascular Disease: The Minnesota Heart Disease Program. *Public Health Reports.* 1998;103(4):360–365.

80. O'Connor P. Is community-oriented primary care a viable concept in actual practice? An opposing view. *J Fam Pract.*28(2):206–209.

81. Sava S, Armitage K, Kaufman A. It's time to integrate public health into medical education and clinical care. *Journal of Public Health Management and Practice.* May/June 2013;19(3):197–198.

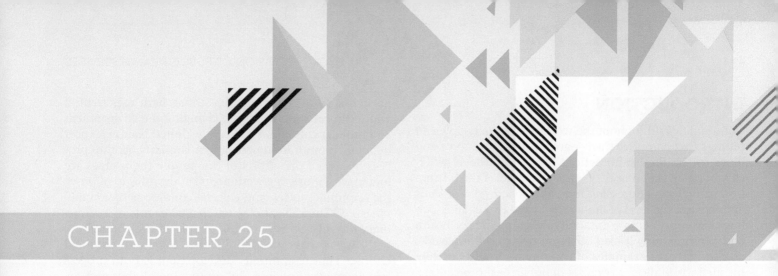

CHAPTER 25

Community Development for Population Health and Health Equity

Stephen Fawcett, PhD • Jerry Schultz, PhD • Vicki Collie-Akers, PhD • Christina Holt, MA • Jomella Watson-Thompson, PhD

LEARNING OBJECTIVES

Upon completion of this chapter, the reader will be able to:

1. Describe key concepts of community health and development such as community development, collaborative action, and community/population health.

2. Differentiate models of community organization practice (i.e., locality development, social planning, social action).

3. Describe three models of community health promotion.

4. Describe the phases and processes of the framework for collaborative action.

5. Discuss the evidence for community development approaches.

6. Understand and apply core competencies for a community health and development workforce.

KEY TERMS

capacity building
community development
community development workforce
community health
health equity
population health

INTRODUCTION

Communities throughout the world—and the people and settings that comprise them—are a primary resource and locus for public health action. In this multilevel work, collaborative action at the community level is the fulcrum between efforts addressing individuals and relationships and those at the level of broader systems. This chapter outlines key concepts in community development for health and health equity. It also offers models and frameworks and several case examples of community health development efforts in diverse contexts of public health practice.

COMMUNITY HEALTH AND ITS DEVELOPMENT

The work of assuring conditions for health and well-being occurs in and with communities; that is, those who share a common place, interest, and/or experience. It occurs in a variety of places—cities and towns, urban neighborhoods, and rural villages. This work engages those with shared interests—for example, people concerned with the incidence of infant mortality or childhood obesity or in addressing health disparities and the conditions that produce them. Community health development engages those with diverse experiences—such as those experiencing violence or exposure to hazards as well as those with technical expertise in community health assessment, planning, and intervention. Exhibit 25-1 describes what community development actually looks like at the ground level.

Some Key Concepts of Community Health and Development

Community development is the process of people working together to affect locally determined issues/goals and the conditions that affect them.[1] An enduring theme is participation of local people—those with experiential and technical knowledge—in changing the environment and broader conditions.[2] An early United Nations report defined community development similarly, as the "process by which the efforts of the people themselves are united with those of governmental authorities to improve the economic, social, and cultural conditions of communities...."[3] The U.N. also stated that a key role of intermediary organizations is to link people of the community with outside resources to advance locally determined efforts.[4] Thus, community development is both process (engagement of people and groups in collaborative action) and product (changed conditions and improved outcomes related to locally determined goals).

In the context of public health practice, the aim of community development is collaborative action for community health improvement.[5] Community/population health improvement requires the engagement of:

a) multiple agents of change (e.g., community residents, local and state organizations),

b) working together across sectors (e.g., governmental units, businesses, faith communities, health and human service organizations),

c) over time (e.g., multiple years), and

d) across ecological levels (e.g., individuals, relationships, community).[6]

Community development is closely related to the work of health promotion at the community level.[7,8] Health promotion refers to the "process of enabling people to increase control over and to improve their health.[2]"An ecological model of health promotion sees population health as an interaction among behavior and personal and environmental factors at multiple ecological levels.[9] As a process of community development, health promotion is ongoing and gradual—unfolding over time, not a one-time response to a

EXHIBIT 25-1 What does the Work of Community Development for Health Look Like?

Media coverage of community health problems shows our city to be lagging far behind others. Childhood obesity and chronic diseases are rising, poverty is high, educational outcomes are low, and access to health services is limited, and some disadvantaged groups are particularly affected. The mayor convened a group—the Healthy City Partnership—to engage community members and organizations in addressing these issues. The county health department agreed to serve as the lead organization—engaging governmental units, schools, health and human service organizations, community organizations, advocacy groups, and local community foundations. Community assessments—using existing data sources, focus groups, and surveys—helped determine the level of particular problems/goals as well as community assets and top concerns. The Partnership's organizational structure reflected its goals: an overall Community Advisory Board and four targeted action committees, including healthy nutrition, physical activity, poverty, and access to health services. Action planning for each goal area (and related committee) helped establish priority strategies and opportunities for assuring environmental conditions needed to meet targeted outcomes. Open monthly meetings—held in a trusted community center—assured space for people and organizations to plan, communicate, and support collaborative action. A monitoring and evaluation system enabled the group to document and systematically reflect on its activities and outcomes, be accountable, and make needed adjustments.

crisis or outbreak. The product of health promotion is a continuum of outputs and outcomes, including:

a) development activities (e.g., planning, training, and capacity building);

b) targeted action (e.g., intervention, advocacy for policy changes);

c) community and systems change (e.g., environmental and policy changes related to targeted goals and objectives);

d) widespread behavior change; and

e) improvement in population-level outcomes (e.g., incidence and prevalence of childhood obesity or violence).[5,6,10]

Social justice and equity demand the elimination of health disparities: going beyond improvement in community-level indicators for the overall population to seek reductions in differences for marginalized groups. Health disparities/inequalities refer to potentially avoidable differences in health (and associated risks) between groups of people who are more and less advantaged socially.[11] A human rights perspective calls for all people and communities to have the right to conditions conducive to health and well-being (e.g., access to healthy food and clean water, education and health services; protection from hazards) and meaningful participation and power in influencing those conditions (e.g., through political rights, fully functioning civil society).[11,12]

The World Health Organization (WHO) reminds us of what is required for health for all: "Without peace and justice, without enough food and water, without education and decent housing, and without providing each and all with a useful role in society and adequate income, there can be no health for the people, no real growth and no social development."[13]

Assuring conditions for health equity requires attention to social determinants of health (SDH).[14,15] The WHO conceptual framework for action on social determinants[16] outlines three levels of determinants that interact to affect equity in health and well-being:

a) structural drivers (e.g., taxation, environmental protections and policies; governance; societal norms);

b) social position and stratification determinants (e.g., social class, race/ethnicity, education, income); and

c) intermediary determinants (e.g., material circumstances, behaviors, and biological factors; psychosocial factors; health care system).

(See Chapter 3 for more detail on social determinants of health.)

Community development approaches for health and health equity seek to change personal and environmental factors related to the priority issues/goals by, for instance, providing information and services, modifying access

and opportunities/exposures, and assuring supportive policies. Community development approaches also seek to change the mechanisms by which social determinants produce inequities. They aim to reduce:

a) differential exposure to intermediary factors (e.g., through policies that reduce exposures to hazards, and assure access to healthy food and decent housing);

b) differential vulnerability to health-compromising conditions (e.g., by enhancing opportunities for early childhood education, training for jobs that pay a sufficient wage); and

c) differential consequences (e.g., assuring access to quality health services for everyone).

When a place has these qualities, WHO refers to it as a healthy community—whether a healthy city, municipality, or village.[13]

MODELS OF COMMUNITY DEVELOPMENT FOR HEALTH

This section leads with several prominent models of community development and health promotion from the fields of community organization and public health. It concludes with a framework for collaborative action for population health and health equity.

Models of Community Organization Practice

Rothman and colleagues[16] differentiate three distinct models of community organization that can be applied to population health improvement: locality development, social planning, and social action (see Table 25-1). The model of *locality development* recognizes the importance of engaging indigenous people, local residents and groups, as the community experts who are well positioned to inform selection of priority goals and development of interventions that fit culture and context. It focuses on building the capacity of individuals (e.g., residents) and groups (e.g., community organizations, nongovernmental organizations) to support community action. Bringing local people together to identify a common vision and shared goals for community health and development is seen as critical for community ownership and sustainability of efforts. The *social planning* model is an expert-based approach for addressing complex community health and development issues.[16] It focuses on providing technical solutions through the development and implementation of plans and policies. The premise is that efforts to influence systems through the community development process should be guided by individuals with established relationships in the community (e.g., elders, trusted leaders) and those with

TABLE 25-1 A Comparison of Three Models of Community Organization Practice

Locality Development	Social Planning	Social Action
Engage local residents and groups	Convene professionals and experts	Mobilize those experiencing the problem
Build capacity to support community action	Develop technical solutions through planning	Ensure disenfranchised groups are heard
Create common vision and shared goals	Focus on getting results	Social justice is a key value

professional expertise and linkages with those systems (e.g., urban planners, agency administrators).

The *social action* model focuses on mobilizing populations and groups experiencing disparities or inequalities in efforts to improve health and development outcomes. It often involves organizing disenfranchised groups to ensure their vision, voice, and power in addressing issues of social injustice and inequities.[16]

Some Models of Community Health Promotion

Healthy Cities and Communities Model

The Healthy Cities and Communities framework was developed by the World Health Organization's Healthy Cities program.[17] It promotes locally determined, comprehensive strategies to enhance overall health and well-being of residents—physical, mental, and social.[13] The Healthy Cities framework provides a step-by-step participatory process for prioritizing and addressing issues, including:

a) getting started (e.g., knowing the context by conducting community assessments);

b) getting organized (e.g., developing a community health plan that summarizes the vision and goals of the project); and

c) taking action (e.g., encouraging community participation; engaging multiple sectors and levels).

Mobilizing for Action through Planning and Partnerships (MAPP)

This approach was codeveloped by the National Association of County and City Health Officials (NACCHO) and the U.S. Centers for Disease Control and Prevention (CDC).[18] MAPP has six phases that structure the process:

1) organizing for success;
2) visioning;
3) assessing (i.e., using a community themes and strengths assessment, a local public health system assessment, a community health status assessment, and a forces of change assessment);
4) identifying strategic issues;
5) setting goals/strategies; and
6) conducting an action cycle.

The planning/implementation/evaluation cycle continues until the community achieves its vision; it then generates a new vision to work toward.

Healthy People 2020 MAP-IT Framework

This is intended to help guide implementation efforts related to achieving health objectives for the nation.[19] The MAP-IT process begins with the **M**obilization of individuals and groups, typically through a coalition or group of individuals and organizations that assemble to address issues in the community. Next, coalition members and community stakeholders work together to **A**ssess the needs and resources/assets present in the community. Based on the assessment, community problems and goals are identified and prioritized. Then, a strategic **P**lan is developed that specifies measurable objectives, which serve as indicators of change and improvement. The plan also identifies clear strategies and action steps necessary to support attainment of the objectives. To **I**mplement the plan, coalition members and key stakeholders work collaboratively to facilitate changes in the community. **T**racking is an ongoing part of the process: data are collected, analyzed, and reviewed to evaluate progress and make adjustments. For tools for implementing MAP-IT, Healthy People 2020 offers links to the Community Tool Box and other resources. (These tools can be accessed at https://www.healthypeople.gov by searching "Mobilize.")

Framework for Collaborative Action for Population Health and Health Equity

The Institute of Medicine's (IOM) report on *The Future of Public Health in the 21st Century* offered a framework for collaborative public health action in communities.[5,10] Figure 25-1 displays an adapted version of this framework for population health and health equity;[6] it includes five phases in this iterative process (see A–E in Figure 25-1), along with 12 associated community development processes. These five phases illustrate a path toward community health improvement—from assessing, prioritizing, and planning, to implementing targeted action, changing conditions and systems, achieving widespread change in behavior, and to improving population health outcomes.

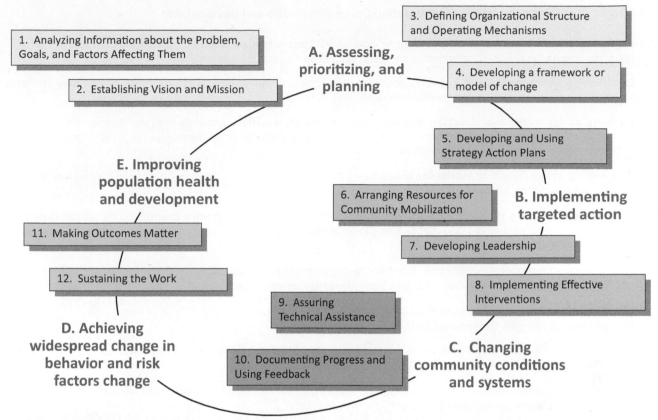

FIGURE 25-1 **Framework for Collaborative Action for Population Health and Health Equity, and Associated Community Development Processes**

Adapted from the "Framework for collaborative public health action," as cited in The Future of the Public's Health in the 21st century.

As referenced in Table 25-2 and outlined in the Community Tool Box (accessed at http://ctb.ku.edu by clicking on the "Help Taking Action" and "Best Change Processes" links), 12 processes are often associated with promoting community health and development.[6,8,20–22]

EVIDENCE BASE FOR COMMUNITY DEVELOPMENT APPROACHES

Do community development approaches work in bringing about community/system change and improvement in population-level outcomes? Under what conditions are changes in communities and systems sufficient to improve population-level outcomes? These are reasonable questions that are easier to ask than to answer.

Evidence Base for Bringing about Community/System Change

The underlying principles of community health[2] and frameworks for collaborative public health action[5] suggest that broad and comprehensive interventions (i.e., multiple community/system changes) are needed to effect widespread behavior change and improvement

in population-level outcomes. Systematic reviews, such as the *Guide to Community Preventive Services*,[23] recommend more comprehensive interventions. Community development approaches—including community mobilization and collaborative planning and implementation—are seen as a way to change conditions in a comprehensive and sustainable way.

There is a modest evidence base for community development processes associated with changes in communities and systems.[22] Since randomized trials—in which some communities engage in community development approaches and others do not—are typically not possible, this evidence is based largely on quasi-experimental designs and the logic of multiple case studies.[24] Using a common measurement system to detect instances of community change (i.e., new or modified programs, policies, and practices), we can look for the strength and prevalence of association between particular development processes—such as action planning—and related accelerations in the rate of community change.[20,25] As noted in the framework for collaborative action (see Figure 25-1), there is modest evidence for some promising community development processes, for instance: analyzing problems and using data to set priorities for targeted action;

TABLE 25-2   Processes Associated with Promoting Community Health and Development

1. **Analyzing information about the problem or goal and factors affecting them**—This enables collaborative efforts to focus on specific goals, risk/protective factors, and targets and agents of change.

2. **Establishing a clear vision and mission**—More focused community efforts are associated with higher rates of change than more diffuse efforts working on multiple outcomes.

3. **Defining an organizational structure and operating mechanisms**—These enhance opportunities for community participation and engagement; they help create a cohesive environment for working together to strengthen implementation and help assure sustainability.

4. **Developing a framework or model for change**—By conveying a presumed pathway, they help guide planning, action, and evaluation phases of the work.

5. **Developing and using strategic and action plans**—Identifying specific community changes to be sought in each relevant sector and who would do what to bring them about has been consistently followed by increases in rates of community change.

6. **Arranging for community mobilizers**—Community organizers help assure better implementation of community-determined action plans than when change efforts rely solely on volunteers.

7. **Developing leadership**—Distributed leadership can protect against the adverse effects of loss of leadership that are typically associated with decreased rates of community change.

8. **Implementing effective interventions**—Collaborative partnerships aim to assure selection and full implementation of evidence-based practices while tailoring interventions to the local context.

9. **Assuring technical assistance**—Training, technical support, and consultation are often needed to build local capacity for what key practices to implement, and under what conditions.

10. **Documenting progress and using feedback**—Documentation and feedback provide information that permits ongoing learning, adjustments, and accountability in the effort.

11. **Making outcome matter**—Contingencies, such as bonus grants for high rates of change and outcome dividends for improvement in population-level outcomes, assure incentives for actual progress.

12. **Sustaining the work**—Improvement in population-level outcomes often requires more time than is funded by external funding agents, making it critical to sustain interventions and the efforts that assure them.

developing leadership and assuring technical assistance; developing and using strategic action plans to guide action; implementing effective interventions that fit the local context; and documenting progress and using the information for accountability and making adjustments.[6,22,26,27,28,29,30,31]

Evidence Base for Improvement in Population-level Outcomes

Community partnerships aim to bring about changes in conditions, such as environmental and policy changes, so that they can effect widespread behavior change (e.g., increased healthy eating, physical activity, reduced tobacco use) and improvements in population-level outcomes (e.g., reduced BMI, incidence of cardiovascular diseases and diabetes). Some recent research suggests that to effect population-level outcomes, community/system changes need to be of sufficient amount and intensity—i.e., strength of intervention strategy, duration, and reach.[32,33]

However, the evidence is mixed as to how well community partnerships improve outcomes at either the level of behavioral risk/protective factors or population-level health outcomes.[34] Some systematic reviews reported that from 9 to 44 percent of the reviewed studies showed improvements that could in some way be attributable to the initiative.[35,36] One plausible explanation is that effect sizes with a whole community or population (e.g., with all children in a city) will likely be much smaller and harder to detect than for more highly specific interventions involving a targeted group (e.g., 50 children enrolled in a school intervention). When the community (not individuals) is the unit of analysis, it is less feasible to engage enough communities in a study (i.e., perhaps 8–10 minimally, for each condition); and this makes it unlikely that statistical analyses will have enough power to detect small differences. The outcomes may take longer to emerge when implemented by community members; yet, most studies are five years or less in duration.

There is broad agreement that more evidence is needed. Yet, there is still a long way to go in producing strong evidence for the community development approach. We need greater support for comprehensive multicommunity studies, improved research designs, and deeper focus and improved analysis that can lead to better understanding of the community development processes that contribute to changes in conditions sufficient to "tip" population-level improvement. Until that time, the logic of multiple case studies can help us address these gaps in evidence- and practice-based knowledge.

THREE CASE EXAMPLES OF COMMUNITY DEVELOPMENT APPROACHES IN PUBLIC HEALTH PRACTICE

This section describes three case studies of community development efforts, each featuring a different approach in public health practice: community health planning and improvement efforts; collaborative partnerships for population health and health equity; and community-based participatory research. Each approach is illustrated with a specific case example with which the authors have been engaged.

Case Example 1: Community Health Planning and Improvement

Background and Context

Accreditation standards for local, state, and tribal health departments, as well as the Patient Protection and Affordable Care Act, call for improved approaches to community health assessment and implementation of planned improvements. These are consistent with the core functions and essential services of public health.[5, 37–39] There are a number of prominent models of community health improvement; they include the MAPP Framework[40] of the National Association of County and City Health Officials (NACCHO/CDC), and those of the Catholic Health Association[41] and the Association for Community Health Improvement[42] (ACHI). This section offers a case example of a community health improvement effort grounded in the Institute of Medicine's framework for collaborative action for population health and health equity. This work began in 2011 and is led by the Lawrence-Douglas County (Kansas)

Health Department (LDCHD), with support from the University of Kansas' Work Group for Community Health and Development.

Core Practices for Community Health Planning and Improvement

This section outlines key implementation tasks for community health planning and improvement efforts based on a report to the CDC on core practice areas.[43] Each of these 11 practices—grounded in the community development approach—is illustrated with implementation examples from the community health improvement effort led by the LDCHD.[44]

1. **Assure shared ownership of the process among stakeholders**. Determining stakeholders' interests and establishing working agreements with clear roles and responsibilities help set the conditions for success. For instance, in the LDCHD effort, the Health Department spearheaded a comprehensive community health assessment. The dual aim was to promote the public's health and to meet NACCHO accreditation standards for a local health department. It engaged a variety of key community stakeholders, including the United Way of Douglas County, the Douglas County Community Health Improvement Partnership, Lawrence Memorial Hospital, Heartland Community Health Center, and the Douglas County Community Foundation.

2. **Assure ongoing involvement of community members**. Seeking involvement of community members and groups through the entire process—from assessment through planning and implementation—is critical for successful efforts. To do so, it is important to make participation and involvement as easy as possible. More than 1,500 community members were involved in the LDCHD community health improvement effort, including: respondents to surveys distributed online and in dozens of locations; participants in focus groups held in community centers, neighborhoods, and places of worship; those in key informant interviews; participants in a Local Public Health System Assessment; and a health-related Photovoice project engaging local youth.

3. **Use small area analysis to identify communities with health disparities**. This method, also known as "spot mapping," helps identify communities with disproportionate unmet health needs in specific geographic locations.[45] This involves geo-mapping of the incidence and prevalence of health issues to help identify places experiencing health disparities. In the LDCHD community health improvement effort, small area analysis was

used to better understand how poverty and outcomes, such as emergency department utilization for particular health conditions, were concentrated in specific areas of the county.

4. **Collect and use information on social determinants of health**. Collecting information related to social determinants of health (e.g., income, education, housing)—and addressing social determinants in the improvement plan—is critical to meaningful and long-lasting improvement efforts. In the LDCHD community health improvement effort, data were collected on rates and concentrations of poverty and educational attainment, and the community health improvement plan set poverty and job creation as a priority issue.

5. **Collect information on community assets**. Community assessment includes working with local partners to identify available community assets and resources for addressing prioritized community needs. In the LDCHD effort, community members identified more than 90 community assets through focus groups and interviews, including the local hospital, public schools, local service agencies, the health department, parks and recreation, local universities, faith communities, mental health center, the United Way, government agencies, the transit system, and features of the built environment.

6. **Use explicit criteria and processes to set priorities**. Priority setting for action involves establishing agreed-upon criteria such as evidence of effectiveness and fit with the local context.[8] It also involves identifying processes, such as community involvement in ranking, to inform prioritization of issues to be addressed in the community health improvement plan. In the LDCHD effort, results from each assessment method were carefully reviewed to find convergence, and a series of local forums were convened for community members to provide input on the results. Community members were invited to participate in priority setting. Five priority issues were chosen to be addressed by the plan: access to health services, healthy foods, mental health, physical activity, and poverty/jobs.

7. **Assure shared investment and commitments of diverse stakeholders**. Shared investment in community health improvement efforts requires shared responsibility. This includes pledges of financial and human resources for implementation of prioritized strategies from stakeholders in different sectors of the community, such as from government, schools, and health organizations. In

the LDCHD effort, many community organizations are helping with implementation of parts of the community health improvement plan. For instance, the United Way of Douglas County has encouraged grantees to report on how they are contributing to implementation of the improvement plan, and the LDCHD has funded new positions to support implementation of the plan.

8. **Participatory monitoring and evaluation of CHI efforts**. In a participatory evaluation approach, stakeholders are involved in identifying indicators of success for each community-determined goal area. This helps to assure measures for accountability—and information for quality improvement—that are accurate, feasible to collect, and sensitive to the context. In the LDCHD effort, community stakeholders from different organizations were trained to systematically document accomplishments related to the community health improvement plan using an online documentation and support system,[46] and to use those data for sense-making, making needed adjustments, and accountability for achieving progress.

9. **Collaborate across sectors to implement comprehensive strategies**. Engaging diverse stakeholders from various sectors—including government, business, education, health, human services, and faith communities—helps ensure implementation of comprehensive strategies for health improvement. In the LDCHD effort, diverse stakeholders have been engaged throughout the process. Continuous communication and outreach efforts are in place to engage partners from all relevant community sectors.

10. **Establish oversight mechanisms**. Once a community health improvement plan is developed, it is important to establish a governance structure and procedures for monitoring effective implementation of the plan. This should include reviewing data periodically and communicating progress to different stakeholders. In the LDCHD effort, the steering committee meets periodically to review progress on implementation of the plan.

11. **Create formal public reporting processes**. Public reporting assures transparency and accountability to the community. It can help raise awareness and build public support for collaborative public health action. In the early implementation of the LDCHD effort, focus groups with community partners were used to assess satisfaction with progress on each prioritized goal area and to obtain community recommendations for improvement.

These steps—from early and ongoing engagement of community members to public accountability—reflect a community development approach to the work of community health improvement.

Case Example 2: Collaborative Partnership for Population Health and Health Equity

Background and Context

Collaborative partnerships are a prominent strategy for intersectoral action for population health and health equity.[6] Established in 2009, the Latino Health for All (LHFA) Coalition is a multisector partnership made up of over 40 community partners. It is supported by a scientific and technical assistance partner, the University of Kansas' Work Group for Community Health and Development. The LHFA Coalition's vision is to "assure health for all"; its mission is to "reduce diabetes and cardiovascular disease among Latinos in Kansas City/Wyandotte County (Kansas) through a collaborative partnership to promote healthy nutrition, physical activity, and access to health services." This ongoing effort has been supported by grants from the National Institute on Minority Health and Health Disparities, the CDC, and community foundations.

Core Elements of the Health for All Model

To address health disparities, the LHFA Coalition implemented the Health for All Model.[47] As depicted in Figure 25-2, this model is also grounded in a community development approach and the Institute of Medicine's Framework for Collaborative Public Health Action.[5,10] The Health for All Model uses five key elements to support community mobilization and community-based participatory research[47] (CBPR). These elements include:

1. **Establishing an organizational structure**. This involves creating organizational arrangements, such as action committees, that promote community participation, decision-making, and targeted action.[48,49] The LHFA Coalition established a Community Advisory Board to provide guidance about the general direction of the coalition, and to make decisions about allocation of funds. The Coalition had three Action Committees, one for each of its goal areas: Healthy nutrition, Physical activity, and Access to health services. The goals were chosen by community representatives based on existing community health assessments and the experience of residents and organizational representatives. Coalition membership has been represented by a broad cross section of people (e.g., members of the local Latino community; agency staff) and community sectors

(e.g., government, health organizations, community and cultural organizations).

2. **Action planning to identify community-determined strategies**. Beginning in 2009 (and periodically thereafter), the membership of the LHFA Coalition developed (and updated) a comprehensive community action plan. Specified for each action committee/goal area, this consisted of a listing of prioritized community/systems changes (programs, policies, and practices) that would be implemented by community partners to enhance health behaviors and reduce health disparities. Examples from among the dozens of priority strategies included:

   a) establishing community gardens (nutrition),
   b) creating more spaces for physical activity/soccer (physical activity), and
   c) increasing the availability of health services for which high-quality translation services were available (access to health services).

The action plan provided multiple niches of opportunity for community engagement; it pinpointed where community members and organizational partners could add their contribution to the shared mission.

3. **Community mobilization to stimulate involvement and action**. Community mobilizers have been employed continuously throughout the LHFA Coalition's operation. The community mobilizers' core tasks included:

   a) creating and maintaining opportunities for engagement of LHFA Coalition members and partners;
   b) supporting partners—including Latinos and Latino-serving organizations—in taking action on community-determined strategies;
   c) serving as the public face and point person for the LHFA Coalition; and
   d) assuring technical support for implementation of the community action plan by LHFA Coalition members and partners.

4. **Distribution of resources to support implementation of the action plan**. To support implementation of the action plan, "mini-grants" were distributed to community partner organizations. The community-determined strategies in the action plan were used by the Action Committees to generate ideas for projects and to identify prospective implementers. LHFA members and other community organizations created proposals (e.g., for community gardens, soccer field). Once reviewed and approved by the Action Committee, applications were forwarded to the Community Advisory Board (CAB). All decisions as to whether to fund, and at what

amount, were made by the CAB. The CAB was composed of cochairs of each action committee and two at-large members; scientific partners did not have a vote. Mini-grants (typically $10,000 or less each) were distributed by the CAB during the Coalition's initial five years in operation, and thereafter when resources were available.

5. **Documentation and feedback on progress to promote understanding and improvement**. As discussed in the third case example (below), participatory research methods were used throughout all phases of the project. Scientific partners and community mobilizers, with input from LHFA Coalition members, were responsible for recording the discrete activities and community/system changes brought about by the Coalition to promote physical activity,

healthy nutrition, and access to health services. The resulting information—for instance, graphs of the amount and kind of community/system changes—was shared regularly with the LHFA Coalition to occasion reflection on what we are seeing, what it means, and implications for adjustment.[46,50] Reports were produced containing information about LHFA Coalition performance and resulting adjustments made by the Coalition.

Case Example 3: Community-Based Participatory Research (CBPR)
Background and Context
Community-based participatory research (CPBR) is a "collaborative approach to research that equitably involves

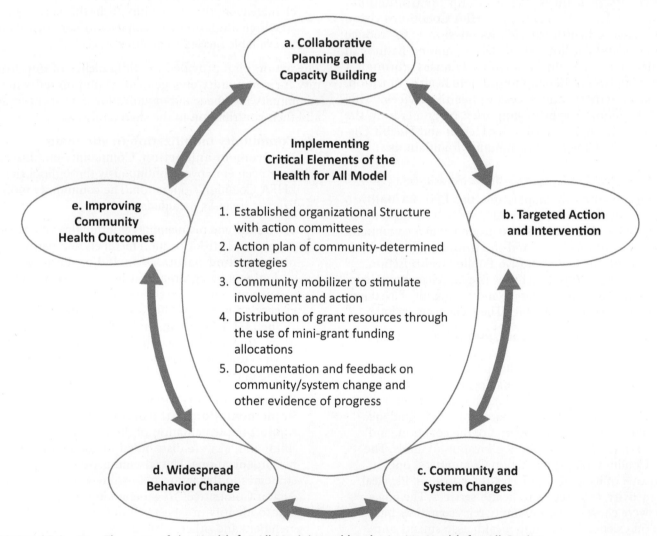

FIGURE 25-2   Five Elements of the Health for All Model Used by the Latino Health for All Coalition

Journal of prevention & intervention in the community by Haworth Press. Reproduced with permission of Haworth Press in the format reuse in a book/textbook via Copyright Clearance Center.

all partners in the research process and recognizes the unique strengths that each brings."[51] Viswanathan and colleagues[52] indicated that essential elements of CBPR include opportunities for colearning by all research partners, a shared role in decision-making, and shared ownership over research processes and products. Researchers have noted that CBPR is a paradigm particularly well-suited to address community development approaches to improve population health and health equity since it helps bridge historical issues, such as distrust, and enhances support for interventions that were codeveloped.[53] CBPR was a key approach used by the Latino Health for All (LFHA) Coalition and its scientific partner (University of Kansas); they worked together in the context of this case example.[26,47]

Principles of Community-Based Participatory Research (CBPR)

Schulz and colleagues[54] articulated a set of principles for CBPR that reflect core aspects of a community development approach. This section outlines how each of the nine CBPR principles was implemented by scientific and community partners as part of the LHFA Coalition's efforts.

1. **CBPR recognizes community as a unit of identity**. Through dialogue, scientific and community partners worked to better understand how Latino community members experienced conditions that put them at risk for health disparities related to chronic diseases, including diabetes and cardiovascular disease. The community was defined as Latino residents residing in a particular low-income area in Kansas City, Kansas. Through years of engagement with community members and partners, scientific partners learned more about how community members perceived and defined their community as shared place, interests, and experiences.

2. **CBPR builds on strengths and resources within the community**. Scientific partners and community members sought to assure engagement of the community in all phases of the community development process, including assessment and collaborative planning, implementation of community-determined strategies, reviewing data and making sense of the findings, and making adjustments. This action cycle was designed to maximize community engagement and utilization of local assets and resources. For example, efforts to assure access to health services benefitted from engagement of existing, highly valued and trusted community health care organizations. Similarly, as part of the nutrition

action committee, a community member with an interest in gardening was identified as a champion, and she ultimately provided leadership for seeing the number of community and residential gardens in the area triple in a three-year period.

3. **CBPR facilitates collaborative, equitable partnership in all phases of research**. The membership of the LHFA Coalition, as well as scientific partners, have been engaged in all phases of participatory research. The Coalition-determined community action plan guided the work of the LHFA Coalition, and the Community Advisory Board made decisions about funding for implementing community-determined strategies. Periodically, members review patterns in the data and reflect on what it means—for instance, what factors (e.g., adding a new community mobilizer) may have led to increases/decreases in activities—and implications for adjustment.

4. **CBPR promotes colearning and capacity building among all partners**. Scientific and community partners contribute in ways that are consistent with their respective strengths. For instance, during the initial development and periodic revisions of the community action plan, scientific partners contributed their knowledge and experience with identifying evidence-based policies and practices; and community members contributed their understanding of the community and local context. This information has been used to prioritize selected strategies and to better understand needed adaptation. Capacity building has occurred through both informal and formal colearning, training, and technical support. The capacity of researchers to understand the complexity of problems has been enhanced by being engaged on the ground and working alongside community members. More formal workshops and technical support were provided to enhance capacity of community members (e.g., to engage in grant-writing or planning for sustainability).

5. **CBPR integrates and achieves a balance between research and action for the mutual benefit of all partners**. Partners balanced the needs of the funded research with the LHFA membership's focus on action to change conditions in the community. Ongoing dialogue among community and scientific partners, including at monthly action committee meetings, helped to bridge potential conflicts. For example, a source of

tension during the first several years of the LHFA Coalition's efforts was the need to designate a clear and somewhat small area within the broader Latino community as the intervention area, according to the design of the initial NIH grant. This supported the research partners' needs to assemble evidence of the Health for All Model's effectiveness, but it seemed artificially bounded by community partners who worked in a broader jurisdiction. As the LHFA Coalition shifted away from being funded solely by the initial grant from the National Institute of Minority Health and Health Disparities, the "target area" expanded to be more inclusive of all areas of Wyandotte County experiencing health disparities, in keeping with the expectations of community partners.

6. **CBPR emphasizes local relevance of public health problems and ecological perspectives that recognize and attend to the multiple determinants of health and disease**. The LHFA Coalition has sought to live up to this principle through collaborative action at multiple ecological levels—including individuals, families/relationships, organizations, and the whole community. The Coalition's community action plan consisted of strategies identified and selected by community members; from local programs (e.g., Zumba classes in the neighborhood) to environmental changes (e.g., establishing new parks and soccer fields in underserved areas). It assured that activities had local relevance through community-determined strategies and mini-grant funding decisions controlled by the Community Advisory Board.

7. **CBPR involves systems development through a cyclical and iterative process**. The LHFA Coalition has been implementing a model, the Health for All Model (described in Case example #2) that is intended to be both interactive and iterative. The phases on the outer section of the model (see Figure 25-2) are intended to assure a cyclical process; for instance, if changes in behavior and outcomes fall short (e.g., as detected in neighborhood-level behavioral surveys), renewed collaborative planning will lead to refined plans for targeted action for changing conditions.

8. **CBPR disseminates findings and knowledge gained to all partners and involves all partners in the dissemination process**. Throughout implementation of the project, the LHFA Coalition has collected different types of data to evaluate its effectiveness. This information is disseminated using multiple means to reach diverse audiences. In periodic sense-making facilitated by scientific partners, community partners use up-to-date information about progress to review what they are seeing, what it means, and implications for adjustment. To promote the activities of the LHFA Coalition, dissemination activities are conducted with local media, and LHFA Coalition members are often part of the communication. Lastly, communications on lessons learned and emerging evidence of effectiveness are delivered to academic and practitioner audiences.

9. **CBPR involves a long-term process and commitment**. The University of Kansas and LHFA Coalition have been working together since 2009, and they have collaboratively generated resources to fully sustain collaborative action through at least 2017. The scientific and community partners share the commitment and responsibility for assuring long-term engagement in the effort to promote healthy behaviors and eliminate health disparities.

Further descriptions of the LHFA Coalition and evidence of effectiveness can be found elsewhere.[26,47]

Sustainability

Sustainability of community development efforts represented in these several case examples have relied on multiple tactics. As described in the Community Tool Box (accessed at http://ctb.ku.edu by searching for "Sustaining the Work or Initiative"), these tactics for sustainability, and examples from these cases, include:

▷ Sharing positions and resources (e.g., Latino Health for All Collaborative partnership—community mobilizer sharing office space within El Centro, a key partner organization);

▷ Becoming a line item in an existing budget of another organization (e.g., LDCHD Community Health Planning and Improvement—the health department provides funding for a dedicated position);

▷ Incorporating the initiative's activities or services into another organization with a similar mission (e.g., LDCHD Community Health Planning and Improvement—the United Way requests that its programs report on contributions to the community health improvement plan);

▷ Applying for grants (e.g., Latino Health for All Collaborative partnership—continuously funded by a series of related grants);

▷ Tapping into available personnel resources (e.g., LDCHD Community Health Planning and Improvement and the Latino Health for All

Coalition—taken together, they have scores of partner organizations that permit staff time to make a contribution).

BUILDING CAPACITY OF THE HEALTHY COMMUNITIES WORKFORCE

Building healthy communities involves people working together to address health and development concerns that matter to them.[10] The community development workforce is necessarily broad and distributed; successful community development efforts extend far beyond the health sector. Sectors essential to community health development include: employers and businesses; academia; the media; governmental public health agencies; the health care delivery system; nonprofit, nongovernmental, voluntary, and social entities, including ethnic and cultural groups; advocacy organizations; and the faith community.[5] Meaningfully engaging various sectors of the community—including people most affected by health disparities—requires a diverse workforce skilled in community development methods.

Community development workers can serve in the role of guide, enabler, or expert.[4] Guides help "the community establish, and find means of achieving, its own goals . . . the choice of direction and method of movement must be that of the community."[4] The enabler helps facilitate the community organization process by focusing discontent, encouraging organization, developing good interpersonal relations, and emphasizing common objectives.[4] The role of the expert is to provide technical assistance, data and evaluation support, and advice on methods. There are outside encouragers or developers—such as university partners or those providing technical support—and indigenous ones—local leaders who support and emerge from the process of community development.[55] The best measure of whether the development effort has been successful is whether it becomes self-perpetuating, as when new generations of developers emerge as the work continues over time.[55]

Core Competencies for the Community Health and Development Workforce

Community development approaches and related skills are critical to assuring conditions for health and well-being for all. Public health essential services—and related standards for a functional local health department—include: monitoring health status through community assessments; supporting community-engaged planning to identify health issues; and mobilizing community partnerships to solve identified problems.[18]

Related core competencies for the community health development workforce can be articulated within the *Healthy People 2020's MAP-IT FRAMEWORK*: *Mobilize* community partners; *Assess* community needs; *Plan* to address these needs; *Implement* the improvement plan; and *Track* the community's progress. Table 25-3 displays core competencies related to this framework, specific skill areas, and available supports for learning these skills, including those available through the Community Tool Box[56] (CTB) (http://ctb.ku.edu/) and other sources.

Capacity Building to Support Community Health and Development

Like other aspects of public health practice, community development requires a prepared workforce.[57] Building the capacity of individuals and groups in the community to come together to organize and take action is part of the community development process.[50,58] Eade and Williams[59] make the case that "strengthening people's capacity to determine their own values and priorities, and to organize themselves to act on these, is the basis of development" (p. 5). Since people, context, and conditions are always changing in communities, capacity building is seen as an ongoing aspect of the community development process.[60] This requires clarity about whose capacities need to be enhanced, what capacities need to be developed, and why or for what purpose.[60] Typically, capacity building needs to occur at multiple levels, including at the organizational and community levels to support change and improvement in both communities and the systems that are supposed to serve them. It is also important to identify what skill or competency areas need to be strengthened among community members and development partners—for instance, in community assessment, planning, intervention, advocacy, leadership development, evaluation, and sustainability.

Often, capacity-building activities include training, technical assistance, and other supports. These are typically offered through intermediaries such as technical assistance providers, universities, government partners, or grantmakers. Workshops, webinars, and online courses are common modes of delivery. Web-based supports, such as the free and open source Community Tool Box[56] (http://ctb.ku.edu/), can help assure affordable and just-in-time supports for implementing community development approaches.[61, 62] In a capacity-building approach, the locus of responsibility for community development is shared among both technical experts and community members, and both are colearners in the community development process.

TABLE 25-3   Core Competencies for Community Development for Health, Related Skill Areas, and Some Available Supports for Workforce Development

Core Competencies for the Public Health Workforce	Some Specific Skill Areas	Some Supports for Workforce Development—from the Community Tool Box (CTB) and Other Sources
Mobilization	• Establishing a vision and mission • Bringing people together • Representing community stakeholders • Building partnerships • Assuring technical assistance • Enhancing cultural competence	• CTB Toolkit: Increasing Participation and Membership • CTB Toolkit: Creating and Maintaining Coalitions and Partnerships • CTB Toolkit: Enhancing Cultural Competence • CTB Chapter 4: Getting Issues on the Public Agenda • CTB Chapter 7: Encouraging Involvement in Community Work • CTB Chapter 12: Providing Training and Technical Assistance • CTB Chapter 27: Cultural Competence in a Multicultural World
Assessment	• Determining community needs • Identifying community assets and resources	• CTB Toolkit: Assessing Community Needs and Resources • CTB Toolkit: Analyzing Problems and Goals • CTB Chapter 3: Assessing Community Needs and Resources • Healthy People 2020 Tool: Brainstorm Community Assets • Healthy People 2020 Tool: Exercise: Prioritizing Issues • CDC CHANGE Action Guide
Planning	• Developing strategic and action plans • Developing objectives • Developing logic models	• CTB Toolkit: Developing Strategic and Action Plans • CTB Toolkit: Developing a Framework or Model of Change • CTB Chapter 8: Developing a Strategic Plan • Healthy People 2020 Tool: Defining Terms • Healthy People 2020 Tool: Setting Targets for Objectives • CDC Evaluation Guide: Developing and Using a Logic Model • CDC Change Community Health Improvement Planning Template
Intervention/ Implementation	• Developing effective interventions that fit local context • Influencing policy development • Developing a plan for communication • Planning for sustainability	• CTB Toolkit: Developing an Intervention • CTB Toolkit: Influencing Policy Development • CTB Toolkit: Sustaining the Work or Initiative • CTB Chapter 6: Promoting Interest in Community Issues • Healthy People 2020 Coalition Self-Assessment
Tracking	• Developing evaluation plans • Documenting progress • Using feedback to improve the effort • Celebrating and communicating progress	• Toolkit: Evaluating the Initiative • CTB Chapter 36: Introduction to Evaluation • CTB Chapter 37: Operations in Evaluating Community Interventions • CTB Chapter 38: Some Methods for Evaluating Comprehensive Community Initiatives • Healthy People 2020: Measuring Progress • CDC Evaluation Guide: Developing an Evaluation Plan

SUMMARY

Community development is integral to the work of assuring conditions for health and well-being for all of us. Its core attributes—community participation, intersectoral action, and locally determined goals—are thoroughly consistent with the theory and practice of public health. With its emphasis on changing communities and systems, it embodies the process and intermediate outcome of collaborative public health action. Selected case examples—from community health planning, collaborative partnerships, and community-based participatory research—illustrate the processes of community development for population health improvement. As the evidence base for implementing community development practices is extended, this approach will be even more vital to efforts to improve population health and health equity. To go to scale, we need to enhance core competencies for community development in a broad and diverse workforce of community members and professionals from different disciplines and sectors. Working collaboratively in the spirit of social justice, we can enable communities—locally and globally—to assure conditions for the health and well-being of all our members.

REVIEW QUESTIONS

1. What is community development?

2. What are community development approaches for health and health equity?

3. Describe three major models of community organization practice.

4. Describe the Institute of Medicine's (IOM) Framework for collaborative public health action and the 12 processes often associated with promoting community health and development.

5. Describe the sectors of the community essential to successful community development for health.

6. Describe the five-phase *Healthy People 2020 MAP-IT Framework* guiding implementation efforts related to achieving health objectives for the nation.

7. Describe the core practices for community health planning and improvement (according to the CDC report on core practice areas).

REFERENCES

1. Murphy FG, Fawcett SB, Schultz JA, Holt C. Fundamental core concepts in the community engagement, organization, and development process. In: Murphy FG, ed. *Community Engagement, Organization, and Development for Public Health Practice.* New York: Springer; 2013: 1–30.

2. World Health Organization. The Ottawa charter for health promotion. http://www.who.int/healthpromotion/conferences/previous/ottawa/en/index.html. Published 1986. Accessed October, 2014.

3. Christenson JA, Robinson JW. *Community Development in Perspective.* Ames, IA: Iowa State University Press; 1989.

4. Ross M. *Community Organization: Theory, Principles, and Practice.* New York: Harper & Row, Publishers; 1967.

5. Institute of Medicine. (2003). The community. In: *The Future of the Public's Health in the 21st Century.* Washington, DC: National Academy Press; 2003: 178–211. http://books.nap.edu/openbook.php?record_id=10548&page=178. Accessed October 2014.

6. Fawcett S, Schultz J, Watson-Thompson J, Fox M, Bremby R. Building multisectoral partnerships for population health and health equity. *Prev Chronic Dis.* 2010; 7(6). http://www.cdc.gov/pcd/issues/2010/nov/10_0079.htm. Accessed October 2014.

7. Bracht N, ed. *Health promotion at the community level.* Newbury Park, CA: Sage Publications, Inc; 1990.

8. Green L, Kreuter M. *Health Promotion Planning: An Educational and Ecological Approach.* 4th ed. Boston: McGraw-Hill; 2005.

9. Green I, Raeburn I. Contemporary development in health promotion—Definition and challenges. In: Bracht N, ed. *Health Promotion at Community Level.* Newbury Park, CA: SAGE Publishing; 1990.

10. Fawcett SB, Francisco VT, Hyra D, Paine-Andrews A, Schultz JA, Roussos S, Fisher JL, Evensen P. Building healthy communities. In: Tarlov A, St. Peters RF, eds. *The Society and Population Health Reader: A State and Community Perspective.* Itasca, IL: F.E. Peacock Publishers; 2000: 314–334.

11. Braveman P. Health disparities and health equity: Concepts and measurement. *Annu Rev Public Health.* 2006; 27: 167–94. doi: 10.1146/annurev.publhealth.27.021405.102103

12. Braveman P, Gruskin S. (2003). Defining equity in health. *J Epidemiol Community Health.* 2003; 57(4): 254–248.

13. Baum FE. *The New Public Health.* 3rd ed. South Melbourne, VIC: Oxford University Press; 2008.

14. Commission on Social Determinants of Health. Closing the gap in a generation: health equity through action on the social determinants of health. Final report of the Commission on Social Determinants of Health. Geneva, Switzerland: World Health Organization; 2008.

15. Jackson S, Birn AE, Fawcett SB, Poland B, Schultz JA. Synergy for health equity: Integrating health promotion and social determinants of health to address health inequity in the Americas. *Rev Panam Salud Publica.* 2013; 34(6): 473–480.

16. Solar O, Irwin A. A conceptual framework for action on the social determinants of health. Social determinants of health discussion paper 2. In: *Policy and Practice*. Geneva, Switzerland: WHO Press; 2010. http://www.who.int/sdhconference /resources/ConceptualframeworkforactiononSDH_ eng.pdf. Published 2010. Accessed 2014.

17. Cox FM, Erlich JL, Rothman J, Tropman JE, eds. *Strategies of Community Organization*. Itasca, IL: F.E. Peacock Press; 1979.

18. Tsouros, A. The WHO Healthy Cities Project: State of the art and future plans. *Health Promot Int.* 1995; 10(2): 133–141.

19. National Association of County and City Health Officials. Operational definition of a functional local health department. http://www.naccho .org/topics/infrastructure/accreditation/upload /OperationalDefinitionBrochure-2.pdf. Published November 2005. Accessed October 2014.

20. Healthy People 2020. Program planning. http: //healthypeople.gov/2020/Implement/MapIt.aspx. Updated November 18, 2014. Accessed November 18, 2014.

21. Fawcett SB, Francisco VT, Paine-Andrews A, Schultz JA. Working together for healthier communities: A research-based memorandum of collaboration. *Public Health Rep.* 2000; 115(2): 174–179.

22. Green L. From research to "best practices" in other settings and populations. *Am J Health Behav.* 2001; 25(3): 165–178.

23. Roussos ST, Fawcett SB. A review of collaborative partnerships as a strategy for improving community health. *Annu Rev Public Health.* 2000; 21: 369–402.

24. Community Preventative Services Taskforce. The guide to community preventative services: The community guide—What works to promote health. http://www.thecommunityguide.org. Published 2013. Updated November 12, 2014. Accessed November 12, 2014.

25. Yin R. *Case Study Research: Design and Methods.* 4th ed. Los Angeles, CA: SAGE Publications; 2009.

26. Watson-Thompson J, Fawcett SB, Schultz JA. Differential effects of strategic planning on community change in two urban neighborhood coalitions. *Am J Commun Psychol.* 2008; 42: 25–38. doi: 10.1007/s10464-008-9188-6.

27. Collie-Akers VL, Fawcett SB, Schultz JA. Measuring progress of collaborative action in a community health effort. *Rev Panam Salud Publica.* 2013; 34(6): 422–428.

28. Guerra N, Backer TE. *Casebook on Youth Violence Prevention Projects—Four Key Elements for Success.* Encino, CA: Human Interaction Research Institute; 2003. http://www.csun.edu/sites/default/files /finalrep130.pdf.

29. Jacobs JA, Jones E, Gabella BA, Spring B, Brownson RC. Tools for implementing an evidence-based approach in public health practice. *Prev Chronic Dis.* 2012. doi: 9:110324. http://dx .doi.org/10.5888/pcd9.110324.

30. Keene Woods N, Watson-Thompson J, Schober DJ, Markt B, Fawcett S. Functioning and sustainability: An empirical case study of the effects of training and technical assistance on community coalition. *Health Promot Pract.* 2014; 15(5): 739–749. doi: 10.1177/1524839914525174.

31. Watson-Thompson J, Fawcett SB, Schultz JA. A framework for community mobilization to promote healthy youth development. *Am J Prev Med.* 2008; 34: S72–S81. http://www.ajpmonline.org/article /PIIS0749379707007581/fulltext.

32. Zakocs RC, Edwards EM. What explains community coalition effectiveness? A review of the literature. *Am J Prev Med.* 2006; 30(4): 351–61.

33. Schultz J, Collie-Akers V, Fernandez C, Fawcett S, Ronan M. Implementing community-based participatory research with two ethnic minority communities in Kansas City, Missouri. *International Journal of Migration, Health and Social Care.* 2009; 5(1): 47–57.

34. Watson-Thompson J, Keene Woods N, Schober DJ, Schultz JA. Enhancing the capacity of substance abuse prevention coalitions through training and technical assistance. *J Prev Interv Community.* 2013; 41(3): 176–187.

35. Hargreaves MB. Using complexity science to improve the effectiveness of public health coalitions. In: Minai A, Braha D, Bar-Yam Y, eds. Online proceedings of the Seventh International Conference on Complex Systems. http://www .necsi.edu/events/iccs7/papers/e839e1bbe9ea54c 690072c99a4b1.pdf. Published 2007. Retrieved 2014.

36. Kreuter MW, Lezin NA, Young LA. Evaluating community based collaborative mechanisms: implications for practitioners. *Health Promot Pract.* 2000; 1(1): 49–63.

37. Merzel C, D'Affitti J. Reconsidering community-based health promotion: Promise, performance, and potential. *Public Health Matters.* 2003; 93(4): 557–574.

38. Institute of Medicine. *The Future of Public Health.* Washington, DC: National Academy Press; 1988.

39. Institute of Medicine. *Improving health in the community: A role for performance monitoring.* Washington, DC: National Academy Press; 1997.

40. Turnock BJ. *Public Health: What It Is and How It Works.* 4th ed. Sudbury, MA: Jones & Bartlett Publishers; 2009.

41. National Association of County and City Health Officials. MAPP Framework. Mobilizing for action through planning and partnerships: Web-based framework tool. http://www.naccho.org/topics /infrastructure/mapp/framework/index.cfm. Published 2001. Accessed 2014.

42. Catholic Health Association. Step 2: Determine the purpose and scope of the community health needs assessment. Assessing and addressing community health needs. http://www.chausa. org/docs/default-source/general-files/cb_assessingaddressing-pdf.pdf?sfvrsn=4. Published 2011. Updated June, 2013. Accessed November 2014.

43. Association for Community Health Improvement. Step 2: Determine the purpose and scope of the community health needs assessment. Community Health Assessment Toolkit. www.assesstoolkit.com. Published 2002. Accessed November 2014.

44. Fawcett S, Holt C, Schultz J. Some Recommended Practices for Enhancing Community Health Improvement. University of Kansas Work Group for Community Health and Development Report to the CDC Office of Prevention through Healthcare. http://ctb.ku.edu/sites/default/files /site_files/recommended_practices_for_enhancing_ community_health_improvement.pdf. Published 2011. Accessed 2014.

45. Lawrence Douglas County Health Department. Community Health Plan. Lawrence Douglas County Health Department website. http: //ldchealth.org/information/about-the-community /community-health-improvement-plan. Published 2013. Accessed 2014.

46. Cutts T, Rafalski T, Grant C, Marinescu R. Utilization of Hot Spotting to Identify Community Needs and Coordinate Care for High-Cost Patients in Memphis, TN. *Int J Geogr Inf Syst.* 2014; 6(1): 23–29. doi: 10.4236/jgis.2014.61003.

47. Fawcett SB, Schultz JA. Using the Community Tool Box's Online Documentation System to Support Participatory Evaluation of Community Health Initiatives. In: Minkler M, Wallerstein N, eds. *Community Based Participatory Research for Health: From Process to Outcomes.* 2nd ed. New York: Jossey-Bass; 2008.

48. Fawcett SB, Collie-Akers V, Schultz JA, Cupertino P. Community-based participatory research within the Latino health for all coalition. *J Prev Interv Community.* 2013; 41(3): 142–154. doi: 10.1080/10852352.2013.788341

49. Mattessich P, Monsey B. *Collaboration: What Makes it Work: A Review of Factors Influencing Successful Community Building.* Saint Paul, MN: Amherst H. Wilder Foundation; 1992.

50. Ploeg J, Dobbins M, Hayward S, Ciliska D, Thomas H, Underwood J. Effectiveness of community development projects. http://web.cche.net /ohcen/groups/hthu/95–5abs.htm. Published 1996. Accessed October, 2014.

51. Fawcett SB, Boothroyd R, Schultz JA, Francisco VT, Carson V, Bremby R. Building capacity for participatory evaluation within community initiatives. In: Suarez-Balcazar Y, Harper G, eds. *Empowerment and Participatory Evaluation of Community Interventions: Multiple Benefits.* New York: Haworth Press, Inc; 2003.

52. W. K. Kellogg Foundation. Definition of CBPR adopted at the spring networking meeting of the Community Health Scholars Program. Ann Arbor, MI; 2001. http://depts.washington.edu/ccph /commbas.html.

53. Viswanathan M, Ammerman A, Eng E, et al. Community-based participatory research: Assessing the evidence: Summary. In: AHRQ Evidence Report Summaries. Rockville, MD: Agency for Healthcare Research and Quality (US); 2004. http://www .ncbi.nlm.nih.gov/books/NBK11852.

54. Wallerstein N, Duran B. Community-based participatory research contributions to intervention research: The intersection of science and practice to improve health equity. *Am J Public Health.* 2010; 100(S1): S40–46.

55. Schulz AJ, Israel BA, Selig SM, Bayer IS. Development and implementation of principles for community-based research in public health. In: MacNair RH, ed. *Research Strategies for Community Practice.* Binghamton, NY: Haworth Press, Inc; 1998: 83–110.

56. Biddle WW, Biddle LJ. *The Community Development Process.* New York: Holt, Rinehart & Winston; 1965.

57. University of Kansas Work Group for Community Health and Development. Community Tool Box. Community Tool Box website. http://ctb.ku.edu. Updated 2014. Accessed November, 2014.

58. World Health Organization. The World Health Report 2006: Working together for health. http: //www.who.int/whr/2006/en/. Published 2006. Accessed 2014.

59. Fawcett SB, Schultz JA, Francisco VT, et al. Using Internet technology for capacity development in communities: The case of the Community Tool Box. In: Rothman J, Erlich JL, Tropman JE, eds. *Strategies of Community Intervention.* 7th ed. New York: Eddie Bowers Publishing; 2008.

60. Eade D, Williams S. *The Oxfam Handbook of Development and Relief.* vol 2. Oxford, UK: Oxfam Publishing; 1995.

61. Eade D. *Capacity-Building: An Approach to People-Centered Development.* Herndon, VA: Stylus Publishing; 1997.

62. Holt CM, Fawcett SB, Schultz JA, Berkowitz B, Wolff T, Francisco VT. Building community practice competencies globally through the Community Tool Box. *The Global Journal of Community Psychology Practice.* 2013; 4(4). http://www.gjcpp .org/en/article.php?issue=16&article=81.

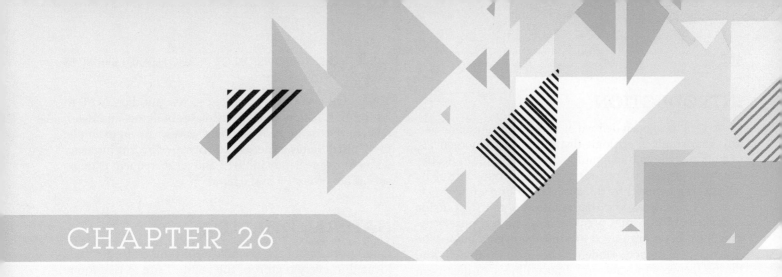

CHAPTER 26

Public Health Preparedness

Linda Young Landesman, DrPH, MSW • Isaac B. Weisfuse, MD, MPH

LEARNING OBJECTIVES

Upon completion of this chapter, the reader will be able to:

1. Describe types of disasters.
2. Identify the types of public health problems caused by disasters.
3. Understand the key components of health systems preparedness.
4. Describe and explain the role of local health departments in preparing and responding to emergencies.

KEY TERMS

disasters
emergency management
first responder
incident command system (ICS)
preparedness
response
National Incident Management System (NIMS)

INTRODUCTION

Disasters have been defined as natural or manmade hazards that result in ecologic disruptions, or emergencies, of such severity and magnitude that they result in deaths, injuries, illness, or property damage that cannot be effectively managed by the application of routine procedures or resources and that result in a call for outside assistance. Historically, preparedness and response activities have been organized around the events before the disaster (preimpact), while it is occurring (impact), and during recovery (postimpact). Injury, illness, or death can be reduced or prevented by the actions taken by public health professionals, emergency management officials, and the population at risk during all three periods.

The basic phases of disaster management include mitigation or prevention, warning and preparedness, response, and recovery. Mitigation includes actions to reduce the harmful effects of a disaster, such as those that may prevent further loss of life, disease, disability, or injury. Warning, or forecasting, refers to monitoring events for indicators that signify when and where a disaster might occur and what its magnitude might be. In preparedness, officials or the public plan a response to potential disasters and, in so doing, lay the framework for recovery.

Across the globe, mankind is experiencing an increase in both natural and technological disasters, as evidenced by events in recent years and statistical trends. A disaster that requires external international assistance occurs, on average, once a day, somewhere in the world. The number of natural disasters worldwide tripled from 1980–1989 to 2000–2009.[1] In 2011 alone, of the 244.7 million people affected internationally, 31,000 people died as a result of 332 natural disasters. The United States ranked sixth among these countries, with 809 deaths.[2] Since the beginning of the twentieth century, 7 of the 10 natural disasters affecting the most people in the United States occurred between 2004 and 2011;[3] 24.3 million people were affected by these top 10 naturally occurring events.[4]

The severity of natural disasters is likely to continue to increase due to climate change. Across the globe, precipitation patterns are changing, sea levels are rising, the oceans are becoming more acidic, and the frequency and intensity of weather events are increasing. Such changes to the climate are likely to result in a multiplication of extreme weather events. Public health professionals are concerned because climate change has multiple impacts on human health, such as heat-related illnesses and deaths due to increasingly frequent and severe heat waves; injuries and increases in waterborne disease due to increased precipitation and associated flooding; and threats to public safety during coastal flooding and storm surges as a result of rising sea levels. As examples, the average temperature in the United States has increased by 1.3°F to 1.9°F since 1895, with most of this increase occurring in the past 45 years.

The global average is projected to rise another 2.0°F to 11.5°F by 2100, with likely increases of illness and death related to extreme heat and heat waves.[5] As an example, the United States experienced increased storm intensity with Hurricane Sandy in 2012 and more frequent extreme storms are projected in the future.[6,7]

NATURAL DISASTERS

Large portions of the population in the United States, located in every region of the country, are at risk today from just three types of natural disasters: earthquakes, floods, and hurricanes. While most people think of California as the most earthquake-prone state, 39 states are seismically active. In 2010, almost 40 percent of the U.S. population (123.3 million people) lived in counties located on the shoreline. Between 2010 and 2020, this population is expected to increase 8 percent.[8] The significance of this concentration is evident when the risk posed just by hurricanes is examined (see Exhibit 26-1). The Center for Climate and Energy Solutions notes that "warmer ocean surface temperatures and higher sea levels are expected to intensify their impacts."[9]

Disasters cause a wide range of morbidity and mortality. As an example, storms, such as hurricanes and tornados, can result in broken bones; crush injuries, and other trauma; dehydration from being trapped without access to drinkable water; injury from clean-up activities; and death. Floods can result in contamination from mold or mildew; drowning, diarrheal, skin, and waterborne diseases due to exposure to contaminated water or hazardous waste; and, vector-borne diseases. In addition, there may be food shortages secondary to flooding. During heat waves people suffer cramps, dizziness, heatstroke, loss of consciousness, myocardial infarction (heart attack), stroke, and even death.

MANMADE OR TECHNOLOGICAL DISASTERS

Like natural disasters, manmade or technological disasters—events caused by human action or technological breakdown—have also increased worldwide with devastating impacts on the public's health. In the past century, the United States alone experienced more than 300 technological accidents that killed 14,558 people and injured 24,481.[10] The aging and crumbling infrastructure of U.S. cities increases our vulnerability for disruptions of daily life that can range from water main breaks, which release asbestos, to bridge collapses. The Deepwater Horizon oil spill in the Gulf of Mexico in 2010 was the largest oil spill in U.S. history, and four years later is still impacting the Gulf Coast. Technological

EXHIBIT 26-1   Natural Disaster: Hurricane Sandy

The 2012 Atlantic hurricane season was particularly devastating to the northeastern Atlantic seaboard. On October 29, 2012, Hurricane Sandy moved up from the Caribbean and first made landfall in New Jersey. Hurricane Sandy affected 24 states, including the entire eastern seaboard from Florida to Maine, with particularly severe damage in New Jersey and New York. The superstorm also moved west across the Appalachian Mountains to Michigan and Wisconsin. The surge of water from the storm flooded streets, tunnels, and subway lines resulting in massive loss of electrical power in the metropolitan area around New York City. New York's governor, Andrew Cuomo, had declared a state-wide state of emergency and asked for a predisaster declaration three days earlier which was signed by President Obama. Preparatory actions in New York and New Jersey were numerous, such as cancelling all air flights in and out of area airports, closing bridges and tunnels, mandatory evacuation of residents in low-lying areas, covering entrances to and closing subways and trains, closing schools and evacuating patients from hospitals and nursing homes in low-lying areas. The East River overflowed its banks, flooding large sections of lower Manhattan. Over 10 billion gallons of raw and partially treated sewage were released by the storm, 94 percent of which went into waters in and around New York and New Jersey[11]

due to an older design of combined sewer and water systems which carries storm water and sewage in the same pipes. When seawater short-circuited the electrical system in a house in New York City's Breezy Point, fire whipped by wind spread to 126 homes. Dozens of fires also occurred in other areas of the region.[12]

Public Health Implications: Despite mitigation procedures, Hurricane Sandy and its associated flooding caused 160 deaths and many injuries. Over 8.6 million households were without power in 21 states and the District of Columbia (some for months, including those needing life support, with the temperature dropping through fall and winter[13]). People living in high rise apartments were trapped, some for days, when elevators did not work. Health care delivery systems were disrupted when hospitals and long-term care facilities were flooded and evacuations required. In addition, many were without medication or medical equipment for both chronic and life-saving conditions.[14]

Public Health Interventions: Three hundred and fifty ambulances were deployed from other areas of the country to New York, and more than 2,300 health care providers were deployed from the National Disaster Medical System and U.S. Public Health Service Commissioned Corps to provide care at hospitals and at shelters in New York and New Jersey.[14]

or industrial accidents, such as the 2011 nuclear accident in Fukushima, Japan, where residents have yet to return to their community, could easily have been as devastating as the nuclear plant meltdown at Chernobyl in 1986. The Midtown Manhattan Con Edison power plant exploded after flooding from Hurricane Sandy, causing a massive blackout for a significant section of the borough. While no one was killed or injured from the explosion, places across the East River in Brooklyn glowed from the blue light emitted from the arc.

Despite previous high-profile disasters in the United States, the most shocking manmade disaster occurred in 2001, when the World Trade Center in New York City and the Pentagon were attacked, resulting in the collapse of the World Trade Center's twin towers. Almost 3,000 people died on September 11, 2001 at the World Trade Center, at the Pentagon, and on the four planes in this coordinated, multipronged attack.

The actual and potential effects of manmade disasters will continue to escalate, generating an increased need for public health intervention as the world's population grows, population density increases, and technology becomes more sophisticated. The need for public health information has spurred the development of readily available guidance.[15]

EMERGING INFECTIOUS DISEASES

Health care professionals around the world are increasingly responding to the potential peril from emerging infectious diseases. Emerging infectious diseases are those which have been identified relatively recently or that have increased in incidence, severity, or geographical distribution.* Diseases of grave concern include those that can be spread:

▸ when an infected person releases tiny airborne droplets through sneezes or coughs, for example, Severe Acute Respiratory Syndrome (SARS) and influenza;
▸ when skin or mucous membranes come in contact with blood or other body fluids or contaminated objects or surfaces, for example, Ebola virus disease (EVD); and
▸ when in close contact, such as living with or caring for an infected person, for example, Middle East Respiratory Syndrome (MERS).

---

*The list of emerging diseases is quite long and a full discussion is beyond the scope of this chapter. Those interested in a comprehensive examination can review Lisa Beltz's *Emerging Infectious Diseases: A Guide to Diseases, Causative Agent, and Surveillance,* Jossey Bass, 2001.

The 2014 epidemic of EVD that spread out of West Africa highlighted the need for those involved in public health preparedness to differentiate between diseases which are spread through the air and those that require direct contact with the virus.

Airborne Diseases: Influenza

Seasonal influenza, a common but frequently serious disease known as "flu," spreads rapidly and can be transmitted by those who are infected but asymptomatic, resulting in simultaneous escalating outbreaks in multiple communities. Influenza infections are responsible for secondary complications such as pneumonia, dehydration, and exacerbations of chronic respiratory and cardiac problems. Most individuals have some immunity to the circulating viruses either from previous infections or from vaccination, often moderating the spread or impact of the seasonal influenza virus.

Pandemic influenza, flu that spreads quickly around the world, occurs, on average, every three to four decades. Pandemics occur when a novel strain of the flu emerges. These unique viral strains are capable of causing significant morbidity and mortality because people have no immunity against them. Three pandemics occurred in the last century—in 1918, 1957, and 1968. In past pandemics, influenza viruses spread worldwide within months. It took two months for the 1918 influenza to spread from American soldiers stationed in Europe to the citizens of their host countries. The 1957 Asian Flu spread to the United States within four to five months after detection in China. The spread of the 1968 pandemic was even quicker—it was detected in the United States only two to three months after being discovered in Hong Kong. In future pandemics, modern travel patterns will result in even faster spread. Importantly, the 2002–2003 pandemic outbreak of SARS, which infected individuals in 37 countries in weeks,[16] demonstrated that countries worldwide must be ready to immediately implement their response plan once pandemic viruses have begun to spread (see Exhibit 26-2).

Contact with Blood or Other Body Fluids: Ebola Virus Disease

Prior to 2014, outbreaks of Ebola virus disease would sporadically occur in rural areas of Africa. The ability to keep the virus from spreading was challenged when EVD reached high population density areas resulting

EXHIBIT 26-2 The 2009 H1N1 Influenza Pandemic in the United States

In the past, new strains of influenza A in humans have been responsible for pandemics (worldwide epidemics) of influenza, including the devastating 1918 pandemic which killed up to 100 million persons across the globe. In April 2009, two children in California were diagnosed as having influenza A that could not be categorized (subtyped) as a previously known influenza strain. Neither of these children had any contact with the other. Soon thereafter, more cases were diagnosed in multiple states. The virus, thought to have originated in Mexico, was a novel strain combining human, avian, and swine influenza viruses.

Public Health Implications: Influenza spreads through respiratory droplets from the coughs and sneezes of persons with the illness. Less commonly, transmission may occur from contaminated surfaces when someone touches them and then touches their nose or mouth. The virus quickly spread across the United States, causing a large number of influenza cases in the spring and fall of 2009. It was estimated that 43 to 89 million cases occurred in the United States, with many cases in children and few in the elderly. The severity of the pandemic as measured by the case fatality rate was less than in prior influenza pandemics. The 2009 H1N1 strain was susceptible to treatment with certain antivirals, but there was no vaccine available at the onset of the pandemic.

Public Health Interventions: A national emergency was declared in the United States, giving the Secretary of Health and Human Services additional powers, such as the power to waive certain federal regulations concerning hospitals. H1N1 influenza strains were rapidly shared with vaccine manufacturers, although because of the length of the current production process, vaccine only became available in the late fall of 2009. Initial efforts in the United States included the creation of a diagnostic test for the strain, which was made available to public health laboratories across the United States. Because children were commonly infected, school closures became an intervention adopted in many U.S. jurisdictions. Alternatively, students or staff with influenza symptoms such as cough and fever were asked to stay home for seven days or until 24 hours had passed since their symptoms had resolved. Other interventions included the creation of clinical guidance for providers, recommendations on infection control, and a public campaign to promote vaccination. When vaccine became available it was distributed to providers, hospitals, and health departments. Many health departments created free vaccination clinics in their jurisdictions. The pandemic subsided and was declared over in August 2010 by the World Health Organization.

in a greater volume of cases which complicated the traditional approach of isolating patients.[17] EVD then spread to the United States when two nurses developed the disease after caring for an infected man who flew from Africa to Dallas. Detailed information about Ebola can be found at http://www.cdc.gov/ebola.

Close Contact: Middle East Respiratory Syndrome

Those who cared for patients with EVD developed the virus because of their direct contact with fluids containing the virus. Middle East Respiratory Syndrome is an example of another virus that has been spread to those caring for patients with this virus.

Other Emerging Threats: Bioterrorism Agents

Terrorist activity both within the United States and globally is increasing, and the likelihood of a chemical or biological warfare (CBW) attack has not diminished since the United States experienced an anthrax attack in 2001. To help prioritize preparedness efforts, the Centers for Disease Control and Prevention (CDC) developed a list of critical agents and grouped them into three categories. Category A agents are those with high impact and require the greatest preparedness. Category B has a lesser requirement for preparedness. Category C can be handled within current public health capacity. Of these diseases, only five Category A agents (anthrax, smallpox, plague, botulism, and tularemia) are considered serious threats. The diseases can be categorized in three ways. The first is those diseases (anthrax, plague, and tularemia) that can be spread by an aerosolized release of bacteria, producing pulmonary disease. The second category includes illness that is transmitted person-to-person, such as smallpox. The last category includes diseases caused by contaminated food, water, or other ingested material, such as botulinum toxin.

The first response to bioterrorism is at the local level, with detection dependent on public health surveillance and the integration of the health care sector. Subsequent public health and health care sector management is coordinated at local, state, and federal levels in predefined plans. For some diseases, early recognition and diagnosis of the disease is essential for preventing devastating outcomes, such as anthrax, for which treatment is usually effective only before the onset of severe symptoms. A release in an airport or among a highly mobile population could disseminate a highly infectious airborne pathogen throughout most of the world before the epidemic would be recognized. To bring such an epidemic under control, a major multifocal international response would need to be activated.

PUBLIC HEALTH CHALLENGES IN DISASTERS

Disasters create public health tasks that require special preparation beyond the routine practice of disease prevention or health care delivery. Some tasks require the provision of emergency health care, such as triage and distribution of casualties, or having to function within a damaged or disabled health care infrastructure. Other tasks, such as warning and evacuating residents and reaching out to those with disabilities or other special needs, involve coordination with both private sector organizations and with multiple jurisdictions at all levels of government. To be effective managers and to respond effectively, public health professionals must work proficiently with emergency management and must be competent in the specialized set of skills needed for disaster related problems. For example, while temporary deficiencies in resources may occur in any disaster, in the United States, the problem with resources during disasters frequently is one of how assets are used or distributed, rather than one of deficiencies.

THE MENTAL HEALTH IMPACTS OF DISASTERS

Responding to mental health issues in populations affected by disaster is a prominent part of emergency response. This is true of any disaster, but it is especially true of crises caused by terrorist attacks, because terrorism often targets the mental health of the affected population. Therefore, strategies to address a community's mental health should be integrated into the initial responses and the public communication used to address the situation. Many emergencies require the provision of crisis counselling to victims and the families of the deceased. Therefore, a cadre of trained mental health providers with expertise in grief counselling needs to be created and maintained. Community mental health providers and the American Red Cross (ARC, discussed below) play a key role in the supply and training of these providers in many communities. Mental health responders should be prepared to mobilize and deploy to sites servicing victims, responders, or the public, such as hospitals or Points of Distribution (PODS). If this is not immediately possible, as may be the case during a large-scale disaster, efforts should be made to ensure that crisis counselling, assessments, and referrals are provided after the event to help identify and treat mental health symptoms among the population.

Members of the public are not the only ones affected by disasters. First responders, including public health staff, may be profoundly affected by their work. Communities, being sensitive to the well-being of all during emergencies, often offer employee counselling to these responders during and after an emergency. Mental health programs and services include informational and educational support about normal reactions, ways to handle reactions, early or long-term treatment where indicated, and services available at family assistance centers.

Community Resilience

For the past several years there has been an increased focus on community resilience as a critical part of emergency preparedness.[19] There are varied definitions of resilience, but it can be thought of simply as the ability of a community to "bounce back" from an emergency event. The National Response Framework encourages improving the resilience of all neighborhoods by reducing negative health and psychological consequences of the disaster and allowing the community services to recover.

Natural Disasters, Manmade Disasters, and Mental Health

Natural and manmade disasters, although differing in origin, have equally profound impacts on the mental health of victims and responders. While both types of events have in common the immediate threat of and the potential for ongoing disruption, there is a huge discrepancy between humans' perceived and actual control over these two kinds of disaster. People tend to see natural disasters simply as part of nature, over which we have no control. In contrast, manmade disasters are, in principle, preventable. Because we expect to be able to control technology, manmade disasters often produce higher levels of anger and distrust than natural disasters, because victims can direct blame and responsibility to those associated with causing the events.[20] Technological acts are also frightening because we may not know when the consequences caused by the event are over, making it difficult for those affected to return to a sense of normality.

THE PUBLIC HEALTH ASPECTS OF ENVIRONMENTAL SERVICES DURING DISASTERS

Following natural disasters, the infrastructure to prevent disease or provide safe water and food may be intact but not working, or it may be destroyed. This is often the result of the destruction or inoperability of barriers, such as sewage plants and water-treatment operations, which protect populations from exposure to environmental hazards. Public health professionals' task is to protect or to restart the protective barriers that exist, or to promote changes in behavior through educational messages that will compensate for the disrupted barriers. Examples of these messages include orders to boil water before using it, warnings about foods that may have spoiled during electrical outages, or announcements regarding where potable water will be provided. For displaced populations, all basic services usually need to be restarted from scratch.

Sanitation and Personal Hygiene

Disasters can disrupt or destroy sewage treatment plants. One of the first activities in disaster response is frequently the reestablishment of a sanitation system. Hand washing, particularly after defecating and before preparing food, has been shown to protect against fecal-oral illnesses, including diarrhea.[21] Therefore, soap should be provided, public education should emphasize the importance of personal hygiene, and a simple monitoring program should be included to ensure that increased hand washing is actually occurring.

Water: Quantity and Quality

After a disaster, ensuring the availability of safe drinking water is critical to preventing disease outbreaks. Once it has been determined that water service to an area has been affected by the disaster, public health professionals can assure that arrangements are made for the water to be lab-tested, for emergency distribution of bottled water, and for the public to be educated about the necessary steps to take to ensure that water is safe.

The United Nations High Commissioner for Refugees (UNHCR) recommends that people need at least 4–5 gallons of water (15–20 liters) per person per day to maintain human health. During a crisis, available water and water consumption by each person should be estimated at least weekly. In areas with piped water, surveys can quickly determine which areas are lacking in water service. Where water service is expected to be inoperable, water often can be transported to the area by vehicle.

Lab testing can determine water quality, usually through detection of fecal coliforms, a bacterial measure that indicates whether water is safe to drink. Although these bacteria may not be pathogenic, their presence is an early indication of fecal contamination and the likely presence of other pathogens. The best way to ensure clean water is to add a chlorine residual to the water. This means that in unsanitary settings, or during times of outbreaks, it may be appropriate to chlorinate safe-source water.

Food and Shelter

Just as with ensuring the availability of safe water, providing food and shelter is also an essential component of disaster preparedness and response. When electrical service is lost, refrigerated food is vulnerable to becoming spoiled. At such times, public health advisories and intervention are critical in protecting a population against foodborne disease. Advisories can be issued about food safety, spoilage, and how to properly handle food to avoid illness. Proper food handling includes correct storage, adequate cooking, and sufficient washing of hands and all utensils.

After a disaster, people who have lost or been evacuated from their homes must be sheltered. Evacuation or establishing shelters will be coordinated with local agencies, such as the American Red Cross (ARC).

Other Issues

Following a disaster, environmental staff should be prepared to mobilize to assess the size of any affected area, help establish or evaluate standards for personal protective equipment for those who enter the affected area, and begin planning for the clean-up and reoccupancy of the area. These are general activities, but other, event-specific responses may include restaurant and food safety inspections (including food service facilities for responders), radiologic assessment, environmental sampling activities, and hazardous waste removal.

HOW DISASTER RESPONSE IS ORGANIZED

In the United States, the response to disasters is organized through multiple jurisdictions, agencies, and authorities that function at local, state, and federal levels. The term emergency management is used to refer to response activities. Emergency management groups organize their activities by sectors, such as fire, police, and emergency medical services (EMS). Public health and health care organizations are part of the health sector.

After a disaster, a multiorganizational public health response is required because disasters typically generate needs beyond the mission of any one health care organization. The response phase of a disaster necessitates relief followed by recovery, including reconstruction of the community. Emergency relief activities include saving lives, providing first aid, restoring emergency communications and transportation systems, and providing immediate care and basic needs to survivors, such as food and clothing or medical and emotional care. Recovery includes actions for returning the community to normal, such as repairing infrastructure, damaged buildings, and critical facilities.

All states and many localities have an emergency management authority (EMA), sometimes called an office of emergency preparedness (OEP). It is the responsibility of the EMA, under the authority of each state's governor's office, to coordinate the use of all state assets during an emergency or disaster. These assets may be expansive and include the state's Department of Health (DOH), housing and social services agencies, and public safety agencies. While the organization of each state's EMA is unique, commonalities exist among EMAs. For example, each EMA coordinates state-wide integration with federal agencies and local governments, and manages and coordinates information needed for response operations. Also, state and local agencies follow the procedures established in their disaster plans. The local and state EMAs establish a command center whose function is to coordinate the response of representatives from each of the numerous pertinent agencies. Called the emergency operations center (EOC), this command center is located away from the disaster site and oversees the emergency response. The DOH participates in the command center activities as a full partner.

The overriding jurisdictional principle in disaster response is that emergencies are local; therefore, localities must have primary responsibility for managing the response unless and until they request assistance or become overwhelmed. When the resources of a local jurisdiction are insufficient to respond to a disaster, the coordinating agency can seek help, called mutual aid, from surrounding jurisdictions or can escalate a request to the state or federal level, or both. States in many regions of the country have formed multistate, regional mutual aid compacts or consortia. These consortia can provide relatively rapid response throughout the area due to geographic proximity. Similar to these consortia, but larger, the Emergency Management Assistance Compact (EMAC) is a mutual aid agreement among all states in the United States. On request by the affected state(s), EMAC can rapidly facilitate the interstate provision of personnel and supplies to the affected areas. Using EMAC, professional liability and reimbursement are worked out in advance.

When response to events requires additional resources, federal aid is available through a presidential disaster declaration, which, since 2000, has been enacted from 45 times (2000) to 99 times (2011) a year. This federal assistance for managing major disasters and emergencies is authorized through the Stafford Act, passed by Congress in 1988 and most recently amended in 2013.[22] Under the Stafford Act, the President may approve allocation of federal resources, medicine, food and other consumables, manpower and services, and financial assistance. Requests for federal assets are initiated at the local level of government and forwarded to the state. The governor of a state makes the formal request for federal assistance, activating the declaration and initiating the flow of federal aid. While most presidential declarations are made immediately after a disaster strikes, a state's governor may submit a request before the disaster has occurred in situations where the consequences are imminent and warrant predeployment of assets to limit catastrophic impacts. Where indicated, the President has the authority to expedite the conveyance of federal resources by declaring a disaster prior to a state's request.

The Emergency Medical Services (EMS) System

For most disasters that occur suddenly, the initial medical response is provided by a local or regional EMS system. In most parts of the United States, EMS is provided by semiautonomous local agencies with regional or state oversight. The EMS includes the prehospital system (e.g., public access, dispatch, Emergency Medical Technicians, Paramedics, and ambulance services) and the in-hospital system (e.g., emergency departments and inpatient care). EMS provides medical care known as basic and advanced life support. Basic life support includes noninvasive first aid and stabilization for a broad variety of emergency conditions, and semiautomatic defibrillation for cardiac arrest victims. Advanced life support, provided by paramedics, includes sophisticated medical diagnosis followed by on-site, protocol-driven medical treatment prior to and during transport to hospitals.

Incident Command Systems

In responding to a disaster, the effective coordination and management of the numerous activities and agencies are crucial. Among the original scholars in the field, Drabek *et al.* found that the coordination of organizations, multiple activities, and local and external resources was among the most difficult and crucial challenges in managing a disaster response.[23] The incident command system (ICS) is the standard management structure used in disaster response across the United States.

The goal of the ICS is to support an efficient and timely response by integrating communication and planning among many agencies, thereby eliminating duplicate efforts. Principles of the ICS include use of a common terminology, a modular organizational approach that may contract and expand depending on the needed response, management by objective, and accountability of personnel and resources. The ICS is flexible enough to be used in any type of incident. Key to the success of the ICS is its organization of tasks and functions into manageable components, known as span of control.

In the ICS, one individual from a facility or from an agency is in charge of the emergency response and decision-making process. This individual is referred to as the incident commander. The person who assumes this responsibility may vary depending on the response skills needed and the time and type of incident. Regardless of the type of incident, someone will assume the role of the incident commander.

Under an ICS framework, a number of additional standardized roles and positions are assigned depending on the incident. This standardization of roles within ICS facilitates effective communication among the different sectors involved in the response. A typical ICS structure includes operations, logistics, planning, and finance sections reporting to an incident commander. Individuals are designated for each function and each function has a predetermined list of duties and responsibilities.

THE PREPAREDNESS OF THE FEDERAL GOVERNMENT

The federal government sets standards for public health emergency preparedness through the legislative process, allocation of funds, and oversight by the Department of Health and Human Services (DHHS) and Department of Homeland Security (DHS). In December 2013, the Pandemic and All-Hazards Preparedness Reauthorization Act (PAHPRA) was passed.[24] The 2013 law authorized funding for public health and medical preparedness programs and amended the Public Health Service Act to allow: (1) flexibility in dedicating Health Department staff resources to meet critical community needs in a disaster; (2) funding through 2018 for buying medical countermeasures under the Project BioShield Act; and (3) BioShield ability to support advanced research and development of potential medical countermeasures and the U.S. Food and Drug Administration to support rapid responses to public health emergencies.

There have been extensive federal preparations for emergency response. The DHS provides the framework for policy and operational directions during an emergency through its National Response Framework (NRF), updated in 2013.[25] The NRF guides the U.S. response to the breadth of disasters and provides a template for the management of incidents and operations called National Incident Management System (NIMS). The NIMS standards, promulgated by the DHS, provide guidance for coordinating all levels of governmental response across the country. Compliance with NIMS standards is a requirement for receipt of any federal funding for emergency preparedness.

Emergency Support Functions (ESF) within the NRF provide detailed guidance for the actual response and delineate the roles and responsibilities of participating federal agencies. ESF 8—the Public Health and Medical Services Annex—covers public health emergencies and is overseen by DHHS, which must assess the need for assistance on a number of issues such as surveillance, deployment of supplemental medical care personnel, worker health and safety, and patient care. Support comes from many other federal agencies.

The Federal Government's Response

In addition to the Strategic National Stockpile (described further below), the federal government has created the National Disaster Medical System (NDMS)[26] which can deploy critical assets during an emergency and has several components. When activated, the NDMS deploys teams that provide emergency medical care at the site of an emergency, set up and run mortuary operations, assist in activities requiring pharmacists, and provide veterinary services during emergencies. Additional resources can be deployed through the Emergency Management Assistance Compact.[27]

Voluntary Agencies

A vast array of voluntary agencies participate in disaster response with functions that contribute significantly to public health outcomes. Under the coordination of the Federal Emergency Management Agency, the ARC provides mass care, which includes providing shelter, food, emergency first aid, and family reunification, as well as distributing emergency relief supplies to disaster victims. ARC responds first through its local chapters, then through state and regional chapters, which may call on national-level ARC resources if necessary. Public health works closely with the ARC in the temporary shelters.

A FRAMEWORK FOR HEALTH SECTOR AND PUBLIC HEALTH PREPAREDNESS

Preparedness begins with planning. This section reviews the planning needed to prepare hospitals and health departments for emergencies.

Risk and Preparedness

Communities, health care providers, and local or state Departments of Health undertake a hazard vulnerability analysis (HVA) to understand the risks that might affect the health and safety of the community. The HVA provides a roadmap for prioritization of planning efforts and projects the response needed and assesses internally and externally available resources. These community assessments enable residents to know in advance of hazards that could affect them. Using the HVA, communities systematically assess the possibility of natural events (e.g., hurricanes), technological events

(e.g., electrical failures), human-related events (e.g., mass casualty incidents), and events involving hazardous materials.

Emergency Management Programs: Emphasis on All-Hazards Planning

Comprehensive emergency plans are often referred to as all-hazards plans because they provide a framework for preparing for and responding to the broadest range of events, disasters, and emergencies. An all-hazards plan can guide the response for unanticipated events or events that unfold in an unanticipated way. Once the probability and the severity of the various hazards are understood, preparedness needs can be addressed. The activities in preparing for and responding to any emergency include:

1. developing the basic emergency management plan
2. ensuring communications to mobilize staff
3. monitoring and evaluating external sources of information
4. addressing staff availability and supporting their needs
5. ensuring effective internal and external communication during the emergency
6. ensuring the availability of equipment, supplies, and services
7. ensuring security (e.g., providers should seek supplemental manpower to deliver care and necessary support, such as medical equipment vendors and pharmaceutical suppliers).

The specific tasks of health care facilities and health departments are different. Hospitals have to be ready to provide medical care to many more people than usual. Sometimes that care is complicated by the type of emergency and the exposures that patients have had. Health departments have to be ready to provide guidance, investigate population-wide issues, and provide preventive care. In all instances, it is critical for health care facilities and health departments to work in partnership to provide an effective and prompt response to the emergencies that they face. The following sections describe specific preparedness activities.

Organizational Preparedness

The single most important resource for the health care and public health systems is an engaged, trained, and well-informed workforce. Therefore, the first task in organizational emergency preparedness is to inform, educate, and test all current employees on their roles and responsibilities during an emergency. The Core Competencies for Emergency Preparedness[28,29] are useful starting points for matching personnel with their emergency roles. Minimum requirements for all staff include having a family plan, understanding the role of their organization during an emergency, basic information on incident command, knowledge of their response role, how to use communication equipment, and how to communicate within the organization. Specific response roles for employees should mirror their everyday tasks as much as possible.

Drills and Exercises

Only after a plan has been written and staff have been educated about it, is it worth spending the time and funds required to conduct exercises to test the plan. Exercises are valuable for testing employee awareness of a plan and for identifying problems by challenging the integrity of the plan. These tests usually are table-top exercises, in which participants are confronted with a hypothetical emergency to which they then need to notionally coordinate a response, or drills which involve actually demonstrating some part of the activity needed for response. A full-scale exercise is often the culmination of previous drills and exercises. It tests the mobilization of all (or as many as possible) of the response components, takes place in real time, employs real equipment, and tests several emergency functions.

HOSPITAL PREPAREDNESS

Hospitals operate under regulations that require emergency preparedness. For example, most states provide direction regarding health care facilities' emergency plans, drills, and general emergency response procedures.[30] Similarly, federal regulations that set forth the conditions for hospitals to participate in the federal Medicare and Medicaid payment programs require that hospitals have certain emergency systems and procedures.[31] Finally, the Joint Commission, a nonprofit nationwide organization that accredits many kinds of health care providers, has specific preparedness requirements.[32] Space constraints do not allow for a full description of hospital-related emergency preparedness roles and responsibilities, and the reader is referred to other sources for additional information.[30–32]

PREPAREDNESS FOR LOCAL AND STATE DEPARTMENTS OF HEALTH

The Oversight Role of Departments of Health

State Health Departments have fiscal and programmatic oversight of the federal cooperative agreements for emergency and health care preparedness within their states, with the exception of the four cities (Washington DC, Los Angeles, Chicago, and New York City) that are directly funded. These appropriations started in 2002, and for fiscal year (FY) 2013 totalled over $611 million for public health emergency preparedness, and $228 million for health care preparedness.[33] Unfortunately these allocations have been decreasing in recent years. It is challenging to provide state-wide solutions to local emergencies because LHDs across a state may vary in size and ability and may serve very different populations, whether rural, suburban, or urban. Because of complicated legal frameworks, state health departments face additional oversight challenges when working with tribal authorities located within the state and with regional metropolitan areas that cross state boundaries. Processes for communication and mutual aid are worked out as part of everyday preparedness. States located on the Mexican or Canadian borders may also need to work with these countries to coordinate emergency response in these cross-border regions.

Surveillance

Surveillance is the backbone of public health. This is especially true during emergencies, where a premium is placed on the earliest possible identification of a threat in order to mitigate its health consequences. Traditional systems that passively collect information from health care providers and laboratories continue to be important parts of emergency preparedness. However, traditional surveillance suffers from a number of deficiencies that create barriers to the rapid diagnosis and reporting needed for quick identification of an outbreak. These deficiencies may include clinicians' lack of understanding of reporting requirements, the lack of a mechanism to report to health departments, and the lack of clinicians' ability to recognize rare infectious diseases or unusual clusters of diseases. Health departments can work with community physicians to resolve these problems by sponsoring educational sessions on the roles of physicians in emergency preparedness, distributing educational materials to clinicians to encourage reporting, and creating 24/7 rapid-response teams who can accept and act on suspicious reports in real time.

Syndromic surveillance systems have been created in part to address the recognition delays inherent in traditional surveillance. These new systems rely on recognizing patterns of symptoms or behavior (such as buying antiflu medications or absenteeism among large groups of people) rather than on diagnoses of specific diseases among individuals (see Chapter 12 for more detail).

A further extension of traditional and syndromic surveillance is biodetection, which uses environmental monitoring to identify the release of bioterrorism agents, in hopes of identifying an attack as early as possible. Several biodetection initiatives have been employed. The first, Biowatch, involves the collection of airborne particles onto filters that are collected and tested for agents of bioterrorism. Biowatch detectors have been deployed in many cities across the United States. A second program, the Bioagent Detection System (BDS), has been deployed in mail-sorting facilities across the United States in an effort to identify any letter containing anthrax as soon as it goes through a sorting machine. BDS enables pathogen testing, using polymerase chain reaction assays, within the system and sets off an alarm when anthrax is detected.[34] When either of these systems is used, public health authorities have to knowledgeably manage a positive laboratory result, through engaging their mandated partners, explaining the result, and acting appropriately on the result.

New surveillance systems may need to be created to enable public health officials to understand the impact of the emergency. Examples of these new surveillance efforts occurred following Hurricane Katrina, when a system was set up to assess the incidence of communicable diseases among evacuation center residents, the mental health needs of returning residents, and the extent of mold problems in homes in New Orleans.[35] Follow-up may be necessary to measure the long-term health effects of the emergency; this may be accomplished through the establishment of a registry. A good example is the World Trade Center Registry,[36] the largest environmental health registry in history, which attempts to identify long-term (20-year) medical and psychological outcomes for building evacuees, first responders, and other groups that were closely associated with the 9/11 disaster.

Monitoring social media or search engine inquiries may be useful as a form of surveillance. For example, analyzing Internet searches for flu or influenza may provide an early indication of the influenza season.[37]

Laboratory Preparedness

In the 2001 anthrax attacks, departments of health were overwhelmed with environmental and clinical specimens for *Bacillus anthracis* screening. This incident focused attention on the fragility of our public health laboratories. Two years earlier, the CDC formed the Laboratory Response Network (LRN), which linked hospital, state and local health, CDC, FBI, local law enforcement, and other reference labs. The LRN was formed to enhance the timeliness of lab testing, to establish common protocols for testing, and to foster communication among the various players involved in emergency response. Specific LRN objectives include

training sentinel, or clinical, labs to rule out, recognize, or refer potential select agents to the Public Health Lab; establishing packaging and shipping requirements between the LRN labs to ensure the safe transport of specimens; establishing Biosafety Level 3 facilities (see Chapter 29) within each state for safe testing of dangerous specimens; and, enhancing security requirements for dealing with bioterrorism agents.

Other preparedness activities may include testing Biowatch specimens, and membership in the Food Emergency Response Network (FERN), which coordinates lab testing in response to a terrorist attack involving the contamination of the food supply.

Communication

Departments of health have a critical role in communicating with the public and with other responding agencies during emergencies. Health departments position themselves as trusted sources of information in everyday situations; this makes it more likely that the public will turn to them during public health emergencies. Risk communications and media relations are critical during emergencies. The tenets of risk communication are sharing information about what is known, acknowledging what is not known, and explaining how the government is working to fill knowledge gaps. Effective risk communication includes delivering what you promise and not over-reassuring people in the face of uncertainty.

Increasingly, health departments are integrating the use of social media into their approach to emergency communications.[38] For example, they use social media to update the public, provide clinical guidance, or to let people know what facilities are open for health care. Alternatively health departments can monitor social media to better understand the needs of the population, learn about local conditions, and to understand if rumors are spreading.

Medical Countermeasures

Departments of health have been tasked with developing strategies to provide medical countermeasures to health threats—in other words, to rapidly treat or provide prophylaxis to large populations during medical emergencies. Such strategies, for example, might include supplying antibiotic prophylaxis following exposure to anthrax, or smallpox vaccination following a smallpox outbreak. The federal government's Strategic National Stockpile (SNS),[39] a federal source of medicine and medical supplies, plays a key role in these strategies. The SNS is maintained at secure locations across the United States and has two components: the first is a "push pack" of antibiotics, and other medicines and medical equipment needed for immediate response. The second is vendor-managed inventory, which provides longer-term support. Push packs can be deployed to any location in the United States within 12 hours after the request from the governor of the affected state. State departments of health need to formally accept the SNS and then develop their own intrastate distribution plan.

Health departments may be involved in other stockpiling and distribution activities. Chempack,[40] for example, is a federal-state initiative to predeploy chemical nerve agent antidotes to hospitals. In addition, several jurisdictions are also considering bolstering supplies of critical-care-related equipment, such as ventilators, by creating stockpiles.

Points of Distribution Sites

Once material reaches the local cities or counties from the Strategic National Stockpile, it is distributed to the affected population. This occurs at Points of Distribution (PODs) sites, which are places where the well public comes to receive preventive medical interventions. Because hospitals' and clinics' capacity is likely to be overwhelmed during a crisis, PODs are usually located in other facilities. POD staff quickly assess attendees and provide the appropriate intervention; however, PODs are not designed to diagnose and treat illness. Because of the enormous difficulties in accessing an entire population for prophylaxis, especially in urban areas with large populations, the CDC has created a City Readiness Initiative to provide increased funding for this activity. In addition, alternatives to PODs are being explored, such as the U.S. Postal Service delivering needed antibiotics through the mail, or working with nursing agencies to provide antibiotic prophylaxis to the homebound.

Volunteers

In an attempt to ensure sufficient personnel during emergencies, the Medical Reserve Corps (MRC) enrolls health care personnel as volunteers, so that they can supplement local workforces during a variety of crises. MRC volunteers were deployed following Hurricane Katrina, for instance. Training MRC volunteers, however, can be a challenge because emergencies, by nature, are unpredictable. The training a volunteer receives may not be appropriate to a specific crisis or may occur far in advance of an emergency and be hard to remember when the crisis occurs. Therefore, many jurisdictions have created "just-in-time" training plans that can be activated when the nature of the emergency and the needed countermeasures are known. A related initiative, the Emergency System for

the Advance Registration of Health Professions Volunteers (ESAR-VHP), has established guidelines to allow states to register, credential, and privilege health professional volunteers to provide a supplemental workforce during an emergency.

Incident-Specific Facility Needs

Both Hurricanes Katrina and Sandy focused attention on evacuation and shelters. Plans for evacuation of facilities, such as hospitals and nursing homes, and of individual persons with disabilities, for example, need to be coordinated with first-responder agencies. Triage protocols to determine whether evacuees require shelters, referral to hospitals, or to other special needs facilities, should be developed and drilled. Public health professionals can work with local providers to support the medical and psychological needs of residents living in evacuation shelters and other housing arrangements.

Health departments must plan for the quarantine of people who are exposed to communicable diseases, such as SARS or pandemic influenza, but who are not yet ill, and for the isolation of those who have become ill. They may need to work with the CDC's Division of Quarantine to identify sick passengers who may arrive in their jurisdiction by airplane or ship. Similarly, medical monitoring systems should be created to identify persons who have been exposed to and have developed an illness, so that they can be isolated from the rest of the population.

Planning for quarantine and isolation must consider a broad range of circumstances, such as identifying facilities to house those who are not from the community (i.e., those on business or visiting). Other scenarios call for caring for people at home. Procedures for the medical, social, and psychological support of these populations should be created.

Community Mitigation

The term *community mitigation* refers to measures that might be instituted to decrease the spread of a highly contagious disease, such as pandemic influenza, usually by discouraging unnecessary gatherings, or, in other words, by encouraging what is called "social distancing." These measures may include cancelling large gatherings such as entertainment events or civic gatherings, or instituting the prolonged closure of schools. This latter measure is difficult to implement, however, because schools supply social support (such as school meals) and because students may recongregate in other settings (such as malls). To successfully carry out a prolonged school closure, LHDs can plan for this contingency with their community's school districts.

Vulnerable Populations

Meeting the needs of vulnerable populations during emergencies cannot occur without prior planning. Vulnerable populations may include the elderly, the homebound, the homeless, immigrants, children, prisoners, persons on renal dialysis, the mentally ill, the chronically ill, and others. These populations may have difficulty in accessing information, resources, or medical care. They may lack the ability to respond to governmental recommendations, such as an order to evacuate, or to report to a POD. Some vulnerable populations, such as children or persons with disabilities, may have medical and emotional needs that are different from those of other vulnerable populations. Health Departments can consult with agencies and individuals who routinely provide care to these populations and with social service providers to create special arrangements for these populations. These providers also need to be prepared to deal with emergencies, to help ensure continuity of services during a crisis, and to better understand effective communication mechanisms and strategies with each of these populations.[41]

Legal Issues

State and local health departments must review their jurisdictions' existing legal authority to determine whether it is adequate to meet the needs of a large-scale emergency, such as one caused by bioterrorism. Specifically, laws covering surveillance (methods as well as specific diseases), isolation and quarantine, and control of property may require revision. Local and state governments need to understand their emergency powers and need to formulate plans for emergency regulatory relief (such as hospital regulations). Because epidemiologic investigations of incidents of terrorism require health departments to coordinate with local law enforcement, agreements on confidentiality, information sharing, and joint investigatory protocols should be formulated and practiced between these agencies. A Model State Emergency Public Health Powers Act has been created that provides a template for comparison to existing legislation, and may enhance the ability of public health authorities to respond to emergencies.[42]

Measuring Preparedness

The National Health Security Preparedness Index[43] was created by a consortium of organizations and individuals involved in preparedness. Its goal is to measure preparedness state by state to assess the levels of national preparedness, improve decision making, promote collaboration, and to create a research agenda for the future. The index is flexible and may be measured over time to better understand progress in preparedness. The 2013 results showed that community engagement and surge management were areas in need of improvement.

SUMMARY

Public health professionals have markedly increased their emergency management expertise since September 11, 2001. Maintaining and enhancing this expertise will be a challenge, however, because of decreased federal funding. Continued federal support, in terms of both leadership and resources, is a critical component of future progress. Likewise, measurable and meaningful benchmarks need to continue to be developed to evaluate future progress. More work needs to be done to meet the needs of society's vulnerable populations and to increase community resilience. Finally, Schools and Programs of Public Health should develop programs to educate their students on emergencies, so that the next generation of public health leadership can further the work of today's leaders.

REVIEW QUESTIONS

1. How should public health professionals prepare for emergency response?
2. What are the potential environmental, behavioral, and physical impacts of disasters?
3. What are incident command systems, and how do they work?
4. What is an all-hazards plan, and why is it useful in disaster response?
5. Which federal assets are utilized in response to an emergency, and when and how are they used?
6. What are the activities carried out by a local department of health in response to an emergency?

REFERENCES

1. Leaning Jennifer and Guha-Sapir Debarati. "Natural Disasters, Armed Conflict and Public Health." *N Engl J Med* 2013; 369:1836–42.
2. Guha-Sapir Debbie; Vos Femke, Below Regina, and Ponserre Sylvain. Annual Disaster Statistical Review 201: The Numbers and Trends; WHO collaborating Centre for Research on the Epidemiology of Disasters (CRED). Universite Catholique de Louvain, Belgium. July 2012.

3. "Top 10 Natural Disasters in United States for the period 1900 to 2014 sorted by numbers of total affected people" http://www.emdat.be/result-country-profile#summtable. EM-DAT. The International Disaster Database. WHO collaborating Centre for Research on the Epidemiology of Disasters (CRED). Universite Catholique de Louvain, Belgium. Accessed August 21, 2014.

4. "Top 10 Natural Disasters in United States for the period 1900 to 2014 sorted by numbers of total affected people." http://www.emdat.be/result-country-profile#summtable. EM-DAT. The International Disaster Database. WHO collaborating Centre for Research on the Epidemiology of Disasters (CRED). Universite Catholique de Louvain, Belgium. Accessed August 21, 2014.

5. Global Climate Change Impacts in the United States, Thomas R. Karl, Jerry M. Melillo, and Thomas C. Peterson (eds.). Cambridge University Press, 2009. www.globalchange.gov/usimpacts Accessed August 21, 2014.

6. Gutowski, W.J., G.C. Hegerl, G.J. Holland, T.R. Knutson, L.O. Mearns, R.J. Stouffer, P.J. Webster, M.F. Wehner, and F.W. Zwiers, 2008: Causes of observed changes in extremes and projections of future changes. In: Weather and Climate Extremes in a Changing Climate: Regions of Focus: North America, Hawaii, Caribbean, and U.S. Pacific Islands [Karl, T.R., G.A. Meehl, C.D. Miller, S.J. Hassol, A.M. Waple, and W.L. Murray (eds.)]. Synthesis and Assessment Product 3.3. U.S. Climate Change Science Program.

7. Kunkel, K.E., P.D. Bromirski, H.E. Brooks, T. Cavazos, A.V. Douglas, D.R. Easterling, K.A. Emanuel, P.Ya. Groisman, G.J. Holland, T.R. Knutson, J.P. Kossin, P.D. Komar, D.H. Levinson, and R.L. Smith, 2008: Observed changes in weather and climate extremes. In: Weather and Climate Extremes in a Changing Climate: Regions of Focus: North America, Hawaii, Caribbean, and U.S. Pacific Islands [Karl, T.R., G.A. Meehl, C.D. Miller, S.J. Hassol, A.M. Waple, and W.L. Murray (eds.)]. Synthesis and Assessment Product 3.3. U.S. Climate Change Science Program, Washington, DC, pp. 35–80.

8. National Oceanic and Atmospheric Administration, National Ocean Service, Ocean Facts, http://oceanservice.noaa.gov/facts/population.html Accessed October 26, 2014.

9. Center for Climate and Energy Solutions, Hurricanes and Climate Change, http://www.c2es.org/science-impacts/extreme-weather/hurricanes Accessed October 26, 2014.

10. EM-DAT The International database, Technological Disaster Trends. World 1900–2011. http://www.emdat.be/technological-disasters-trends. Accessed October 26, 2011.

11. Michael Schwirtz, "Report Cites Large Release of Sewage From Hurricane Sandy" New York Times, April 30, 2013, http://www.nytimes.com/2013/05/01/nyregion/hurricane-sandy-sent-billions-of-gallons-of-sewage-into-waterways.html?_r=1&. Accessed October 28, 2014.

12. John Manuel. "The Long Road to Recovery: Environmental Health Impacts of Hurricane Sandy." *Environ Health Perspect* 121:A152–A159 (2013). http://dx.doi.org/10.1289/ehp.121-a152 [online 01 May 2013]. Accessed August 22, 2014.

13. Cowan AL, et al. Hurricane Sandy's deadly toll. The New York Times, NY/Region section, online edition (17 Nov 2012). Available: http://goo.gl/SrIIU [accessed 8/22/14].

14. Hurricane Sandy–Public Health Situation Updates, December 4, 2012, U.S. Department of Health and Human Services, Office of the Assistant Secretary for Preparedness and Response, http://www.phe.gov/newsroom/Pages/situpdates.aspx. Accessed August 22, 2014.

15. Landesman LY. Public Health Management of Disasters: The Practice Guide. 3rd ed. Washington, DC: American Public Health Association, 2012.

16. Smith, R.D. (2006). "Responding to global infectious disease outbreaks, Lessons from SARS on the role of risk perception, communication and management." *Social Science and Medicine* 63 (12): 3113–3123.

17. Bill Foege Global Health Op-Ed: Bill Foege on how to make Ebola worse, 29 October 2014, http://www.humanosphere.org/basics/2014/10/op-ed-bill-foege-make-ebola-worse/. Accessed October 30, 2014.

18. World Health Organization, Media Center, Ebola Fact Sheets, http://www.who.int/mediacentre/factsheets/fs103/en/. Accessed November 2, 2014.

19. At-Risk, Behavioral Health & Community Resilience (ABC). Office of the Assistant Secretary for Preparedness and Response. U.S. Department of Health and Human Services. http://www.phe.gov/Preparedness/planning/abc/Pages/community-resilience.aspx. Accessed November 21, 2014.

20. Green BL, Solomon SD. The mental health impact of natural and technological disasters. In Freedy JR, Hobfoll SE eds. *Traumatic Stress: from Theory to Practice*. New York: Plenum Press; 1995: 163–80.

21. Gerald T. Keusch, et.al., Chapter 19 Diarrheal Diseases. In Jamison DT, Breman JG, Measham AR, et al., editors. Disease Control Priorities in Developing Countries. 2nd ed. Washington (DC): World Bank; 2006.

22. Robert T. Stafford Disaster Relief and Emergency Assistance Act, as amended, and Related Authorities as of April 2013, http://www.fema.gov/media-library-data/1383153669955-21f970b19e8eaa67087b7da9f4af706e/stafford_act_booklet_042213_508e.pdf. Accessed November 3, 2014.

23. Drabek TE, et al. Managing Multiorganizational Emergency Response: Emergency Research and Rescue Networks in Natural Disaster and Remote Area Setting. Boulder, CO: Natural Hazards Information Center, University of Colorado; 1981.

24. Public Law 113–5, Pandemic and All-Hazards Preparedness Reauthorization Act of 2013. http://www.gpo.gov/fdsys/pkg/PLAW-113publ5/pdf/PLAW-113publ5.pdf. March 13, 2013. Accessed November 2, 2014.

25. National Response Framework. Federal Emergency Management Agency. Department of Homeland Security. https://www.fema.gov/national-response-framework. July 31, 2014. Accessed November 2, 2014.

26. National Disaster Medical System. Office of the Assistant Secretary for Preparedness and Response. http://www.phe.gov/Preparedness/responders/ndms/Pages/default.aspx. October 2, 2014. Accessed November 18, 2014.

27. Emergency Management Assistance Compact. Federal Emergency Management Web site. http://www.fema.gov/pdf/emergency/nrf/EMACoverviewForNRF.pdf. Accessed November 18, 2014.

28. Public Health Preparedness & Response Core Competency Model. Centers for Disease Control and Prevention Web site. http://www.cdc.gov/phpr/documents/perlcPDFS/PreparednessCompetencyModelWorkforce-Version1_0.pdf. December 17, 2010. Accessed November 18, 2014.

29. Disaster-Related Competencies for Health Care Providers. United States Department of Health & Human Services Web site. http://sis.nlm.nih.gov/dimrc/professionalcompetencies.html. September 5, 2013. Accessed November 18, 2014.

30. 10 New York State Code, Rules and Regulations Section 405.24(g) Environmental Health. New York State Department of Health Web site. http://w3.health.state.ny.us/dbspace/NYCRR10.nsf/56cf2e25d626f9f785256538006c3ed7/55a72e625f3c49cb8525677c006f7cf9?OpenDocument&Highlight=0,405.24. November 17, 2004. Accessed November 18, 2014.

31. 42 Code of Federal Regulations Section 482.41, Condition of Participation: Physical Environment. Government Publications Office Web site. http://www.gpo.gov/fdsys/granule/CFR-2011-title42-vol5/CFR-2011-title42-vol5-sec482-41/content-detail.html. October 1, 2011. Accessed November 18, 2014.

32. Joint Commission on Accreditation of Healthcare Organizations. Comprehensive Accreditation Manual for Hospitals: The Official Handbook (EC 1.6, EC 2.5, EC 2.9, EC-5, EC-6, EC-12, EC-13, EC-25, EC-26, EC-49, EC-50, HR 1.25 (draft), HR 4.35 (draft), Oakbrook Terrace, IL: 2005.

33. HHS grants bolster health care and public health disaster preparedness. United States Department of Health & Human Services Web site. http://www.hhs.gov/news/press/2014pres/07/20140701a.html. July 1, 2014. Accessed November 18, 2014.

34. Centers for Disease Control and Prevention. Responding to detection of aerosolized Bacillus anthracis by autonomous detection systems in the workplace. *MMWR*. 2004;53(RR-7):1–11.

35. Centers for Disease Control and Prevention. Assessment of Health-Related Needs After Hurricanes Katrina and Rita—Orleans and Jefferson Parishes, New Orleans Area, Louisiana, October 17–22, 2005. *MMWR*. 2006;55(02): 38–41.

36. Weisfuse IB, Marsik T, Brackbill RM. The Public Health Response to the World Trade Center Attack and Its Aftermath by the New York City Department of Health and Mental Hygiene. In: Terrorism and Public Health, 2nd ed. V. Sidel and B. Levy, eds. Oxford University Press: 2011, New York.

37. Explore flu trends—United States. Google Web site. http://www.google.org/flutrends/us/#US. Accessed November 18, 2014.

38. Merchant Raina M, Elmer S, Lurie N. Integrating Social Media into Emergency-Preparedness Efforts. *NEJM* 2011, 356;4: 289–291.

39. Strategic National Stockpile. Centers for Disease Control and Prevention. http://www.bt.cdc.gov/stockpile. Accessed November 18, 2014.

40. Chempack. United States Department of Health & Human Services. http://chemm.nlm.nih .gov/chempack.htm. June 25, 2011. Accessed November 18, 2014.

41. Eisenman DP, Cordasco KM, Asch S, Golden JF, Glik D. Disaster planning and risk communication with vulnerable communities: lessons from Hurricane Katrina. *Am J Public Health*. 97(Suppl 1):S109–15.

42. The Model State Emergency Health Powers Act (MSEHPA). The Center for Law & the Public's Health Web site. http://www.publichealthlaw.net /ModelLaws/MSEHPA.php. January 27, 2010. Accessed November 18, 2014.

43. NHSPI: A New Way to Measure and Advance Our Nation's Preparedness. National Health Security Preparedness Index Web site. http://www.nhspi .org/. Accessed November 18, 2014.

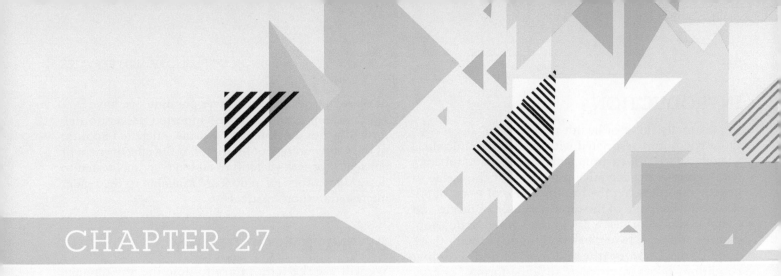

CHAPTER 27

Injury Prevention and Control

María Seguí-Gómez, MD, ScD • Keshia M. Pollack, PhD, MPH • Susan P. Baker, MPH, ScD (Hon.)

LEARNING OBJECTIVES

Upon completion of this chapter, the reader will be able to:

1. Describe the term *injury* and the importance of energy.

2. Summarize the dimension and magnitude of injury as a public health problem, and its relationship with other public health problems.

3. Explain the application of the public health model to injuries.

4. Describe William Haddon's framework and proposed countermeasures.

5. Outline other conceptual frameworks for injury prevention.

6. Recognize the axioms guiding injury prevention.

7. Explain the role of individual public health practitioners and agencies in preventing injuries.

KEY TERMS

accidents
countermeasures
energy
event
injuries
injury prevention
vehicles (or vectors)

INTRODUCTION

We normally think of health problems or diseases as those conditions associated with exposure to infectious agents (e.g., HIV), environmental agents (e.g., tobacco, lead), chronic degenerative processes, or those due to genetic disorders. Yet the leading cause of years of potential life lost, one of the top five causes of death, and a major source of disability in the United States population and worldwide, has nothing to do with those conditions. These deaths and morbid and disabling conditions relate to exposure to some form of energy (kinetic, potential, electrical, or other) in amounts that exceed the individual's tolerance threshold or in amounts released in too short a time period, therefore resulting in injuries. Injuries are a major health problem as old as humankind.

Given the magnitude of this problem, it seems natural, then, that as public health practitioners we should turn our attention to injuries and their prevention and control. Unfortunately, this has not always been the case. Injuries, and their prevention and control, have not traditionally been embraced as a public health issue. One obstacle has been the belief that injuries are the result of accidents, which has caused them to be considered by many as unpredictable and therefore unpreventable. In the instances in which they were "investigated," the conclusion was often that they were primarily due to some irresponsible behavior on the part of the injured individual or someone else. As a result, injury control has been stymied by the "accident" folklore, including the notion of reckless, selfish, careless, and intoxicated people as primarily responsible for injuries.[1] Thus, until the last quarter of the twentieth century, the field of injury prevention and control was characterized by misunderstanding, lack of progress, and scarcity of relevantly trained scientists.

Fortunately, current public health thinking embraces injury prevention and control. In fact, all of the 10 Essential Public Health Services and the Core Competencies for Public Health Professionals are applicable to this major public health problem.[2,3] In this chapter, we will provide a brief overview of the injury problem and some solutions. The chapter is designed to provide a general orientation, rather than an exhaustive discussion. The goal is to facilitate a clearer understanding of the role of the public health practitioner and public health agencies in the reduction of the burden related to injuries. To achieve that goal, we will present useful definitions and conceptual frameworks, a summary of the magnitude of the problem, and examples of the use of public health tools in injury prevention. Emphasis is placed on the preventability

of these injuries, and wherever possible, we have provided examples of evidence-supported prevention efforts. It is not our intent to provide a detailed account of the epidemiology of injuries, nor the effectiveness or efficiency (or lack thereof) of all interventions tested to date. Many other references are available to the reader interested in those matters.[4–7]

DEFINITION OF INJURY

We will use the term *injury* to describe any damage to the body due to acute exposure to amounts of thermal, mechanical (kinetic or potential), electrical, or chemical energy that exceed the individual's tolerance for such energy, or to the absence of such essentials as heat or oxygen. We have, therefore, adopted the broad definition described in *Injury Prevention*[8] and endorsed by the Institute of Medicine (IOM),[9] which includes intentional injuries (e.g., homicide, suicide) as well as unintentional injuries (e.g., falls, burns). This chapter also encompasses injuries regardless of where they occur (e.g., outdoors, at home, or at school), the activity that was taking place when the injurious event happened (e.g., occupational, recreational, sports-related), and the object that was involved in the energy transfer (e.g., motor vehicle, gun). The chapter does not address psychological damage as a result of, for example, violence or motor vehicle crashes.

Table 27-1 lists energy types, their frequency as the source of fatal injuries in the United States population, the vehicles (or vectors) that most frequently transfer the energy, and the most common types of resulting injuries.

DIMENSIONS AND MAGNITUDE OF THE PROBLEM

In the United States in 2010, 180,811 people died because of injuries, amounting to a rate of 58.6 per 100,000. Injuries are among the five leading causes of death in our population, right behind heart, cancer, respiratory diseases, and cerebrovascular disease. As seen in Table 27-2, unintentional injuries are the fifth leading cause of death for individuals of all ages combined, and the leading cause of death for individuals ages 1 through 44. Intentional injuries (whether suicide or homicide) are the second to fifth leading causes of death for ages 1 to 54. Therefore, injuries are the leading cause of years of potential life lost (YPLL, see Chapter 12) amounting to 35.2 percent of YPLL before aged 65—a proportion twice that of

TABLE 27-1 Examples of Energy, Vehicle, Injury Types, and Their Proportion of Injury Deaths in the United States, 2010, Fatally Injured Population (N = 180,811)

Etiology of Injury	Vehicle (vector)	Type of Injuries	Percentage of Deaths
Kinetic energy	Motor vehicle, train, other vehicles, bullets, knives, machinery	Abrasions, contusions, sprains, strains, dislocations, fractures, concussion, blunt, open wounds (cuts, piercing), crushing	40.0%
Chemical energy	Drugs, cleaning products, poisonous animals	Poisonings, chemical burns	23.7%
Absence of oxygen	Water, foreign objects	Drowning, strangulation, suffocation	11.5%
Potential energy*	Falling person	Same as kinetic	15.4%
Thermal energy	Fire, heat	Burns, heat stroke	1.7%
Other (electrical, absence of heat, ionizing radiation)	Wire, radioactive materials	Electrocution, frostbite, burns	7.6%

*It has been argued, however, that potential energy causes injury only when transformed into kinetic energy.

SOURCE: CDC NCHS, Underlying Cause of Death File, 1999–2010. CDC WONDER On-line Database. Available at: http://wonder.cdc.gov.

YPLL to malignant neoplasms, the next most common condition (see Figure 27-1).[10]

In addition to deaths, injuries result in some 2 million hospital admissions and 29 million emergency-department-only visits every year.[10] The relationship between mortality and morbidity (or different degrees of severity) is referred to as the "iceberg" or "pyramid" of injury (Figure 27-2); the actual ratio between the levels of that pyramid varies depending on the specific injury or the specific injury mechanism because some injuries are more lethal than others. Table 27-3 further illustrates this point by presenting the crude death and hospitalization rates per 100,000 population by several mechanisms of injury. As shown in the table, drowning/near drowning has a death:hospitalization ratio of 1:0.5, whereas the ratio for homicide/legal interventions is 1:7.5, and fall-related injuries, 1:35.7. All injuries combined have an average death:hospitalization ratio of 1:12.8.

Injuries are also a leading source of short- and long-term disability.[11] Globally, estimates are that up to 25 percent of disabilities may result from injuries and violence. In the United States alone, approximately 5 million people suffer from chronic, injury-related disabilities.[12]

When one combines mortality, morbidity, and disability in a metric such as Disability Adjusted Life Years (DALYs; see Chapter 12), injuries are responsible for approximately 11 percent of all DALYs lost in the world.[13] According to 2010 data documenting the 30 leading conditions contributing the most to DALYs lost in the United States, injuries due to motor vehicle crashes, suicide, falls, and interpersonal violence ranked 9th, 14th, 15th, and 22nd, respectively.[11] Poisoning from prescription overdose, an emerging injury issue, was not in the top 30, but its contribution to DALYs increased by more than 30 percent in the past two decades.[13] If this trend continues, it is likely that prescription drug overdose will join the list of other pressing injury issues contributing the most to DALYs lost in the United States.

The economic impact of injuries is also significant. It is estimated that the aggregate lifetime cost of all fatal and nonfatal injuries produced in 2005 amounted to $404 billion dollars; $80 billion of which resulted from health care, and the remainder from lost productivity resulting from premature death and disability.[14] In the last Global Burden of Disease publication, injuries rank among the highest as death and disability-inducing conditions when compared to any other health problem.[13]

Finally, a summary of the impact of injuries cannot be complete without reference to the largely unmeasured but immense burden that they impose on families and communities. The literature in this field provides evidence of higher divorce rates among parents of injury victims, higher school dropout rates among siblings of victims, and higher alcohol and drug involvement among relatives and others.[15]

TABLE 27-2   Five Most Common Causes of Death by Age Group, United States 2010, All Races, Both Sexes

Rank						Age Groups						
	<1	1-4	5-9	10-14	15-24	25-34	35-44	45-54	55-64	65+	Total
1	Congenital Anomalies 5,107*	Unint. Injuries 1,394	Unint. Injuries 759	Unint. Injuries 885	Unint. Injuries 12,341	Unint. Injuries 14,513	Unint. Injuries 14,792	Malignant Neoplasms 50,211	Malignant Neoplasms 109,501	Heart Disease 477,338	Heart Disease 597,689
2	Short Gestation 4,148	Congenital Anomalies 507	Malignant Neoplasms 439	Malignant Neoplasms 477	Homicide 4,678	Suicide 5,735	Malignant Neoplasms 11,809	Heart Disease 36,729	Heart Disease 68,077	Malignant Neoplasms 396,670	Malignant Neoplasms 574,743
3	SIDS 2,063	Homicide 385	Congenital Anomalies 163	Suicide 267	Suicide 4,600	Homicide 4,258	Heart Disease 10,594	Unint. Injuries 19,667	Chronic L. Resp. Disease 14,242	Chronic L. Resp. Disease 118,031	Chronic L. Resp. Disease 138,080
4	Maternal Pregnancy Comp. 1,561	Malignant Neoplasms 346	Homicide 111	Homicide 150	Malignant Neoplasms 1,604	Malignant Neoplasms 3,619	Suicide 6,571	Suicide 8,799	Unint. Injury 14,023	Cerebrovascular 109,990	Cerebrovascular 129,476
5	Unint. Injuries 1,110	Heart Disease 159	Heart Disease 68	Congenital Anomalies 135	Heart Disease 1,028	Heart Disease 3,222	Homicide 2,473	Liver Disease 8,651	Diabetes Mellitus 11,677	Alzheimer's Disease 82,616	Unint. Injury 120,859

*Numbers indicate counts of deaths.

SOURCE: CDC NCHS, Office of Statistics and Programming. National Vital Statistics Systems. WISQARS™. Available at: http://www.cdc.gov/ncipc/wisqars/

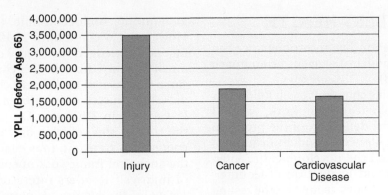

FIGURE 27-1   Years of Potential Life Lost by Cause of Death Before Age 65

Adapted from the CDC NCIPC National Center for Health Statistics Vital Statistics System, U.S., all genders, both sexes, 2004.

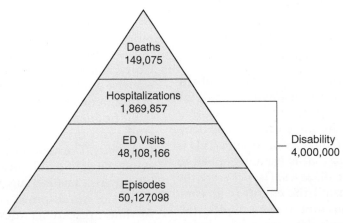

FIGURE 27-2   The Pyramid of Injury, U.S. 2000

Adapted from Finkelstein EA, Corso PA, Miller TR, et al. *The Incidence and Economic Burden of Injuries in the United States.* New York: Oxford University Press; 2006.

TABLE 27-3   Crude Rates of Deaths and Hospitalizations Due to Injury per 100,000 Population, United States 2010, All Ages, Both Sexes

	Deaths per 100,000	Hospitalizations per 100,000	Ratio of Death : Hospitalizations
Motor vehicle	11.5	102.8	1:8.9
Falls	8.7	310.7	1:35.7
Drowning/near drowning	1.5	0.7	1:0.5
Fires/flames	1.0	3.8	1:3.8
Poisonings	13.9	122.7	1:8.8
Homicide/legal intervention	5.4	40.3	1:7.5
Suicide/self-harm	12.4	69.5	1:5.6
Total	58.6	747.8	1:12.8

SOURCE: Office of Statistics and Programming. National Vital Statistics Systems. WISQARS™. Available at: http://www.cdc.gov/ncipc/wisqars/

THE ROLE OF PUBLIC HEALTH

As with any other population health problem, we can apply the public health model of a scientific approach to prevention (Figure 27-3).

For the remainder of this chapter we will follow this model. Under "Epidemiological Framework," we will discuss issues related to the definition of the problem: data collection and surveillance, the identification of causes and risk factors, and the development of interventions. Under "Choice and Evaluation of Countermeasures," we will present issues related to the testing and selection of interventions. Issues that relate to the last step of the public health model will be presented in the "Axioms to Guide Injury Prevention" section and in our discussion of the roles of public health practitioners and public health agencies.

Epidemiological Framework

Injury epidemiology allows for investigation of the interaction among the host (or individual injured), the etiological agent (energy), the vehicle or vector that transmits the energy, and the physical and sociocultural environment where the interaction occurs. This is the same *epidemiologic triad* that is usually applied to infectious or communicable diseases. (*Vehicles* are the inanimate objects that transmit the energy [e.g., cars, flames, bullets], whereas *vectors* are the plants, animals, or persons that transmit the energy [e.g., biting animals, poisonous snakes, human fists].) The use of epidemiology has helped demonstrate that injuries, like diseases, display long-term trends and demographic,

geographic, socioeconomic, and seasonal patterns. However, it was not until 1949 that Dr. John Gordon first acknowledged that injury occurrence and severity, much like any other health condition, could be measured and related to different characteristics of individuals, the sources of injuries, and their environments. It was only in 1961 that Dr. James Gibson separated the role of the vehicles or vectors from that of the energy they transmit, thus enabling the application of the analytical framework of epidemiology to the study of injuries. (Readers interested in a more extensive review of the history of injury control are referred to the work of J. A. Waller.[16])

Data Collection and Surveillance

As identified in the essential public health services[17] and in several of the specific competencies outlined in the first domain (Analytic Assessment Skills) of the Core Competencies for Public Health Professionals,[18] effective control of injury (or any other disease, for that matter) requires collection of appropriate detailed data (e.g., frequency, location) related to the injury under study and the events or circumstances surrounding that injury. The analysis of such data helps us to understand the epidemiological patterns of these problems, identify risk factors, suggest causal factors, and guides us in the development of preventive interventions. At times, researchers develop unique data collection efforts to better address the issues under investigation. Most commonly, however, existing datasets are used, despite the fact that most of these datasets are administrative in nature and tend to be oriented either

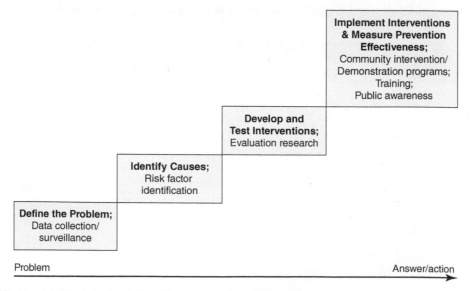

FIGURE 27-3   Public Health Model of a Scientific Approach to Prevention
Adapted from the National Center for Injury Prevention and Control, Centers for Disease Control and Prevention

toward the injuries (i.e., the medical aspects) or toward the events (i.e., the circumstances), and rarely include enough detailed information for both. Several U.S. government and private agencies maintain data systems that collect injury data on a continuous basis as part of their public health practice. Table 27-4 lists some of the most commonly used data systems, as well as their website addresses.

Identification of Causes and Development of Interventions

We have indicated, thus far, that injuries involve an unfavorable interaction between etiologic agents and the individual. Therefore, the essence of injury prevention involves keeping the etiologic agent from reaching the potential host (i.e., preventing the interaction) or from

TABLE 27-4   Selected Surveillance Systems Used in Injury Control

Federal Agency	Data System	Acronym	Web Address
National Institute of Drug Abuse	Monitoring the Future Study	MTFS	http://monitoringthefuture.org
Substance Abuse and Mental Health Services Administration	Drug Abuse Warning Network	DAWN	http://samhsa.gov/ (Search "DAWN")
Bureau of the Census	Census of Agriculture	BCCOA	http://www.agcensus.usda.gov/
Agency for Health Care Policy and Research	Healthcare Cost and Utilization Project	HCUP	http://www.ahrq.gov/data/hcup
Bureau of Justice Statistics	National Crime Victimization Survey	NCVS	http://www.bjs.gov
Bureau of Labor Statistics	Census of Fatal Occupational Injuries	CFOI	http://www.bls.gov
	Survey of Occupational Injuries and Illnesses	SOII	http://www.bls.gov
	Survey of Workplace Violence Prevention	—	http://www.bls.gov
Centers for Disease Control and Prevention	Behavioral Risk Factor Surveillance System	BRFSS	http://www.cdc.gov/brfss
	Youth Risk Behavioral Surveillance System	YRBSS	http://www.cdc.gov/yrbs
	Web Based Injury Statistics Query and Reporting System*	WISQARS	http://www.cdc.gov/injury (Search "WISQARS")
	National Ambulatory Medical Care Survey	AMCS	http://www.cdc.gov/nchs
	National Health Interview Survey	NHIS	http://www.cdc.gov/nchs
	National Hospital Ambulatory Medical Care Survey	NHAMCS	http://www.cdc.gov/nchs
	National Hospital Discharge Survey	NHDS	http://www.cdc.gov/nchs
	National Vital Statistics Systems—Current Mortality Sample	NVSSS	http://www.cdc.gov/nchs
	National Vital Statistics Systems—Final Mortality Data	NVSSF	http://www.cdc.gov/nchs/deaths.htm

(Continued)

TABLE 27-4   (Continued)

Federal Agency	Data System	Acronym	Web Address
	National Traumatic Occupational Fatality Surveillance System	NTOF	http://www.cdc.gov/niosh/
Consumer Product Safety Commission	National Electronic Injury Surveillance System	NEISS	http://www.cpsc.gov/
Federal Bureau of Investigation	Uniform Crime Reporting System—Supplemental Homicide Report	UCRSHR	http://www.fbi.gov
	Law Enforcement Officers Killed and Assaulted	LEOKA	http://www.fbi.gov/
	National Incident Based Reporting System	NIBRS	http://www.fbi.gov/
National Center for Child Abuse and Neglect	National Data Archive On Child Abuse and Neglect	NDACAN	http://www.ndacan.cornell.edu
Fire Administration	National Fire Incident Reporting System	NFIRS	http://www.nfirs.fema.gov
National Highway Traffic Safety Administration	Fatality Analysis Reporting System	FARS	http://www.nhtsa.gov/FARS
	National Automotive Sampling System—Crashworthiness Data System	NASS CDS	http://www.nhtsa.gov/NASS
	National Automotive Sampling System—General Estimates System	NASS GES	http://www-nrd.nhtsa.dot.gov
	National Occupant Protection Use Survey	NOPUS	http://www-nrd.nhtsa.dot.gov (Search "NOPUS")
Federal Highway Administration	National Household Travel Survey	NHTS	http://www.rita.dot.gov (Search "NHTS")

*It contains multiple data sources identified in this table and provides user-friendly access to its data.

reaching it at rates and in amounts that would produce damage (i.e., minimizing the consequences). Under some circumstances, prevention is aimed at modifying the agents; under others, at reducing exposure to the agent or the susceptibility of individuals. Several conceptual models have been developed over the past 40 years to facilitate the understanding of injury-producing events and possible **countermeasures**. Before we present these models, let us revisit the sequence of injury events.

We live in a particular environment. In this environment, we conduct our lives: we walk, drive, exercise, prepare meals, and do countless other things. On each occasion, we are exposing ourselves to the possibility of experiencing an event that may lead to an injury. This is what could be referred to as the *exposure* component of the chain of events. For example, consider every minute a child spends enjoying a playground. Every so

often, a potentially injurious **event** may happen. Following our example, the child falls from the swing; but only a fraction of such falls lead to any *injury*. Some of these injuries, however, may be severe enough to cause death or disability. This chain of events is depicted in Figure 27-4. This sequence of events is very similar to what is known as the Domino Model[19] because of the temporal relationship between the different components of this model. **Injury prevention** and control consists of intervention(s) aimed at blocking the progression of the events. In our example, we could have prevented the event from happening by eliminating the swings from the playground area or by designing them in such a manner that prevents ejection of the child. We could have minimized the impact of the fall by using energy-absorbing flooring underneath the swing. Finally, we could have minimized the consequences of the injury by providing timely care at a pediatric trauma center with expertise in head injury.

The Haddon Matrix

Dr. William Haddon, Jr., a pioneer in the field of injury prevention, proposed a framework that integrates the role of the individual, the vehicle or vector conveying the energy, and the environment in the sequence of events associated with the injury.[20]

Individuals, vehicles (or vectors), and environments play different roles at different times. The sequence of events over time is divided into three phases: *pre-event* (i.e., preventing the event or incident from occurring),

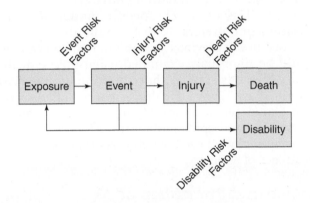

FIGURE 27-4 Sequence of Injury Incidence and Outcomes

event (i.e., preventing injury while the event is happening), and *postevent* (i.e., minimizing the adverse results after the event has occurred). For example, interventions aimed at preventing motor vehicle crashes or falls, suicide attempts, or shootings are pre-event interventions. Event-phase interventions are aimed at either preventing the injury or at reducing the resulting injury by minimizing its severity. Examples of interventions at this stage include bicycle helmets, bullet-proof vests, or pills with smaller medication doses so that they are not as toxic if ingested. The variety and effectiveness of countermeasures at this event stage highlight the point that even if the event (e.g., crash) is not prevented, damage to passengers and occupants can be reduced or eliminated. Postevent interventions can be directed to two goals: reducing any further damage or restoring the health of the individual who sustained injury.

In Table 27-5, we have listed potential interventions to reduce motor vehicle-related injuries using the Haddon Matrix.

Haddon's 10 Basic Strategies

In addition to developing the matrix, Haddon described 10 basic strategies for injury control, presented here with examples relating to injury produced by chemicals:

1. Prevent the initial production of the agent. (Do not produce lead paint.)

2. Reduce the amount of the agent produced. (Package medicine in small quantities.)

3. Prevent release of the agent. (Use childproof caps on bottles of medicine.)

TABLE 27-5 Haddon Matrix with Selected Examples of Motor Vehicle Occupant Injury Prevention Interventions

	Host (Child and Adult Occupants)	Vehicle (Car)	Environment Physical (Road)	Socioeconomic
Precrash	Avoid distracting technology and behaviors Driver's drug or alcohol use, and fatigue	Antilock brakes Speed control Daytime running lights	Improve traffic patterns Increase visibility of hazards	Children in rear seats Legislation regarding child restraint Speed limits Licensing laws
Crash	Use adequate child restraint Use safety belts, airbags	Seating position Built-in child car seats Vehicle speed, size, and mass Interior surfaces	Separation from other lanes Energy-absorbing roadside fixtures	
Postcrash	Exercise and other health enhancement to reduce comorbidity	Crash detection systems that notify EMS (and indicate type of occupants on board) Designs to facilitate extrication Improve location of fuel tank	Designated lanes for emergency vehicles Reduce distance from EMS	Trauma system EMS system prepared to handle children Societal acceptance of residual disabilities

4. Modify the rate or spatial distribution of release of agent from its source. (Devise containers that release poison at limited rates.)

5. Separate, in space or time, the agent from the susceptible person. (Keep children out of orchards while spraying.)

6. Separate the agent from the susceptible person with a material barrier. (Use personal protective equipment such as gas masks.)

7. Modify the contact surface, subsurface, or basic characteristics of the agent. (Reformulate detergents to make them less caustic.)

8. Strengthen the resistance of the person who might otherwise be damaged. (Immunize susceptible people against insect stings.)

9. Counter the continuation and extension of the damage. (Provide and make use of first-aid treatment and poison control centers.)

10. Repair and rehabilitate. (Institute intermediate and long-term therapy.)

Human Performance and Environmental Demands Model

Another system-oriented model was described in the ergonomics literature by Blumenthal.[21] His model focuses on the dynamic interaction between the subject and the environment (Figure 27-5). The lower line represents the variable demands of a particular task, for example, driving a car, and includes the limitations and deficiencies in the vehicle and the environment (including other drivers). The upper line represents the performance of the subject of interest. The injurious event occurs when the system demands increase or the subject performance decreases simultaneously to levels at which they overlap. At times, it is the individual's behavior that fails

dramatically, such as in the situation of a driver who suffers a myocardial infarction or stroke. At other times, it is the system that becomes overwhelming, as in the case where another vehicle on the road has a tire blowout. The third, and most common situation, involves neither cataclysmic human failure nor overwhelming demands but rather a simultaneous decrease in performance and increase in task demand. Such would be the situation where an intoxicated driver (who may be able to drive in a straight line) fails to negotiate an unexpected curve, or a teenager who is distracted by a passenger.

Historically, efforts in injury prevention have focused on the individual's performance. It is only recently that attention has been focused on reducing demands of the task—for example, by using automated lighting systems that do not require drivers to remember to turn on their vehicle lights at dawn or dusk.

Regardless of which specific model of injury causation one prefers, data from the data systems described in the previous section (and others) can and should be rigorously examined using public health science methods such as those listed under the sixth domain (Basic Public Health Sciences Skills) of the Core Competencies,[3] for example, social sciences, biostatistics, and epidemiology, to better characterize the contribution of each possible factor involved in the occurrence of an injury.

Choice and Evaluation of Countermeasures

The role of epidemiology in identifying modifiable risk factors is closely related to the identification of countermeasures. Modifiable risk factors become the basis for intervention design. Note that factors playing an important role in minor injuries are not necessarily the same as factors that are important in severe or fatal injuries. Consequently, the choice of countermeasures may

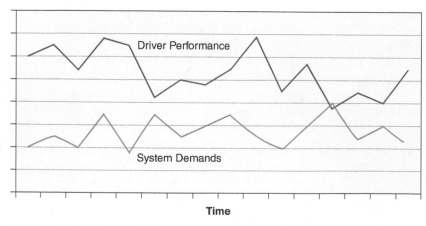

FIGURE 27-5 Hypothetical Localized System Failure
Adapted from Blumenthal 1968.

change as the severity of injuries changes. Also, counter-measures should not be determined by the relative importance of causal or contributing factors or by their earliness in the sequence of events. Rather, priority and emphasis should be given to measures that will most effectively and efficiently reduce injury losses. For example, although psychological factors may be important in the initiation of motor vehicle crashes, it does not follow that psychological screening of drivers would be fruitful.

It is also important to discuss the assumption that anything that sounds reasonable will be effective; this assumption has been the rationale for countless programs, from "defensive driving" training to holiday death counts. Safety programs may not only lack effectiveness, but also may even increase the number or severity of injuries under certain circumstances. One example of this is the case of driver education programs that enable teenagers to drive at an earlier age than they otherwise would.[22]

Numerous safety measures have been adopted without proof of their real-world effectiveness. In many such cases there was only efficacy or laboratory-tested effectiveness data, which turned out to be insufficient when actually applied—for example, Antilock Brake Systems in motor vehicles when first adopted. In other cases, not even efficacy data were available at the time of implementation. The resulting entrenchment of untested measures makes improvement difficult and comparison with alternatives impossible. Millions of dollars can be wasted in unsuccessful safety campaigns, and without adequate preplanned evaluation, no one will ever know whether a campaign was effective and guidance for the future will be lost. The importance of effectiveness evaluation across all public health problems is emphasized both in the Essential Services[17] and as "monitoring program performance" under the seventh domain of the Core Competencies.[3]

In contrast, many other interventions have been evaluated. Table 27-6 lists selected injury control interventions that have been proven effective. For a review of the issues involved in evaluating more detailed prevention interventions, refer to Dannenberg and Fowler's article in the journal *Injury Prevention*.[23]

Another issue to keep in mind when selecting countermeasures is that, very frequently, a "mixed strategy" should be employed, incorporating countermeasures that address complementary aspects. Here the challenge will be in choosing the right type, intensity, and order of interventions to make the "combined" countermeasures most efficient. For example, whether airbags should be designed to protect even unbelted occupants in a frontal collision or as a supplement to safety belts became the issue of a long and

intense dispute among motor vehicle safety specialists in the early 1980s. After it was decided that they should be supplemental restraints, the issue of which crashes were severe enough to warrant airbag deployment in a belted occupant became the new topic of debate.[24] Fortunately, current thorough reviews of countermeasure effectiveness are available to public health practitioners, particularly in the area of motor vehicle safety.[25]

Choices must be made, consciously or by default, on such matters as these or on the question of how many dollars to spend in preventing a given number of lost days or injury hospitalizations or deaths. More complicated still are decisions as to how many hundreds of drivers a state will attempt to take off the road in an effort to prevent one of them from killing himself or herself or someone else. This conscious weighing of alternatives is often lacking in the safety field.

AXIOMS TO GUIDE INJURY PREVENTION

Over the years, enough experience has been gathered to establish several axioms that can help guide efforts in controlling injuries.

Injury Results from Interactions between People and the Environment

The agent of injury will cause little damage if the amount of energy reaching tissues is below human tolerance levels. For example, limited exposure to tap water temperature of less than 49°C (120°F) is not likely to acutely damage human tissue, although higher temperatures or lengthy immersion may. The importance of this interaction is reflected in approaches that control the environment by reducing hot water temperatures at the tap and that simultaneously target the parents of small children for education about hot water scald risk.

Injury-Producing Interactions Can Be Modified through Changing Behavior, Products, or Environments

Modifying the immediate or most adaptable link in the chain of causation can reduce injuries. For example, placing an isolation fence or barrier between a child and a residential pool more easily reduces unsanctioned swimming than by supervising the child's behavior all the time. During sanctioned swimming, supervision is the most important strategy. Changing the environment, policies, the person, or the product can each lead to reductions in injuries.

TABLE 27-6   Examples of Injury Prevention Strategies of Known Effectiveness

Type of Injury	Effective Prevention Strategies	Type of Injury	Effective Prevention Strategies
Motor vehicle	Child passenger restraint	Recreational	Four-sided barriers around swimming pools
	Child passenger restraint laws		Bicycle helmet use
	Safety belts		Promoting bicycle helmet use (e.g., laws)
	Safety belt laws		Breakaway bases for softball
	Sobriety check points	Sports injuries	Mouthguards
	Laceration protective windshields		
	Nighttime curfews for teenage drivers		Protective equipment (e.g., knee and elbow pads, wrist pads for inline skating)
	Pedestrian-friendly front end of automobiles	Falls	Window guards in high-rise buildings
	Minimum drinking age laws		Weight-bearing exercise among elderly
	Breakaway utility poles		Fall-cushioning materials underneath playground equipment
Firearm	Absence of handguns in homes		Protective hip pads for elderly
	Police efforts to target persons illegally carrying guns in high-risk places		Prevention or treatment of osteoporosis in women
	Programs integrating mentoring of at-risk youth, violence interruption, workers and community mobilization	Poisonings	Packaging of children's aspirin in sublethal doses; Implement Prescription Dug Monitoring Programs (for prescription drug misuse/overdose)
	Restricting gun access with child access protection laws and universal background check laws	Farm	Rollover protective structures on farm tractors
Fires/burns	Manufacture of fire-safe cigarettes	Choking and suffocation	Legislation and product design changes (e.g., safe refrigerator disposal, warning labels on thin plastic bags)
	Smoke detectors		
	Automatic sprinklers	All injuries	Minimum drinking age of 21
	Fire-resistant clothing for children		Increase in excise tax for alcohol
	Legislation regulating flammability of children's clothing		911 response systems
	Fire exits and fire drills		

Environmental Changes Have the Potential to Protect the Greatest Number of People

Changes to the environment that automatically provide protection to every person have the potential to prevent the most injuries. Automatic protection includes, for example, bullet-proof windows in liquor stores, automatic sprinkler systems in buildings or homes, energy-absorbing steering wheel columns in vehicles, fuses in homes, and child-resistant packaging of consumer products.

Effective Injury Prevention Requires a Mixture of Strategies and Methods

The primary strategies—behavior change (whether by education or by legislation) and technology/engineering are widely recognized as potentially effective in preventing injuries. Strategies such as individual behavior change, product engineering, public education, legal requirements, law enforcement, and changes in the physical and social environment work together to reduce injuries. The challenge in intervention planning is to select the most effective combination of strategies to produce the desired results. Identifying target populations and deciding on the proper combination of strategies are not exclusive to injury prevention but are part of the fundamental competencies of a public health professional, as outlined in several of their second domain (policy development/program planning) skills.[3]

Further supporting a need for interventions that involve multiple strategies is the concept of the "Three E's" of injury prevention: education, enforcement, and environment.[26] Modifying the design of products and the environment, enforcing laws, educating the public about risk factors and policies—all of these strategies together can be effective. Fully as important is the "Fourth E"—evaluation—without which we cannot move forward with proven preventive measures.

Public Participation Is Essential for Community Action

Effective public policy requires the support and participation of community members. This is, again, reflected both in the 10 Essential Public Health Services[17] and under the fifth domain (Community Dimensions of Practice Skills) of the Core Competencies.[3] Local conditions and resource availability often determine the direction of injury prevention programs. Injury prevention is most successful when there is public participation, support for, and understanding of injury prevention methods. Without public support, laws that are designed to protect the public, such as laws requiring the use of bicycle or motorcycle helmets or safety belts, may be ignored or repealed. This was clearly seen in the Massachusetts legislature regarding mandatory safety belt use; the law was repealed by popular vote in 1986, 11 months after the legislation had been enacted, and then reenacted in 1994.

Cross-Sector Collaboration Is Necessary

Injury prevention requires coordinated action by many groups. Participation by community leaders, in addition to health officials, is necessary in planning and implementing injury prevention programs. Behavior and environmental modification to large numbers of people and sustained through time, together with coordinated postevent responses, require the participation of all. If, as suggested by James Reason's Human Error Model,[27] injury prevention is about ensuring that no holes are permitted through the always imperfect slices of life's whereabouts, everybody needs to be doing their part.

There are a number of ways that other community members can contribute to a program's success, ranging from identifying problems to mobilizing community action and evaluating intervention effectiveness.

THE ROLE OF THE PUBLIC HEALTH PRACTITIONER

Public health professionals can play a vital role in injury prevention from a variety of positions. One of the earliest examples of the role that public health practitioners may have in reducing injuries is the 1980s development and establishment of the Massachusetts Statewide Injury Prevention Program, where public health-trained professionals in government-related public servant roles set up a surveillance system from which they derived information as to what risks were larger to the pediatric population in the state, developed an intervention to address them, and evaluated and disseminated their findings.[28]

Research

Public health practitioners are particularly well positioned to collect and analyze local data to identify injury patterns, trends, and risk factors. They are also well positioned to introduce scientific methods to injury control by insisting that new countermeasures be evaluated and that, where relevant, they first be subjected to testing in the field.

Service

Public health practitioners can assist community organizations in analyzing data and choosing countermeasures that are known to be effective. They can also help conduct surveillance of important injury problems.

Education

It is essential to educate not only individuals in the community but also the public and private decision makers (e.g., legislators, designers, executives, builders) whose decisions affect the risk of injury for large numbers of individuals. Every day, these decision makers are confronted with issues such as whether to delay implementation of vehicle standards; whether to make an appliance safer or depend upon users to always follow directions; or whether to promote products on the basis of their potential for reducing injury, as opposed to assuming that "you can't sell safety." Public health practitioners can be of great assistance in these processes. It is also particularly important to educate the members of the media who, in their reporting of injury stories, inform public opinion and shape our understanding of health issues.[29]

Influencing Legislation and Regulation

Public health practitioners are particularly well-positioned to assist (or initiate) local policy discussions and assist in evaluating the validity or quality of the facts presented by the different parties involved in policy discussions. For a public health practitioner to be successful in all these areas, he or she must also be aware of the barriers to the implementation of injury prevention activities, including funding limitations, organizational difficulties, and turf battles.[7]

THE ROLE OF PUBLIC HEALTH AGENCIES

The growing awareness that injuries can be reduced through the application of public health principles to populations has expanded expectations for national, state, and local public health agencies to increase their activities in injury control.

National Leadership

A good example of national leadership is the 1986 enactment by the U.S. Congress of legislation creating the Division of Injury Control within the CDC's Center for Environmental Health; in 1992, the Division became the National Center for Injury Prevention and Control (NCIPC). The NCIPC supports both extramural and intramural research that is essential to advancing the science and prevention strategies for violence and injury.[30] Research has been supported through several mechanisms, including funding for Injury Control Research Centers (ICRCs). ICRCs are centers for excellence in injury research and they not only study prevention, acute care, and rehabilitation, but also train the next generation of injury prevention specialists. NCIPC's support has also guided the field through landmark documents including the Injury Research Agenda.[31]

Information Collection

Effective injury control depends on adequate information systems. National agencies play a major role in the response to injury-related issues, but the quality of their basic data is determined, predominantly, at the local level. Health departments can stimulate uniform reporting and prompt analysis of injury data and make appropriate use of injury data in administration. Numerous issues that are related to injury definition, coding, case inclusion criteria, event definition and coding and its standardization, remain unresolved and prevent further advancement of the injury field.

National public health agencies can also reinforce these activities by ensuring that information developed from local data eventually gets back to the local level.

Regulation and Legislation

Safety standards have long been applied to many kinds of products and operations. Standards may be descriptive in nature, specifying such things as materials, design, and process, or they may be performance standards, indicating what a product should do (and what it should never do) no matter how it is made. For safety purposes, performance standards are generally preferable, although both types sometimes contribute little except a false sense of security. Most commonly, standards are voluntary and industry-wide. Yet voluntary standards are often insufficient. When public attention is drawn to an industry's failure to keep its products from being unreasonably hazardous, the government may consider issuing regulatory standards.

In addition to product and environmental standards, laws regulating human behavior are also intended to reduce injuries. As with other regulations, whether they succeed depends upon whether they are enforced, whether the penalties are effective, and whether the basic assumptions underlying the regulations and their enforcement are valid. State-level safety belt laws provide a wonderful example of this point. By 2007, all states except New Hampshire had established some form of safety belt law for motor vehicle occupants. (As of 2015, New Hampshire remained the only state without a primary or a secondary seat belt law for adults, although it does have a primary child passenger safety law that covers all drivers and passengers under 18.) The degree of coverage, details, and enforcement of these laws varies widely from state to state; however, one of the most distinguishing factors of these laws' effectiveness is whether they are primary (e.g., not wearing safety belts is reason enough for arrest and punishment) or secondary (i.e., some other offense is needed for the safety belt regulation to be enforced). Figure 27-6 shows safety belt use as reported from observational surveys by state. States with secondary safety belt laws have significantly lower safety belt use.

The ability to regulate is one key characteristic of government structures, and these structures are critical for injury prevention. For instance, the United Nations Decade of Action for Road Safety, an effort to stabilize and reduce global road traffic fatalities by 2020, underscores the importance of government structures. This initiative's activities revolve around five strategies, one of which, Road Safety Management, emphasizes stronger institutions to prevent injury.[32] Specifically: "Designation of national lead agencies with the capacity to develop and lead the delivery of national road safety strategies, plans, and targets, underpinned by the data collection and evidential research to assess countermeasure design and monitor implementation and effectiveness."

Emergency Systems

When primary prevention strategies fail to accomplish needed injury reduction, secondary and tertiary strategies become imperative. These emergency systems are governed by agencies at the local, state, and

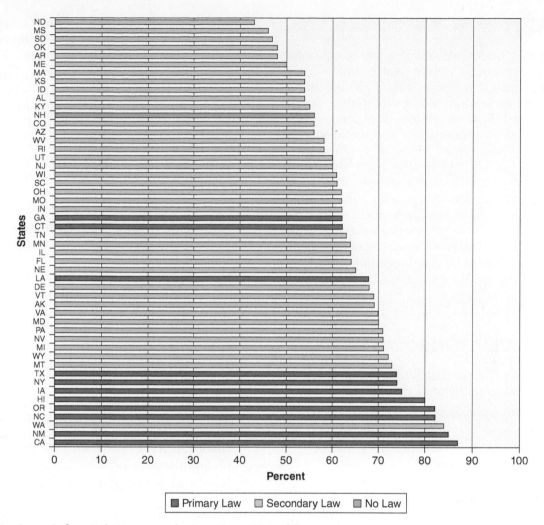

FIGURE 27-6   State Safety Belt Use Rates by Law Type. United States, 2006

SOURCE: National Highway Traffic Safety Administration. Traffic Safety Facts: Safety Belt Use in 2006--Use Rates in the States and Territories. DOT HS 810690. Washington, DC; 2007.

federal levels. Local and regional planning is required for successful organization of emergency communication systems, transportation, trauma units, poison control centers, and specialized units such as those for burns. Public health agencies have a role in organizing such systems, for example, by categorizing emergency facilities on the basis of what kind of injury cases they are equipped and staffed to treat, so that seriously injured persons can have the optimum chance of receiving adequate care. Lately, this role has expanded into development of triage criteria and establishment of regionalized trauma systems where not only the emergency facilities are categorized, but hospitals are too.

Education

Even though it has been earlier stated that priority in injury prevention should be given to measures that require little or no human action or cooperation, education must supplement some forms of injury control.[33] Public health agencies must devise and implement educational efforts directed to the general public that address all three phases of the injury sequence: pre-event, event, and postevent. Another very important function of education is to convince the public as well as private and public organizations that the hazards of their environment can be controlled, reduced, or eliminated. Public support is often needed before a preventive measure can be introduced; for example, people must be persuaded of the benefits of a motorcycle helmet law before they support it. Finally, individuals (e.g., legislators, regulators, administrators) whose decisions can determine the likelihood of injury to thousands of people need to be educated to take advantage of their role in injury prevention.

SUMMARY

Injury is a public health problem that can be controlled with the application of public health tools such as epidemiology, program design, policy change, implementation, and evaluation. Major achievements of the field over the past 30 years reinforce this point. Further reductions in both unintentional and intentional injuries and their associated medical, psychological, and economic burden will require continued efforts by the public health community in surveillance and research, in building partnerships with public and private organizations, and in the development of state and local health department injury control programs. Those public health practitioners who understand the issues and scientific concepts involved in injury occurrence can contribute effectively to substantially reducing this huge problem.

REVIEW QUESTIONS

1. If the bumper of a car strikes a pedestrian, fracturing the femur, what is the etiologic agent?

2. Name the three phases of the injury sequence.

3. What is the most important criterion when choosing among possible countermeasures to reduce an injury problem?

4. Give an example of automatic ("passive") protection from electrical injuries.

5. Seat belts are an example of what type of protection of automobile passengers?

6. What is the difference between a primary and secondary seat belt law?

ACKNOWLEDGMENTS

Partial support for writing this chapter was provided by Grant Number 5R49CE001507 from the Centers for Disease Control and Prevention to the Johns Hopkins Center for Injury Research and Policy. The findings and conclusions are those of the authors and do not necessarily represent the official views of the U.S. Centers for Disease Control and Prevention.

REFERENCES

1. Baker SP. Injury control. In: Rosenau MJ, Maxcy KF, Sartwell PE, eds. *Preventive Medicine and Public Health*. 10th ed. New York: Appleton Century-Crofts; 1973.

2. Public Health Functions Steering Committee. Public Health in America. 1995; http://www.health.gov/phfunctions/public.htm.

3. Council on Linkages Between Academia and Public Health Practice. Core Competencies for Public Health Practice. Vol Available at: http://www.phf.org/link/corecompetencies.htm. Washington, DC; 2001.

4. Baker SP, O'Neill B, Li G, Ginsberg M. *The Injury Fact Book*. 2nd ed. New York: Oxford University Press; 1992.

5. Gielen AC, Sleet DA, DiClemente RJ. *Injury and Violence Prevention: Behavioural Science Theories, Methods and Applications*. San Francisco: John Wiley & Sons; 2006.

6. Laflamme L, Svanstrom L, Schelp L, eds. *Safety Promotion Research: A Public Health Approach to Accident and Injury Prevention*. Stockholm, Sweden: Karolinska Institute; 1999.

7. Christoffel T, Gallagher SS. *Injury Prevention and Public Health: Practical Knowledge, Skills and Strategies*. 2nd ed. Gaithersburg, MD: Aspen Publishers; 2006.

8. National Committee for Injury Prevention and Control. Injury prevention: meeting the challenge. *Am J Prev Med*. 1989;5 (3, Supplement):1–303.

9. Bonnie RJ, Fulco CE, Liverman CT. *Reducing the Burden of Injury: Advancing Prevention and Treatment*. Washington, DC: Institute of Medicine, National Academy Press;1999.

10. Centers for Disease Control and Prevention/ National Center for Health Statistics Office of Statistics and Programming. Vital statistics system for numbers of deaths. http://www.cdc.gov/ncipc/wisqars/. Accessed June 10, 2014.

11. U.S. Burden of Disease Collaborators. The state of US health, 1990–2010: burden of diseases, injuries, and risk factors. *JAMA*. 2013;310(6):591–608. DOI: 510.1001/jama.2013.13805.

12. National Center for Injury Prevention and Control. CDC Injury Research Agenda, 2009–2018. Atlanta, GA: Centers for Disease Control and Prevention, US Department of Health and Human Services; 2009:Available at: http://www.cdc.gov/ncipc.

13. Murray CJ, Vos T, Lozano R, et al. Disability-adjusted life years (DALYs) for 291 diseases and injuries in 21 regions, 1990–2010: a systematic analysis for the Global Burden of Disease Study 2010. *Lancet*. December 15, 2012;380(9859): 2197–2223.

14. Centers for Disease Control and Prevention/ National Center for Health Statistics Office of Statistics and Programming. Cost of Injury Reports. http://www.cdc.gov/ncipc/wisqars/. Accessed June 10, 2014.

15. Segui-Gomez M. *Literature Search for Psychological and Psychosocial Consequences of Injury (Report # NHTSA DOT HS 808 527)*. National Highway Traffic Safety Administration, US Dept of Transportation;1996.

16. Waller JA. Public health then and now: reflections on a half century of injury control. *Am J Public Health*. 1994;84:665–670.

17. CDC National Public Health Performance Standards (NPHPS). The Public Health System and the 10 Essential Public Health Services. Updated May 29, 2014; http://www.cdc.gov/nphpsp/ essentialservices.html.

18. Calhoun JG, Ramiah K, Weist EM, Shortell SM. Development of a core competency model for the master of public health degree. *Am J Public Health*. September 2008;98(9):1598–1607.

19. Heinrich HW. *Industrial Accident Prevention. A Scientific Approach*. 4th ed. New York: McGraw-Hill; 1980.

20. Haddon W. A logical framework for categorizing highway safety phenomena and activities. *J Trauma*. 1972;12:193–207.

21. Blumenthal M. Dimensions of the traffic safety problem. *Traffic Safety Research Review*. 1968;12: 7–12.

22. Vernick JS, Li G, Ogaitis S, MacKenzie E, Baker SP, Gielen AC. Effectiveness of high school driver education on motor vehicle crashes, violations, and licensure. *Am J Prev Med*. 1999;16 (1 Suppl):40–46.

23. Dannenberg AL, Fowler CJ. Evaluation of interventions to prevent injuries: an overview. *Inj Prev*. June 1998;4(2):141–147.

24. Graham JD. *Preventing Automobile Injury: New Findings from Evaluation Research*. Dover, MA: Auburn House Publishing Co; 1988.

25. Elvik R, Hoye A, Vaa T, Sorensen M. *The Handbook of Road Safety Measures*, 2nd ed. Wagonlane, Bingley, U.K. : Emerald Group Publishing Limited; 2009.

26. Standfast SJ. Prevention of motor vehicle injuries in state and local health departments: the New York model. *Bull NY Acad Med*. 1988;64(7):846–856.

27. Reason J. Human error: models and management. *BMJ*. 2000;320(7237):768–770.

28. Guyer B, Gallagher SS, Chang B-H, Azzara CV, Cupples LA, Colton T. Prevention of childhood injuries: evaluation of the Statewide Childhood Injury Prevention Program (SCIPP). *Am J Public Health*. 1989;79(11): 1521–1527.

29. Smith KC, Girasek DC, Baker SP, et al. It was a freak accident': an analysis of the labelling of injury events in the US press. *Injury Prevention*. 2012;18(1):38–43. DOI: 10.1136/ip.2011.031609.

30. Gielen A, Runyan C, Pollack K, Mickalide A, Baker S. Reflections on NCIPC's 20 Years of Injury Control.......Then...... Now...... Imagine. *Journal of Safety Research*. 2012;43(4):319–321.

31. National Center for Injury Prevention and Control. *CDC Injury Research Agenda, 2009–2018*. Atlanta, GA: US Department of Health and Human Services, Centers for Disease Control and Prevention;2009.

32. World Health Organization. Global Plan for the Decade of Action Road Safety. 2011–2020. 2014; http://www.who.int/roadsafety/decade_of_action/.

33. Sleet DA, Gielen AC. Behavioral interventions for injury and violence prevention. In: Doll LS, Bonzo SE, Mercy JA, Sleet DA, eds. *Handbook of Injury and Violence Prevention*. New York: Springer; 2007.

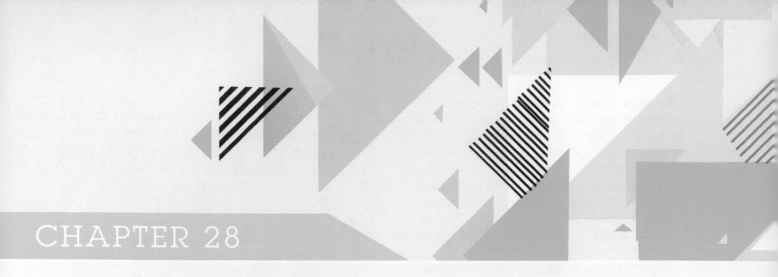

CHAPTER 28

Behavioral Health and Substance Abuse

C.G. Leukefeld, DSW • Katherine Marks, PhD • April Young, PhD •
Danelle Stevens-Watkins, PhD • Rice Leach, MD

LEARNING OBJECTIVES

Upon completion of this chapter, the reader will be able to:

1. Describe behavioral health and substance abuse practice issues.

2. Identify ways to explore processes in behavioral health decision making using substance abuse as an example.

3. Discuss behavioral health implications for public health practice using substance abuse as an example.

4. Assess the overall effects of substance abuse (including prevalence, mortality, disparities, and health problems) for public health practice.

KEY TERMS

addiction
behavioral health
epidemiological triad
harm reduction
illegal use
illegal recreational use
legal use
legal recreational use
substance abuse
supply reduction

INTRODUCTION

Most public health practitioners agree that local health departments (LHDs) in the United States provide limited behavioral health and substance abuse prevention and treatment services. This opinion is supported by recent data from the 2013 National Profile of Local Health Departments.[1] Perhaps it is associated with the idea that it is difficult to change health behaviors because they are chronic and relapsing.[2] This reality is now supported by both brain and behavioral research, particularly in the area of drug abuse.[3] Recognizing the reality of chronicity and relapse, this chapter focuses on introducing behavioral health and substance abuse issues within a public health context. We include incidence and prevalence data and policy information for substance abuse as examples to understand the high levels of behavioral health-related issues in the general U.S. population. Likewise we suggest that places such as prisons and jails may allow for interactions with the same individuals as local public health service providers.

Because avoiding behavioral health issues in public health settings can be common, we look forward to future changes in public health policy and practice on behavioral health. Policy is also an arena where local public health practitioners can impact behavioral health with changes in prevention and treatment practice. Public health adds an approach to behavioral health and substance abuse interventions, which incorporates the interaction of the agent, the host (the individual), and the environment (the community)—the classic epidemiologic triad often used only for infectious/communicable diseases. These interventions can include biological, psychological, social, cultural and spiritual factors. For example, a community intervention focused on only the agent, the host, or the environment separately may be useful; however, the more useful and successful interventions systematically target all three simultaneously. For this chapter, behavioral health is defined as a focus on lifestyles that are associated with preventable and premature deaths including substance abuse, tobacco use, physical inactivity, unhealthy dietary habits, risky sex, and violence.

DEFINITION OF SUBSTANCE USE

There are a variety of definitions of substance abuse. Each definition includes the use of psychoactive substance for a nontherapeutic effect. Medical definitions include the two most commonly used diagnostic tools, the American Psychiatric Association's (APA) *Diagnostic and Statistical Manual of Mental Disorders* and the World Health Organization's (WHO) *International Statistical Classification of Diseases and Related Health Problems* (ICD). The medical or disease model defines addiction as a chronic relapsing medical condition in which a user/abuser does not have control over his or her drug or alcohol use.

Substance use, abuse, and dependence are prominent in the United States. Effective substance use prevention and treatment intervention can reduce problems associated with use, which includes harmful consequences such as relapse, criminal justice involvement, economic instability, and mental health disorders. Drug and alcohol use is the ingestion of a substance that can be distinguished across two dimensions: legal status and purpose of use.[4] The combination of these two dimensions produces four types of use: (1) legal use, (2) illegal use, (3) legal recreational use, and (4) illegal recreational use. Legal use includes over-the-counter or prescription drugs, whereas, legal recreational drug use is the use of government-sanctioned psychoactive substances to achieve a specific mental or psychic state (e.g., drinking alcohol to get intoxicated). Illegal use refers to taking drugs without a prescription for some socially sanctioned purpose (e.g., using an amphetamine to work all night). Illegal recreational use includes taking drugs without a prescription to achieve a specific mental or psychic state (e.g., taking heroin to get high). Public health practitioners focus on the latter three combinations; however, illegal recreational use currently receives the most attention.

PREVALENCE OF SUBSTANCE USE

Alcohol and other drug use are present throughout the U.S. society among all social and economic classes, ethnic/racial groups, and geographic regions. Rates of use vary by type of drug, with alcohol the most commonly used drug. The use of other drugs varies by group and availability; however, marijuana, psychotherapeutics (nonmedical use), and cocaine use represent the most frequently used drugs in the United States.[5]

According to the 2012 National Survey on Drug Use and Health (NSDUH),[5] nearly 52 percent of the population over 12 years of age uses alcohol at least once a month, compared to 9.2 percent for those who report illicit drug use (see Table 28-1). Marijuana accounts for the majority of illicit drug use, with approximately 7 percent of the population reporting current use in the past month. The prevalence of other illicit drug use (3.4 percent) is lower and relatively stable over several years.

Drug use among high school seniors has been reported for about 40 years with the Monitoring the Future (MTF) Survey. This survey examines prevalence of drug use and trends in drug use, and provides a picture of emerging illicit drug use among U.S. youth. According to the 2013 MTF Survey, alcohol is the most

TABLE 28-1   Past Month Use of Alcohol and Selected Illicit Drugs by Those Age 12 or Older for 2010, 2011, and 2012

Substance	Percent of Age 12 or Older		
	2010	2011	2012
Alcohol	51.8%	51.8%	52.1%
Any illicit drug	8.9%	8.7%	9.2%
Marijuana	6.9%	7.0%	7.3%
Cocaine	0.6%	0.5%	0.6%
Heroin	0.2%	0.3%	0.3%
Methamphetamine	0.1%	0.2%	0.2%
Hallucinogens	0.7%	1.0%	1.1%
Psychotherapeutics*	2.7%	2.4%	2.6%
Pain relievers	2.0%	1.7%	1.9%
Tranquilizer	0.9%	0.7%	0.8%
Stimulants	0.4%	0.4%	0.5%
Sedatives	0.1%	0.1%	0.1%

*"Nonmedical" use of prescription pain relievers, tranquilizers, stimulants, or sedatives, defined as use without a prescription of the individual's own or simply for the experience or feeling the drugs caused.

SOURCE: Substance Abuse and Mental Health Services Administration. Results from the 2010, 2011, and 2012 National Survey on Drug Use and Health. Substance Abuse and Mental Health Services Administration.[5–7]

TABLE 28-2   High School Seniors: Past Month Alcohol and Selected Illicit Drug Use for 2011, 2012, and 2013

Substance	Percent of High School Seniors		
	2011	2012	2013
Alcohol	40.0%	41.5%	39.2%
Any illicit drug	25.2%	25.2%	25.5%
Marijuana	22.6%	22.9%	22.7%
Ecstasy (MDMA)	2.3%	0.9%	1.5%
Cocaine	1.1%	1.1%	1.1%
Inhalants	1.0%	0.9%	1.0%
Methamphetamine	0.6%	0.5%	0.4%
Heroin	0.4%	0.3%	0.3%
Prescription drugs*	7.2%	7.0%	7.0%
Amphetamines	3.7%	3.3%	4.1%
Sedatives	1.8%	2.0%	2.2%
Narcotics	3.6%	3.0%	2.8%
Tranquilizers	2.3%	2.1%	2.0%

*Prescription drugs used without a prescription.

SOURCE: Johnston LD, O'Malley PM, Bachman JG, Schulenberg JE, Miech RA. Monitoring the Future national survey results on drug use, 1975–2013. 2014.[8]

commonly used drug among these youth, albeit at a lower rate than overall U.S. levels. In addition, higher percentages of high school seniors report current illicit drug use, specifically marijuana, cocaine, prescription narcotics, and tranquilizers, than the U.S. population and these rates have remained relatively stable over the past few years (see Table 28-2).

Table 28-3 shows 2012 data on rates of use by ethnic and racial group. Between 2002 and 2012, there were statistically significant increases in current illicit drug use among whites (8.5 percent to 9.2 percent) and blacks (9.7 percent to 11.3 percent) aged 12 and older. Whites and individuals reporting two or more races were significantly more likely to use alcohol than other racial/ethnic groups.[5] Researchers are growing increasingly concerned about the alarming prevalence of drug use among native Hawaiians/Pacific Islanders and mixed-race people.[9] Research based on NSDUH data has shown that whites had a lower prevalence of past-year marijuana use compared to multiracial individuals but a higher prevalence compared to Asian Americans and Hispanics.[10]

Similar racial/ethnic variability has been observed in rates of substance use disorders, with substance dependence and/or abuse being lower among Asians (3.2 percent) and native Hawaiians or Pacific Islanders (5.4 percent) than among whites (8.7 percent), Hispanics (8.8 percent), blacks (8.9 percent), multiracial individuals (10.1 percent), and American Indians/Alaskan Natives (21.8 percent).[5] Interestingly, recent research identified no significant disparity in past-year participation in substance abuse treatment in comparisons of black and Latino adults with whites; however, when analyses were adjusted for socioeconomic factors and criminal history, significant disparities became apparent.[11] These studies and others underscore the importance of contextualizing racial/ethnic substance use disparities within the milieu of individual, familial, sociocultural, and economic factors.

The 2012 National Survey (NSDUH) estimated that 22.2 million individuals were dependent on or abusing illicit drugs or alcohol, which is 8.5 percent of the U.S. population age 12 or older. In addition, 14.9 million Americans were dependent on or abusing alcohol but

TABLE 28-3 Past Month Use of Alcohol and Selected Illicit Drug Use Among Persons Aged 12 or Older by Selected Race/Ethnicity for 2012

Substance	Percent of Use by Race/Ethnicity Group					
	White	Black	Hispanic	American Indian or Alaskan Natives	Asian	Two or more races
Alcohol	57.4%	43.2%	41.8%	41.7%	36.9%	51.9%
Any illicit drug	9.2%	11.3%	8.3%	12.7%	3.7%	14.8%
Marijuana	7.4%	9.1%	6.2%	9.4%	2.5%	13.1%
Cocaine	0.6 %	1.1%	0.4%	1.6%	0.5%	1.2%

SOURCE: Substance Abuse and Mental Health Services Administration. Results from the 2012 National Survey on Drug Use and Health: Summary of National Findings, NSDUH Series H-46, HHS Publication No. (SMA) 1304795. Substance Abuse and Mental Health Services Administration, 2013.[5]

not illicit drugs in 2012, whereas 4.5 million were dependent on or abusing illicit drugs but not alcohol. Approximately 2.8 million individuals were dependent on or abusing both illicit drugs and alcohol with illicit drug dependence or abuse for marijuana at 4.3 million, prescription pain relievers at 2.1 million, and cocaine at 1.1 million. Young adults (i.e., ages 18–25) were more likely to be dependent on or to abuse illicit drugs or alcohol (18.9 percent) compared to those age 12–17 (6.1 percent) and age 26 and over (7.0 percent). In addition, the overall prevalence of substance dependence or abuse among males (11.5 percent) was nearly double that of females (5.7 percent); however, there was no gender difference in prevalence for youth ages 12–17.[5]

Excluded Groups

As noted above, the NSDUH and Monitoring the Future surveys are the primary sources for U.S. data on alcohol and other drug use; however, these data sources do not reflect the entire U.S. population. The NSDUH does not include individuals who are in-patients or are entering in-patient treatment or those who reside in hotels, hospitals, and prisons/jails, or who are without a home. In addition, the school-based surveys do not include those who dropped out of school before graduation or who were absent the day of the survey. This is important to keep in mind because other studies suggest that alcohol and other drug use within these populations is significantly higher than in the general population.[12–14]

BEHAVIORAL HEALTH

A major public health milestone was the 1979 Surgeon General's Report on health promotion and disease prevention, titled *Healthy People*, which is updated approximately every 10 years as a set of health objectives for the nation (see http://www.healthypeople.gov). This initial report encouraged a second public health revolution in the United States that emphasized prevention and extended the first revolution that targeted infectious diseases.[15] **Behavioral health**, including substance abuse prevention, was identified as one of the challenges for public health, with high prevalence among U.S. youth. The initial report established five major goals that focused on lifecycle stages (i.e., healthy infants, healthy children, healthy adolescents/young adults, healthy adults, and healthy older adults). Early successful smoking prevention efforts were identified as a key factor for prevention.[16] *Healthy People 2020* provides a comprehensive set of 10-year national goals and objectives for improving the health of all Americans.[17] *Healthy People 2020* includes 42 topic areas with over 1,200 objectives. A smaller set of objectives, called Leading Health Indicators, has been selected to communicate high-priority health issues and actions with twelve Leading Health Indicator Topics. Of these 12 the following Leading Health Topics are clearly in the behavioral health arena:

1. Injury and Violence—including motor vehicle crashes, homicide, domestic and school violence, child abuse and neglect, suicide, and unintentional drug overdoses;

2. Mental Health—which has a serious impact on physical health and is associated with the prevalence, progression, and outcome of chronic diseases, including diabetes, heart disease, and cancer;

3. Nutrition, Physical Activity, and Obesity—which are essential to a person's overall health including conditions such as high blood pressure, high cholesterol, diabetes, heart disease, stroke, and cancer;

4. Reproductive and Sexual Health—which is key to eliminating health disparities, reducing rates of infectious diseases and infertility, and increasing educational attainment, career opportunities, and financial stability;

5. Social Determinants—which incorporate the critical role of home, school, workplace, neighborhood, and community in improving health;

6. Substance Abuse—which is associated with cardiovascular conditions; pregnancy complications, teenage pregnancy, human immunodeficiency virus/acquired immunodeficiency syndrome (HIV/AIDS), sexually transmitted infections (STIs); domestic violence, child abuse, motor vehicle crashes, homicide, and suicide; and

7. Tobacco Use—which is the single most preventable cause of disease, disability, and death in the United States.

THEORY AND FRAMEWORKS

There are gaps in the public health literature on theoretical factors impacting behavioral health and substance abuse. For example, the majority of public health theories are not specific to understanding drug and alcohol use, but focus on explaining health behaviors in a broader context. Although public health practice is, to a large extent, biomedically grounded, drug and alcohol use interventions can be enriched with the integration of a variety of psychological[18-20] and multilevel socioecological theories[21-26] to broaden the traditionally individual-level perspective of behavioral health. Focusing on individual factors alone can promote victim-blaming[27] and personal failure. Research should consider interpersonal processes, organizational factors, and regulatory perspectives.[27-29] Table 28-4 presents examples of two multilevel theoretical frameworks for addressing factors that influence health behaviors associated with substance use and abuse.

A PUBLIC HEALTH PARADIGM

Using the three key components (the epidemiologic triad) of understanding a public health problem (i.e., host, agent, and environment), drug and alcohol use/abuse can be better understood in the context of behavioral health. The *host* is the individual with the problem, and the *agent* is the substance. The *environment* includes social, economic, physical, political, and cultural settings in which the host and agent interact.[33] Drugs and alcohol can play differing roles within this public health paradigm. For example, with drug-related illnesses such as cirrhosis of the liver, the agent or vector can be alcohol. However, for alcohol-related trauma, the agent is the impact of an automobile hitting an object, with alcohol as a significant environmental factor increasing the likelihood of injury. A high-risk environment creates opportunities for harm. Importantly, environmental change can provide protection to large numbers of people by helping to prevent the agent and host from interacting. A comprehensive public health strategy focuses on all three components.

Community prevention, which includes primary, secondary, and/or tertiary prevention, is unique to public health. For example, primary prevention is directed

TABLE 28-4   Frameworks and Theories for Studying and Intervening on Health Behaviors Associated with Substance Use and Abuse

Theoretical Framework	Factors	Processes Influencing Behavior
Social Ecological Model[27,30]	• Intrapersonal / • Individual[18,31,32] • Interpersonal • Institutional • Community • Public Policy	• Demographics and individual characteristics (knowledge, attitudes, behavior, self-concept, and skills) • Formal/informal social networks and support systems • Organizational climate and operational regulations • Relationships among organizations, institutions, and informal networks with defined boundaries, community norms • Policies, procedures, and laws designed to protect the community
Bio/Psycho/ Social/Spiritual Interaction[28]	• Biological/Genetic • Psychological • Social/Environmental • Spiritual	• Heritability and biologically conditioned aspects of addiction • Individual characteristics (expectancies to use, personality factors, and individual risk and protective factors) • Laws, culture, family norms, customs, peer associations and consequences associated with social learning • Spiritual beliefs

at preventing the initial use of drugs (e.g., drug-related education programs or antidrug advertising). Secondary prevention focuses on early identification of drug use and intervention before the progression to drug or alcohol dependence (e.g., drug testing). Tertiary prevention includes substance abuse treatment.

A SHIFT IN ALCOHOL POLICY

Until recently, public health principles applied to alcohol and other drug problems have focused on the host and the agent to the exclusion of environmental risk factors. For example, during the late 1800s and early 1900s, alcohol policy was dominated by a focus on the individual immorality of drinking and the need to restrict and/or prohibit the availability of "demon" alcohol.[34] Following the repeal of Prohibition in 1933, policy shifted to a medical and predominantly host perspective. This primary focus was on identifying and treating alcoholics, not prevention. With this perspective, policies to address environmental risk factors and controls on alcohol were irrelevant. In fact, these policies were perceived as potentially harmful because they could lead to increased criminal activities and create a "forbidden fruit" status for alcohol.

In the past 35 years, a public health perspective to alcohol use/abuse brought a dramatic shift in assumptions.[35] In part, this shift was associated with prevalence data that alcohol problems were not experienced by a small, discrete subpopulation of alcoholics, but others as well. Researchers also pointed to the health problems associated with alcohol in addition to alcoholism, including trauma, alcohol-related birth defects, sexual assaults and other violence, cirrhosis of the liver and other long-term health problems, and workplace/school problems.[36-40] The diversity of alcohol problems also led to realizing the complexity since alcohol interacts with and contributes to a variety of social and health problems; that these problems occur in the context of a complex system; and strategies for addressing them must take into account the interaction of diverse risk factors.

As a result of these shifts in perspective, there is more concern with alcohol availability, drinking environments, and environmental risks. The focus shifted to population-based alcohol policies rather than individual-based strategies. In contrast to prohibition policies, the current focus is reducing problems and harm associated with alcohol use.

DRUG POLICY

The U.S. illicit drug policies have been dominated by the Prohibition perspective. The focus has been on individual deviance and immorality, and the need to abolish the illicit drug trade. Historically and during the late 1800s, opiate and cocaine preparations were inexpensive and were widely used in over-the-counter preparations including Bayer aspirin®, Coca-Cola®, and patent medicines. Beginning in the early 1900s, there was increased government regulation to decrease physician-prescribing practices to reduce opiate and cocaine use. Early U.S. illicit drug policies targeted minorities to eradicate recreational use. The 1937 Marihuana Tax Act essentially banned the possession and sale of marijuana products until 1970 when it was replaced with the passage of the Comprehensive Drug Abuse Prevention and Control Act.[41] In sum, these licit-illicit drug policies have had little or no relationship to the relative risks to public health that the drugs pose.[42]

Illicit drug use peaked in the general population during the 1970s and the abuse of most drugs remained elevated during the 1980s. However, there was increased crack/cocaine use in the mid-1980s and increased heroin use in the 1990s. This was also the case for methamphetamine (meth) and prescription drugs into the 2000s with raves, club drugs, meth cooking, and the abuse of prescription drugs such as OxyContin® and a "lock them up" approach. In response to sustained illicit substance use, drug policies continued to evolve. For example, the passage of the Fair Sentencing Act of 2010 reduced the disparity in federal criminal penalties between cocaine and crack cocaine.

For fiscal year 2014, the President's National Drug Control Strategy budgeted $25.4 billion for drug control, a more than two-fold increase from 2007.[43,44] Because the United States incarcerates drug abusers, nearly 60 percent of that budget was allocated for law enforcement costs, drug interdiction (stopping drugs at the border), and other Department of Justice activities.[44] However, recently there has been an increase in the percentage of federal funding dedicated to behavioral health prevention and treatment initiatives. Despite this financial investment, past month, or "current" use, of illegal drugs has remained stable since 2009.[5]

Decriminalizing and Legalizing Marijuana

There is almost universal agreement that marijuana should not be used by children and adolescents as they develop physically and emotionally. Beginning in 1996, marijuana possession was legalized for medical purposes, including for cancer treatment-associated nausea, in several states (http://www.norml.org/index). In 2012, Washington and Colorado approved legalized possession, sales, and taxation of small amounts of marijuana for personal recreational use along with taxing marijuana dispensaries, which are significant departures from the 1937 Marihuana Tax Act.

An argument for legalization is that it saves taxpayers money with the current minimum-mandatory sentencing of marijuana users contributing to the crowded prisons and jails. On the other side of the issue, legalizing marijuana gives the wrong message to adolescents and others—that it is okay to use a mind-altering drug. Opponents of legalization point out that marijuana is a "gateway" drug to the use of other illegal drugs, or "hard drugs" such as cocaine and heroin.

Drug Policy Strategies

U.S. drug policies have changed in the past several decades, sometimes dramatically, from an emphasis on law enforcement strategies to lock-up drug users, to an emphasis on drug prevention/treatment. Drug policies have been shaped by planned as well as spur-of-the-moment political, moralistic, and media-inspired responses to three major illicit drugs—heroin, marijuana, and cocaine—and to a lesser extent, two legal drugs—alcohol and nicotine. From one point of view, the U.S. drug policy has been successful with only marginal increases and decreases in overall use. However, from another point of view, increased use of stimulants, particularly cocaine/crack use, marijuana, and prescription opioids like OxyContin®, is helping to fill U.S. prisons and jails. Opioid overdose is also a burden to the health care system. Drug abuse has been a major national issue for more than 30 years with the rhetoric of using the "War on Drugs." Congresses, presidents, and both major political parties have fought the war, with increased federal spending as the armament to change the chronic and relapsing nature of drug misuse.

The federal drug czar, a cabinet-level official, coordinates federal law enforcement and drug prevention/treatment activities. The drug czar's Office of National Drug Control Policy (ONDCP) is responsible for developing and updating the *National Drug Control Strategy*, which can be accessed at http://www.whitehouse.gov by searching under "National Drug Control Strategy." The federal drug strategy incorporates *supply reduction* (law enforcement) and *demand reduction* (prevention and treatment). Current national priorities are (1) preventing use before it starts, (2) expanding access to treatment, (3) reforming the criminal justice system to break the cycle of drug use, crime, and incarceration, and (4) reducing the stigma associated with substance use disorders.

Different ideas and approaches continue to influence drug policy. *Public health officials* generally encourage **harm reduction**. An example of harm reduction is to make needles available to injectors via needle and syringe provision programs. Needle exchange programs have been demonstrated to decrease the spread of HIV/AIDS, though opponents continue to voice concerns that it encourages drug abuse.[45] *Enforcement/police approaches* focus on arresting and locking up drug pushers and users. *Treatment providers* emphasize helping users become drug free. *Social scientists* employ an environmental approach, which focuses on two overall risk factors: the availability of illegal drugs, and the broader family, community, social, cultural, and political contexts in which illegal drug problems occur. *Educators* have historically denied there is a drug problem in their school and have developed drug-free zones around schools to prevent school drug use. *Employers* of pilots, police officers, military personnel, and production workers support and use drug testing to monitor employee drug use. However, drug testing remains controversial due to the difficult balance of protecting individual rights and protecting society from harms. Proponents of drug testing say that individuals should not be on drugs while on duty or on the job. Nonsupporters of drug testing advocate individual rights and stress that what a person does when not at work should not be "controlled" by an employer. Courts support employment-related drug testing with analysis of urine, blood, breath, saliva, and hair samples with subsequent legal sanctions. There are also those who support the idea that drugs should be legalized to eliminate profits from drug sales while others say that drug abusers need to "pull themselves up by their bootstraps." The media also continues to have a powerful and sometimes controversial role in shaping perceptions about drugs and drug use. This is underscored by advertising and product promotion for alcohol and prescription drugs. Controversy, however, surrounds the degree to which advertising should be controlled. Given the changing consensus about drug abuse and the lack of quick fixes or instant cures, shifting U.S. drug policies remains a reality.

Harm Reduction Is a Public Health Tradition

Harm reduction is a set of practical strategies and ideas to reduce the negative consequences associated with drug use (http://harmreduction.org/about-us/principles-of-harm-reduction/). Harm reduction approaches for disease prevention and health promotion, such as distributing bleach to drug injectors to clean needles, are limited in the United States by federal policy, but have roots in Britain and in the Netherlands. More common harm reduction approaches in the United States include designated drivers, cigarette-warning labels, smoke-free areas, and seat belts. Harm reduction is particularly relevant to reduce the spread of HIV and hepatitis C virus (HCV), which are transmitted with contaminated drug injection equipment or sharing needles, syringes, water, cotton, and cookers.

Disease prevention and health promotion continue today as key approaches for major public health advances which have included safe water, sanitation, and air quality. For behavioral health, using substance abuse as the example, lifestyle risk reduction can be a major approach for promoting health. Lifestyle risk reduction for alcohol and drug problems emphasizes that risk is a result of the interaction between biological/genetic risk, quantity of substance used, and frequency of use within a social or peer use context (including encouragement to use).[46] Prevention includes both no use (abstinence), as well as reducing high-risk choices and use (harm reduction). Individual choices about quantity and frequency are a key to preventing alcohol and drug problems. Quantity/frequency choices determine how much a person uses, how often alcohol or drugs are used, and whether a person's threshold for alcohol (biologic/genetic) is reached. Environmental, social, and psychological factors establish risk by influencing whether, how much, and how often a person uses alcohol or drugs. This interaction among biology, individual choice, and setting/environment determines the degree of intoxication, risk for problems, and the degree of later physiological damage or risk. Lifestyle risk reduction approaches incorporate five conditions for effective prevention: (1) It could happen to me—my choices matter; (2) I know what to do to reduce my risk; (3) People around me support low-risk choices; (4) I want to make low-risk choices; and (5) I have the skills I need to make lower risk choices. Biology establishes an individual threshold for intoxication, addiction, and diseases such as liver damage. Prevention strategies including harm reduction strategies can be most effective if they first target personal vulnerability by establishing the belief that high-risk choices are likely to cause alcohol/drug-related personal health or impairment problems.

Drug Supply and Demand

Supply reduction policies in the United States target two major approaches to reduce drug supply: law enforcement to arrest drug dealers, and border control. Law enforcement policies include searches and seizing drug dealers' property, as well as mandatory sentencing. Federal efforts target reducing drugs from other countries, which is called *interdiction*. Interdiction includes interrupting the flow of drugs high in the drug-dealing pyramid to decrease sales. The intent is that large-scale arrests of drug dealers increase the street price of illicit drugs, which then lowers the demand and use of illicit drugs. Several federal agencies are involved in supply reduction and interdiction, including the Bureau of Alcohol, Tobacco, Firearms and Explosives (ATF), the Drug Enforcement Agency (DEA), U.S. Customs, the Food and Drug Administration (FDA), Homeland Security, and, for some cases, the Federal Bureau of Investigation (FBI).

During the past 30 years, U.S. national strategies to increase interdiction and related law enforcement efforts have been implemented. These supply-reduction policies, although generally politically popular, have not been as effective in reducing overall drug use in the United States as expected while most other developed countries with similar drug problems have enacted risk reduction and harm reduction policies. However, U.S. lawmakers have traditionally supported "get tough" enforcement policies to increase the street prices of illicit drugs, even though the relationship between increasing illicit drug costs and overall drug use is not as clear.[47]

Treatment Approaches for Substance Use

Decreasing use during a drug abuser's addiction career can include community treatment, coerced treatment, incarceration, pharmacotherapy, 12-step self-help, and other self-help groups, all of which are considered to be drug demand strategies. Research has consistently supported the effectiveness of drug abuse treatment. For example, the National Institute of Drug Abuse (NIDA) reported that drug treatment reduces drug use by 40 to 60 percent.[48] Effective drug abuse treatment can also reduce related public health issues such as the spread of HIV among people who inject drugs.

Drug abuse treatment can be as effective as other treatments for long-term, relapsing diseases, if it is well delivered and targeted. Intervention options can range from drug testing, intensive behavioral/pharmacological treatment, self-help groups such as Alcoholics Anonymous, relapse prevention, and follow-up supervision. However, without treatment follow-up or continuing treatment, former users can return to drug use.

Drug abuse treatment generally begins with detoxification. Detoxification can be either medical with medication for withdrawal, or social detoxification without medication, depending on withdrawal-related medical complications. Because detoxification time is short with limited success alone, patients are usually referred to treatment. *Residential treatment* can include social skills training, relapse prevention, individual/group counseling/education, and/or family therapy. Treatment facilities can be public or private. *Therapeutic communities* incorporate a community approach that focuses on changing behaviors over a longer period to "graduation." *Halfway houses* are less structured than therapeutic communities and are generally a transition between institutions, such as prisons, and independent living to help individuals reenter the community. *Outpatient treatment* is the most common setting for drug treatment, with individual and/or group sessions.

Pharmacotherapy, or medication-assisted therapy, approaches incorporate using prescribed drugs to maintain illicit drug abstinence and reduce drug craving. The most commonly used pharmacotherapy is methadone, a synthetic opioid primarily for heroin/opioid detoxification and replacement therapy. Disulfiram (Antabuse) is often used for alcohol. If alcohol is consumed, disulfiram produces a severe reaction including nausea and irregular heartbeat. Compliance with taking disulfiram, however, is often minimal. Other currently approved pharmacotherapies for alcohol and opioid dependence include naltrexone, buprenorphine, and acamprosate (Campral). There are no currently approved pharmacotherapies for cocaine or methamphetamine dependence, although naltrexone and d-amphetamine have shown promise. It is important to note that the combination of pharmacotherapy and counseling is often more effective than either treatment alone. Although clinical and randomized studies report the utility of pharmacotherapies, their use in the United States is more limited than in other countries.

Using physician-prescribed drugs to treat drug and alcohol abuse has been controversial in the United States. Controversy centers on the idea that drug abusers should abstain from drug use; this idea is generally supported by law enforcement, judges, and some self-help groups. The *diversion* (using prescription medication for recreational purposes) of methadone and Suboxone (a combination of buprenorphine and naloxone) has also presented challenges.[49,50]

The distribution of naloxone (Narcan) to first responders and family members has also been controversial. Naloxone, an opioid antagonist, rapidly reverses the effects of heroin/opioid overdose. The primary argument for the widespread distribution of naloxone is that it saves lives. Opponents of the naloxone distribution say that its availability will encourage dangerous use by eliminating the natural consequences of drug use. Naloxone is not designed to prevent or reduce drug use, rather, it is considered to be a harm reduction approach due to its tertiary application (i.e., to mitigate effects of overdose).

THE SPECIAL BEHAVIORAL HEALTH NEEDS OF WOMEN

Several studies have reported gender differences for behavioral health including mental health and substance use disorders. "Telescoping" has been a term historically used to describe the biological and psychosocial factors among substance use in women.[51] Specifically, women tend to advance more rapidly than men from use, to problematic use, to treatment. Women also average more medical, mental health, and adverse social consequences than men.[52] However, a study of nationally representative data from the National Longitudinal Alcohol Epidemiologic Survey (NLAES, 1991–1992) and the National Epidemiologic Survey on Alcohol and Related Conditions (NESARC, 2001–2002) found no gender-specific differences in alcohol use disorders in the U.S. population.[53]

Women can experience a complexity of maternal, behavioral, and other health issues that are compounded by substance use. Women who come into contact with local health departments (LHDs) may have needs that require gender-specific services to address special issues, including mental health, victimization and violence, relationship issues, and physical health. These specialized services should incorporate continuing care tailored to behavioral health needs. One approach is to identify at-risk women as they enter public health care through targeted assessments and outreach at entry. Increased community linkages with other community treatment should be a priority. For example, the additional focus can be behavioral interventions for HIV/STI prevention and risky sex. Interventions for substance abuse should target decreasing behavioral health risks including sex in exchange for drugs, sex with multiple partners, inconsistent condom use, and unprotected oral sex.[54]

Women appear to be less likely to enter treatment for a substance use disorder than men, although study findings differ. Reasons cited for lower rates of treatment involvement include stigma, lack of a partner or family support, lack of child care, pregnancy, fears related to child custody issues, and complexities associated with treatment for co-occurring mental health, and substance abuse.[55] Treatment outcomes depend on individual, family, interpersonal, and community factors.

In addition, children with prenatal drug exposure are at increased risk for health, developmental, and substance use disorders.[56,57] In particular, neonatal abstinence syndrome (NAS), a withdrawal syndrome following prenatal opioid exposure, has increased five-fold since the year 2000 due to the increasing rates of opioid misuse among women.[58] NAS produces a range of symptoms from feeding difficulty to seizures and results in extended postnatal hospitalization.[57] Services to address the acute medical needs of the child as well as the long-term services to support both mother and child are indicated.

Mental Health

A mental health disorder tends to be an antecedent to a substance use disorder.[52] For example, an early study reported that women who experienced a major depressive episode were more than seven times likely to have alcohol dependence while men with a major depressive episode were not at risk for alcohol dependence.[59]

Women, as well as men, who report past suicide attempts and/or serious plans of suicide with a history of depression, substance use disorders, and episodes of interpersonal violence are at a significant elevated risk for future suicidal behavior.[60] In addition, a multisite study of randomly selected women in urban and rural jails found that about 53 percent of the women met criteria for Post-Traumatic Stress Disorder (PTSD) and 38 percent met criteria for a serious mental illness with a co-occurring substance use disorder.[61] It is often difficult to assess and determine whether a mental health disorder preceded a substance use disorder, particularly when a person has a significant history of victimization.

Victimization and Violence

Many drug-abusing women have histories of physical, mental, and sexual abuse.[62-64] For example, over half (57 percent) of incarcerated women reported experiencing at least one lifetime incidence of physical or sexual assault.[65] Among U.S. female prisoners, it has been estimated that 33 percent of females reported intimate partner abuse, while other studies reported that 72 percent of women reported being beaten by a boyfriend or a spouse, and 44 percent were abused by one or both parents.[63] The association between experiences of victimization and violence, particularly as a child, significantly impacts adult experiences of behavioral health and health problems.[66] Women exposed to violence as adults also present a higher risk for drug and/or alcohol use disorders, and substance abuse placed women at risk for repeated victimization, perpetuating a cycle of substance use and victimization.[67]

BEHAVIORAL HEALTH AND INCARCERATION

Since other community services including welfare and mental health are limited, many of the same individuals who contact LHDs also come into contact with jails and prisons. Perhaps the deficiency in such community services is the reason that the number of individuals involved in the U.S. criminal justice system has grown significantly over the past three decades. Criminal justice involvement includes those who are incarcerated or on community supervised release including parole or probation.[68] In the 1980s, approximately 1 in 77 adults were involved in the criminal justice system, which increased to approximately 1 in 30 in 2005.[68] Drug and alcohol use is significantly higher among offenders compared to the general population with about 80 percent involved in the criminal justice system committing crimes to support a substance use disorder, being charged with a drug-related crime, and/or possession

of illegal substances. According to the Bureau of Justice statistics, 21 percent of state prisoners and 18.5 percent of federal prisoners reported alcohol use at the time they committed a drug-related offense.[69] Alcohol use was reported by 37 percent of state prisoners convicted of a violent crime and 29 percent convicted for a property crime.[69] However, the proportion of violence-related alcohol use declined over the past decade and recent alcohol-related crime was less likely to involve juveniles or weapons.[69] Furthermore, a large study of over 40,000 state prisoners reported that those with co-occurring psychiatric and substance use disorders were at substantially higher risk for multiple incarcerations over a six-year period than those with psychiatric disorders or only substance use disorders.[70]

Data from 2007 to 2012 in selected U.S. cities found agreement between self-reported drug use and positive urine screens among 2012 arrestees, by drug, with 83 percent agreement for marijuana, 63 percent for methamphetamine, 50 percent for heroin, and 43 percent for cocaine.[71] Marijuana was the drug most often found while cocaine and crack were the second most commonly used at arrest. There was also a statistically significant increase in arrestees testing positive for opiates, specifically heroin. In addition, the proportion of offenders receiving treatment while incarcerated in prison or jail increased.[68]

The relationship between drugs and crime remains controversial in spite of the documented association. An early survey of inmates in state and federal correctional institutions found that 80 percent of state prisoners reported drug use in their lifetime and over 50 percent reported using a drug other than alcohol at the time of arrest.[72] Controversy focuses on how law enforcement officials and community treatment providers think about drug abuse treatment as control versus treatment. However, drug offenders, under criminal justice authority, usually remain in substance abuse treatment as long as or longer than those not under court-ordered treatment. There are other ways of thinking about treatment and control because interventions can incorporate both approaches. For example, a therapeutic community/residential treatment facility has a very high level of both treatment and control with judicial referrals, whereas outpatient drug treatment is usually low in both treatment and control unless treatment is court-ordered. Nevertheless, treatment and control are usually discussed as opposites, which depend upon ideology, perceived public interest, and political needs. Part of the controversy is the idea that drug abusers have limited internal motivation and need to be externally motivated to enter drug treatment in order to change. Behavior change is expected to include reduced arrests, reduced crime, reduced recidivism, and no drug use. It is important to keep in mind that, from both a criminal justice point of view and the treatment point of view, no illicit drug use is expected. Unlike the earlier "Just Say No" campaign, the benefits of drug courts have been described in the research literature as reduced recidivism, decreased drug use, increased birth rates of drug-free babies, high program retention, and cost-efficient treatment.[73]

Special Populations Within Prisons

Racial and ethnic minority men and women are disproportionately incarcerated in the United States compared to white males. According to the 2010 U.S. Census, African Americans comprised 13 percent of the U.S. population, but were 37 percent of the jail inmates in 2012.[74,75] Hispanics comprise 16 percent of the population, but are 2.5 times as likely as white males to be incarcerated.[75,76] In their lifetime, African American men are incarcerated at least four times the rate of white males, and African American men age 39 or younger are more than six times more likely than white males to be incarcerated.[76,77] At the end of 2010, African Americans comprised 44.6 percent of state prisoners convicted of offenses involving illegal drugs, compared to 29.3 percent of non-Hispanic whites and 20 percent of Hispanics.[74] African American women are incarcerated at two to three times the rates of white women, and Hispanic women are incarcerated between one and three times the rate of white women.[74] African American children are seven and a half times more likely than white children to have a parent in prison while Hispanic children are two and a half times more likely than white children to have a parent in prison.[78] In other words, 1 in 15 African American children and 1 in 42 Hispanic children have a parent in prison compared to 1 in 111 for white children.[79]

Women are being incarcerated at higher rates than ever before with drug law violation as the most serious offenses for 60 percent of women in federal prisons and 25 percent of women in state prisons.[74,80] Recently, the growth in the adult female jail population outpaced males with an increase of 10.9 percent between midyear 2010 and 2013.[81] Since more than 70 percent of women in prison have children, many of these children will have or will experience emotional hardship and instability. While incarceration rates for substance related offenses have significantly increased among women, there has not been a significant difference in overall substance use reported by women in recent years.[5] Nationally, a higher percentage of men reported alcohol use (58 percent) compared to women (47 percent).[5] In addition, the rate of illicit drug use by men is currently higher compared to women for marijuana (9.3 percent vs. 4.9 percent), prescription drugs (2.6 percent vs. 2.2 percent), and cocaine (0.7 percent vs. 0.4 percent).

SEXUALLY TRANSMITTED INFECTIONS, HIV, AND HARM REDUCTION

Drug and alcohol use can indirectly contribute to the transmission of sexually transmitted infections (STIs) and HIV.[82,83] For example, drug use can reduce the likelihood of using condoms and/or ability to negotiate condom use with partners in some contexts.[84–86] Stigma associated with substance use can also discourage individuals from seeking HIV and STI testing, which has been shown to reduce transmission.[87] Substance use can also affect an individual's willingness to seek treatment for STIs/HIV[88] and can negatively impact treatment adherence.[83,89–91] These studies highlight the importance of integrating HIV and STI services in LHDs as well as with drug treatment strategies for those who use drugs.

HIV and viral hepatitis, particularly HCV, can be transmitted by sharing contaminated drug injection equipment, including needles, syringes, rinse water, cotton, and cookers. In 2011, injection drug use accounted for an estimated 6 percent of new HIV infections among men and 14 percent of new infections among women in the United States.[92] Moreover, HCV incidence has been increasing among young people who inject drugs in the United States,[93,94] where 50 to 80 percent of people who inject drugs are infected.[95] Harm reduction approaches such as needle and syringe provision programs and opiate substitution therapy are effective in reducing HIV and HCV transmission.[96–101] However, the implementation of these prevention initiatives has been limited by U.S. state and federal policies, as many states continue to prohibit establishing harm reduction programs such as needle and syringe provision programs.

IMPLICATIONS FOR PUBLIC HEALTH PRACTICE

The public health practice implications for behavioral health seem clear. Simply stated, more LHD attention and involvement is needed to provide leadership and to help shape approaches to addressing behavioral health concerns, including substance abuse policy and practice. At the operational level, using Kentucky as an example, LHDs recognize the need to work with local groups and providers involved with mental health and substance abuse. The result is an increasing recognition that more can be accomplished together. Findings from an informal survey of Kentucky LHDs indicate that most health departments participate in local groups focused on substance abuse issues, report observing the impact of mental illness on their clients, see benefits from working with mental health and substance abuse professionals, and make referrals to substance abuse and mental health community agencies. Specific examples in Kentucky of building on common strengths include:

▶ A statewide program called HANDS (Health Access Nurturing Development Services), which provides home-based support services for first time mothers, including screening for depression, referral when appropriate, and counseling during home visits.[102] This program has been shown to reduce child neglect and child abuse and improve infant and child health and development.[103]

▶ Most health departments completed community assessments or a community health improvement plan that includes substance abuse as a major issue.[104]

▶ School health nursing staff have increased their knowledge of mental health issues which is attributed to working with mental health professionals who visit students at school.

▶ Local health departments increasingly include mental health or substance abuse educational topics and speakers for field staff.[105]

▶ Several health departments provide major leadership roles in their local community substance abuse activities.

▶ Some health departments provide public health services within group homes serving mental health or substance abuse clients.

▶ Many health departments report significant benefits when mental health or substance abuse teams share thoughts on new approaches, which is more likely to occur when the representatives are colocated.

This involvement must not only focus on behavioral health issues broadly, but also on behaviors that are associated with a constellation of problems such as accidents, STIs, maternal and child health-related problems, violence, and criminality, which are often influenced by national, state, and local politics. High-risk behaviors deserve community-based attention by LHDs as a partner so the "whole person" is targeted rather than disassociated community interventions for each behavioral health and health issue. This focus includes tailored community-wide policy developments such as enhancing disease prevention and community health promotion activities. However, these kinds of holistic behavioral public health approaches are generally limited and fractured by funding, and statutory and traditional agency responsibilities.

Local health department funding for individual level behavioral health preventive services to at-risk populations expanded from nearly nothing in the 1960s to significant amounts in the late 1990s. According to the NACCHO Profile, however, in 2013 only 10 percent of LHDs reported providing any behavioral health/mental health services, while only 7 percent reported providing any services for substance abuse.[1] Since 2000 there have been declines in the financial resources available to LHDs while state and federal programs expanded patient medical care coverage for increasing numbers of patients. For example, while Kentucky had a little over 500,000 patients enrolled in Medicaid in 1997, the state added 400,000 more in 2013, with well over a million covered as of 2014.[106–108] Specifically, state and federal funding for the Lexington-Fayette County (Kentucky) Health Department contributed about two-thirds of the revenue in fiscal year 2011 while those funding sources contributed only one-third in fiscal year 2015.[109] Consequently, the response of many LHDs across the country has been to refer patients in need of care for behavioral health-related problems to primary care providers and to focus on population-based mission critical issues. This focus includes programmatic activities that may impact behavioral health and substance abuse problems, but are not necessarily specific to them, e.g., communicable disease control and a focus on individuals at high risk for substance abuse, including those with TB, STI, or HIV; epidemiology and surveillance; regulatory activities; public health education and policy development. This mission focus is exemplified by the Lexington-Fayette County Health Department's active involvement in the local heroin task force by providing health education and primary prevention leadership.

Public health practice at the local level has not comprehensively addressed behavioral health—including substance abuse as a priority—in part because states and communities historically developed separate categorically funded intervention systems. In recent years public health leaders have estimated that socioeconomic status and behavioral health patterns contribute about two-thirds to health status while access to medical care and environmental factors contribute about one-third. This awareness coupled with resource reallocations across the health care spectrum can provide opportunities for LHDs, together with community behavioral health and substance abuse organizations, to develop ways to build on each other's strengths to prevent, detect, and intervene in behavioral health including substance abuse-related problems at the earliest and most effective point.

This chasm for public health practice is deepened by U.S. prevention and intervention policies that largely do not focus on harm reduction approaches, which are perceived to be and can be controversial. Disrupting the illicit drug market is very important; however, there is also a need for additional resources to support behavioral health prevention and intervention initiatives through public health practice. For example, as noted earlier, there are few needle and syringe provision programs to reduce the spread of STIs, HIV, and HCV in the United States. Likewise, there are limited intervention and health promotion interventions in jails and prisons to prepare for behavioral health related issues at community reentry. Local public health practitioners can identify and target at-risk women and their children—who often receive LHD services—who can be at high risk for a variety of behavioral health related issues.

Increasing the behavioral health knowledge base in public health practice would be enhanced by thinking and planning to develop multidisciplinary and comprehensive practice as well as explanatory theories that can be used to better examine health-related behaviors and to implement policy and practices. This enhanced and broadened theoretical foundation will facilitate support to target and tailor behavioral health interventions for the whole person, including biological, psychological, social, and spiritual factors. One possibility to consider, for example, is additional public health education and training for community leaders as well as cross-training public health practitioners on behavioral health consequences.

Behavioral health policies and practices can be controversial both within and across communities, as noted above. Controversies include real and perceived differences. Clearly, a challenge for public health policy and practitioners is not only how to provide holistic behavioral health services but also how to cooperatively work with others in the behavioral health community to enhance overall local and national public health.

abuser does not have control over his or her drug or alcohol use. Alcohol and other drug use are present throughout the U.S. society among all social and economic classes, ethnic/racial groups, and geographic regions. Women, in particular, tend to experience a complexity of maternal, behavioral, interpersonal (victimization and violence), and other health issues that are compounded by substance use. The federal drug policy strategy addresses supply reduction (law enforcement) and demand reduction (prevention and treatment). Demand reduction can include community treatment, coerced treatment, incarceration, pharmacotherapy, 12-step self-help, and other self-help groups. The public health strategy expands this approach by addressing the interaction of the agent, the host (the individual), and the environment (the community)—the classic epidemiologic triad often used only for infectious/communicable diseases. These interventions can include biological, psychological, social, cultural and spiritual factors. Addressing organizational factors and regulatory perspectives also broaden the traditionally individual-level perspective of behavioral health. Public health officials generally encourage harm reduction to reduce the negative consequences associated with drug use. Effective drug abuse treatment can reduce related public health issues such as the spread of HIV among people who inject drugs. More local health department involvement is needed to provide tailored, community-wide policy development to help shape approaches to addressing disease prevention and community health promotion activities.

RECOMMENDED WEBSITES

Centers for Disease Prevention and Control—Substance Abuse Risks
    http://www.cdc.gov/hiv/risk/behavior/substanceuse
.html
National Institute on Drug Abuse
    http://www.drugabuse.gov/
Substance Abuse and Mental Health Services Administration
    http://www.samhsa.gov/
National Institute on Alcohol Abuse and Alcoholism
    http://www.niaaa.nih.gov/
NLM MedlinePlus Substance Abuse Problems
    http://www.nlm.nih.gov/medlineplus/
substanceabuseproblems.html

REVIEW QUESTIONS

1. Describe behavioral health from a public health perspective.
2. Using a theoretical framework (e.g., as shown in Table 28-1), review factors that influence health behaviors, with substance abuse as the example.
3. Discuss the prevalence of behavioral health in the United States using alcohol and drug use as the example.
4. How can an understanding of the criminal justice system be useful for public health practitioners?
5. Discuss an individual harm reduction approach to prevent alcohol and drug problems.

SUMMARY

The medical or disease model defines addiction as a chronic relapsing medical condition in which a user/

REFERENCES

1. National Association of County & City Health Officials. *2013 National Profile of Local Health Departments.* Washington, DC; 2014.

2. Institute of Medicine. *Pathways of Addiction: Opportunities in Drug Abuse Research.* Washington, DC: National Academy Press; 1996.

3. Leshner AI. Addiction is a brain disease, and it matters. *Science.* Oct 3 1997;278(5335):45–47.

4. Goode E. *Drugs in American society.* 6th ed. Boston: McGraw-Hill; 2005.

5. Substance Abuse and Mental Health Services Administration. Results from the 2012 National Survey on Drug Use and Health: Summary of National Findings, NSDUH Series H-46, HHS Publication No. (SMA) 1304795. *US Department of Health and Human Services.* 2013.

6. Substance Abuse and Mental Health Services Administration. Results from the 2010 National Survey on Drug Use and Health: Summary of National Findings, NSDUH Series H-41, HHS Publication No. (SMA) 11-4658. *US Department of Health and Human Services.* 2011.

7. Substance Abuse and Mental Health Services Administration. Results from the 2011 National Survey on Drug Use and Health: Summary of National Findings, NSDUH Series H-44, HHS Publication No. (SMA) 12-4713. *US Department of Health and Human Services.* 2012.

8. Johnston LD, O'Malley PM, Bachman JG, Schulenberg JE, Miech RA. Monitoring the Future national survey results on drug use, 1975–2013. Vol Volume I, Secondary school students. Ann Arbor: Institute for Social Research, The University of Michigan; 2014:630.

9. Wu LT, Blazer DG, Swartz MS, Burchett B, Brady KT. Illicit and nonmedical drug use among Asian Americans, Native Hawaiians/Pacific Islanders, and mixed-race individuals. *Drug Alcohol Depend.* 2013;133(2):360–367.

10. Wu LT, Brady KT, Mannelli P, Killeen TK. Cannabis use disorders are comparatively prevalent among nonwhite racial/ethnic groups and adolescents: a national study. *J Psychiatr Res.* 2014;50:26–35.

11. Cook BL, Alegria M. Racial-ethnic disparities in substance abuse treatment: the role of criminal history and socioeconomic status. *Psychiatr Serv.* Nov 2011;62(11):1273–1281.

12. Fazel S, Bains P, Doll H. Substance abuse and dependence in prisoners: a systematic review. *Addiction (Abingdon, England).* Feb 2006;101(2):181–191.

13. Fazel S, Khosla V, Doll H, Geddes J. The prevalence of mental disorders among the homeless in western countries: systematic review and meta-regression analysis. *PLoS Med.* Dec 2 2008;5(12):e225.

14. Townsend L, Flisher AJ, King G. A systematic review of the relationship between high school dropout and substance use. *Clin Child Fam Psychol Rev.* 2007;10(4):295–317.

15. United States. *Healthy People: The Surgeon General's Report on Health Promotion and Disease Prevention.* Washington, DC: U.S. Department of Health, Education, and Welfare, Office of the Assistant Secretary for Health and Surgeon General; 1979.

16. Evans RI, Rozelle RM, Maxwell SE, Raines BE, Dill CA, Guthrie TJ. Social modeling films to deter smoking in adolescents: results of a three-year field investigation. *Journal of Applied Psychology.* 1981;66(4):399–414.

17. U.S. Department of Health and Human Services. Healthy People 2014; http://www.healthypeople.gov/2020/default.aspx. Accessed September 25, 2014.

18. Bandura A. *Social Foundations of Thought and Actions: A Social Cognitive Theory.* Englewood Cliffs, NJ: Prentice-Hall; 1986.

19. Jessor R, Jessor S. *Problem Behavior and Psychosocial Development: A Longitudinal Study of Youth.* New York: Academic Press; 1997.

20. Kaplan HB. *Self-attitudes and deviant behavior.* Pacific Palisades, Calif: Goodyear Pub. Co.; 1974.

21. Akers RL, Krohn MD, Lanza-Kaduce L, Radosevich M. Social learning and deviant behavior: a specific test of a general theory. *Am Sociol Rev.* 1979;44(4):636–655.

22. Becker H. *Outsiders: Studies in the Sociology of Deviance.* New York: Free Press; 1963.

23. Hirschi T. *Causes of Delinquency.* Berkeley: University of California Press; 1969.

24. Gottfredson MR, Hirschi T. *A General Theory of Crime.* Stanford, CA: Stanford University Press; 1990.

25. Lindesmith AR. A sociological theory of drug addiction. *Am Journal Sociol.* 1938;43:593–613.

26. Merton RK. *Social theory and social structure.* New York: Free Press; 1968.

27. McLeroy KR, Bibeau D, Steckler A, Glanz K. An ecological perspective on health promotion programs. *Health Educ Q.* Winter 1988;15(4):351–377.

28. Leukefeld CG, Leukefeld S. Primary socialization theory and a bio/psycho/social/spiritual practice model for substance use. *Subst Use Misuse.* Jun 1999;34(7):983–991.

29. Stokols D. Translating social ecological theory into guidelines for community health promotion. *Am J Health Promot.* 1996;10(4):282–298.

30. Bronfenbrenner U. *The Ecology of Human Development.* Cambridge, MA: Harvard University Press; 1979.

31. Janz NK, Becker MH. The Health Belief Model: a decade later. *Health Educ Q.* Spring 1984;11(1):1–47.

32. Ajzen I, Fishbein M. *Understanding Attitudes and Predicting Social Behavior.* Englewood Cliffs, NJ: Prentice Hall; 1980.

33. Mosher JF, Yanagisako KL. Public health, not social warfare: a public health approach to illegal drug policy. *J Public Health Policy.* 1991;12(3):278–323.

34. Levine HG. The alcohol problem in America: from temperance to alcoholism. *Br J Addict.* Mar 1984;79(1):109–119.

35. Center for Substance Abuse Prevention. *Environmental Prevention Strategies: Putting Theory into Practice. Training and Resource Guide.* Rockville, MD: Center for Substance Abuse Prevention, Substance Abuse and Mental Health Services Administration; 2000.

36. Cahalan D. *Problem Drinkers: a National Survey.* San Francisco, CA: Jossey-Bass; 1970.

37. Humphreys K, Tucker JA. Toward more responsive and effective intervention systems for alcohol-related problems. *Addiction (Abingdon, England).* Feb 2002;97(2):126–132.

38. Moore M, Gerstein D, eds. *Alcohol and Public Policy: Beyond the Shadow of Prohibition.* Washington, DC: National Academy Press; 1981.

39. Walters GD. Spontaneous remission from alcohol, tobacco, and other drug abuse: seeking quantitative answers to qualitative questions. *Am J Drug Alcohol Abuse.* 2000;26(3):443–460.

40. Wechsler H, Davenport A, Dowdall G, Moeykens B, Castillo S. Health and behavioral consequences of binge drinking in college. A national survey of students at 140 campuses. *Jama.* 1994;272(21):1672–1677.

41. Musto DF. *The American Disease: Origins of Narcotic Control.* New York: Oxford University Press; 1999.

42. Mosher JF. Drug availability in a public health perspective. In: Resnik H, ed. *OSAP Prevention Monograph 6 Youth and Drugs: Society's Mixed Message.* Rockville, MD: Office of Substance Abuse Prevention; 1990:129–168.

43. National Drug Control Strategy. FY 2007 Budget Summary. *Office of National Drug Control Policy.* 2006.

44. National Drug Control Strategy. FY 2014 Budget and Performance Summary. *Office of National Drug Control Policy.* 2013.

45. Office of National AIDS Policy. National HIV/AIDS Strategy for the United States. 2010.

46. Daugherty RP, Leukefeld C. Reducing the Risks for Substance Abuse: A Lifespan Approach New York and London: Plenum Press; 1998.

47. Musto DF. *The American Disease.* 2nd ed. New York: Oxford University Press; 1987.

48. National Institute on Drug Abuse. *Principles of Drug Addiction Treatment: A Research-Based Guide. NIH Publication No. 06–5316.* 1999.

49. Dasgupta N, Bailey EJ, Cicero T, et al. Post-marketing surveillance of methadone and buprenorphine in the United States. *Pain Medicine.* 2010;11(7):1078–1091.

50. Johanson CE, Arfken CL, di Menza S, Schuster CR. Diversion and abuse of buprenorphine: findings from national surveys of treatment patients and physicians. *Drug Alcohol Depend.* Jan 1 2012;120(1–3):190–195.

51. Piazza NJ, Vrbka JL, Yeager RD. Telescoping of alcoholism in women alcoholics. *Int J Addict.* 1989;24(1):19–28.

52. Back SE, Contini R, Brady KT. Substance abuse in women: Does gender matter? *Psychiatric Times.* 2007;24:48–51.

53. Keyes KM, Martins SS, Blanco C, Hasin DS. Telescoping and gender differences in alcohol dependence: new evidence from two national surveys. *Am J Psychiatry.* Aug 2010;167(8):969–976.

54. Brewer VE, Marquart JW, Mullings JL, Crouch BM. AIDS-related risk behavior among female prisoners with histories of mental impairment. *The Prison Journal* 1998;78(2):101–118.

55. Greenfield SF, Brooks AJ, Gordon SM, et al. Substance abuse treatment entry, retention, and outcome in women: a review of the literature. *Drug Alcohol Depend.* Jan 5 2007;86(1):1–21.

56. Newcomb MD, Huba GJ, Bentler PM. Mothers' influence on the drug use of their children: Confirmatory tests of direct modeling and mediational theories. *Developmental Psychology.* 1983;19(5):714–726.

57. Logan BA, Brown MS, Hayes MJ. Neonatal abstinence syndrome: treatment and pediatric outcomes. *Clinical obstetrics and gynecology.* Mar 2013;56(1):186–192.

58. Patrick SW, Davis MM, Lehman CU, Cooper WO. Increasing incidence and geographic distribution of neonatal abstinence syndrome: United States 2009 to 2012. *Journal of perinatology: official journal of the California Perinatal Association.* Aug 2015;35(8):667.

59. Gilman SE, Abraham HD. A longitudinal study of the order of onset of alcohol dependence and major depression. *Drug Alcohol Depend.* Aug 1 2001;63(3):277–286.

60. Ilgen M, Kleinberg F. The link between substance abuse, violence and suicide. *Psychiatric Times.* 2011;28(1):25–27.

61. Lynch SM, Dehart DD, Belknap JE, et al. A multisite study of the prevalence of serious mental illness, PTSD, and substance use disorders of women in jail. *Psychiatr Serv.* May 1 2014;65(5):670–674.

62. Bond L, Semaan S. At risk for HIV infection: incarcerated women in a county jail in Philadelphia. *Women Health.* 1996;24(4):27–45.

63. Liebling A. Suicide amongst women prisoners. *Howard J Crim Justice.* 1994;33(1):1–9.

64. Sheridan MJ. Comparison of the life experiences and personal functioning of men and women in prison. *Families in Society: The Journal of Contemporary Human Services.* 1996;77:423–434.

65. Hammett TM, Harmon, P. Sexually transmitted diseases and hepatitis: burden of disease among inmates. 1996–1997 Update: HIV/AIDS, STDs, and TB in correctional facilities. In: Statistics BoJ, ed. Washington, DC1999.

66. Staton M, Leukefeld C, Logan TK. Health service utilization and victimization among incarcerated female substance users. *Subst Use Misuse.* 2001;36(6–7):701–716.

67. Widom CS, Marmorstein NR, White HR. Childhood victimization and illicit drug use in middle adulthood. *Psychol Addict Behav.* 2006;20(4):394–403.

68. Feucht TE, Gfroerer J. Mental and substance use disorders among adult men on probation or parole: some success against a persistent challenge. In: Administration SAaMHS, ed2011.

69. Bureau of Justice. Alcohol and Crime: Data from 2002 to 2008. 2010; http://www.bjs.gov/content/acf/29_prisoners_and_alcoholuse.cfm.

70. Baillargeon J, Penn JV, Knight K, Harzke AJ, Baillargeon G, Becker EA. Risk of reincarceration among prisoners with co-occurring severe mental illness and substance use disorders. *Adm Policy Ment Health.* 2010;37(4):367–374.

71. Office of the National Drug Control Policy. Arrestee Drug Abuse Monitoring Program II (ADAMII): 2012 Annual Report. 2013; http://www.whitehouse.gov/sites/default/files/ondcp/policy-and-research/adam_ii_2012_annual_rpt_final_final.pdf.

72. Mumola CJ. Substance Abuse and Treatment of State and Federal Prisoners, 1997. 1999; http://www.bjs.gov/index.cfm?ty=pbdetail&iid=1169. Accessed September 25, 2014.

73. Belenko S. Research on Drug Courts: A Critical Review. *National Court Institute Review.* 1998;1:1–30.

74. Carson AE, Sabol WJ. Prisoners in 2011. In: Statistics UDoJBoJ, ed2012.

75. United States Census. 2010 Census Shows America's Diversity. 2011; https://http://www.census.gov/2010census/news/releases/operations/cb11-cn125.html.

76. Carson AE, Golinelli D. Prisoners in 2012: Trends in Admissions and Releases, 1991–2012. In: Statistics UDoJBoJ, ed2013.

77. Drake B. Incarceration gap widens between whites and blacks. In: Center PR, ed2013.

78. Glaze LE, Maruschak LM. Parents in prison and their minor children. In: Statistics UDoJ, ed2008.

79. The Pew Charitable Trusts. Collateral Costs: Incarceration's Effect on Economic Mobility. In: Trusts TPC, ed. Washington, DC; 2010.

80. Bureau of Justice Statistics. Federal Criminal Case Processing Statistics Online Analysis Tool. In: Center FJSR, ed2012.

81. Bureau of Justice Statistics. Jail Inmates at Midyear 2013: Statistical Tables. 2014.

82. Cook RL, Clark DB. Is there an association between alcohol consumption and sexually transmitted diseases? A systematic review. *Sex Transm Dis.* Mar 2005;32(3):156–164.

83. Shuper PA, Neuman M, Kanteres F, Baliunas D, Joharchi N, Rehm J. Causal considerations on alcohol and HIV/AIDS—a systematic review. *Alcohol Alcohol.* 2010;45(2):159–166.

84. Mansergh G, Shouse RL, Marks G, et al. Methamphetamine and sildenafil (Viagra) use are linked to unprotected receptive and insertive anal sex, respectively, in a sample of men who have sex with men. *Sex Transm Infect.* Apr 2006;82(2):131–134.

85. Leigh BC. Alcohol and condom use: a meta-analysis of event-level studies. *Sex Transm Dis.* Aug 2002;29(8):476–482.

86. Halpern-Felsher BL, Millstein SG, Ellen JM. Relationship of alcohol use and risky sexual behavior: a review and analysis of findings. *J Adolesc Health.* Nov 1996;19(5):331–336.

87. Weinhardt LS, Carey MP, Johnson BT, Bickham NL. Effects of HIV counseling and testing on sexual risk behavior: a meta-analytic review of published research, 1985–1997. *Am J Public Health.* 1999;89(9):1397–1405.

88. Calsyn RJ, Klinkenberg WD, Morse GA, Miller J, Cruthis R. Recruitment, engagement, and retention of people living with HIV and co-occurring mental health and substance use disorders. *AIDS Care.* 2004;16 Suppl 1:S56–70.

89. Mills EJ, Nachega JB, Bangsberg DR, et al. Adherence to HAART: a systematic review of developed and developing nation patient-reported barriers and facilitators. *PLoS Med.* 2006;3(11):e438.

90. Malta M, Strathdee SA, Magnanini MM, Bastos FI. Adherence to antiretroviral therapy for human immunodeficiency virus/acquired immune deficiency syndrome among drug users: a systematic review. *Addiction (Abingdon, England).* Aug 2008;103(8):1242–1257.

91. Wolfe D, Carrieri MP, Shepard D. Treatment and care for injecting drug users with HIV infection: a review of barriers and ways forward. *Lancet.* 2010;376(9738):355–366.

92. Centers for Disease Control and Prevention. HIV Surveillance Report. 2011; http://www.cdc.gov/hiv/topics/surveillance/resources/reports/. Accessed July 2, 2014.

93. Centers for Disease Control and Prevention. Use of enhanced surveillance for hepatitis C virus infection to detect a cluster among young injection-drug users—New York, November 2004–April 2007. In: report MMamw, ed. Vol 572008.

94. Centers for Disease Control and Prevention. Hepatitis C virus infection among adolescents and young adults: Massachusetts, 2002–2009. *MMWR Morbidity and mortality weekly report.* 2011;60:537–541.

95. Williams IT, Bell BP, Kuhnert W, Alter MJ. Incidence and transmission patterns of acute hepatitis C in the United States, 1982-2006. *Arch Intern Med.* 2011;171(3):242–248.

96. Strathdee SA, Vlahave D. The effectiveness of needle exchange programs: A review of the science and policy. *AIDScience.* 2001;1(16):1–31.

97. Palmateer N, Kimber J, Hickman M, Hutchinson S, Rhodes T, Goldberg D. Evidence for the effectiveness of sterile injecting equipment provision in preventing hepatitis C and human immunodeficiency virus transmission among injecting drug users: a review of reviews. *Addiction (Abingdon, England).* 2010;105(5):844–859.

98. Hurley SF, Jolley DJ, Kaldor JM. Effectiveness of needle-exchange programmes for prevention of HIV infection. *Lancet.* Jun 21 1997;349(9068):1797–1800.

99. Aspinall EJ, Nambiar D, Goldberg DJ, et al. Are needle and syringe programmes associated with a reduction in HIV transmission among people who inject drugs: a systematic review and meta-analysis. *Int J Epidemiol.* Feb 2014;43(1):235–248.

100. Turner KM, Hutchinson S, Vickerman P, et al. The impact of needle and syringe provision and opiate substitution therapy on the incidence of hepatitis C virus in injecting drug users: pooling of UK evidence. *Addiction (Abingdon, England).* 2011;106(11): 1978–1988.

101. MacArthur GJ, Minozzi S, Martin N, et al. Opiate substitution treatment and HIV transmission in people who inject drugs: systematic review and meta-analysis. *BMJ (Clinical research ed.).* 2012;345:e5945.

102. Kentucky Cabinet for Health and Family Services. Health Access Nurturing Development Services. 2014; http://chfs.ky.gov/dph/mch/ecd/hands.htm. Accessed October 10, 2014.

103. Illback RJ, Sanders, D., Pennington, M., Sanders III, D., Kilmer, A. Health Access Nurturing Development Services (HANDS) Kentucky's Home Visiting Program for First Time Parents Program Evaluation Findings. 2008; http://www.greatkidsinc.org/research/Eval KY HANDS 1-08 Report 8-6-08.pdf. Accessed October 10, 2014.

104. National Association of County & City Health Officials. Community Health Assessment and Improvement Planning. http://www.naccho.org/topics/infrastructure/CHAIP/. Accessed October, 13, 2014.

105. Lexington-Fayette County Health Department. Tobacco Use Cessation and Prevention Program. http://www.lexingtonhealthdepartment.org/ProgramsServices/TobaccoUseCessationand Prevention/tabid/79/Default.aspx. Accessed October, 13, 2014.

106. Kentucky Cabinet for Health and Family
     Services. MS 264 Reports Medicaid in Kentucky
     Fiscal Year 1997. http://chfs.ky.gov/NR
     /rdonlyres/85902C69-9E92-40E3-BEC7
     -214307C03BE1/15214/ms2641997.pdf.
     Accessed October, 13, 2014.

107. The Henry J. Kaiser Family Foun-
     dation. Total Medicaid and CHIP
     Enrollment February—July, 2014. 2014;
     http://kff.org/health-reform/state-indicator
     /total-monthly-medicaid-and-chip-enrollment/.

108. Kynect. Kynect Statistics. 2014; http://governor
     .ky.gov/healthierky/Pages/default.aspx.

109. Lexington-Fayette County Health Department.
     Lexington-Fayette County Health Department
     2011 Annual Report.

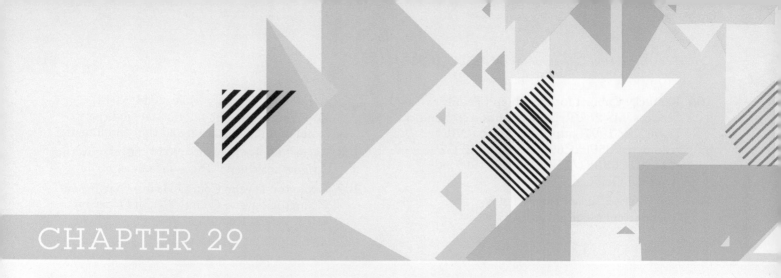

CHAPTER 29

The Public Health Laboratory

Eric C. Blank, DrPH • Scott J. Becker, MS • Ralph Timperi, MPH

LEARNING OBJECTIVES

Upon completion of this chapter, the reader will be able to:

1. Summarize the history of public health laboratories and impetus for their creation.

2. Describe the core functions of public health laboratories.

3. Explain the unique role of public health laboratories vis-à-vis other governmental laboratories and the private sector.

4. Explain public health laboratories' role in infectious and environmental disease surveillance, prevention, and control.

5. Describe technology's impact on current public health laboratory practices, diagnostic testing, and future trends in laboratory science.

6. Explain the role of U.S. public health laboratories in the international arena, including support for national laboratory systems, global health security, and global public health surveillance and research. Explain why this role is important.

KEY TERMS

Biosafety Level (BSL)
Clinical Laboratory Improvement Amendments Act of 1988 (CLIA '88)
core functions
emerging infectious diseases
laboratory information management system (LIMS)
metabolic disease
newborn screening
public health laboratory system
quality assurance

INTRODUCTION

The public health laboratory has been a driving force behind the development and evolution of public health practice. The discoveries of the late nineteenth century linking microorganisms to disease, coupled with the basic epidemiologic principles developed by John Snow and others form the foundation on which public health practice is built.[1] Over time, public health laboratories have expanded their roles from infectious disease surveillance and outbreak investigations to such varied public health programs as emergency response, newborn screening, and environmental health monitoring and assessment. In essence, public health laboratories provide objective, scientific data upon which public health agencies rely to meet their core responsibilities of assessment, assurance, and policy development.[2] In this chapter, we describe the evolving role of public health laboratories throughout their history, describe the core functions of public health laboratories, how they relate to public health practice, and discuss the alignment of public health laboratory services with public health agency needs. We conclude with a discussion of the public health laboratory system. Throughout the chapter, we discuss current scientific and technological trends and their impacts on laboratory practice, as well as the potential impact of changes in the U.S. health care delivery and payment system on public health laboratories.

A BRIEF HISTORY OF THE EVOLVING ROLE OF PUBLIC HEALTH LABORATORIES

Public health laboratories emerged in concert with the establishment of public health departments in the late nineteenth century. The demographic shift from a largely agrarian society to an industrialized and more urban and densely-populated society facilitated the spread of the common infectious diseases of the day such as cholera, diphtheria, tuberculosis, and typhoid fever. At the same time there was growing understanding of the nature of these infectious diseases and their modes of transmission. In many instances, as demonstrated by Snow in the famous 1854 Broad Street cholera investigation in London, a fairly simple intervention, such as the removal of a pump handle to prevent further exposure to a contaminated water supply, had immediate and highly beneficial effects on community health. From these beginnings, public officials recognized the need to provide for a safe drinking water supply and, equally important, to assure proper disposal of human waste. Thus, beginning in the late 1800s, as the establishment of boards of health were expanding, there

are many instances in which those agencies included a laboratory.[1]

By World War II, further scientific advances led to the discovery of antibiotics. Vaccines were developed for childhood diseases such as measles, diphtheria, and whooping cough. The public health laboratory identified the diseases and the health department could now treat those diseases and implement preventive measures to limit further disease transmission. While public health officials' early focus was on sanitation and hygiene, by the middle of the twentieth century, the focus broadened to include the control of sexually transmitted diseases and establishment of vaccination programs. As public health practitioners began developing better tools for community-wide communicable disease surveillance and outbreak detection and investigation, the public health laboratories provided the often sophisticated and complex testing services needed to support those vital activities.

Since their beginnings, public health laboratories have tested water and dairy products for infectious disease agents associated with diarrheal illnesses. In the early 1970s, with passage of the federal Clean Air Act, Clean Water Act, and Safe Drinking Water Act,[3-5] public health and environmental protection agencies relied on public health laboratories to test for a wide range of chemical contaminants, in addition to the traditional tests for bacterial water contaminants. This development introduced advanced analytical equipment capable of detecting chemical elements in infinitesimal quantities. With that instrumentation also came automation and the need for analyzing and managing large amounts of data.

In the mid-1960s a test was developed to detect phenylketonuria (PKU), a metabolic disease affecting one out of every 15,000 infants.[6] Without initiation of appropriate treatment within the first weeks of life, the affected infants experience stunted physical and mental development and a life expectancy of 35 years or less. However, with a relatively simple change in diet and appropriate medical management the consequences of this disorder are drastically ameliorated. By the mid-1970s, states began passing laws requiring the testing of infants for PKU, as policy makers recognized that early intervention not only gave the infant the opportunity to live a long and productive life, but also negated the need for costly, lifelong institutional and medical services required by those with untreated PKU. Public health laboratories were the natural institutions to provide the testing to support these new metabolic disease programs. As time passed, these programs grew to include newborn screening for sickle cell disease and other hemoglobinopathies. By the late 1990s, a host of other metabolic disorders were added to newborn screening panels. All are characterized by the need for early postpartum detection so appropriate medical and, often dietary, treatment can be implemented to prevent serious, possibly life-threatening consequences for affected individuals.

From the 1980s to the present, public health laboratories have been on the frontline of efforts to detect and characterize emerging infectious diseases. Public health laboratories were the first laboratories to employ a serologic test for HIV, first known as HTLV-III, and supported public health clinics and programs focused on containing the spread of the disease. This *modus operandi*—adopting and employing testing methodologies for emerging illnesses—continued through the hantavirus outbreaks in the early 1990s and the emergence of West Nile virus in the late 1990s, SARS (Severe Acute Respiratory Syndrome) in 2003, novel influenza strains H5N1 and H7N9 in the late 2000s, and MERS-CoV (Middle Eastern Respiratory Syndrome Coronavirus) and Ebola in 2014. Finally, the need for public health laboratories to fulfill one of their traditional roles— rapid detection of an infectious disease threat—was publicly demonstrated during the high-profile anthrax attacks of 2001.

In the span of just over 100 years, the public health laboratory has grown and developed into an organization with a breadth of analytical and diagnostic capabilities; however, for all the evolving technology and science, at its core, public health laboratories remain remarkably true to their original role. They are institutions where testing is done to support public health services and activities.

THE CORE FUNCTIONS OF PUBLIC HEALTH LABORATORIES

Throughout their history, public health laboratories have had to explain their role to the public and its elected representatives. In particular, they have often been asked: What distinguishes a public health laboratory from any other clinical or analytical laboratory? In 2002, the Centers for Disease Control and Prevention (CDC) publication, *Morbidity and Mortality Weekly Report*, published a paper from the Association of Public Health Laboratories (APHL) detailing the core functions and capabilities of public health laboratories.[7] This article describes in plain language what public health laboratories do and how they relate to the broader laboratory community. The latest version of the core functions of public health laboratories is presented in Figure 29-1. In Figure 29-2, the core functions of public health laboratories are aligned with the 10 essential services of public health.[8] This "cross walk" between the core functions of public health laboratories and the 10 essential services of public health was done to show

	11 CORE FUNCTIONS OF STATE PUBLIC HEALTH LABORATORIES
1	Disease prevention, control, and surveillance
2	Integrated data management
3	Reference and specialized testing
4	Environmental health and protection
5	Food safety
6	Laboratory improvement and regulation
7	Policy development
8	Emergency response
9	Public health-related research
10	Training and education
11	Partnerships and communication

FIGURE 29-1   11 Core Functions of State Public Health Laboratories

Adapted from Core Functions and Capabilities of Public Health Laboratories, MMWR 51 (RR14); 1–8, September 20, 2002.

how the laboratory functions are integrated with the broader public health services.

It should be noted that not all core functions are conducted in all public health laboratories. Instead, the jurisdictions they serve determine the level and scope of public health laboratory services. At the local level, a public health laboratory may provide sexually transmitted diseases (STDs) testing to support STD clinics, while others may also provide water bacteriology testing and basic microbe culture work (i.e., growing colonies of pathogens in Petri dishes so they can be identified and further characterized) to support outbreak investigations, with microbial isolates sent to a state laboratory for definitive identification and further characterization. At the state level, roughly half of the public health laboratories provide all required regulatory testing—chemical, radiological, and biological—for the environmental programs noted above. Thirty-eight states perform newborn screening, and the remaining states and territories contract with either one of those 38 states or with a private commercial laboratory for

10 ESSENTIAL PUBLIC HEALTH SERVICES	VS.	11 CORE FUNCTIONS OF STATE PUBLIC HEALTH LABORATORIES	
1	Monitor health status to identify community health problems	▶	1	Disease prevention, control, and surveillance
2	Diagnose and investigate health problems and health hazards in the community	▶	2	Integrated data management
			3	Reference and specialized testing
			4	Environmental health and protection
			5	Food safety
			8	Emergency response
3	Inform, educate, and empower people about health issues	▶	10	Training and education
			11	Partnerships and communication
4	Mobilize partnerships to identify and solve health problems	▶	11	Partnerships and communication
5	Develop policies and plans that support individual and community health efforts	▶	7	Policy development
6	Enforce laws and regulations that protect health and safety	▶	6	Laboratory improvement and regulation
7	Link people to needed personal health services and assure provision of health care when unavailable	▶	3	Reference and specialized testing
8	Assure a competent public and personal health care workforce	▶	10	Training and education
9	Evaluate effectiveness, accessibility, and quality of personnel and population-based services	▶	3	Reference and specialized testing
			6	Laboratory improvement and regulation
10	Research for new insights and innovative solutions to health problems	▶	9	Public health-related research

FIGURE 29-2   10 Essential Public Health Services vs. 11 Core Functions of State Public Health Laboratories

Adapted from Ten Essential Services of Public Health, http://www.cdc.gov/od/ocphp/nphpsp/essential services.htm

this testing. In eight states, the state public health laboratory also provides alcohol and drug testing to support state laws governing driving while under the influence of alcohol or certain drugs.[9]

Other factors that determine the scope and level of services a public health laboratory provides are federal and state laws and regulations and local ordinances. When national environmental legislation was passed

in the 1970s, some states split out the environmental responsibilities from the health agency and created a separate department for environmental protection. Often that department established its own laboratory to provide the analytical services necessary for the newly required environmental monitoring.

Demographics and jurisdictional size also influence what a public health laboratory does. Less populous states and territories do not have enough live births to sustain a newborn screening laboratory and find it more cost-effective to contract with another state for those services. Similarly, many local public health agencies find it too costly to maintain a laboratory, even one with a limited test menu, and rely on the state public health laboratory for their testing services.

Although few public health laboratories directly conduct all of the core functions outlined by APHL, the leaders of those institutions are responsible for knowing where, within a state or region, those functions are conducted. For example, if the state public health laboratory does not perform environmental regulatory testing, its director should be familiar with the testing performed by the state environmental laboratory and know how those services are provided and can be accessed.

Core Functions and Biosafety Level Designations

Not only do the core functions describe the work of public health laboratories, they form the basis of the organization and even dictate the design of public health laboratories. For example, the essential public health services related to disease prevention, control, and surveillance are directly supported by the core public health laboratory functions of reference and specialized testing and emergency response. At the federal, state, and large municipality levels, the public health laboratories are required to handle dangerous infectious disease agents in a safe and secure manner. Thus, public health laboratories are designed with these particular needs in mind. In the United States, laboratory facilities are designated as Biosafety Level (BSL) 1, 2, 3, or 4 according to safety practice guidelines and standards, and guidelines for air handling systems and construction.[10] These levels are distinguished by the ability of laboratory practices and building design to control exposure to hazardous biological, chemical, and radiological agents. The small laboratory area set aside in a physician's office or in a small clinic is certain to be rated BSL-1. It is essentially an office environment, but removed from public areas and equipped with the means to safely dispose biological waste.

BSL-2 laboratories are discrete laboratory areas, either stand-alone facilities or within larger buildings. Access to the laboratory is restricted. The laboratory areas or rooms are closed off from halls and other public areas. Some work is done under biosafety cabinets to contain infectious agents and prevent them from contaminating the surrounding work area or room. Chemical preparations are often performed under fume hoods to control noxious odors and the caustic effects of the fumes. Air handling systems, at the very least, exhaust air from the laboratory to the outside and do not recirculate it in the building. BSL-2 laboratories are most common, as the majority of laboratory work can be safely conducted in this type of physical environment.

BSL-3 laboratories require special construction. They are, in effect, laboratory rooms within the laboratory. A special feature of these self-contained areas is that air can only go one way. Clean air comes into the BSL-3 area and is exhausted only after it passes through a high-efficiency particulate air (HEPA) filter. Ceilings must be solid, not tiled, and there can be no seams where the walls meet the floors to facilitate decontamination of the area should there be an accidental release of infectious material. Access to BSL-3 laboratories is restricted to those authorized to work in that area. All materials, including lab gowns and other coverings, are sterilized before leaving the BSL-3 area. The causative agents of anthrax, tuberculosis, tularemia, plague, and novel influenza viruses, among many others, can only be safely handled in BSL-3 (or higher-level) facilities. Thus, public health laboratories that conduct testing for disease prevention, control, surveillance, reference and specialized biological testing, and emergency response have BSL-3 facilities.

The final laboratory safety category is BSL-4. The public is familiar with BSL-4 facilities because they are often highlighted in popular television series and movies. These are the facilities whose workers are outfitted with self-contained suits connected to an independent air supply. Exit and entrance to BSL-4 facilities are done through multiple steps, including final access via an airlock. These laboratories handle the most infectious and hazardous biological agents known. Exposure to such agents often results in death. Hemorrhagic fever viruses, such as Ebola or Marburg, are perhaps the best known agents handled in these facilities. There are only a handful of BSL-4 laboratory facilities in the United States, and most are administered by the federal government.

Public Health Laboratories and the Environment

The core functions also reflect an ingrained understanding of the relationship between the environment and public health. The core functions related to environmental health and protection, food safety assurance, and even emergency response are rooted in the early history of public health and the public health laboratory. The quality of the water we drink and the food we eat greatly influences population health. As noted earlier, current public health practice grew out of concern for the spread of disease from contaminated water. From the earliest times in their history, public health laboratories analyzed water samples and specimens from ill and exposed persons for disease agents. That is still true today. Yet, as scientists and clinicians learn more about adverse health effects from exposure to chemical and biological agents in the environment, the breadth of testing in public health laboratories has grown exponentially. Many state and large municipal public health laboratories have long been involved in foodborne disease outbreak investigations, testing both suspected foods and specimens from those exposed to the foods for the same causative disease agents, much as was done 100 years ago. Today, however, public health laboratory work goes well beyond that. The first biomonitoring programs—focused on blood lead screening and environmental mitigation—began in the late 1970s as the effects of childhood exposure to lead from lead-lined water pipes and lead-based paint were recognized. Once again public health laboratories provided critical testing services, in this case testing blood specimens from potentially exposed populations and environmental samples taken from suspected sources of exposure. In the early twenty-first century, public health laboratories expanded their environmental test repertoire to respond to the 2001 anthrax attacks. Not only did public health laboratories identify *Bacillus anthracis* in individual cases in Connecticut, Florida, and Washington, DC, they also quantified the extent of environmental contamination at postal facilities in the Washington, DC, area through the examination of environmental swab samples.

Unlike a century ago, test methods no longer rely on a multistep, multiday process to identify the causative agent. With current molecular methods, identification of a causative agent can be accomplished in hours or a day or so, at most. In 1993, the Jack-in-the-Box *E. coli* outbreak that sickened more than 700 people (mostly children) took 39 days before public health investigators determined the source of contamination—tainted "Monster Burger" sandwiches that were on sale at the restaurant chain.[11] In 2011, the source of a multistate *Listeria* outbreak was identified in 12 days.[12] In 2014, the CDC launched its Advanced Molecular Detection (AMD) initiative, focused on employing whole genome sequencing technology to detect and identify infectious disease agents. This technology holds the promise of being able to identify and fully characterize an infectious disease agent to the molecular level within hours in clinical or environmental specimens and samples.

Laboratory Regulation

The adoption of new technologies is necessary to fully carry out the function of reference and specialized testing. Because of their role as a reference laboratory for their jurisdiction, public health laboratories hold themselves to a high standard of quality and have had a historic interest in improving the quality of laboratory testing and practice generally. The core functions related to laboratory improvement and regulation, public health-related research, and training and education are the direct expressions of that interest. In order to perform their reference functions effectively, public health laboratories require hospital and private laboratories to submit quality specimens on a timely basis to assure rapid analysis, avoid delay due to an inadequate specimen, and provide early warning for emergency response. To that end, public health laboratories have traditionally been involved in improving laboratory practice in hospitals and private laboratories and, by extension, regulating laboratories.

Laboratory regulation stems from the state and federal levels and encompasses clinical and environmental testing. At the federal level, the **Clinical Laboratory Improvement Amendments of 1988 (CLIA '88)** require all laboratories conducting testing on human specimens to be licensed.[13] States that have assumed responsibility for implementing provisions of the federal Safe Drinking Water Act are required to have a program that regulates laboratories that perform testing used to meet the act's monitoring requirements. A number of states have additional requirements for certification of laboratory personnel over and above CLIA requirements. In some states, the public health laboratory administers these regulatory programs; in others the administration of these programs may be conducted by another organizational unit within the public health agency or administered by other state agencies.

Training and Workforce Development

Because of the serious nature of laboratory work and the link between a well-trained workforce and an effective regulatory program, public health laboratories value training and education for their workers and for the broader laboratory community. In fact, public health laboratories have traditionally conducted training for laboratorians in their jurisdictions, especially in their principle area of scientific expertise of infectious diseases. In the past, this training may have focused on the culturing and biochemical identification of bacteria—so-called bench work because it is performed at the laboratory bench. Today, the training may be focused on the safe and proper handling and shipping of biological or chemical agents. Newborn screening laboratories regularly provide training on the proper technique for collecting the bloodspot specimen that is captured on filter paper and used for testing. In some states, the public health laboratory is responsible for overseeing the training and certification of law enforcement officers in the administration of breath alcohol tests.

Data and Information Management to Support Public Health Decision Making

In many jurisdictions, the public health laboratory's primary role is to provide accurate and reliable diagnostic and analytical data to support public health programs. As discussed, the scope of public health laboratory services is extensive. Consequently, the amount of data and information they produce is considerable. Consider an average size state that has between 75,000 and 80,000 live births a year. That birth rate translates into an average of between 260 to 330 bloodspots submitted per day for newborn screening. Each of those bloodspots are screened for a minimum of 29 conditions using three or four different testing platforms, and many newborn screening laboratories report results for 50 or more conditions. Thus, on any given day there can be 10,000 or more data points generated just from this one laboratory activity. While not all laboratory sections generate the same volume of data, there is the additional challenge of managing data from so many varied activities. Thus, public health laboratories have come to increasingly rely on **laboratory information management systems (LIMS)**. These systems can take data directly from the instrumentation that is used for testing and, in addition to providing results, provide the **quality assurance** information needed to initiate results reporting and package the data for the initial laboratory analysis performed before a report is issued.

Translating laboratory data into useful information for clinicians, epidemiologists, policy makers, and others, and moving that information to the appropriate places in the public health system, is a primary laboratory role. In addition to reporting to the appropriate public health program, the public health laboratory has the legal and ethical responsibility to report to the provider or institution that originally submitted the specimen. Consequently, like any other clinical laboratory in the private sector, public health laboratories must meet the meaningful use standards for electronic laboratory reporting established under the 2010 Patient Protection and Affordable Care Act (ACA).[14] The LIMS is instrumental to meeting these requirements.

The Public Health Laboratory and Research

Public health research is perhaps one of the more challenging core functions for public health laboratory leaders. First, there is the challenge of defining what is meant by *research*. The evaluation and implementation of new technologies is often considered an inherent, natural part of a laboratory's work and in some circles is not viewed as research in the conventional sense. Nevertheless, in addition to "bringing up" new technology, public health laboratories work collaboratively with epidemiologists and other public health practitioners to study populations selected for particular public health interventions or programs, to examine the effects of exposure to environmental contaminants, and increasingly, to determine how new and emerging laboratory technologies can be employed to advance public health practice generally.

In some cases, public health laboratory research directly impacts policy development. For example, the expansion of newborn screening over the past 15 years from a small number of treatable metabolic disorders to testing for upwards of 50 conditions showcases how advances in laboratory science can drive public health policy.

Policy Impact and Implications

Laboratory activities can, in and of themselves, also raise policy questions. The posttesting retention of newborn screening bloodspot specimens (which are used for quality control and, sometimes, research purposes) is one example. Researchers value newborn screening specimens because they are derived from the entire population in a given geographic area and are thus extremely useful for studying population genetics. However, given the increasing ability to identify genetic markers for infectious or chronic disease susceptibility, there is growing public concern about the privacy of the genetic information in those bloodspots. Consequently, states have had to develop policies governing bloodspot storage, disposal, and availability for researchers. More states, for example, now require parents' tacit or explicit consent before researchers can access bloodspots, and, even then, they must be used only under specified conditions, generally including deidentification and Institutional Review Board oversight.

This interaction between science, technology, and policy development occurs with more frequency than is often thought. The rise of so-called culture-independent tests is a current example. Because these tests enable laboratory technicians to identify pathogens without preserving the patient specimen, they could seriously hamper notifiable disease reporting and the molecular characterization of infectious agents, which depends upon specimens being forwarded to public health laboratories for specialized analysis. How disease surveillance and outbreak detection activities will be conducted in the future will depend on the public health policies that emerge in response to this development, and public health laboratories will need to be involved in those discussions.

Another policy area involving public health laboratories is the implementation of the ACA. Among the emerging issues is billing for public health services, including laboratory testing. Does the public health agency have the authority to bill for services? If so, does the money generated through billing go back to the public health agency, the public health laboratory, or the state's general fund? At present, the answers are unclear.

Newborn screening, culture-independent diagnostic testing, and ACA implementation are just a few examples of the many areas, some not patently evident, in which the public health laboratory contributes to public health policy. Public health practitioners and public health laboratory leaders must be open and proactive in identifying areas where the laboratory can and should contribute to the development of sound public health policy.

Partnership Development

The final core function of public health laboratories is developing partnerships and communicating with partners, including health departments, federal agencies, law enforcement agencies, elected officials, the public, and others. Of note, it is a consistent observation of the authors that the public health laboratories with the best reputations are virtually always in agencies with strong public health programs. These successful organizations are characterized by a collaborative agency culture, open lines of communication at the leadership and program levels, and an openness to forming new partnerships and adopting new or different approaches to public health service provision. The link between strong public health laboratories and strong public health programs makes sense, since the value of laboratory data lies in its application to community health. Thus, a public health program will suffer if the laboratory data it depends upon are tardy or of poor quality. While technology has become more complex and sophisticated, these basic principles of public health practice remain fundamentally unchanged.

THE PUBLIC HEALTH LABORATORY SYSTEM

From the previous section, it should be clear that public health laboratories do not work in a vacuum. They are an intrinsic part of the broader public health system of local, state, and federal agencies and structure their testing services to meet the public health needs of the jurisdictions they serve. However, as also noted above, few public health laboratories directly perform all the core functions outlined by APHL. From the perspective of the public health laboratory, the laboratory system includes all institutions and organizations that contribute to fulfillment of those roles. For a local public health laboratory, that system may include the

state public health laboratory or a local hospital laboratory that may provide additional testing services. In states where environmental monitoring is conducted by another state agency, the public health laboratory system includes that agency's laboratory. In states that do not perform newborn screening, the external newborn screening laboratory is part of their public health laboratory system.

The public health laboratory system then includes laboratories that provide services or perform testing for biological, chemical, and radiological agents of public health significance. Thus, even laboratories in the private sector are part of the broader **public health laboratory system**, as graphically illustrated in the pyramid diagram in Figure 29-3. Their role, from a public health perspective, is that of the proverbial "canary in the coal mine." Hospitals will see the first patients exposed to an emerging infectious agent, whether it is naturally occurring or intentionally released. The first specimens will be examined at those hospital laboratories. To minimize the risk of further disease spread, potentially infectious specimens and isolates need to be moved safely and securely to the public health laboratory, or as shown in the pyramid, the reference laboratory for the given jurisdiction. We see here the intersection of two core functions: (1) training and education (especially with regard to specimen packaging and safe handling) and (2) communication and partnerships (between sentinel and reference laboratories). Finally, at the national level, the agents are submitted to appropriate federal laboratories for further characterization and study.

It is important to note that while the samples and specimens are shown flowing in one direction, from the sentinel laboratories to the national laboratories, data and information flow in both directions. In part, this bidirectional flow is essential to assure the laboratory system is functioning effectively. Laboratories need to know that their analysis was correct. The sentinel laboratories need information that validates their appropriate recognition of a public health threat, which they properly handed off to the public health laboratory. The public health laboratories, in turn, need information that confirms that their methods and procedures accurately identified or characterized the threat sufficiently to initiate an appropriate public health response. Thus, the bidirectional data flow is also of critical importance to the broader public health system.

Any response to a public health threat, whether biological, chemical, or radiological, requires identification of that threat. In many instances, the identification will be made in a laboratory, often a public health laboratory. To mount an effective public health response then requires an effective public health laboratory system that is seamlessly integrated into the public health system.

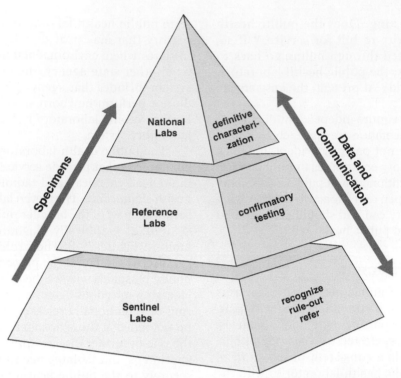

FIGURE 29-3   Depiction of Laboratory Response Network with specimen and information flows
Adapted from the Centers for Disease Control and Prevention

While it is easy to see how the public health laboratory system should be integrated within the broader public health system during a threat event, this systemic approach is practiced on a daily basis. Consider influenza surveillance. In the United States, each state develops and implements an influenza surveillance program. A certain number of specimens from symptomatic individuals in a geographic region are sent to municipal and state public health laboratories, which process the specimens for the influenza viruses known to be circulating. Many of these laboratories also participate in the World Health Organization's (WHO's) global influenza surveillance program. Influenza viruses identified in these specimens often are characterized down to the molecular level and reported nationally to the CDC. Representative isolates are also sent to the CDC—one of six WHO International Collaborating Centers for global influenza surveillance—for further characterization. Not only does this global surveillance system track circulating influenza virus, it actively looks for the emerging influenza strains which inform vaccine production for the next influenza season. Finally, this system actively looks for emerging novel influenza viruses, such as H5N1 or H7N9, which have potential to pose significant public health threats should they become more transmissible from person to person.

The influenza surveillance system demonstrates the value of an international network of laboratories capable of conducting highly specialized testing. The system works because the laboratory data produced are managed and moved rapidly and efficiently, often electronically, throughout the laboratory and public health systems.

The 2005 revisions of the WHO's International Health Regulations (IHR) require signatory nations to report "public health events of international concern," but do not specify diseases, agents or conditions that would trigger an international public health alert.[15] Part of the reporting process requires that signatory countries have laboratories capable of verifying the nature of the event. Consequently, it is in the interests of the developed countries of the world to work with their counterparts in less developed countries to build laboratory systems that can fulfill the IHR requirements. In the United States, the Global Health Security Agenda is meant to do that. Organizations such as APHL, in concert with the CDC and other federal partners, have been working internationally to develop laboratory systems that can consistently produce high quality public health data, develop organizations that are sustainable and support high quality testing, and develop data management systems to assure laboratory data and information are effectively reported to appropriate health authorities. In North America, APHL and the Canadian Public Health Laboratory Network have a formal memorandum of understanding facilitating communication and promoting the coordination of laboratory activities among their members on both sides of the border. Efforts are underway to develop a similar relationship with Mexico. As can be seen, the pyramid depicting laboratory systems applies at any geographical level, national, regional or international, and, as can be seen from the preceding discussion, the systems and networks are set up to fulfill the core functions of public health laboratories.

SUMMARY

Public health laboratories played a central role in the development of public health practice. They have evolved along with the rest of the public health system to meet the dynamic public health challenges of our era. Public health laboratories integrate the latest scientific findings and technologic advances into public health practice. They are at the forefront of public health's most publically visible essential services related to surveillance and community assessment, and emergency response and outbreak investigation. Yet, public health laboratories do not work alone. They work within the larger public health system in partnership and collaboration with other public health practitioners, such as epidemiologists, disease control investigators, biostatisticians, public health nurses, and environmental health specialists. They also work within laboratory systems at the jurisdictional, national, and even international levels. They build networks that function to provide core public health laboratory functions, which in turn support the 10 essential services of public health now and into the future.

REVIEW QUESTIONS

1. Describe testing conducted by public health laboratories since 2000.
2. List out the 11 core functions of public health laboratories.
3. What relationship is there between the WHO's International Health Regulations and public health laboratories?
4. List the other public health professions and settings that public health laboratories work with closely.

REFERENCES

1. Becker, S.J., Blank, E.C., Martin, R and Skeels, M. (2001). Public Health Laboratory Administration. In L.F. Novick and G.P. Mays (Eds.), *Public Health Administration: Principles for Population-Based Management* (pp 623–627). Gaithersburg, MD: Aspen Publishers.
2. Institute of Medicine. (1988). *The Future of Public Health* Washington, DC: U.S. Government Printing Office.
3. Safe Drinking Water Act, 42 USC 300 et. seq., 1974 (amended 1986 and 1996).
4. Clean Water Act, 33 USC 1251-1387, 1972 (amended 1977 and 1987).
5. Clean Air Act, 42 USC 7401 et seq., 1963 (amended 1967, 1970, 1977 and 1990).
6. PKU: Screening and Management, NIH Consensus Statement, October 16–18, 2000, 17 (3): 1–27 or NIH Consensus Statement on-line reference http://consensus.nih.gov/2000/2000phenylketonuria 113html.htm
7. Core Functions and Capabilities of Public Health Laboratories, MMWR 51 (RR14); 1–8, September 20, 2002.
8. Ten Essential Services of Public Health, http://www.cdc.gov/od/ocphp/nphpsp/essential services.htm
9. APHL Survey Resource Center, Laboratory Profiles, 2013.
10. Biosafety in Microbiological and Biomedical Laboratories, 5th ed. L. Casey Chosewood, M.D. and Deborah E. Wilson, Dr.P.H., CBSP, eds. HHS Publication No. (CDC) 20-1112, Rev. 12/09.
11. Summary of Jack-in-the-Box outbreak, 1993, MMWR April 16, 1993 42 (14); 258–263.
12. Multistate Outbreak of Listeriosis Linked to Whole Cantaloupes from Jensen Farms, CO, August 27, 2012, http:/www.cdc.gov.listeria/outbreaks /cantaloupes.
13. Clinical Laboratory Improvement Act, 1988, 42 USC 201, sec. 263a.
14. Patient Protection and Affordable Care Act, 42 USC 300 et. seq.
15. International Health Regulations, http://www .who.int/topics/international_health_regulations

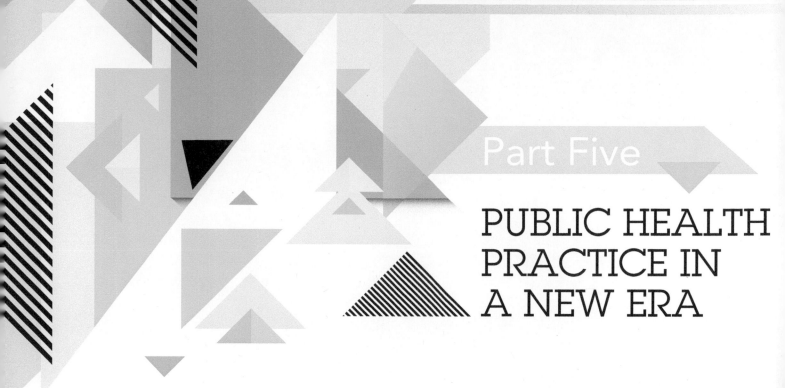

PUBLIC HEALTH PRACTICE IN A NEW ERA

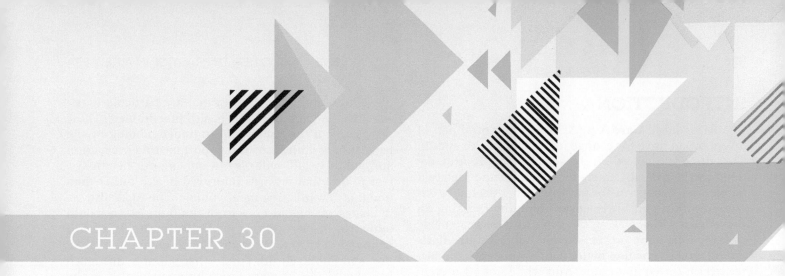

CHAPTER 30

The Affordable Care Act and Public Health

Naomi Seiler, JD • Mary-Beth Malcarney, JD, MPH • Jeffrey Levi, PhD

LEARNING OBJECTIVES

Upon completion of this chapter, the reader will be able to:

1. Summarize how the Affordable Care Act (ACA) promotes health and prevention efforts across the federal government.

2. Demonstrate how insurance coverage of clinical preventive services is enhanced under the ACA and potential implications for public health agencies providing these services.

3. Describe how the ACA supports increased funding for prevention and public health through a mandatory funding stream.

4. Explain how the ACA supports community-level prevention efforts.

5. Discuss how health system and financing changes within and beyond ACA may affect population health activities.

KEY TERMS

accountable care organization (ACO)
Center for Medicare and Medicaid Innovation
clinical preventive services
Health in All Policies
Medicaid expansion
National Prevention, Health Promotion and Public Health Council (NPC)
National Prevention Strategy
Prevention and Public Health Fund (PPHF)
Section 2713
triple aim

INTRODUCTION

The Affordable Care Act (ACA) is the central part of a very broad drive for change in the U.S. health system. That drive is centered on the so-called triple aim, defined by the federal Centers for Medicare and Medicaid Services as "better care for patients, better health for our communities, and lower costs." Only by focusing on prevention will achieving the triple aim be sustainable over the long term: prevention and public health efforts are integral to creating better care for patients and better health for communities. And while not all prevention efforts will lower costs, many will.[1] Achieving the triple aim, therefore, will require a strong partnership between the health care delivery system and the public health community, including both governmental public health and community-based organizations working on prevention at all levels.

Achieving the triple aim will also require a strong partnership between the health community and non-health sectors. As the health care sector takes on long-term financial risk for the health of the populations it serves, it is beginning to embrace the "Health in All Policies" concept that has become so fundamental to public health over the last decade. Health in All Policies is an approach that aims to incorporate health considerations into decision-making across all policy areas—from transportation, to housing, to education policies—ensuring that decision makers are informed about the health consequences of policy options. Together with public health, the health care system must address the social determinants of health through a range of clinical and community responses. In this process, public health serves several essential roles—in understanding the full breadth of the needs of the populations being served, in offering preventive and other public health services that are important to the health care system, and in being the "integrator" among the various contributors to health in a community. Indeed, public health can become what some are calling the "chief health strategist" for the community.

From a 30,000-foot perspective, the ACA can be described as achieving three main things: mandating insurance coverage for almost all individuals; expanding access to public and private health insurance coverage so individuals can fulfill this mandate; and reforming the health insurance market to make these expansions sustainable. In the process, the ACA also makes significant changes to the scope of what insurance plans must cover, as well as myriad other changes to Medicaid, Medicare, and the private market.

A full discussion of the ACA's significance to public health is beyond the scope of this chapter. Instead, we highlight here the ACA's investments and initiatives in prevention and public health that are particularly relevant to the work of public health practitioners. These provisions of the law reflect an understanding by the legislation's drafters of the important role prevention and public health will play in moving our health system to one that rewards improved health rather than one that rewards treatment volume. The ACA also establishes various levers—from the population health initiatives of the Center for Medicare and Medicaid Innovation to new programs funded under the Prevention and Public Health Fund—that promote this much broader vision of what contributes to health in the United States.

THE NATIONAL PREVENTION COUNCIL AND STRATEGY

Within the ACA, the vision of public health and prevention's fundamental role is most clearly articulated in the *National Prevention Strategy: America's Plan for Health and Wellness*. The ACA mandated the creation of a National Prevention, Health Promotion, and Public Health Council (NPC), comprising agency heads from across the federal government. The NPC is chaired by the Surgeon General, who leads the U.S. Public Health Service, and includes representatives from the following agencies:

- Department of Health and Human Services
- Department of Agriculture
- Department of Education
- Federal Trade Commission
- Department of Transportation
- Department of Labor
- Department of Homeland Security
- Environmental Protection Agency
- Office of National Drug Control Policy
- Domestic Policy Council
- Bureau of Indian Affairs, Department of the Interior
- Department of Justice
- Corporation for National and Community Service
- Department of Defense
- Department of Veterans Affairs
- Department of Housing and Urban Development
- Office of Management and Budget
- Department of the Interior
- General Services Administration
- Office of Personnel Management

The NPC was charged with issuing a National Prevention Strategy within one year of enactment of the ACA, and now meets regularly to oversee agency initiatives that are associated with implementation of the Strategy.[2-4] The Strategy reflects a very broad notion of what contributes to health outcomes, as articulated by then-Surgeon General Regina Benjamin in the Strategy's introduction:

> We know that preventing disease before it starts is critical to helping people live longer, healthier lives and keeping health care costs down. Poor diet, physical inactivity, tobacco use, and alcohol misuse are just some of the challenges we face. We also know that many of the strongest predictors of health and well-being fall outside of the health care setting. Our housing, transportation, education, workplaces, and environment are major elements that impact the physical and mental health of Americans. This is why the National Prevention Strategy helps us understand how to weave prevention into the fabric of our everyday lives.

Thus, all of the actors in the National Prevention Strategy look across government and across sectors of society to see how they can contribute to improved health, whether it is in providing better education, stable housing, more employment, or simply having people more engaged in their communities. Figure 30-1 shows the four strategic directions (the inner circle) and seven priority areas (the outer circle) of the National Prevention Strategy, all leading to the goal of increasing the number of Americans who are healthy at every stage of life.

In short, the National Prevention Strategy makes clear that achieving health and wellness, including addressing the prevention needs of Americans, includes, but also goes far beyond, insurance and coverage.

THE PREVENTION AND PUBLIC HEALTH FUND

The ACA created the **Prevention and Public Health Fund (PPHF)**, a historic allocation of reliable, mandatory funding designated specifically for public health and prevention, in addition to the funds made available through the regular appropriations process. Funds are available automatically at the beginning of each fiscal year. Congress or the Secretary of Health and Human Services may allocate these funds across existing and new public health programs. The PPHF has been used to fund a range of new and ongoing community prevention activities across the country as well as to support development of a stronger public health infrastructure and workforce.

The Fund is a reflection of Congress's belief that investment in prevention and public health can contribute to lower costs and better health outcomes. As defined by the law, the purpose of the Fund is "to provide for expanded and sustained national investment

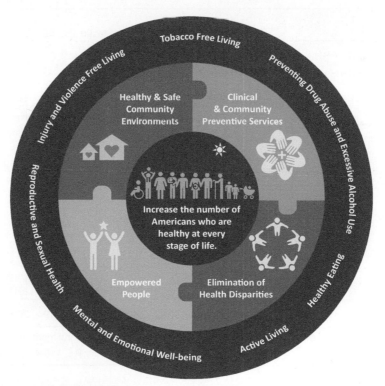

FIGURE 30-1   Strategic Directions and Priority Areas of the National Prevention Strategy
Courtesy of U.S. Department of Health and Human Services

in prevention and public health programs to improve health and help restrain the rate of growth in private and public sector health care costs."[5]

As seen in Figure 30-2, the Fund was scheduled to start at $500 million in FY 2012 and was to rise to $2 billion in FY 2015. Because Congress reduced the number of dollars available in the early years of the Fund as an offset to pay for a short-term fix for physician payment rates under Medicare, the ramp-up of funds was slowed, with funding at only $927 million in FY 2015 (after $73 million was deducted due to sequestration) and rising to $2 billion by FY 2022, remaining at that level annually thereafter. In addition, on several occasions, the administration diverted part of the Fund to pay for other ACA-related activities.

EVIDENCE-BASED PREVENTION

The ACA authorizes the U.S. Preventive Services Task Force (USPSTF) and the Community Preventive Services Task Force, panels of independent experts who make evidence-based recommendations regarding preventive services in clinical and community settings, respectively. The former is staffed by the Agency for Healthcare Research and Quality; the latter is staffed by the Centers for Disease Control and Prevention (CDC). As noted below, the USPSTF's recommendations carry great weight in terms of insurance coverage: any recommendation carrying an A or B grade in its *Guide to Clinical Preventive Services* must now be covered by most health insurers.[6] The Community Task Force produces the *Community Guide to Preventive Services*, which includes its findings on the evidence base for community-based interventions; however, the Community Guide's recommendations have no impact on insurance coverage under the ACA.[7] The Prevention and Public Health Fund has been used to expand the capacity of both task forces from time to time since passage of the ACA.

CLINICAL PREVENTION UNDER THE ACA

The ACA contains provisions significantly expanding insurance coverage of **clinical preventive services**, creating opportunities for public health practitioners to promote increased uptake of these services.

ACA's Insurance Expansions

The preventive services expansions must be understood against a backdrop of expanded insurance coverage overall. The ACA established an individual requirement to maintain adequate insurance coverage.[8] The law creates two main new sources of insurance coverage:

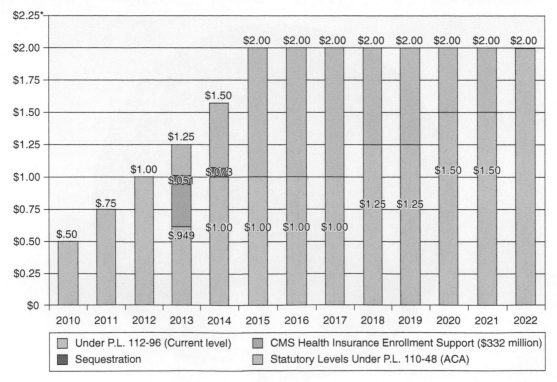

* in $U.S. billions

FIGURE 30-2   Prevention and Public Health Fund
DATA SOURCE: Trust for America's Health (2015)

state-level Exchanges, or "marketplaces" (referred to here as Exchanges), and Medicaid expansions. In Exchanges, individuals and small businesses can compare coverage and costs and purchase health insurance policies.[9] People with household incomes between 100 and 400 percent of the federal poverty level (FPL) can receive a federal tax credit to help pay premiums, and those with income under 250 percent of the federal poverty level are also eligible for cost-sharing assistance.[9]

Medicaid is a federal-state program of health insurance for low-income individuals. Prior to the ACA, most states only offered coverage to low-income people in certain categories, such as children, pregnant women, and people with disabilities; for the most part, childless adults were categorically excluded from Medicaid. The ACA gives states the ability to expand Medicaid to cover *all* adults up to 138 percent of the federal poverty level.[10] The Supreme Court's 2012 decision in *NFIB v. Sebelius* made this expansion optional for states; as of September 2015, 31 states and the District of Columbia were implementing expansions of their Medicaid programs under ACA.[11]

In those states that are not expanding Medicaid, very low-income people will likely be left uninsured. In those states, people with income between 100 and 400 percent FPL are eligible for premium support to purchase plans on the Exchange. However, people with income below 100 percent FPL are *not* eligible for premium support, meaning that the poorest of the poor in these states will likely not be able to get insurance. As of July 2015, an estimated 6.5 million adults would have no access to Medicaid and are likely to remain uninsured in nonexpansion states.[12] (See also http://familiesusa.org/product/50-state-look-medicaid-expansion.)

The ACA contains additional provisions broadening access to health insurance. Young adults can remain on their parents' insurance up until age 26;[13] large employers may face penalties for not providing adequate health coverage.[14] In addition, the law contains important insurance market reforms, such as preventing individual and small group plans from excluding people based on preexisting conditions, and prohibiting them from charging higher premiums based on gender or health status (other than tobacco use).[15] From a public health standpoint this continuity of coverage is critical, both to assure timely receipt of clinical preventive services and to assure that those in treatment for communicable diseases, such as HIV, continue to receive care that is critical to preventing further spread of the disease.

Section 2713 of ACA: Coverage of Clinical Preventive Services

In addition to these insurance expansions, ACA includes specific coverage requirements for clinical preventive services. As discussed in detail below, the requirements

vary across different types of insurance; however, they are all based on a set of preventive services defined in Section 2713 of the law[16] to include:

(a) U.S. Preventive Services Task Force (USPSTF) items or services with a grade of "A" or "B" (the ACA recodifies this Task Force and authorizes continued funding);

(b) Immunizations recommended by the CDC's Advisory Committee on Immunization Practices (ACIP);

(c) Evidence-informed preventive care and screening guidelines for infants, children, and adolescents recommended by the Health Resources and Services Administration (HRSA)[17]; and

(d) Additional preventive care and screening services for women recommended by HRSA.[18] The initial list of preventive services for women was prepared by a committee of the Institute of Medicine and included comprehensive sexually transmitted infection and family planning services, which has raised some legal challenges.[19]

A full description of clinical preventive services may be found at the Kaiser Family Foundation website (www.kkf.org) by searching under "preventive services covered."

The ACA applies the requirements of Section 2713 to different insurance types as follows:

▸ *Private Employer-Based Plans*: Most employer-based plans must cover *all* Section 2713 services with no cost-sharing imposed on the enrollee (no deductible, copayments, or coinsurance).[20,21]

▸ *Individual and Small-Group Plans*: Most individual plans, whether or not purchased through an Exchange, must cover *all* Section 2713 services with no cost-sharing.[22]

▸ *Medicaid*:
  • The *"Expansion population"*: In states expanding Medicaid, the newly-eligible population is entitled to *all* Section 2713 services without cost-sharing.[23]
  • The *"traditional" population*: In all states, people in traditional eligibility categories are not automatically entitled to any of the Section 2713 services, and even if these preventive services are covered, beneficiaries may be responsible for copayments or other forms of cost-sharing. Studies indicate that coverage of preventive services in traditional Medicaid varies significantly.[24] However, ACA did create an incentive: states that cover *all* USPSTF- and ACIP-recommended services for all of their Medicaid enrollees will receive a 1 percent boost in the federal contribution to their Medicaid costs for those services.[25] Note that the

ACA does not give states any incentive to provide traditional Medicaid coverage of the preventive services recommended by HRSA.

▸ *Medicare*: The Medicare program does not have to cover Section 2713 services. However, if Medicare does cover a USPSTF-recommended service, ACA requires that it do so with no cost-sharing imposed on the beneficiary.[26]

Implications for Public Health Practice

Along with expansions in insurance coverage, the ACA's preventive services coverage provisions have significant implications for population health and for public health practice. The provisions may have the most direct effects on public health departments that directly provide clinical services. Many of the services traditionally offered by health departments, such as sexually transmitted infections (STIs) screenings, are included in the list of Section 2713 services because they are recommended by the USPSTF. Under the ACA, the patient populations that health departments serve are more likely than before to have insurance. Health departments that are not already billing for services may need to consider whether they should initiate billing—of Medicaid, private insurance, and/or Medicare—to support their provision of clinical services. It is quite possible that federal grant programs will begin to establish "payer of last resort" requirements similar to those that already exist in statute for the Ryan White program, allowing public health departments to provide free clinical services only if no source of insurance reimbursement is available. It is also possible that newly insured patients will begin seeking clinical care from other providers, changing the health department's role. And it is quite possible that categorical funding for clinical preventive services may decline—whether because of expanded insurance coverage or because of budgetary pressures—further changing the role of public health departments that have traditionally provided clinical services. In Massachusetts, for example, funding cuts for state STI clinics combined with increased insurance coverage across the state have significantly changed the health department's role with regard to STI services.[27]

Public health practitioners who do not directly provide clinical services often still engage in efforts to promote awareness and uptake. The ACA's new coverage requirements create an opportunity for improved uptake, and health departments' education and outreach efforts to providers and to patients should emphasize this new coverage—and particularly the lack of cost-sharing.

Despite ACA's efforts to expand coverage of preventive services, the law's requirements pose a number of key challenges for professionals focused on population health. First, the recommendations on which the coverage guidelines are based focus on a finite set of "clinical" services. As discussed further below, the ACA also includes attention to, and funding for, "community-based" services. But the insurance coverage requirements only apply to the services that USPSTF and the other relevant bodies deem "clinical." This draws a bright line between preventive services that health insurance should reimburse and those it should not, based solely on a definition of "clinical" that does not necessarily align with patient, or population, interests. Second, the coverage requirements are stronger for some populations than others, in ways that do not necessarily track the need for zero-cost preventive services. For example, most people in private insurance have access to all Section 2713 services without cost-sharing, but low-income people who are in "traditional" Medicaid eligibility categories, such as children and pregnant women, may not. Finally, gaps in Medicare coverage of preventive services remain. For example, Medicare only covers some recommended vaccines without cost-sharing.[28] It will likely fall to public health practitioners to assess coverage gaps among Medicare-eligible seniors and people with disabilities, particularly vaccination coverage gaps, and focus programs on responding to this unmet need.

Despite these challenges, the expanded preventive service requirements represent a crucial step for population health. In addition to promoting awareness and uptake of these benefits, public health practitioners can serve as front-line monitors of how the provisions are implemented, measuring not only process but also impact on population health.

COMMUNITY PREVENTION UNDER THE ACA

While definitions of "community-based prevention" vary, for purposes of understanding the ACA, a helpful framework is to think of community-based prevention as any preventive health intervention taking place outside of a clinical setting, regardless of who the provider is.

Community Prevention in the Law

The ACA authorizes new community prevention initiatives. Its largest investment in community prevention is in fact a continuation and expansion of a program created under a 2009 stimulus bill.[29] That bill created Communities Putting Prevention to Work (CPPW), a CDC-administered program that awarded competitive funding to jurisdictions across the country for community-based programs to address obesity and tobacco use.[30] The ACA expanded on this effort by creating a program of Community Transformation Grants (CTGs) using Prevention Fund dollars. Also administered by the CDC, the CTG program funded state and local agencies, nonprofits, and coalitions to implement community-based interventions that focus on chronic disease prevention. In FY 2014, Congress ended funding for the CTG program; however, even higher levels of funding were made available for a series of community-oriented prevention efforts focusing on policy and systems change, including the Partnerships to Improve Community Health (PICH).

Other ACA provisions supporting community-based prevention include the codification and authorization of funds for the Task Force on Community Preventive Services, the community-based counterpart to the USPSTF (as noted above); the establishment of a national Diabetes Prevention Program that includes community-based diabetes prevention programs; federal nutrition labeling requirements for chain restaurants; and provisions for adequate break time and coverage of breast pumps for breastfeeding mothers.

Implications for Public Health Practice

The community prevention provisions of the ACA create enormous opportunities for public health practitioners, but also highlight existing challenges. The opportunities lie in the funding and attention that the law, and ARRA before it, brought to community prevention. The Community Transformation Grants, as well as the broader National Prevention Strategy, focus on "community prevention" in ways that recognize two key points: first, that some of the most important determinants of health are structural or "upstream," and second, that addressing these factors requires a cross-sector "Health in All Policies" approach with a particular focus on policy and systems to create long-lasting "environmental" change. These points may be obvious to public health experts, but in a national health system so focused on medical care and the clinical settings, community prevention efforts may be novel. These efforts also provide policy and financial support for building the partnerships across sectors that are essential to a Health in All Policies approach.

Another opportunity under the ACA is the possibility of better integrating public health with the clinical health system. While such integration could and did occur prior to the passage of ACA, the law contains several specific provisions promoting such partnerships. For example, ACA revises the requirements for nonprofit hospitals to maintain their tax status.[31] The new requirements include an enhanced "community health needs assessment," or CHNA, that assesses the health needs of the hospital's entire community, not just of the patients it serves. The hospital must report on how it will provide a "community benefit" to address needs identified in the CHNA, thus acting not only as a clinical provider but also as a monitor and improver of population health in the community.[32,33] Agency guidance implementing the rule explicitly requires the inclusion of public health officials in the CHNA process. There is also strong potential for partnership between these hospitals and community-based governmental and nongovernmental organizations as they implement their community benefit plans.

Another change subsequent to the ACA involves broader provider eligibility for preventive services under Medicaid. In rules implementing some of the law's Medicaid provisions, CMS also modified an existing rule to allow states to reimburse a broader range of nonlicensed health professionals for providing preventive services.[34] This new flexibility allows states to opt to reimburse a range of qualified practitioners—such as community health workers, many of whom may work for health departments—to provide preventive services. This change has the potential to expand the reach of preventive services, better reaching enrollees who need it most.[35]

DELIVERY SYSTEM REFORMS AND THE ACA

Beyond raising the profile of public health through clinical and community prevention initiatives, a number of ACA provisions and programs are focused on realigning the health care system in ways that emphasize community-based prevention and population health outcomes. While the efforts described below are primarily focused on transforming the clinical health care system, they offer key opportunities for the public health system to leverage clinical care to promote population health. Through these initiatives, providers, insurers, states and communities are experimenting with alternative health care delivery system and payment models that reward and incentivize prevention practice, holding promise for promoting disease prevention and population health.

Medicaid Health Homes

The concept of a "patient-centered medical home" (PCMH) was first described by the American Academy of Pediatrics in 1967, and has evolved since then to define a model of primary care that is "patient-centered, comprehensive, team-based, coordinated, accessible, and focused on quality and safety."[36] The ACA embraces these efforts by providing a framework for states to adopt medical home models for high-risk populations served by Medicaid.

Termed Medicaid "health homes", the new state Medicaid option allows eligible individuals to seek care through a PCMH-like model.[37] To qualify for health home services, eligible Medicaid enrollees must meet one of three requirements:

a) have a serious and persistent mental illness; or

b) have two chronic conditions (qualifying chronic conditions are specified by the law); or

c) have one chronic condition and be at risk of developing a second.

Under the law, a Medicaid health home is responsible for providing or coordinating all patient care, as well as performing a set of health home services including care management, coordination and health promotion, patient and family support, and referral to community and social support services. For these specific "health home" services, the federal government will pay an enhanced federal Medicaid match rate of 90 percent during the first eight quarters (two years) of state participation.

Implications for Public Health Practice

While states have discretion to determine the range of health home participating providers and treatment settings, federal guidance emphasizes that a health home must contain sufficient providers to deliver a "whole-person approach to care," including promotion of disease self-management, access to preventive and health promotion services, and coordination with community-based services.[38] As a result, public health practitioners and programs have an opportunity to be designated as part of the "health team" responsible for the care of health home participants. For example, through a health home model, primary care practitioners may refer patients to smoking cessation support or diabetes education offered by a local health department or community-based organization. The health home structure could also encourage collaborations between primary care and public health to support immunization efforts, disease identification and control, or health education.

At the time of writing, 15 states have created Medicaid Health Homes, and several other states have received planning grants to explore health home implementation.[39] As Medicaid Health Homes develop, states may see this ACA initiative as a desirable way to integrate community-based public health services into new health care delivery models. In addition, states may have the opportunity to invest any Medicaid savings generated by the health home model back into public health to further address population-level health concerns among disadvantaged residents.

Accountable Care Organizations (ACOs)

An **accountable care organization (ACO)** is a network of doctors and hospitals that agrees to be held accountable for improving the health of its patients while reducing the rate of growth in health care spending. In an ACO model, providers keep a share of financial savings they generate from better-than-expected health care performance, but may also share risk for financial loss. Providers are also held accountable for certain quality and outcomes standards, and shared savings may be contingent on meeting these standards. Much like the medical home model described above, ACOs are built around a strong primary care core. By including specialists, hospitals, and other providers in the care team, ACOs go further than the medical home to address health outcomes across the entire care continuum.

While the ACO model has existed in some form for nearly a decade,[40] health reform puts ACOs at center stage by encouraging Medicare fee-for-service program providers to form ACOs under the *Medicare Shared Savings Program*,[41] or through one of two ACO models being tested through the Center for Medicare and Medicaid Innovation (CMMI) (described in further detail below).[42,43] While provider participation is completely voluntary, as of December 2013, more than 360 ACOs had been established through the shared savings program, serving over 5.3 million Americans with Medicare.[44]

Implications for Public Health Practice

Under these various Medicare ACO models, payment is linked directly to quality of care; before an ACO can share in any savings, it must meet over 30 quality performance measurements.[45] Many of these quality measures implicate public health, including measures related to health promotion and education, preventive screenings, and various care coordination metrics. ACOs may also look to employ specific community-based, population-level interventions as a cost-effective way of managing chronic disease, preventing avoidable illness, and reducing unnecessary care for the populations they serve.

Regardless of the outcome of the particular ACO programs being pushed forward by ACA, the notion of providers participating in systems that require accountability for care coordination and quality of care is a concept that is likely here to stay as governmental payers, the employer community, and commercial health insurance companies all push for more integrated health care delivery systems. Public health can have a significant role collaborating with ACOs—or other ACO-like structures that evolve—to produce

EXHIBIT 30-1 Case Study: Hennepin Health, a Social Accountable Care Organization

Hennepin Health is a Medicaid demonstration project formed in January 2012 by a cooperative network of health care organizations in Hennepin County, Minnesota, including a health plan, a health care system, a federally qualified health center, and the county's Human Services and Public Health Department.

Hennepin Health serves approximately 6,100 local adults enrolled in the state's Medicaid expansion (18- to 64-year-old adults with no dependent children, with income < 75 percent of the federal poverty line) under a care model that is built on the concepts of a primary care medical home. The model promotes a strong continuum of care coordination and emphasizes the importance of addressing the social determinants of health, such as housing, substance abuse, and joblessness. Hennepin Health receives a capitated per-member, per-month payment from the state Medicaid office and shares any savings with the state at the end of the year.

Early results have been positive: in its first year of operation, Hennepin Health reduced emergency department visits by more than 20 percent, increased primary care visits and linkages to social services, and decreased spending for many of the program's top users of medical services. In total, the county has been able to reinvest more than $1 million in savings toward filling service gaps and providing higher-quality, cost-saving care. For example, the county has used savings to invest in a sobering center and vocational services support program and plans to use future savings to provide interim housing for patients who are ready to leave the hospital but do not have access to stable housing.[46]

innovative models of clinical-public health integration that foster health and wellness while reducing expenditures (see Exhibits 30-1 and 30-2).

Center for Medicare and Medicaid Innovation

Established by the ACA, the Center for Medicare and Medicaid Innovation (Innovation Center) is a testing ground for innovative payment and service delivery models. The goal of testing these new models of care is to reduce Medicare and Medicaid expenditures while preserving or improving the quality of care provided to beneficiaries under these public health insurance programs. The Innovation Center has the flexibility to rapidly test innovative care and payment models and encourage widespread adoption of practices that deliver better health care at lower cost.

Implications for Public Health Practice

One of three areas of Innovation Center focus is the Community and Population Health Models group, which focuses on community prevention as a core element of its work. This group has offered up to $1 billion in Health Care Innovation Awards to community-based organizations that are implementing the most compelling new ideas to deliver better health, improved care, and lower costs to people enrolled in Medicare and Medicaid. Through this funding, the Innovation Center is seeking to award projects that will improve the health of populations through prevention, wellness, and comprehensive care that extends beyond the clinical service delivery system setting and addresses the social determinants of health.

EXHIBIT 30-2 Health Care Innovation Award: Optimizing Health Outcomes for Children with Asthma in Delaware

Nemours/ Alfred I. duPont Hospital for Children received over $3.6 million from the Innovation Center to enhance family-centered medical homes in their community by adding community-based services for children with asthma. The goal of this model is to reduce asthma-related emergency room use and asthma-related hospitalization among pediatric Medicaid patients in Delaware by 50 percent by 2015. This goal will be accomplished by focusing on three distinct strategies:

(1) Enhancement of the family-centered medical home by adding new services for children with asthma and developing a well-coordinated interdisciplinary approach to managing asthma care;

(2) Development of a sustainable network of evidence-based supports and services surrounding each of the three targeted primary care sites, using the "integrator" model that Nemours has already adopted; and

(3) Deployment of a "navigator" workforce that incorporates nonmedical needs into the provision of care for children with asthma that promotes respiratory health and addresses environmental asthma triggers throughout the target communities.[47]

Another signature Innovation Center program is the State Innovation Models (SIM) Initiative. The SIM awards are grants to states to support the development and testing of state-based models for multipayer payment and health care delivery system transformation efforts.[48] Funding through SIM offers states the resources to plan, design, test, and evaluate new payment and service delivery models in the context of larger health system transformation, with the goal of improving health outcomes for the state's population. CMS has required SIM grantees to specifically address population health concerns.

Implications for Public Health Practice

As SIM projects develop, and as additional states are awarded funding through this initiative, the public health system has an opportunity to become integrated into emerging state-wide models of care, such as the examples described in Table 30-1.

Medicaid Health Homes, ACO models promoted by the ACA, and the range of programs sponsored by the Innovation Center present unprecedented opportunities to integrate population health principles into evolving delivery system and payment models. Indeed, the larger systemic changes in the financing of health care—moving toward reward for outcomes rather than volume—provides an opportunity for new partnerships between public health and the health care system if public health can demonstrate its added value in moving toward achieving the triple aim.

OTHER ACA PROVISIONS OF INTEREST TO PUBLIC HEALTH PRACTITIONERS

The ACA includes numerous additional provisions with implications for public health practice and for population health, including:

▷ *Essential Health Benefits*: The ACA requires all individual and small group plans to include ten categories of "Essential Health Benefits":
  - ambulatory patient services;
  - emergency services;
  - hospitalization;
  - maternity and newborn care;
  - mental health and substance use disorder services, including behavioral health treatment;
  - prescription drugs;
  - rehabilitative and habilitative services and devices;

TABLE 30-1   State Innovation Models: Snapshots

State Innovation Models: Snapshots	
Minnesota: Model-Testing State	Minnesota plans to use SIM funding to test new ways of delivering and paying for health care using the *Minnesota Accountable Health Model* framework. This model expands patient-centered, team-based care through service delivery and payment models that support integration of medical care, behavioral health, long-term care, and community prevention services. The Accountable Health Model will include the establishment of up to 15 *Accountable Communities for Health* which will develop and test strategies for "creating healthy futures for patients and community members."[49]
Oregon: Model-Testing State	Prior to receiving the SIM grant, Oregon had created coordinated care organizations (CCOs) within their Medicaid program. CCOs are local health entities delivering care to Medicaid beneficiaries within the state that are accountable for health outcomes of the population they serve. The SIM grant will support the state in strengthening the CCO model and to begin to make some of the model's key elements, such as patient-centered primary care homes, available to other populations such as public employees and Medicare beneficiaries.[50]
California: Model-Design State	California plans to use SIM funding to support development of 2-3 *Accountable Care Community pilots*, "which will model how population health can be advanced through collaborative, multi-institutional efforts that promote a shared responsibility for the health of the community. Pilots will include a Wellness Trust, which will serve as a vehicle to pool and leverage funding from a variety of sources for long-term sustainability."[51]
Maryland: Model-Design State	With SIM dollars, Maryland is engaging in a planning process to develop a *Community-Integrated Medical Home* model. "This model of care will integrate patient-centered medical care with community-based resources while enhancing the capacity of local health entities to monitor and improve the health of individuals and their communities as a whole."[52] Maryland included local health improvement coalitions (panels of local health departments, hospitals, physicians, community organizations, and other local entities) in a stakeholder engagement process to help the state develop plans for integrating community health and clinical care in the state's medical home model.

- laboratory services;
- preventive and wellness services and chronic disease management; and
- pediatric services, including oral and vision care.

▶ *Essential Community Providers*: To assure that low-income, medically underserved populations eligible for essential health benefits have access to providers who address their care needs, the law includes a requirement that health plans in the exchange include certain "essential community providers" within provider networks.[53] These include Ryan White clinics, STI clinics, community health centers, and other important safety net providers.

▶ *Public Health Workforce*: Recognizing the need for a larger and better trained health care and public health workforce, the law includes a set of provisions designed to increase the supply and enhance the training of the health workforce across a variety of disciplines. Loan repayment provisions, training grants, fellowship opportunities, and other programs aim to address critical workforce shortages to ensure that the health system is adequately staffed and prepared to meet new demands in a posthealth reform era.

- *Public Health Infrastructure*: The ACA also invests in the public health infrastructure through changes in the structure of the U.S. Public Health Service Commissioned Corps, new grants to enhance public health epidemiology and laboratory capacity, and grants to fund construction and operations of school-based health centers.

It is also important to note the role of health information technology (HIT) in creating the connections between public health and the health care system under ACA. While the ACA did not itself make major revisions to HIT policy, the adoption and use of HIT by all facets of the health care and public health system—including by public health institutions—is foundational to the implementation of many aspects of health reform. For example, the federal "meaningful use" program, which gives financial incentives payments under Medicare and Medicaid to providers who adopt electronic health records, includes the requirement that providers' systems be capable of transmitting immunization and syndromic surveillance data to public health departments. Public health practitioners need to be aware of such policies and work to develop sufficient capacity on the public health side to make use of such information (see Chapter 12 for more detail on emerging surveillance systems).

It is important to acknowledge that implementation of the ACA has been the subject of highly partisan debates. Yet, critical elements of the ACA's reforms are very popular with the public—including coverage of clinical preventive services without cost sharing, elimination of the preexisting condition exclusions in insurance policies, and allowing children under age 26 years to remain on their parents' insurance plans. Even the controversial Medicaid expansion is gaining support, as states previously opposed to the option negotiate new arrangements with the federal government over the terms of the expansion.

We cannot predict the outcome of these partisan debates, but these and other popular reforms are likely to remain central to a reformed system. And, perhaps more importantly, the push in our health care system to move away from volume-driven financial incentives to approaches that reward health outcomes will be a constant in the years ahead. This movement started before passage of the ACA, has been strengthened by the experiments and demonstrations that have been supported under the ACA, and is central to the financial viability of our health system and federal and state budgets. These financing and structural reforms will help incentivize a prevention and early intervention approach to health care and will thus form the basis for a continuing and growing relationship between public health and the health care system.

SUMMARY

Taken together, the various public health and prevention related provisions of the ACA, along with the coverage and delivery system reforms that it authorizes, offer new opportunities to integrate a population health approach into our health care system. Indeed, from the creation of the National Prevention Council and its "Health in All Policies" approach, to the new funds available through the Prevention and Public Health Fund, and the experiments in taking a comprehensive approach to the health-related needs of patients, public health officials have a tremendous opportunity to become the "chief health strategists" in their communities. Now, more than ever, resources and financial incentives are in place to create new partnerships across many sectors that can improve the health of the public.

REVIEW QUESTIONS

1. How does the ACA embrace a "Health in All Policies" approach to prevention and public health?

2. How does the ACA expand insurance coverage of clinical preventive services?

3. How might changes in insurance access under ACA affect public health departments that provide clinical services?

4. How does the ACA promote community-based preventive services?

5. What new funding stream does the ACA create for prevention and public health, and how is it different from usual funding for public health?

6. How do financing and structural changes in the health care system create new opportunities for partnership between public health and the health care system?

ACKNOWLEDGMENT

The authors would like to thank Rosalind Fennell for her assistance in the development of this chapter.

REFERENCES

1. *Prevention for a Healthier America: Investments in Disease Prevention Yield Significant Savings, Stronger Communities.* Washington, DC: Trust for America's Health; February 2009.

2. National Prevention Council: National Prevention Council Members. Accessed October 13, 2014 (http://www.surgeongeneral.gov/initiatives/prevention/about/npcouncilmembers.html).

3. National Prevention Council Action Plan: Implementing the National Prevention Strategy. June 2012. Accessed October 13, 2014 (http://www.surgeongeneral.gov/initiatives/prevention/2012-npc-action-plan.pdf).

4. *National Prevention, Health Promotion, and Public Health Council: Annual Status Report.* Washington, DC: Office of the Surgeon General, US Department of Health and Human Services; July 2014.

5. Patient Protection and Affordable Care Act, Public Law No. 111-148. § 4002(a).

6. US Preventive Services Task Force: What Is the Task Force and What Does It do? http://www.uspreventiveservicestaskforce.org/Page/Basic OneColumn/28. Accessed October 13, 2014.

7. The Guide to Community Preventive Services: What is the Community Guide? Accessed October 13, 2014; http://www.thecommunityguide.org/about/index.html.

8. Patient Protection and Affordable Care Act, Public Law No. 111-148.§ 1501(b).

9. Patient Protection and Affordable Care Act, Public Law No. 111-148.§ 1311(b).

10. Patient Protection and Affordable Care Act, Public Law No. 111-148.§ 2001.

11. Kaiser Family Foundation, "Status of State Action on the Medicaid Expansion Decision, 2014" October 13, 2014 http://kff.org/health-reform /state-indicator/state-activity-around-expanding-medicaid-under-the-affordable-care-act/.

12. Urban Institute, "In States That Don't Expand Medicaid, Who Gets New Coverage Assistance Under the ACA and Who Doesn't?" Oct 2014; Accessed October 13, 2014 (http://www.urban.org/uploadedpdf/413248-Who-Gets-New-Coverage-Assistance-Under-the-ACA-and-Who-Doesnt.pdf).

13. Patient Protection and Affordable Care Act, Public Law No. 111-148.§ 1001.

14. Patient Protection and Affordable Care Act, Public Law No. 111-148.§ 1513.

15. Patient Protection and Affordable Care Act, Public Law No. 111-148.§ 1201.

16. Public Health Services Act §2713. *as added by the Patient Protection and Affordable Care Act §1001.*

17. Bright Futures / AAP Periodicity Schedule. *The category of preventive services for children is reflected in the "Bright Futures" recommendations developed by HRSA in cooperation with the American Academy of Pediatrics.* Accessed October 13, 2014 (Available at: http://brightfutures.aap.org/clinical_practice.html).

18. The preventive services for women are based on a set of recommendations made by an Institute of Medicine panel and adopted by HRSA in 2011. *Institute of Medicine, "Clinical Preventive Services for Women: Closing the Gap."* July 2011; Accessed October 13, 2014 (Available at: http://www.iom.edu/Reports/2011/Clinical-Preventive-services-for-Women-Closing-the-Gaps.aspx); Health Resources and Services Administration, "Women's Preventive Services Guidelines" (available at http://www.hrsa.gov/womensguidelines/).

19. Burwell v. Hobby Lobby Stores, Inc. *573 U.S. — (2014).*

20. The requirement applies to self-insured or fully insured employer plans governed by the Employee Retirement Income Security Act (ERISA). *"Grandfathered" plans are excluded, but as they make certain changes to coverage or cost sharing they lose their exemption.*

21. Patient Protection and Affordable Care Act, Public Law No. 111-148.§1563 (e).

22. Grandfathered plans are exempted; however, a large and growing majority of individual plans are not grandfathered.

23. Patient Protection and Affordable Care Act, Public Law No. 111-148.§2001.

24. Wilensky S. Existing Medicaid Beneficiaries Left Off The Affordable Care Act's Prevention Bandwagon. *Health Affairs.* July 2013;32: 71188–71195.

25. Patient Protection and Affordable Care Act, Public Law No. 111–148.§4106.

26. Patient Protection and Affordable Care Act, Public Law No. 111–148.§4104.

27. Drainoni ML, Sullivan M, Sequeira S, Bacic J, Hsu K, Fagain M, Morgan J, Iliaki E. *Evaluating the Impact of Changes in Funding for Sexually Transmitted Infection Services in Massachusetts: A Two-Phase Study. Boston University PowerPoint Presentation.* Feb. 2013. Accessed October 13, 2014 (Available from: http://www.bu.edu/sph /files/2010/2011/STD_slides_for_2012-2021- 2013_BU_presentation.ppt).

28. U.S. Government Accountability Office, "Medicare: Many Factors, Including Administrative Challenges, Affect Access to Part D Vaccinations" 2011. Accessed October 13, 2014 (Available at: http:// www.gao.gov/products/GAO-12-61).

29. American Recovery and Reinvestment Act of 2009.

30. Division of Community Health, National Center for Chronic Disease Prevention and Health Promotion. Communities Putting Prevention to Work. *Centers for Disease Control and Prevention.* Accessed October 13, 2014 (Available at: http://www.cdc.gov/nccdphp/dch/programs /CommunitiesPuttingPreventiontoWork/).

31. Internal Revenue Services: New Requirements for 501(c)(3) Hospitals Under the Affordable Care Act. March 2014. http://www.irs.gov /Charities-&-Non-Profits/Charitable-Organizations /New-Requirements-for-501%28c%29%283%29- Hospitals-Under-the-Affordable-Care-Act. Accessed October 13, 2014.

32. Internal Revenue Services: Hospitals and Community Benefit-Interim Report. April 2014; Accessed October 13, 2014 (http://www.irs.gov/ Charities-&-Non-Profits/Charitable-Organizations /New-Requirements-for-501%28c%29%283%29- Hospitals-Under-the-Affordable-Care-Act).

33. Somerville M, Nelson GD, Mueller CH. Community Benefits After the ACA: The State Law Landscape. The Hilltop Institute. March 2013; Accessed October 13, 2014 (http://www.rwjf.org/content/dam /farm/reports/issue_briefs/2013/rwjf408711).

34. Final Rule: Medicaid and Children's Health Insurance Program: Essential Health Benefits in Alternative Benefits Plans, Eligibility Notices, Fair Hearing and Appeal Processes, and Premiums and Cost Sharing, Exchanges: Eligibility and Enrollment. Centers for Medicare & Medicaid Services. *Section 42 CFR §440.130. 78 Federal Register 42160.* July 2013.

35. Trust for America's Health and Nemours. *Medicaid Reimbursement for Community-Based Prevention: Based on Convening Held October 31, 2013.* May 2014 (Available from: http://healthyamericans .org/health-issues/wp-content/uploads/2014/07 /Medicaid-and-Community-Prevention-Final -Revised-5-15-14.pdf).

36. Patient-Centered Primary Care Collaborative. *Defining the Medical Home.* Accessed October 13, 2014 (Available at: http://www.pcpcc.org/about /medical-home).

37. Social Security Act § 1945, added by the Patient Protection and Affordable Care Act. *Public Law No. 111-148.*§2703, 124 Stat. 855 (March 2010).

38. Health Homes for Enrollees with Chronic Conditions: SMDL# 10-024. *Centers for Medicaid and Medicare Services, Center for Medicaid, CHIP and Survey & Certification.* November 16, 2010 (Accessed October 13, 2014).

39. Approved Health Home State Plan Amendments. *Centers for Medicare & Medicaid Services.* Accessed October 13, 2014 (Available at: http://www.medicaid.gov/State-Resource- Center/Medicaid-State-Technical-Assistance/ Health-Homes-Technical-Assistance/Approved- Health-Home-State-Plan-Amendments.html).

40. Fisher ES, et al. *Creating Accountable Care Organizations: The Extended Hospital Medical Staff.* Health Affairs (2007;26(1):w44–w57).

41. Social Security Act § 1899, added by the Patient Protection and Affordable Care Act. *Public Law No. 111-148.*§3022, 124 Stat. 855 (March 2010).

42. Center for Medicare & Medicaid Innovation. *Pioneer ACO Model. Centers for Medicare and Medicaid Services.* Accessed October 13, 2014 (Available at: http://innovation.cms.gov/initiatives /Pioneer-ACO-Model/).

43. Center for Medicare & Medicaid Innovation. *Advance Payment ACO Model. Centers for Medicare and Medicaid Services.* Accessed October 13, 2014 (Available at: http://innovation .cms.gov/initiatives/Advance-Payment-ACO- Model/).

44. Centers for Medicare and Medicaid Services. *Press release: More partnerships between doctors and hospitals strengthen coordinated care for Medicare beneficiaries.* December 23, 2013 Accessed October 13, 2014 (Available at: http:// www.cms.gov/Newsroom/MediaReleaseDatabase /Press-Releases/2013-Press-Releases-Items/2013- 2012-2023.html).

45. Medicare Shared Savings Program Quality Measure Benchmarks for the 2014 and 2015 Reporting Years. *Centers for Medicare and Medicaid Services.* Accessed October 13, 2014 (http://www.cms.gov /Medicare/Medicare-Fee-for-Service-Payment /sharedsavingsprogram/Downloads/MSSP-QM -Benchmarks.pdf).

46. Garrett N. *How a Social Accountable Care Organization Improves Health and Saves Money and Lives.* Nov 2013 Accessed October 13, 2014 (Available at: http://healthyamericans.org/health-issues /prevention_story/how-a-social-accountable-care -organization-improves-health-and-saves-money -and-lives).

47. Health Care Innovation Awards: Project Profile; Nemours/ Alfred I. duPont Hospital for Children. *Center for Medicare and Medicaid Innovation.* Accessed October 13, 2014 (Available from: http://innovation.cms.gov/initiatives/participant /Health-Care-Innovation-Awards/Nemours -Alfred-I-Dupont-Hospital-For-Children.html).

48. State Innovation Models Initiative: General Information. Center for Medicare and Medicaid Innovation. Accessed October 13, 2014 (Available at: http://innovation.cms.gov/initiatives /state-innovations/).

49. State Innovation Model Grant: Minnesota Accountable Health Model. *Minnesota Department of Human Services.* Accessed October 13, 2014 (Available at: http://www.dhs.state.mn.us/main /idcplg?IdcService=GET_DYNAMIC_CONVERSION &RevisionSelectionMethod=LatestReleased&dDocNa me=SIM_Home).

50. Oregon Health Policy and Research: State Innovation Model Grant. Accessed October 13, 2014 (Available at: http://www.oregon.gov/oha/OHPR/Pages/sim /index.aspx).

51. California State Health Care Innovation Plan. *California Health and Human Services Agency.* March 2014. Accessed October 13, 2014 (Available at: http://www.chhs.ca.gov/ PRI/CalSIM%20State%20Health%20Care%20 Innovation%20Plan_Final.pdf).

52. State Innovation Model (SIM). *Maryland Department of Health and Mental Hygiene.* Accessed October 13, 2014 (Available from: http://hsia. dhmh.maryland.gov/SitePages/sim.aspx).

53. Patient Protection and Affordable Care Act, Public Law No. 111-148.§1311(c)(1)(C).

CHAPTER 31

Public Health in the Global Context

Didier Wernli MD, MA • Antoine Flahault, MD, PhD

LEARNING OBJECTIVES

Upon completion of this chapter, the reader will be able to:

1. Understand the practice of public health in the global context, referred to here as global health.

2. Describe how globalization has impacted health and how health is related to socio-economic development.

3. Provide an overview of the distribution of disease across the world.

4. Describe the main actors involved in the global governance of health.

5. Define global health innovation, including its two main components, technological and social innovation.

6. Elaborate on the concept of reverse innovation as well as the role of academic institutions.

KEY TERMS

economic globalization
epidemiological transition
global burden of diseases (GBD)
global health
global health governance
globalization
health equity
human mobility
innovation

INTRODUCTION

Dramatic improvements in health have taken place across the world during the last century, including a considerable increase in life expectancy in all regions of the world.[1] Almost everywhere, population health has been profoundly impacted by globalization, and many of today's multifaceted health challenges are influenced by its processes. Two main transitions—demographic and epidemiologic—are under way, and large variations in countries' socio-economic development levels are present throughout the world. On the one hand, communicable diseases and problems associated with reproductive health remain major causes of morbidity and mortality in low income countries. On the other hand a shift has occurred toward noncommunicable diseases which today account for the biggest burden of diseases worldwide.

To be relevant to today's challenges, the practice of public health needs to take into account the global forces that shape health across the world. This changing context of health in the last few decades has often been labelled global health. The concept captures the idea that, in our interdependent world, health is influenced by many factors beyond national borders and socio-economic sectors, and that many contemporary health issues cannot be fully understood without examining the global forces that influence them. Public health professionals working at any level, including local, national, or regional, should have the tools to understand these issues. In this chapter, we use "global health" to describe the practice of public health in the global context.

We start by providing an overview of the global context of public health by exploring how globalization impacts health. We then discuss the relation between economic development and health and introduce the concepts of sustainable development and health equity. We present the current state of world health and provide an overview of the main challenges across the world. Furthermore we look at the implications of today's global nature of health on the governance processes across the world. Finally, we discuss the nature of innovation in global health.

GLOBALIZATION AND HEALTH

Understanding global health requires one to examine how the present era of globalization has been impacting health during the last several decades. Although the process of globalization and its impact on health is not new, as the emergence of modern public health is precisely the result of events in one part of the world having health effects in countries far away at the end of the nineteenth century, it is, however, undisputable that the acceleration of globalization dating from the 1980s has had dramatic consequences on how the world is interconnected. Economic globalization, which can be understood as the growing interdependence of economies across the world through reductions in trade barriers between countries and the resulting increased flow of goods, services, and capital across countries, has been the "fundamental driving force behind the overall process of globalization" over the last decades.[2]

However, globalization cannot be reduced to a unique economic dimension and, for the purpose of this chapter, we use a multidimensional definition from McMichael and Beaglehole, which reads as follows: "[Globalization] refers to the increasing interconnectedness of countries through cross-border flows of goods, services, money and people, information and ideas; the increasing openness of countries to such flows; and the development of international rules and institutions dealing with cross-border flows."[3] According to this definition, globalization is not only concerned by different flows (e.g., people, goods, money and information, see Exhibit 31-1, "Flows Associated with Globalization") around the world but also with institutional arrangements that seek to deal with these flows (discussed later in this chapter).

Overall Impact of Globalization on Health

The relation between globalization and health is complex because of the growing integration and interdependence of societies in multiple domains. The effects of the flows that are constitutive of contemporary globalization on health can be summarized as either direct (or proximal), affecting individuals, populations, and health systems, or indirect (distal) through global markets and the institutions that are responsible for global governance.[2] The magnitude of the spread of infectious diseases around the world with increasing flows of goods (trade) and people (tourism and migration), the influence of multilateral trade agreement on the cost and availability of drugs, and the rapid diffusion of medical knowledge and research worldwide, are examples of direct effects. By contrast, the impact of the liberalization of trade on socioeconomic development and on the rise of social and health inequities is an example of an indirect effect of globalization on health. In a not so distant past, society used to produce, trade, and consume goods and services on a dominantly local or national basis and, for this reason, the determinants of health were mostly national; increasingly, though, within the processes of globalization, the wider determinants of health (social, environmental, political)

EXHIBIT 31-1 Flows Associated With Globalization

Human Mobility

Contemporary globalization is associated with an unprecedented velocity and scope of human mobility. It is estimated that each year more than 2 billion people travel on long geographic distances[4] of which more than 1.2 billion cross national borders. This includes:

- international tourism—1,087 million arrivals in 2013, according to the United Nations World Tourism Organization[5]
- migration for economic, environmental, and other reasons—globally there are 232 million international migrants in 2013, a 50 percent increase since 1990[6]
- global forced displacement—refugees, asylum-seekers, and internally displaced people, which amounts to 51.2 million in 2013, corresponding to the highest number in the post-World War II era.[7]

Flow of Money

Flows of money between countries have been one of the main components of contemporary globalization. For example, Foreign Direct Investment (FDI), defined as "an investment made to acquire lasting interest in enterprises operating outside of the economy of the investor,"[8] has increased more than seven times between 1990 and 2013 (FDI peaked in 2007 but has not yet recovered from the global slump). Another indicator of interest is official development assistance (ODA) which measures aid flows between high income countries (HIC) and low- and middle-income countries (LMIC). After rising steadily during the last decade, ODA has slightly receded in 2011–2012, given austerity measures in high income countries, but rebounded to an all-time high in 2013.[9] Within the health sector, development assistance for health, which can be defined as "all flows for health from public and private institutions whose primary purpose is to provide development assistance to

low-income and middle-income countries"[10] has proved resilient to the financial and economic crisis, reaching U.S. $31.3 billion in 2013 from U.S. $5.6 billion in 1990.[11]

Flow of Commodities

International trade has been a major driver of economic globalization, pushed by the reduction in tariffs through the General Agreement on Tariffs and Trade, and from 1995 onward, by the World Trade Organization. According to World Bank data, the volume of the world merchandise exports has increased more than nine fold from 1980 to 2012.[12] The globalization of production means that commodities produced in one part of the world are often consumed at long distances from their origin. Services are also increasingly traded between countries, including services in the health sector, for example, through the cross border supply of services (e.g., telemedicine) and the supply of services abroad (e.g., medical tourism).

Flow of Information and Ideas

Another dominant force that shapes the present era of globalization is the growth in information and communication technology, which allows us to communicate globally and share information easily. Improvement in communication capacities—in particular the Internet, with almost 3 billion people having access in 2014, and mobile phone networks, with almost 7 billion mobile phone subscriptions worldwide[13]—has resulted in a global network which has an impact in many sectors, including trade and health. Increasingly, these sources of "big data" contribute to disease surveillance (e.g., aggregated data from Google search for flu symptoms are good indicators of flu activity), disease management, and health systems management. Furthermore, with the improvement of access to education, the increase of revenues, and with more than 7 billion inhabitants, the potential for new innovation has dramatically increased.

transcend the borders of countries and are situated beyond the health sector.

The overall effect of globalization on health is difficult to assess and remains debated; Table 31-1 summarizes some positive and negative effects of globalization on health. On one hand, globalization may exacerbate health inequalities and leads to the spreading of culture and unhealthy lifestyles such as lack of physical activity and poor diet. Globalization also increases the international spread of health risks.[14] For example, human mobility and flow of goods and commodities make the transmission of infectious diseases easier, although mortality due to infectious diseases has continuously decreased during the last decades. On the other hand, technological globalization can also facilitate diffusion of knowledge and adoption of new technologies that improve health and the management of health systems.

In addition, globalization increases economic growth, which in turn promotes development, reduces poverty, and improves health and education.[15] In the next section, we examine in more detail the links between economic growth, poverty, and the burden of diseases, and outline the challenges associated with different levels of socio-economic development as well as the common challenge of sustainable development.

DEVELOPMENT AND HEALTH

During the last century, dramatic economic growth has allowed many countries to escape from economic hardship and poverty. Improvements in the material conditions of life have led to a demographic transition from high birth and death rates to low birth and death

TABLE 31-1   Positive and Negative Health Impacts of Globalization

Factor	Positive Health Impacts	Negative Health Impacts
Flow of people	Enhanced transmission of ideas, values, knowledge, skills, and habits	Spread of infectious diseases (e.g., HIV, influenza); Brain drain of health workers and researchers
Flow of goods	Better availability of supplies such as medicine and food through free trade	Spread of infectious diseases or vectors (e.g., food borne diseases) Spread of unhealthy lifestyles (e.g., tobacco and unhealthy food)
Flow of information	Better disease surveillance and control; Improved access to knowledge (e.g., Massive Open Online Courses and online database)	Spread of fear through media and social networks
Flow of money	Increased investments in health care sectors and companies active in Research and Development	Decreased government spending on public services due to, for example, structural adjustment programs

Adapted from Martens et al. 2010

TABLE 31-2   Country Levels of Socio-economic Development and Health, World Bank Numbers 2013

	High Income	Middle Income	Low Income
Population	~1 billion	~5 billion (2.5 billion in upper middle income countries)	~1 billion
GDP per capita	> 12,746 US$	> 1,045 and < 12,746 US$	Less than 1,045 US$
Main burden of diseases	Noncommunicable diseases	Noncommunicable diseases and communicable diseases	Communicable and noncommunicable diseases
Welfare system	Generally good	Limited but improving	Most often absent

rates in most regions of the world.[16] Globally, life expectancy at birth is today more than twice as high as it was in 1900, and the world population has quadrupled from around 1.7 billion in 1900 to 7.2 billion in 2014. However, the benefits of these changes have not been universally and equally shared between and within countries.

Countries' Levels of Socio-economic Development and Health

Based on the World Bank classification of countries, it is useful to distinguish three categories of countries with regard to their income and associated health challenges. Table 31-2 summarizes some key features of these groups of countries.

High Income Countries

In high income countries (North America, Western Europe including Israel, Australia, New Zealand, Japan,

South Korea), which together represent approximately 1 billion people out of 7.2 billion, the last century has seen tremendous progress in the social and material conditions of life. Improved education, nutrition, and sanitation, but also progress in biomedicine and public health, have resulted in a dramatic reduction in infant and child mortality and a progressive rise in life expectancy. These countries have, to various extent, social systems that protect their citizens from the hardships of life, such as the consequences of diseases and injuries. In these countries, as the population ages, noncommunicable diseases have become the main cause of morbidity and mortality. Most of these countries are facing escalating health care costs due to multiple drivers, including expensive technologies, population ageing, and the shift from communicable to noncommunicable diseases.[17] They struggle to keep the benefits of the welfare system within the challenging context of the global financial and economic crisis since 2008, which seems to have exacerbated inequalities and poverty in some regions, including Europe.

Lower and Upper Middle Income Countries

There has been significant progress in countries such as China, Brazil, India, and Mexico, which were predominately poor 30 years ago and are now growing middle-income countries. Together these countries that are split by the World Bank between lower and upper middle income countries represent the category where the highest number of people live today (approximately 5 billion). Their health indicators have been improving for many years due to economic reforms and ensuing economic growth associated with concomitant investments in education and health. However, significant pockets of poverty remain in these countries, which means that growing inequalities are present. These countries typically exhibit a large array of health issues, from infectious diseases to noncommunicable diseases, the latter of which tend to predominate.[17] Many middle income countries have engaged in developing universal health coverage with notable successes, for example, in Mexico,[18] Costa-Rica, and Thailand. Amid the expansion of health coverage, some middle income countries have seen a steep rise in health care costs.

Low Income Countries

Poverty and its extreme form (extreme poverty) remain a huge challenge in the world and in particular in low income countries and some lower middle income countries such as India. Although the proportion of people living in extreme poverty has been diminishing and is today concentrated in sub-Saharan Africa and some countries in Southeast Asia, including Bangladesh and Nepal, and Haiti in the Caribbean, overall more than 1 billion people in the world struggle for daily survival in impoverished rural communities and in slums in urban areas. These people live without the commodities and amenities such as food, electricity, safe water, and sanitation that would allow them to satisfy basic needs. Lack of access to education and basic health services are also characteristics of extreme poverty. These people remain largely excluded from the benefits of modern medicine, and experience a high burden from neglected tropical diseases. People living in countries where poverty rates are very high are prone to epidemics, violence and war, environmental hazards, and political instability. Pollution of water, vector-borne diseases such as malaria, and lack of hygiene are responsible for many diseases of poverty, and the burden of disease is the highest in these populations.

Growth, Health, and Human Development

Despite the benefits of economic growth on world health, the persistence and even deepening of health inequalities within the three categories of countries call into question how the benefits of growth and globalization are distributed across the population. In most countries, these inequalities result in a huge gap in life expectancy between the poor and the rich. As noted by Paluzzi and Farmer, "many of the most devastating problems that plague the daily lives of billions of people are problems that emerge from a single, fundamental source: the consequences of poverty and inequality."[19]

This calls into question our appraisal of the relation between development and health. In the 1980s and the early 1990s, the dominant development model—often called the Washington consensus—contended that market liberalization and budgetary rigor were essential interventions to promote growth and development among poor countries, especially in Latin America.[20] The main idea was that economic growth alone was sufficient to take countries out of poverty. As some developing countries failed to grow despite adopting policies that seek to stimulate growth, it has been increasingly recognized that targeting only economic growth is not sufficient to address the problem of poverty. Ill health on a large scale hinders the capacity to fulfill educational potential and productivity at work. In turn this reduces the potential for economic growth. This vicious circle, sometimes called the "poverty trap," tends to cause the persistence of poverty in these countries, meaning that illness and poor health is both a cause and consequence of poverty. As health and development are intimately linked, health has become central to development.[21,22]

Because of interdependence between development and health, measuring development is oversimplified when considering GDP only. Instead, indicators such as the Human Development Index (HDI) provide a more holistic account of human development by combining measures of health, education, and income. By combining three dimensions, the HDI emphasizes "that people and their capabilities should be the ultimate criteria for assessing the development of a country, not economic growth alone."[23] The HDI helps also to "question national policy choices, asking how two countries with the same level of GNI [Gross National Income] per capita can end up with such different human development outcomes."[24] In other words, the use of an indicator such as HDI might be helpful in designing social policies which aim at limiting the social gradient and health inequalities.

Sustainable Development

It is increasingly recognized that, facing the ever-growing demands on a crowded planet whose population is expected to reach 9 billion by 2100, humanity has to find a way to live sustainably within its boundaries. Sustainable development is defined as "development that meets the needs of the present without compromising the ability of future generations to meet their own needs."[25] It is sometimes said that sustainable development calls for socially inclusive and environmentally sustainable economic growth. Amid this broader agenda, health has a double function. It is first a prerequisite to sustainable development: good health is required for people to achieve their full potential. Second, health is an outcome of sustainable development. Beyond the intrinsic value of health, health is influenced by the physical environment (e.g., pollution and climate change due to greenhouse gas emissions) and the social environment (e.g., social determinants of health).[26] With the end of the Millennium Development Goals (MDGs) in 2015, sustainable development goals will have to offer the broad framework for development for the next several decades.

GLOBAL BURDEN OF DISEASES AND THE EPIDEMIOLOGICAL TRANSITION

To establish policy priorities, allocate resources, and address health challenges, data based on evidence are highly needed to measure the state of world health. Margaret Chan, Director General of the World Health Organization (WHO), which is based in Geneva, Switzerland, states that "accurate assessment of the global, regional, and country health situation and trends is critical for evidence-based decision making for public health."[27] Except for high income countries, health-related data collection is still poor and not systematic in most of the world, and closing the data gaps represents a priority.[27]

At the global level, the global burden of diseases (GBD) approach was launched by the WHO in 1991 with the aim of collecting and assessing comprehensively epidemiological data on the main diseases (291) and injuries and risks.[28] As the main investigator of the GBD explains: "the advantage of the GBD approach is that consistent methods are applied to critically appraise available information on each condition, make this information comparable and systematic, estimate results from countries with incomplete data, and report on the burden of disease with the use of standardized metrics."[28] Although it has to be recognized that these data are often only rough estimates, especially with regard to LMIC, these are currently the best available data to understand the global burden of diseases (see Exhibit 31-2 for further discussion on the GBD). We present here the results of GBD 2010 and when available those from GBD 2013.

The results of the last estimates from the GBD study indicate overall significant progress in the state of world health in the last decades, including rising life expectancy

and reduction of child and maternal mortality (see the "Measuring Health, Disability, and Well-being" box for explanations on how health is measured). In 40 years (from 1970 to 2010), worldwide life expectancy at birth increased from 61.2 to 73.3 years for females and from 56.4 to 67.5 years for males.[29] The reduction of child mortality is also significant: there are fewer deaths occurring in children younger than 5 years, with almost a 60 percent decline since 1970 (16.4 million vs 6.8 million in 2010).[29] In addition, more deaths occur at an older age than before. For example in 2010, 42.8 percent of deaths occurred at age 70 years versus 33.1 percent in 1990, while deaths at 80 years or older increased from 15.9 percent to 22.9 percent during this same timeperiod.[29]

Overall, progress has been made with regard to the control of communicable diseases, even though they still account for 4 of the 10 leading causes of Disability-Adjusted Life Years (DALYs) (see below and Chapter 12 for more information on DALYs). While lower respiratory tract infections were the leading cause in 1990, ischemic heart disease ranks first in the 2010 GDB study. Murray et al. note that in 2010 "54% of all DALYs [are] due to noncommunicable diseases, compared with 35% due to communicable, maternal, neonatal, and nutritional disorders, and 11% due to injuries."[30] These numbers reflect the so-called "epidemiological transition" from infectious diseases to noncommunicable diseases as the main causes of mortality worldwide. With people living longer, there has also been a shift "from premature death to years lived with disability."[31] In other words what affects the quality of daily life of people is not necessarily what kills them (e.g., mental and musculoskeletal disorders have greater impact on morbidity than mortality).[28]

TABLE 31-3   10 Leading Causes of Disability-Adjusted Life Years (DALYs), Diseases and Injuries, in 2010

1. Ischemic heart disease
2. Lower respiratory tract infection
3. Stroke
4. Diarrhea
5. HIV-AIDS
6. Malaria
7. Low back pain
8. Preterm birth complication
9. Chronic obstructive pulmonary disease
10. Road-traffic injury

Adapted from Murray et al.

EXHIBIT 31-2 The Use of the Global Burden of Disease Approach to Measuring Global Health

In this chapter, we use and present data calculated by the GBD study because they are the most comprehensive data available. As noted by Polinder et al., "a major strength of the burden of disease concept is that it allows comparison between different health problems, between different years, and between countries."[32] It is, however, important to recall that the GBD study uses estimates, not direct measurements.[33] In addition, there are criticisms about the GBD and how these estimates are calculated, including:

- Lack of transparency: all data and estimates are not publicly available.[33]
- Lack of comprehensiveness: The missing data in low-income countries are filled by complex estimation techniques. The data presented amount to less than a third of global deaths.[33]
- The choice of metrics: the use of DALYs is controversial because it involves some subjective evaluation with regard to the calculation of disability.[34]

Other sources of estimates include those compiled by WHO. Interestingly, the estimated leading cause of DALYs is not the same between different sources of data, which means that the results have to be considered with caution. The use of DALYs and the GBD study is recognized as a monitoring tool but it remains more controversial when it comes to policymaking and resource allocations.[34]

Measuring Health, Disability, and Well-being

Several metrics are usually used to measure world health. The list below describes some of the most commonly used indicators (by alphabetical order):

- Cause-specific mortality rate is the mortality attributable to a specific disease (e.g., diabetes or malaria).
- Child mortality, most often referred to as the *under-5 mortality*, corresponds to the mortality of children under the age of 5 years.
- Disability-adjusted life years (DALYs): DALYs is a measure that combines measurement of premature mortality and disability weighted for the severity of the conditions.[34] One DALY can be considered as one lost year of healthy life. It is calculated by computing the sum of the years of life lost (YLL) due to premature mortality and adding the years lost due to disability (YLD) for those affected by a disease and its consequences. As people are living longer it has become essential to measure the burden of disease in terms of disability rather than simply reviewing causes of mortality. However, the measure of disability is made complicated and controversial by subjective assessment, cultural differences, and the attribution of a weighting factor according to the severity of the conditions, although efforts have been made by the GBD study team to address these issues.[35] As the authors of the GBD note, "quantifying health loss in terms of DALYs has led to increased attention to mental health problems and injuries, nonfatal health effects of neglected tropical diseases, and more generally noncommunicable diseases (NCDs)."[30]
- Life expectancy at birth is measured by computing the mortality table of all age groups in a given year. According to the World Bank definition, "life expectancy at birth indicates the number of years a newborn infant would live if prevailing patterns of mortality at the time of its birth were to stay the same throughout its life."[36]
- Maternal mortality rate is generally expressed as the number of women who die from pregnancy or childbirth related complications out of 100,000 women in a given country or region.
- Potential Years of Life Lost corresponds to the number of years of potential life not lived when a person dies before a specified "standard" age (usually age 75 or 65). The earlier a death occurs, the higher are the potential years of life lost.
- Premature mortality is defined as the proportion of deaths occurring before the age of 75. The premature death rate is generally expressed as the number of people who die before the age of 75 out of 100,000 people in a given country or region. High premature mortality can result from high infant mortality and high death rates in children and younger adults. This measure is less prone to biases or error in its estimation than other measures such as DALYs, and provides a good insight into the investments dedicated to public health and prevention.

The Unfinished Agenda of Communicable Diseases

Due to general improvements in the material conditions of life during the twentieth century (such as sanitation and the availability and quality of food) and to the progress in biomedicine (including development of vaccines and antimicrobials, better hygiene in hospitals, and improved surveillance), infectious diseases have receded globally. Notable successes of public health include the eradication of smallpox and the control of polio and measles virus. However, the burden of infectious diseases remains high, particularly in LMIC where the aforementioned progress has been slower. For example, pneumonia and diarrheal diseases, which have declined from 1990 to 2010, still accounted for an estimated 4.2 million out of 52.8 million deaths globally in 2010[37] and are among the leading causes of deaths in sub-Saharan Africa. According to the GBD study, globally HIV-AIDS is the 6th leading cause of death, tuberculosis the 10th, and malaria the 11th. HIV-AIDS killed 1.5 million people in 2010 (from 0.3 million in 1990 and a peak of 1.7 million in 2006). The burden from tuberculosis and malaria has been reduced but they were still responsible for approximately 1.2 million deaths each in 2010.[37] Although dramatic progress has been made in the control of preventable infectious diseases around the world, communicable diseases cannot be considered as diseases of the past. Indeed, "changes in environment and human behavior due to the globalization of the world and the evolutionary dynamics of microbial agents may, furthermore, produce new ecological niches that enable the emergence or reemergence of infections, thus posing a persistent threat to the developed world too."[38] The rise of antimicrobial resistance as a significant contributing factor to infections worldwide represents a growing concern for the control of infectious diseases.

Maternal, Infant, and Child Mortality

Maternal and child health have also improved during the past two decades. Maternal mortality has receded from about 376,034 deaths in 1990 to about 292,982 in 2013, which amounts to a 28.3 percent reduction during the last 20 years.[39] These reductions are even more significant when we consider that the global population has increased by about 2 billion during the last two decades. There are, however, considerable variations across the world, as well as within countries. While 16 countries had maternal mortality ratios above 500, 15 countries, all in high income countries, had a maternal mortality ratio below 5.[39] Further reduction in maternal mortality will require commitment to prevent conditions such as anemia and other nutritional deficiencies, as well as to improve the response to complications during and after delivery, most importantly through skilled birth attendance. With regard to child mortality, fewer children are dying than 40 years ago, down from 17.6 million in 1970 to 6.3 million in 2013, which amounts to a significant reduction of 64 percent.[40] In this evaluation, neonatal deaths (occurring in the first 28 days of life), which have been reduced from 5.9 million in 1970 to 2.6 million in 2013, represent the largest proportion of child mortality (41.6 percent).[40] Sub-Saharan Africa

TABLE 31-4 The Eight Millennium Development Goals (Each Goal has Specific Targets and Indicators for Monitoring Progress)

1. Eradicate extreme poverty and hunger
2. Achieve universal primary education
3. Promote gender equality and empower women
4. Reduce child mortality
5. Improve maternal health
6. Combat HIV/AIDS, malaria, and other diseases
7. Ensure environmental sustainability
8. Develop a global partnership for development

SOURCE: United Nations Millennium Development Goals; available at http://www.un.org/millenniumgoals/

bears the brunt of the child burden of diseases, claiming the 10 last places in the ranking of under-5 mortality, with 80 percent of child deaths occurring in only 26 countries in the world.[40]

The considerable progress with regard to infectious diseases and child and maternal mortality described above is due in part to political commitment and increased attention; however, despite this progress it is expected that the MDGs (see Table 31-4) will be met only in a minority of LMIC. According to the GBD study, "communicable, maternal, neonatal, and nutritional causes of deaths are responsible for three-quarters of premature mortality in sub-Saharan Africa and the main cause of YLL [years of life lost] in 2010."[37] MGD-4 (reduction by two-thirds of child mortality from 1990 levels by 2015) will be met in only 27 LMIC out of 138 for which data are available, although an acceleration of the reduction of mortality rates is noted since 2000.[40] MDG-5 (reduction of maternal mortality ratio by three-quarters between 1990 and 2015) is likely to be met in only 16 countries[39] while important progress has been made toward MDG-6 (whose targets are to begin to reverse by 2015 the incidence of HIV/AIDS, malaria, and other major diseases and achieve by 2015 universal access to treatment for HIV/AIDS for all those who need it).[41] The conditions related to MDG 4-5-6 represent together 29.8 percent (equivalent to 742 million DALYs in 2010) of the global burden of disease, down from 43.8 percent in 1990.[30]

The Rise of Noncommunicable Diseases

With people living longer, particularly in high and middle income countries, there has been a shift toward noncommunicable diseases as the main causes of death. In 2010, approximately two-thirds of the world mortality was attributable to noncommunicable diseases. Chronic conditions represent today's main causes of ill health across the world. This shift from infectious, maternal, and child mortality to chronic conditions in older people is described as the "epidemiological transition." Starting first in industrialized countries, the epidemiological transition continues today in LMIC. Globally, one in four deaths is caused by ischemic heart disease (13.3 percent) and stroke (11.1 percent), resulting in 12.9 million deaths in 2010, a considerable increase from one in five deaths in 1990.[37] Ischemic heart disease and cerebrovascular disease are also major causes of YLL and YLD, ranking respectively first and third as the causes of DALYs in 2010.[30] With an ageing population, deaths from neurodegenerative diseases such as Alzheimer's disease and Parkinson's disease have increased substantially. Diabetes, a major cause of cardiovascular complications, caused twice as many deaths in 2010 as in 1990.[37] Cancers were responsible for 15.1 percent of all deaths globally (equivalent to 8 million deaths).[37] The main sites of cancer are those of the respiratory system, including lung cancer—which increased between 1990 and 2010—liver, and stomach cancer, mostly avoidable through prevention.

The causes of chronic diseases are complex and encompass a wide set of determinants across sectors and countries. Distal determinants of chronic conditions include the socio-economic environment, and trade and food policies across the world. Proximal determinants are mainly risk factors associated with lifestyle. According to the results of the GBD study, "high blood pressure is the biggest global risk factor for disease, followed by tobacco smoking, excess in alcohol consumption, and poor diet."[42] High blood pressure, which is associated with stress, obesity, and high consumption of salt, accounts for an estimated 7 percent of global DALYs and is responsible for ischemic heart attack, stroke, and other cardiovascular disorders.[43] Smoking tobacco, which accounts for around 6.3 percent of global DALYs in 2010, is a major risk factor for arteriopathies and respiratory disorders, including chronic obstructive pulmonary disease and cancer, especially lung cancer. The abuse of alcohol is the third leading global risk factor for chronic diseases and the main risk factor in some regions, including Eastern Europe, Andean Latin America, and southern sub-Saharan Africa.[43] Poor diet (low in vegetables and fruits, and high in sugar, salt, and fat) along with lack of physical activity, represent the main drivers of overweight, obesity, and metabolic disorders. "Taken together, all components of diet and physical inactivity accounted for 10.2% of global DALYs in 2010."[28] Globally, there are around 1.5 billion overweight people (BMI > 25) including

500 million people who are obese (BMI > 30). In some countries obesity rates reach more than 35 percent of the population. Overweight and obesity are associated with disorders such as insulin resistance, dyslipidemia, and hypertension, which are risk factors for cardiovascular diseases, diabetes, and some cancers. It has to be noted that some recent studies have found that people who are overweight or have nonsevere obesity (30 < BMI < 35) might have a better prognosis in terms of mortality than leaner people, in particular with regard to cardiovascular diseases and diabetes, a controversial phenomenon called the obesity paradox.[44-46]

The Growing Agenda of Mental Health Problems

Falling within the scope of noncommunicable diseases, mental health conditions contribute significantly to the global burden of disease. According to the WHO, mental health "is a state of well-being in which an individual realizes his or her own abilities, can cope with the normal stresses of life, can work productively and is able to make a contribution to his or her community."[47] The determinants of mental health are wide and encompass a set of biological, psychological, environmental, and social factors. The factors which may contribute to mental health problems include, but are not limited to, conflicts and human rights violations, job stress, social exclusion, gender discrimination, and substance abuse, including excessive alcohol consumption. People with mental health problems are subject to stigma resulting from stereotypes, prejudice, and discrimination.[48] Services for mental health have been especially neglected in LMIC where there is a vicious cycle between poverty and mental health problems.[49] As noted by Whiteford et al., "in many countries [they] were segregated from mainstream health care with resourcing not commensurate with the burden."[50]

Using DALYs to quantify health loss has increased the prominence of mental health as a cause of ill health.[30] In terms of morbidity, mental health problems are responsible for a large proportion of years lived with a disability, amounting to approximately 7.4 percent of all global DALYs, especially in adults between the ages of 15 and 39.[50] Although mental health issues account for only 0.5 percent of all YLLs, since mortality due to mental disorders is low, they represent 22.7 percent of YLDs worldwide and the main cause of YLDs.[51] Depressive disorders, anxiety disorders—including stress-related disorders—and illicit drug and alcohol use disorders are the main causes of mental health problems.[50] Murray et al. note that: "self-harm is a top ten cause of burden in high-income Asia Pacific (rank 5), eastern Europe (rank 6) and central Europe (rank 11)."[30]

GLOBAL HEALTH GOVERNANCE AND POLICIES

While global forces and processes increasingly influence health across countries, responsibilities for health care and public health remains mainly at the national and local level. The diversity of economic, political, and social contexts means that the practice of public health requires examining the interplay between the global, the regional, the national, and the local environments. For example the rising prevalence of obesity and diabetes results from the complex interrelationships between multiple factors at the local, national, regional, and global level. Cross-border issues such as rapid transmission of emerging infectious diseases can disrupt countries' health systems and cause social, economic, and political problems as it has been seen with the Severe Acute Respiratory Syndrome (SARS) outbreak in 2003, pandemic influenza in 2009, and Ebola in 2014. To be effective, interventions and policies that seek to address these issues need to be coherent between levels. Importantly, with health issues increasingly transcending national borders, no one country and no one sector acting alone can address these issues effectively on its own. As we live in a world of health interdependence, international and intersectoral collaboration is required, and there is a common interest to provide health at the global level in a context where the capacity to address health risks varies greatly between countries.[52]

Health issues cross not only national borders but they also cross sectors of activities, as illustrated by HIV-AIDS or climate change, which means that the health sector cannot address these issues alone. As McMichael and Beaglehole state: "the public health endeavor is thus a broad and inclusive enterprise that extends to political, social and environmental leadership and management."[53] In a globalized world, the practice of public health is not only a challenge of framing health issues so that it can generate momentum but also of coordination and collective action among multiple actors which are part of the global health system. This challenge is even made harder by the proliferation of actors including public-private partnerships, NGOs, and the private sector in the last two decades (see Table 31-5 for a summary of actors and their role in global health). All these

TABLE 31-5   Actors in the Global Health System

Type of Actor with Examples	Role in the Global Health System
National Governments Bilateral development cooperation agencies; Ministries of foreign affairs; Ministries of Health; CDC (U.S.)	As health is primarily a national responsibility, Nation states are the traditional actors in global health. Donor countries are involved in development assistance for health through their bilateral development cooperation agencies. National, and to some extent international public health, depends on Ministries of Health (who, for example, vote at the World Health Assembly of the World Health Organization). Recently, as health has gained political prominence as "soft" power, Ministries of Foreign Affairs have been increasingly involved in global health policymaking.
United Nations System World Health Organization; Joint United Nations Program on HIV/AIDS; UNICEF; World Bank; World Intellectual Property Organization; World Trade Organization	The United Nations System is composed of one institution dedicated to health (WHO) with a universal membership of 194 countries and a broad institutional mandate. In addition, there is one specific U.N. program dedicated to HIV-AIDS (UNAIDS) and a multitude of multilateral institutions whose health is not the first domain, but the decisions of which influence health to various extent.
Global Health Initiatives Drugs for Neglected Diseases; Global Fund to Fight AIDS, Tuberculosis, and Malaria; GAVI Alliance; UNITAID	Global health initiatives are hybrid organizations or public-private partnerships which mix elements of the private and public sectors. They are typically programs targeted at specific diseases that were created to address major communicable diseases in LMIC. Their number has risen sharply since 2000 with now about 100 organizations active in global health. They can be a finance mechanism—such as the Global Fund—an implementation program, or product development partnership which aims to research and develop new products such as drugs for neglected tropical diseases.
Philanthropic Organizations Bill and Melinda Gates Foundation; Rockefeller Foundation; Welcome Trust; Aga Khan Foundation	Philanthropic organizations have contributed significantly to the increase in funding in global health in the last 20 years. Founded in 2000, the Bill and Melinda Gates Foundation has become a prominent player with an annual budget of more than $3 billion and total payments of more than $30 billion. With their huge financial means, the biggest philanthropies have the ability to set priorities and influence the global health agenda.

TABLE 31-5 (Continued)

Global Civil Society Organizations Care International; Doctors Without Borders (*Médecins sans Frontières*); OXFAM International; Save the Children; People Health Movement	Global Civil society organizations are nongovernmental, nonbusiness organizations or movements that are active across borders. International NGO's have been an important player in global health in implementation programs as well as in advocacy (e.g., the Campaign for access to essential medicines by Doctors Without Borders, which aims at increasing the availability of drugs in LMIC). Global civil society also encompasses networks such as the People Health Movement, which focuses on health equity and plays a critical role in advocacy and scrutiny of health policy.
Private Industry Pharmaceutical companies; medical devices companies; biotechnology, information, and communication companies, such as Google or Microsoft	Private industry develops and disseminates products such as drugs, diagnostics, and technologies through global markets. Some private companies have set up their own foundations and/or participate in public private partnerships.
Academic Institutions and Professional Associations Consortium of Universities for Global Health; World Medical Association; Association of Schools and Programs of Public Health; World Federation of Academic Institutions for Global Health; The European Academic Global Health Alliance	Academic institutions and networks play an essential role in global health education and research. Professional societies gather members of the same profession such as physicians or nurses and usually set professional standards. In global health, professional societies can enact recommendations for best practices and play a role in global health education.
Regional Organizations European Union; Association of Southeast Asian Nations (ASEAN); CARICOM (Caribbean Community); Organization for Economic Co-operation and Development (OECD)	Regional organizations are international organizations whose membership is constrained by boundaries such as geography, economics (e.g., Europe and the European Union), or geopolitics. Increasingly, regional organizations have a voice in global health as their economies have become more deeply integrated with health.

Adapted from Frenk & Moon 2013

actors contribute to global health but also compete and pursue their own interests, which do not necessarily converge. Overall, **global health governance** can be understood as "the use of formal and informal institutions, rules, and processes by states, intergovernmental organizations, and nonstate actors to deal with challenges to health that require crossborder collective action to address effectively."[54] With this definition, as noted by Kickbusch et al., "the challenges facing the ever-expanding global public health domain are therefore less of a technical nature—in many areas we already have the knowledge and the technologies—but require political will and the willingness of states and other actors to prioritize health."[55] We analyze the governance of global health issues according to three main angles.[55]

Health for All at the Local and National Level

As states are the main actors in the global health arena, it is critical to assess their role with regard to governance of global health issues. This angle of analysis encompasses all processes at local or national levels that seek to respond to global health challenges. At the local level, public health authorities are responsible for prevention, promotion, and protection of public health. Collective problem-solving often requires the involvement of many actors across sectors. Initiatives such as Healthy Cities illustrate how local governments can contribute to put health high on the agenda by committing to "continually creating and improving those physical and social environments and expanding those community resources which enable people to mutually support each other in performing all the functions of life and developing to their maximum potential."[56] An example is the area of transport, which plays a significant role in traffic injuries, but also in air pollution and noise, especially in urban areas, all having a negative impact on health. The design of urban transport policies that incorporate health as an objective can mitigate these adverse health effects and promote healthier behaviors such as cycling and walking. At the national level, the same challenge of intersectoral coordination arises between the health ministry and ministries whose health is not the first priority, such as the Ministry of Foreign Affairs or the Ministry of Agriculture. Some countries such as Norway and Finland have endorsed a "Health in All Policies" approach, which has been defined as an "approach to public policies across sectors that systematically takes into account the health implications of decisions, seeks synergies, and avoids harmful health impacts, in order to improve population health and health equity."[57] As governments increasingly pursue their health interests abroad, giving way to some countries enacting a health foreign policy including the United Kingdom,[58] Germany[59] or Switzerland,[60] policy coherence—better coordination of policies across sectors of activities and between domestic and foreign policy—will become even more challenging. With the integration of health concerns into foreign policy agendas, which traditionally focus on security and economic interests, there are additional concerns about the instrumentalization of health for objectives other than health itself.

Institutions with an International Health Mandate

Beyond the role of local and national health systems and public authorities in the global health arena, there is a challenge to ensure health and health security at the global level where there is no government. This angle of analysis encompasses "those institutions and processes of governance which are related to an explicit health mandate, such as the World Health Organization (WHO), hybrid organizations such as the GAVI Alliance (GAVI) and the Global Fund to Fight AIDS, Tuberculosis, and Malaria (GFATM), as well as health-focused networks and initiatives and nongovernmental organizations."[55] Many of these organizations are based in Geneva, Switzerland. In this regard, the WHO, with its representation of 194 Member States, has the broadest mandate that comes from its constitution established in 1948: "the objective of the World Health Organization shall be the attainment by all peoples of the highest possible level of health."[61] Indeed, one of the main WHO functions conferred by its constitution "shall be to act as the directing and co-ordinating authority on international health work."[61] International treaties can be concluded under the auspices of WHO by member states.[62] In recent decades, this treaty-making power has been used to fight against tobacco (Framework Convention on Tobacco control) and to prevent the international spread of infectious diseases (the International Health Regulations).

Health in All International Policies

This angle of analysis "refers mainly to those institutions and processes of global governance which have a direct and indirect health impact" but without a direct health mandate.[55] Other sectors essential to human activity such as agriculture and trade are represented by international institutions such as the World Trade Organization, the World Bank, World Organization for Animal Health, or the Food and Agriculture Organization, which impact health and health governance. This means that part of global health policy is made in, or at least influenced by, sectors traditionally outside the health sector. An example is the Sanitary and Phytosanitary Agreement at the World Trade Organization which governs how WTO member states can restrict international trade for health reasons. Knowledge of the rules that govern these institutions has become essential to address global health issues. A challenge of representation and coordination exists within the international system as decisions taken in one international organization can have a broad impact on other sectors.

INNOVATION EVERYWHERE

Innovation in global health "encompasses the entire process—from idea to implementation—for new products, services, processes, practices, and policies."[63] On the technological side, innovation is concerned with health technologies (e.g., drugs, vaccines, diagnostic tests, medical devices) and with devising and implementing solutions to strengthen health systems and improve the wider determinants of health, including sanitation, access to water, communication, food systems, or road safety.[64] The broad use of technologies in global health stems from the fact that "most health problems are best addressed by a combination of technologies, some of which are specific to health, such as drugs and medical devices, whereas others have health benefits that arise from use outside of health, such as the Internet or irrigation."[64]

Social Innovation

Innovation in global health is also concerned with social innovation which has been defined as "new ideas (products, services, and models) that simultaneously meet social needs (more effectively than alternatives) and create new social relationships or collaborations."[65] Social innovation plays a pivotal role both in health care and in population health.[63] In health care, social innovation can facilitate the adoption and uptake of new drugs, medical devices, and diagnostics. In population health, social innovation is needed in health policy and health promotion, for example, to find ways to reduce sedentary behavior and favor physical exertion in the population. Groups of citizens, as well as NGOs, play a pivotal role in social innovation. They not only scrutinize health policy but also advocate for change. An example is the HIV-AIDS epidemic in which AIDS activists, including patients, helped to shape the debate and campaigned to provide access to medicine in developing countries.[66] A similar phenomenon of citizen involvement is observable within the current shift from tobacco to electronic cigarettes in high income countries. Today's social networks facilitate the emergence and the involvement of a global citizen who is aware of global health challenges. Social networks also offer means of engagement between public health researchers and practitioners and the community.

Reverse Innovation

One important feature in global health is the changing locus of innovation. Both technological and social innovations are no longer the privilege of high income countries: innovation also happens in LMIC. As the need to develop practical and effective local solutions can benefit health systems in high income countries, these countries will increasingly benefit from innovations in LMIC, a process described as reverse innovation or mutual learning. Beyond improved skills and competencies for those working abroad, examples of reverse innovation include improvements in health systems, and research and development for new drugs to fight against tuberculosis in India.[67,68] The flows of global innovation across the world will in particular benefit from ideas with an extended scope, such as universal health coverage. As Nigel Crisp notes: "whilst many countries are seeking to create or expand universal health coverage for their people, others in Europe and the west are struggling to find ways to maintain it. The issues they are facing are the same: how to emphasize health promotion and disease prevention, how to involve other sectors in health, how to engage citizens and patients in their own health and health care, and how to do so in an affordable and sustainable way."[69]

Academic Institutions: Education and Research in Global Health

As places of knowledge production and transmission, academic institutions play a significant role with regard to innovation, education, and practice in global health. Academic institutions first bear a social responsibility to be relevant and to address societal challenges. During the last two decades, academe has done so by shedding light on huge health inequalities both between and within countries.[70] Second, as a narrow biomedical and technical focus has predominated within the health sector,[71] both in health care and to a lesser extent in public health, academic institutions have a responsibility to endorse, develop, and promote interdisciplinary

and systems thinking which are critical to tackling contemporary health challenges and devising sustainable solutions in our interdependent world. This calls for engaging all relevant academic disciplines in global health so that knowledge can be integrated to provide a better understanding of health issues. An example of such an approach includes "One Health", which seeks to make the human, animal, and environmental sectors work more closely in tackling global health challenges such as emerging infectious diseases and antimicrobial resistance.[72] Third, within the globalization of education and research, the production of knowledge increasingly entails collaboration between academic institutions across the world. It is important that all collaborating institutions from the North and the South benefit from their engagement in partnerships. Any research project requires ethical evaluation that takes into account the local context. Fourth, within the global health context, the role of academic institutions is not only to produce basic science but also to reflect on how to implement solutions as a way to translate science into practice and reduce the science-to-policy gap.

SUMMARY

As globalization profoundly affects health and health systems across the world and makes the world more interdependent than ever, public health practice is increasingly shaped by the global context. This means that public health practitioners and researchers need to understand the global context even when they work in the local context. Health plays an essential role in socio-economic development in LMIC and HIC, but global health is not limited to development aid from HIC to LMIC. Rather, it encompasses the health of all people in all countries and seeks to tackle complex health issues which cross national borders and require international cooperation within a quickly evolving burden of diseases worldwide. To achieve better health for all, global health requires intersectoral and integrated approaches which tackle distal social determinants as a well as proximal ones such as lifestyle. Global health improvement is dependent on implementation science, looking for evidence-based solutions to improve health for all, through changes in policies, behaviors, or practices.

REVIEW QUESTIONS

1. How does globalization impact health?
2. What is the relationship between development and health?

3. What is the global burden of diseases approach, and how might this be applied to a specific public health issue?

4. Who are the main actors in global health governance?

5. What is innovation in global health and how has innovation contributed to solving problems in global health?

REFERENCES

1. Riley JC. Estimates of Regional and Global Life Expectancy, 1800–2001. *Population and Development Review.* 2005;31(3):537–543.

2. Woodward D, Drager N, Beaglehole R, Lipson D. Globalization and health: a framework for analysis and action. *Bulletin of the World Health Organization.* 2001;79(9):875–881.

3. McMichael T, Beaglehole R. The global context for public health. In: Beaglehole R, ed. *Global Public Health: A New Era.* Oxford; New York: Oxford University Press; 2003:xx, 284 p.

4. MacPherson DW, Gushulak BD, Baine WB, et al. Population mobility, globalization, and antimicrobial drug resistance. *Emerging Infectious Diseases.* Nov 2009;15(11):1727–1732.

5. World Tourism Organization. International tourism exceeds expectations with arrivals up by 52 million in 2013. 2014; http://media.unwto.org/press-release/2014-01-20/international-tourism-exceeds-expectations-arrivals-52-million-2013. Accessed 12/08/2014.

6. United Nations. Department of Economic and Social Affairs. Population Division. International migration report 2013. 2013.

7. Office of the United Nations High Commissioner for Refugees. *War's Human Cost—Global Trends 2013.* Geneva, Switzerland: UNHCR; 2014.

8. UNCTAD. Foreign Direct Investment. 2014; http://unctad.org/en/Pages/DIAE/Foreign-Direct-Investment-(FDI).aspx. Accessed 12/08/2014.

9. OECD. Aid to developing countries rebounds in 2013 to reach an all-time high 2014; http://www.oecd.org/newsroom/aid-to-developing-countries-rebounds-in-2013-to-reach-an-all-time-high.htm. Accessed 12/08/2014.

10. Ravishankar N, Gubbins P, Cooley RJ, et al. Financing of global health: tracking development assistance for health from 1990 to 2007. *The Lancet.* Jun 20 2009;373(9681):2113–2124.

11. Institute for Health Metrics and Evaluation. *Financing Global Health 2013.* Seattle, WA: IHME;2014.

12. World Bank. World merchandise exports. 2014; http://data.worldbank.org/indicator/TX.VAL .MRCH.CD.WT. Accessed 11/08/2014.

13. International Telecommunication Union. The World in 2014—ICT Facts and Figures. 2014; http://www.itu.int/en/ITU-D/Statistics/ Documents/facts/ICTFactsFigures2014-e.pdf. Accessed 07/08/2014.

14. Pang T, Guindon G. Globalization and risks to health. *EMBO Reports.* 2004;5:S11–S16.

15. Feachem RG. Globalisation is good for your health, mostly. *British Medical Journal.* Sep 1 2001;323(7311):504–506.

16. Hunter DJ, Fineberg HV. Convergence to Common Purpose in Global Health. *New England Journal of Medicine.* 2014;370(18):1753–1755.

17. Jamison DT, Summers LH, Alleyne G, et al. Global health 2035: a world converging within a generation. *The Lancet.* Dec 7 2013;382(9908): 1898–1955.

18. Knaul FM, Gonzalez-Pier E, Gomez-Dantcs O, et al. The quest for universal health coverage: achieving social protection for all in Mexico. *The Lancet.* Oct 6 2012;380(9849):1259–1279.

19. Paluzzi JE, Farmer PE. The Wrong Question. *Development.* //print 2005;48(1):12–18.

20. Williamson J. Democracy and the "Washington consensus." *World Development.* 1993;21(8): 1329–1336.

21. *World Development Report 1993.* The World Bank; 1993.

22. Sen A. Health in development. *Bulletin of the World Health Organization.* 1999;77(8):619–623.

23. UNEP. Human Development Index. 2014; http:// hdr.undp.org/en/content/human-development-index-hdi. Accessed 12/08/2014.

24. UNEP. Frequently Asked Questions - Human Development Index (HDI). 2014; http://hdr.undp. org/en/faq-page/human-development-index-hdi. Accessed 12/08/2014.

25. World Commission on Environment and Development. *Our Common Future.* Oxford: Oxford University Press; 1987.

26. Haines A, Alleyne G, Kickbusch I, Dora C. From the Earth Summit to Rio+20: integration of health and sustainable development. *The Lancet.* 2012;379(9832):2189–2197.

27. Chan M. From new estimates to better data. *The Lancet.* Dec 15 2012;380(9859):2054.

28. Murray CJ, Lopez AD. Measuring the global burden of disease. *New England Journal of Medicine.* Aug 1 2013;369(5):448–457.

29. Wang H, Dwyer-Lindgren L, Lofgren KT, et al. Age-specific and sex-specific mortality in 187 countries, 1970–2010: a systematic analysis for the Global Burden of Disease Study 2010. *The Lancet.* Dec 15 2012;380(9859):2071–2094.

30. Murray CJ, Vos T, Lozano R, et al. Disability-adjusted life years (DALYs) for 291 diseases and injuries in 21 regions, 1990–2010: a systematic analysis for the Global Burden of Disease Study 2010. *The Lancet.* Dec 15 2012;380(9859):2197–2223.

31. Murray CJ, Ezzati M, Flaxman AD, et al. GBD 2010: design, definitions, and metrics. *The Lancet.* Dec 15 2012;380(9859):2063–2066.

32. Polinder S, Haagsma JA, Stein C, Havelaar AH. Systematic review of general burden of disease studies using disability-adjusted life years. *Population Health Metrics.* 2012;10(1):21.

33. Byass P, de Courten M, Graham WJ, et al. Reflections on the global burden of disease 2010 estimates. *PLoS Medicine.* 2013;10(7):e1001477.

34. Voigt K, King NB. Disability weights in the global burden of disease 2010 study: two steps forward, one step back? *Bulletin of the World Health Organization.* Mar 1 2014;92(3):226–228.

35. Salomon JA, Vos T, Hogan DR, et al. Common values in assessing health outcomes from disease and injury: disability weights measurement study for the Global Burden of Disease Study 2010. *The Lancet.* Dec 15 2012;380(9859):2129–2143.

36. World Bank. Life expectancy at birth. 2014; http://data.worldbank.org/indicator/SP.DYN.LE00.IN. Accessed 11/08/2014.

37. Lozano R, Naghavi M, Foreman K, et al. Global and regional mortality from 235 causes of death for 20 age groups in 1990 and 2010: a systematic analysis for the Global Burden of Disease Study 2010. *The Lancet.* Dec 15 2012;380(9859):2095–2128.

38. Krämer A, Akmatov M, Kretzschmar M. Principles of Infectious Disease Epidemiology. *Statistics for biology and health, Modern infectious disease epidemiology : concepts, methods, mathematical models, and public health.* 1st ed. New York: Springer; 2010.

39. Kassebaum NJ, Bertozzi-Villa A, Coggeshall MS, et al. Global, regional, and national levels and causes of maternal mortality during 1990–2013: a systematic analysis for the Global Burden of Disease Study 2013. *The Lancet.* May 2 2014;384, no. 9947 (2014): 980–1004.

40. Wang H, Liddell CA, Coates MM, et al. Global, regional, and national levels of neonatal, infant, and under-5 mortality during 1990–2013: a systematic analysis for the Global Burden of Disease Study 2013. *The Lancet.* May 2 2014;384, no. 9947 (2014): 957–979.

41. Murray CJ, Ortblad KF, Guinovart C, et al. Global, regional, and national incidence and mortality for HIV, tuberculosis, and malaria during 1990–2013: a systematic analysis for the Global Burden of Disease Study 2013. *The Lancet.* Jul 21 2014;384, no. 9947 (2014): 1005–1070.

42. Horton R. GBD 2010: understanding disease, injury, and risk. *The Lancet.* Dec 15 2012;380(9859): 2053–2054.

43. Lim SS, Vos T, Flaxman AD, et al. A comparative risk assessment of burden of disease and injury attributable to 67 risk factors and risk factor clusters in 21 regions, 1990–2010: a systematic analysis for the Global Burden of Disease Study 2010. *The Lancet.* Dec 15 2012;380(9859):2224–2260.

44. Romero-Corral A, Montori VM, Somers VK, et al. Association of bodyweight with total mortality and with cardiovascular events in coronary artery disease: a systematic review of cohort studies. *The Lancet.* Aug 19 2006;368(9536): 666–678.

45. Lavie CJ, Alpert MA, Arena R, Mehra MR, Milani RV, Ventura HO. Impact of obesity and the obesity paradox on prevalence and prognosis in heart failure. *Journal of the American College of Cardiology. Heart Failure.* Apr 2013;1(2):93–102.

46. Lavie CJ, Milani RV, Ventura HO. Obesity and cardiovascular disease: risk factor, paradox, and impact of weight loss. *Journal of the American College of Cardiology.* May 26 2009;53(21):1925–1932.

47. World Health Organization. Mental health: strengthening our response. 2014; http://www.who.int/mediacentre/factsheets/fs220/en/. Accessed 11/08/2014.

48. Corrigan PW, Watson AC. Understanding the impact of stigma on people with mental illness. *World Psychiatry.* Feb 2002;1(1):16–20.

49. Lund C, De Silva M, Plagerson S, et al. Poverty and mental disorders: breaking the cycle in low-income and middle-income countries. *The Lancet.* Oct 22 2011;378(9801):1502–1514.

50. Whiteford HA, Degenhardt L, Rehm J, et al. Global burden of disease attributable to mental and substance use disorders: findings from the Global Burden of Disease Study 2010. *The Lancet.* 2013;382(9904):1575–1586.

51. Vos T, Flaxman AD, Naghavi M, et al. Years lived with disability (YLDs) for 1160 sequelae of 289 diseases and injuries 1990–2010: a systematic analysis for the Global Burden of Disease Study 2010. *The Lancet.* Dec 15 2012;380(9859):2163–2196.

52. Frenk J, Moon S. Governance Challenges in Global Health. *New England Journal of Medicine.* 2013;368(10):936–942.

53. Beaglehole R. *Global Public Health : A New Era.* Oxford; New York: Oxford University Press; 2003.

54. Fidler D. *The Challenges of Global Health Governance.* Washington DC: Council on Foreign Relations;2010.

55. Kickbusch I, Szabo MM. A new governance space for health. *Global Health Action.* 2014;7:23507.

56. World Health Organization. Types of Healthy Settings. 2014; http://www.who.int/healthy_settings/types/cities/en/. Accessed 12/08/2014.

57. World Health Organization, Ministry of social affairs and health of Finland. Health in All Policies 2013; http://www.healthpromotion2013.org/health-promotion/health-in-all-policies. Accessed 12/08/2014.

58. HM Government. Health is global: a UK Government strategy 2008–2013. 2008.

59. The Federal Government. Shaping global health—taking joint action—embracing responsibility: the federal Government's strategy paper. Berlin: The Federal Government; 2013.

60. Federal Department of Foreign Affairs, Federal Department of Home Affairs. *Swiss Health Foreign Policy.* 2012.

61. World Health Organization. WHO constitution. 2006; http://www.who.int/governance/eb/who_constitution_fr.pdf.

62. Gostin LO. *Global Health Law.* Cambridge, MA: Harvard University Press; 2014.

63. Gardner CA, Acharya T, Yach D. Technological and social innovation: A unifying new paradigm for global health. *Health Affairs.* July 1 2007;26(4):1052–1061.

64. Howitt P, Darzi A, Yang GZ, et al. Technologies for global health. *The Lancet.* Aug 4 2012;380(9840): 507–535.

65. European Commission. Social innovation. 2014; http://ec.europa.eu/enterprise/policies/innovation/policy/social-innovation/index_en.htm. Accessed 12/08/2014.

66. Brandt AM. How AIDS invented global health. *New England Journal of Medicine.* 2013;368(23): 2149–2152.

67. Syed SB, Dadwal V, Martin G. Reverse innovation in global health systems: towards global innovation flow. *Globalization and Health.* 2013;9:36.

68. Chakma J, Chakma H. Developing countries can contribute to global health innovation. *Nature Medicine.* Feb 2013;19(2):129.

69. Crisp N. Mutual learning and reverse innovation–where next? *Globalization and Health.* 2014; 10:14.

70. Merson MH. University engagement in global health. *New England Journal of Medicine.* May 1 2014;370(18):1676–1678.

71. Frenk J, Chen L, Bhutta ZA, et al. Health professionals for a new century: transforming education to strengthen health systems in an interdependent world. *The Lancet.* Dec 4 2010;376(9756):1923–1958.

72. Zinsstag J, Schelling E, Waltner-Toews D, Tanner M. From "one medicine" to "one health" and systemic approaches to health and well-being. *Preventive Veterinary Medicine.* Jan 9 2011;101(3–4): 148–156.

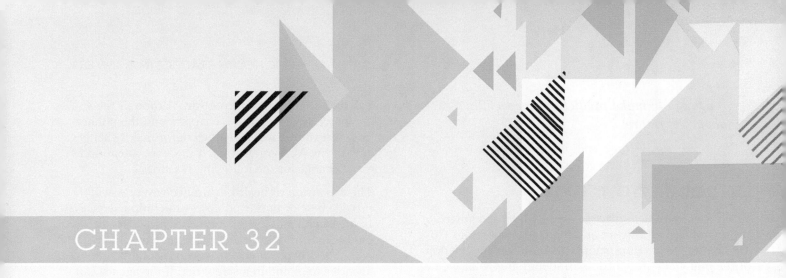

CHAPTER 32

The Future of Public Health Practice

Paul C. Erwin, MD, DrPH • Ross C. Brownson, PhD

LEARNING OBJECTIVES

Upon completion of this chapter, the reader will be able to:

1. Recognize the major forces of change which will likely impact the future of public health practice.

2. Define the necessary approaches to measuring, tracking, and understanding the impact of the forces of change on public health practice.

3. Describe the likely impact of the major forces of change on the preparation of the public health practitioner of the future.

4. Illustrate the critical capacities and capabilities that public health practitioners can build upon to successfully prepare for and respond to the forces of change.

KEY TERMS

accreditation
Affordable Care Act
climate change
evidence-based public health (EBPH)
forces of change
Health in All Policies (HiAP)
informatics
practice-based research
social media

It's tough to make predictions, especially about the future.

—Yogi Berra

INTRODUCTION

While we are reluctant to go against the sage advice of the great baseball catcher and manager, we see this closing chapter as an opportunity to build on the wisdom of the many chapter authors in identifying what we describe as the "forces of change" which have potential to significantly impact public health practice well into the future. By "forces of change" we draw from the MAPP Framework (Mobilizing for Action through Planning and Partnerships),[1] which includes "Forces of Change" as one of the four assessment processes, described as:

> ... changes that affect the context in which the community and its public health system operate ... The Forces of Change Assessment is designed to help answer the following questions: "What is occurring or might occur that affects the health of our community ..." and "What specific threats or opportunities are generated by these occurrences?"

We identify seven such forces of change for the future of public health practice: the Patient Protection and Affordable Care Act (ACA), accreditation, climate change, Health in All Policies, social media and informatics, demographic transitions, and globalized travel. We next describe possible approaches to measuring, tracking, and understanding the impact of these forces of change on public health practice, including the use of evidence-based public health (EBPH), practice-based research, and policy surveillance. Finally, we end with a consideration of what these forces of change, and approaches to addressing them, will mean for the public health practitioner of the future.

FORCES OF CHANGE

The Patient Protection and Affordable Care Act

In Chapter 30, Drs. Seiler, Malcarney, and Levi describe the ACA as "the central part of a very broad drive for change in the U.S. health system,"[2] with the ambitious goal of achieving what had been previously posed as the necessary triple aim of health reform: improving the experience of care, improving the health of populations, and reducing per capita costs of health care.[3] The chapter authors describe implications for public health practice for several major aspects of ACA, including the National Prevention Council and Strategy, the Prevention and Public Health Fund, and evidence-based, clinical, and community prevention. Although the gap in time between writing these chapters and the publication of this textbook will be sufficient for major changes in many of the ACA provisions, it deserves attention as a force of change for the following reasons:

1. The expansion of health insurance coverage will provide new or improved access to clinical services. In areas with adequate health care providers, capable of absorbing the increased demand, there will be less dependency on governmental health agencies to maintain a safety net. If the agency can manage without the revenue generated through fee-for-services, this lessened dependency will in turn allow such agencies to focus on broader community preventive services. In areas with an inadequate supply of providers, the demand on governmental health agencies to establish, continue, or expand both clinical preventive services and primary care will increase, straining already scarce resources and limiting the capacity of such agencies to address community-level, "upstream" concerns.

2. The requirement of insurance carriers to provide "first dollar" coverage for primary and secondary preventive services such as immunizations, cervical cancer screening, and other preventive services recommended by the U.S. Preventive Services Task Force will change the nature of what health departments provide (and the funding support for this) and how they may bill for such services. For example, as a result of the ACA, changes in the federally-funded Vaccines for Children program and the so-called Section 317 program (under the Public Health Services Act) will result in families being steered to sources other than health departments for childhood immunizations.[4,5] Funding support for clinical services such as treatment for sexually transmitted diseases (STDs) and tuberculosis (TB)—for decades traditionally provided through most health departments—will decrease as insurance coverage increases, further changing not only the array of services provided, but also impacting the surveillance capacities that also rely on this same funding support. Some health departments will adapt by billing "third party" providers, while others will relinquish these services to the private sector.

3. The Internal Revenue System (IRS) requirements for community benefit by nonprofit hospitals codify both community health assessments and the engagement of health departments in this process. As described in Chapters 7–10 (federal, state, local, tribal and territorial public health practice) and reinforced in Chapter 13 on community health planning, most health departments are already leading or participating in community health assessments. The IRS rules will increase demand for expertise

in community health assessments, which in many places may reside only in health departments; however, such demand will also increase opportunities for graduates of academic programs in public health, as Drs. Boulton, Baker, and Beck describe in Chapter 18 on the public health workforce. When resources are focused on addressing prioritized strategic issues at the community level, there will be a heightened demand for accountability, thus evaluation, as Drs. Leviton and McGeary describe in Chapter 15. Unlike competencies in community health assessment, however, competencies in a full range of evaluation activities among public health practitioners are often lacking—increased demand will place an added strain on this.

Accreditation

The voluntary national accreditation program administered by the Public Health Accreditation Board (PHAB) has come to fruition following decades of attempts to improve the performance of governmental public health agencies by developing standardized measures of accountability. The prerequisites for accreditation—a community health assessment, a community health improvement plan, and an agency strategic plan—will by themselves increase public health performance capacity. Perhaps to a degree not previously experienced, these prerequisites will necessitate the establishment of productive community partnerships, the sustainability of which will be imperative for making substantive improvements in population health outcomes. In order to enhance community participation and sustainability, health departments will increasingly be called upon to engage in the work of community development, as Dr. Fawcett and colleagues describe in Chapter 25. Health departments pursuing accreditation will, by the nature of the process, be in a stronger position to engage with non-profit hospitals in assuring community benefit.

Along with the benefits of accreditation, as with most such initiatives, there will be unintended consequences. If funding streams for local and state public health agencies become earmarked for or restricted to agencies which have achieved accreditation, then the aphorism "The rich get richer and the poor get poorer" will become a reality for the many agencies which do not have the capacity to meet accreditation standards. In what many already see as a two-tiered health system in the United States—high value and quality for those who have insurance or can afford to pay, limited access and availability for those who cannot—a two-tiered *public health* system will lead to worsening health inequities. The Institute of Medicine's (IOM's) recent efforts to establish a "minimum package of public health services"[6]—the foundational capabilities and an array of basic programs that no health department can be without—may help to ensure that local and state health departments do not become even more fractured and differentiated as accreditation (and health reform) evolves.

Climate Change

In 2006, Dr. Poki Namkung, upon her installment as the president of the National Association of County and City Health Officials (NACCHO), declared that global warming would be the most important public health challenge that *current* and future practitioners would face [personal communication from Dr. Poki Namkung 11/24/2014 to Paul Erwin]. Although debates about the causes of climate change (as global warming has been recoined) will continue with the increasingly polarized politicization of the issue, the *fact* of climate change as a real, experienced phenomenon is clearly established. As a force of change, climate change will impact public health practice in several ways, as described by Drs. Hatcher and Tarver in Chapter 21; we focus on just five.

First, unpredictable and often catastrophic weather or weather-related events—flooding, tornadoes, drought (and drought-associated fires), and heat waves—will require greater emergency preparedness by governmental health agencies. This will continue to shape the evolution of health department capacities and capabilities from the occasional connection to emergency management (pre-mid-1990s), to bioterrorism preparedness (mid-1990s to mid-2000s) to what Drs. Landesman and Weisfuse describe (from mid-2000s forward) more broadly in Chapter 26 as *public health preparedness*. Second, climate change will impact the ecology and evolution of infectious diseases, including vector-borne and zoonotic diseases, by increasing the range or abundance of animal reservoirs or insect vectors, and by prolonging transmission cycles.[7] A third impact of climate change on public health practice is more long-range: rising sea levels and the movement of populations through "forcible displacement by climate impacts, resettlement schemes, and migration as an adaptive response."[8] The displacement of thousands of people due to Hurricane Katrina in 2005—and the public health response—is a foreshadowing of this impact of climate change. Fourth, weather extremes—particularly drought and flooding—will impact food production, security, and costs. Finally, because we are already experiencing the direct effects of air pollution on cardiovascular and pulmonary health (including childhood asthma), and direct effects of temperature extremes (both cold and heat-related morbidity and mortality), health promotion and disease prevention efforts will require new knowledge and skill sets in public health practice. As the climate change issue unfolds, it is likely to illustrate how a combination of policy and politics shapes public health practice, as outlined by Dr. Ricketts in Chapter 6.

Health in All Policies

Health in All Policies (HiAP) was first popularized in Scandinavia in the mid-2000s as an approach to increase multisectoral coordination across countries of the European Union. As defined by the World Health Organization,

> Health in All Policies is an approach to public policies across sectors that systematically takes into account the health and health systems implications of decisions, seeks synergies, and avoids harmful health impacts, in order to improve population health and health equity. A HiAP approach is founded on health-related rights and obligations.
>
> It emphasizes the consequences of public policies on health determinants, and aims to improve the accountability of policy-makers for health impacts at all levels of policy-making.[9]

More succinctly, HiAP is a recognition that economic policy is health policy, that transportation policy is health policy, that tax policy is health policy. In the United States, the IOM has highlighted HiAP in reports[10] and discussion papers.[11] In 2012 NACCHO became the first national association to adopt a position statement on HiAP,[12] recognizing that policy decisions made outside the health sector impact the determinants of health, and that governmental health agencies at all levels have a leadership role to play. In many ways, MAPP, with its focus on the Local Public Health *System* (all organizations, groups, and individuals which impact the public's health at the local level), embodied the HiAP concept even earlier. The creation of the National Prevention, Health Promotion, and Public Health Council as part of the ACA, is perhaps the best example of the application of the HiAP approach at the federal level. An increasing demand for community health assessments, whether through the IRS requirements for nonprofit hospitals or through PHAB for accreditation, will provide public health practitioners unparalleled opportunities to apply the HiAP approach to partnership development. Public health practitioners who have understood the social determinants of health and the socioecological model of health, intuitively understand that cross-sectoral, multidisciplinary policy engagement requires a HiAP approach in order to "move the needle" on population health outcomes.

Social Media and Informatics

The use of social network analysis to investigate or track the spread of infectious diseases,[13] particularly STDs,[14] was just a foreshadowing of the explosion in social media beginning in the mid-2000s. When the first edition of this textbook was published in 1996, e-mail and Internet access were still not available in many public health practice locations, Facebook and Twitter had yet to be founded, and smart phones were well beyond the horizon. As of the writing of this fourth edition, the social media and informatics landscape and its impact on public health practice looks revolutionary by comparison, for example:

▶ Since the first state health department adoption of Twitter (2008) and Facebook (2009), by 2012 the use had expanded to 41 states for Twitter and 28 states for Facebook.[15]
▶ By 2012, 24 percent of local health departments had Facebook, 8 percent had Twitter, and 7 percent had both.[16]
▶ In 2012, the New York City Department of Health and Mental Hygiene began extracting information from Yelp—which publishes crowd-sourced reviews about local restaurants—and Twitter to detect real or potential foodborne outbreaks.[17]
▶ The Chicago Department of Public Health and its civic partners established "FoodBorne Chicago", a community approach to detecting disease outbreaks by monitoring Twitter feeds.[18]

As a force of change, the expanded use of social media and informatics will compress the time between exposure to illness and source identification, placing added demands for quick resolution onto public health practitioners. Syndromic surveillance systems, as described by Dr. Shih and colleagues in Chapter 12, once the "cutting edge" of public health informatics, may be replaced by automated surveillance systems which monitor an array of social media sources, the use of which will expand to noninfectious diseases and conditions.

Demographic Transitions

As Dr. Elder and colleagues note in Chapter 14, "in 2011 the first members of the large Baby Boom generation turned 65." From 4.1 percent of the population in 1900, those 65 years and over comprised 13 percent of the U.S. population in 2010, and by 2050 are projected to be 20.9 percent of the total U.S. population. Although there are continued improvements in the major causes of mortality—cardiovascular disease and cancer—the sheer number of older people with chronic conditions will result in much higher prevalence rates for these and related conditions.

Yet, chronic disease prevention and related health promotion activities have been slow in coming to (particularly, local) public health practice. As earlier chapters chronicle so well, the establishment of maternal and child health, infectious/communicable diseases, and environmental health programs at the local and state levels all predated a public health practice focus on chronic diseases. The first National Conference on Chronic Disease Prevention and Control was held in 1985, and it was only in 1988 when the CDC established the National Center for Chronic Disease Prevention and Health Promotion.[19] At the state level, it was not until 1993 when all states had established tobacco control and prevention programs, and 1995 when all states had established screening programs for breast cancer.[19]

Despite the major causes of mortality now being chronic diseases, the predominant focus at the local level remains on the care of mothers and babies, outbreak investigation, and environmental health. To some degree there is significant justification for this, i.e., getting the best start in life is perhaps the most important first milestone on the path to chronic disease prevention. But, as mentioned above, the overall burden of chronic disease with the aging of the U.S. population will necessitate an added focus within public health practice. The practical implications will be borne out most likely through health departments' engagement in community health assessments and in their responses to the ACA. Using skills to effect both individual and community-level behavioral change, public health practice will be increasingly called on to develop, implement, and evaluate programs that impact older populations, as Dr. Elder and colleagues describe in Chapter 14 in assessing a program to prevent falls in the elderly. Public health practice, while coming to chronic disease prevention relatively late, has, nevertheless, a significant headstart in creating and using evidence-based public health (EBPH) to optimize community-level impact, as seen through the *Guide to Community Preventive Services*.[20]

In addition to the changing age structure of the population, the demographic transition includes changes in the racial and ethnic make-up of the population. Between 1990 and 2010, persons identified as Hispanic (regardless of race) surpassed the percentage identified as black or African-American (regardless of ethnicity). The U.S. Census Bureau projects that by 2043, the United States is projected to become a majority-minority nation; while the non-Hispanic white population will remain the largest single group, no group will make up a majority.[21] Since risk factors, access to care, and approaches to primary, secondary, and tertiary prevention all impact and are impacted by race and ethnicity, these demographic changes will profoundly affect public health practice at all levels.

Globalized Travel

In October 2014, several west-African countries were in the throes of the largest-ever Ebola outbreak, and the first cases to be diagnosed in the United States were headline news. With the first U.S. case diagnosed in a Liberian man who traveled to the United States during the incubation period of Ebola, the fact that apparently well individuals could be infected and yet make their way to the United States in less than 24 hours from their places of exposure, highlighted in a way not previously appreciated that globalized travel is a public health issue. Certainly there have been many examples of people traveling during the incubation period of various diseases (which are not endemic in the United States), only to become symptomatic and subsequently diagnosed here–from malaria (with the United States experiencing a 40-year high of 2000 cases in 2011),[22] to Chikungunya,[23] and even Yellow Fever.[24] Globalized travel, however, is also to "blame" for importation of diseases that are at relatively low levels in the United States, which can subsequently result in outbreaks of disease—for example, measles[25] and multidrug resistant tuberculosis.[26] Moreover, globalized travel—of both vectors as well as human hosts—can give rise to the establishment of diseases not previously seen in the United States—the West Nile Virus being perhaps the best recent example.

As a force of change, globalized travel will increasingly impact public health preparedness and response at all levels. With the 2014 Ebola outbreak as an example, however, public health practitioners will be called upon to not only contribute to the scientific understanding of such exotic diseases, but equally importantly to communicate this understanding to the public in such a way that fear and anxiety are replaced with knowledge and awareness. This will be more difficult when science becomes the victim of partisan politics, when the politicization of the tools of the public health practitioner—surveillance, isolation, and quarantine—results in a worsening of fears and negative repercussions. The acts of governors in New York, New Jersey, and Illinois to quarantine anyone arriving at its airports who had had direct contact with Ebola patients was met with resistance by the public health/scientific community; among other issues, this created the unintended consequence of dissuading U.S. health care workers from traveling to and working in Ebola-affected countries.[27] Public health practitioners, therefore, will be expected to contribute to policy formulation to address issues stemming from globalized travel, even as they work to strengthen their own preparedness and response capabilities.

APPROACHES TO MEASURING, ADDRESSING, TRACKING, AND UNDERSTANDING THE IMPACT OF THE FORCES OF CHANGE

While describing real or potential forces of change is a first-order challenge for public health practice, developing or augmenting methods to measure, track, and understand these forces will be an even greater challenge. We believe there is a certain logic to this approach through strengthening the evidence-base of public health and through policy surveillance.

Evidence-Based Public Health and Practice-Based Research

Evidence-based public health (EBPH) has made its way in this textbook from being an appendix in the third edition to one of the prominent new chapters in this fourth edition. As described in Chapter 11, EBPH is defined as the integration of science-based interventions with community preferences to improve population health.[28] The *Guide to Community Preventive Services*[20] and the *Guide to Clinical Preventive Services*[29] are the best examples of the process of examining existing evidence and making scientifically-justifiable recommendations on the basis of such evidence. Addressing the forces of change described above will certainly require greater use of these guidelines, for example:

- in response to the ACA as a force of change, using the guidelines to decide which primary and secondary preventive services should be provided and covered by insurance;
- in response to Health in All Policies as a force of change, using the guidelines to implement smoke-free policies in the worksite;
- and, in response to demographic transitions as a force of change, using the guidelines to address obesity and other chronic diseases at the community level, being sensitive to and knowledgeable about the influence of age, race, and ethnicity.

Evidence also exists at the level of evidence-based administrative practices within public health (described in Chapter 11),[30] and wider implementation of such practices will facilitate addressing several forces of change, for example:

- in-service training in quality improvement or evidence-based decision making as a response to accreditation as a force of change;
- access and free flow of information, and conscious creation of environments conducive to innovation as a response to social media and informatics as a force of change;

- and, building and/or enhancing partnerships with schools, hospitals, community organizations, social services, private businesses, universities, and law enforcement as a response to HiAP as a force of change.

Measuring, tracking, addressing, and understanding several of the above-described forces of change, however, will necessitate the creation of new knowledge and the development of new evidence through research. Drs. Scutchfield and Ingram describe the research agenda for the emerging field of public health services and systems research (PHSSR) in Chapter 17, which has direct relevance to several forces of change; for example, specific research questions from this agenda include:

- What conditions and strategies facilitate productive inter-organizational relationships and patterns of interaction among organizations that contribute to public health strategies at local, state, and national levels?
- How do public health agency accreditation programs influence the effectiveness, efficiency, and outcomes of public health strategies delivered at local, state, and national levels?
- What policy, system, and administrative strategies are most effective in reducing disparities in the effectiveness, efficiency, and outcomes of public health strategies delivered to racial and ethnic minority and low-income populations?
- How do funding formulae, payment methods, policy decisions, and community health needs and risks influence the levels of investment made in public health strategies at local, state, and national levels?
- How do health information and communication technologies influence the effectiveness, efficiency, and outcomes of public health strategies delivered at local, state, and national levels (e.g., electronic health records, mobile health technologies, social media, electronic surveillance systems, Geographic Information Systems, network analysis, predictive modeling)?

Exploring these and related research questions will be important means for addressing forces of change. A critically important aspect of EBPH, especially as it relates to building the evidence related to forces of change, is the locus of such research endeavors. Dr. Lawrence Green summed it best by stating, "If we want more evidence-based practice, we need more practice-based evidence."[31] A primary challenge to addressing this relates to the relevance of public health research. Public Health Practice-based Research Networks (as described in Chapter 17) hold much promise in heeding Dr. Green's call, as these networks require engagement and full participation from both practitioners as well as academicians, increasing the potential that the research conducted, and its findings, will be more relevant to the practice setting. There remains, however, a tension that will continue to challenge such collaboratives: even if the research is practice-based, if it only answers the questions posed by academicians—or their funders—it runs the risk of being irrelevant to practice.

Policy Surveillance

A common public health adage is "what gets measured, gets done."[32,33] In public health, this measurement largely occurs via public health surveillance (i.e., the ongoing systematic collection, analysis, and interpretation of outcome-specific health data[34]). For example, we now have excellent epidemiologic data for estimating which population groups and which regions of the United States are affected by which diseases, and how patterns are changing over time.

The power of public health surveillance is apparent across a vast array of topics in public health. For example, in tobacco control, agreement on a common metric for tobacco use enabled comparisons across the states and an early recognition of the doubling and then tripling of the rates of decrease in smoking in California after passage of its Proposition 99,[35] and then a quadrupling of the rate of decline in Massachusetts compared with the other 48 states.[36]

To supplement these routine surveillance data, we need better information on a broad array of environmental and policy factors that influence the patterns of risk factors and diseases. This shifts the focus from downstream endpoints (diseases, risk factors) to upstream determinants (physical environments, policies). When implemented properly, policy surveillance systems can be an enormous asset for policy development process and evaluation. It allows us to examine time trends in policies; to conduct more sophisticated research on the determinants, implementation, and effectiveness of policies; and by triangulating various surveillance data, hypotheses can be developed which can in turn be tested in intervention studies. A few efforts are underway to develop public health policy surveillance systems. For example, a group of federal and voluntary agencies have developed policy surveillance systems for tobacco, alcohol, and more recently, school-based nutrition and physical education.[37] Since so many of the forces of change involve policy, a stronger policy surveillance system will be essential in tracking the process, content, and outcomes of these macro-level changes.

THE PUBLIC HEALTH PRACTITIONER OF THE FUTURE

If, despite Yogi Berra's warning at the opening of this chapter, the evolution of public health practice takes place as described above, what are the implications for the public health practitioner of the future? We believe there are five critical capacities and capabilities that public health practitioners can build upon to successfully prepare for and respond to these forces of change.

#1: Systems Thinking

Peter Senge popularized this phrase over two decades ago in *The Fifth Discipline*:

> Systems Thinking is a discipline for seeing wholes. It is a framework for seeing interrelationships rather than things, for seeing patterns of change rather than static "snapshots"….[it is] a sensibility—for the subtle interconnectedness that gives living systems their unique character.[38(pp 68–69)]

Paramount to systems thinking is the shift in thinking from a reaction to the present, to creating the desired future. Three decades before Senge, though, René Dubos described systems thinking without ever naming it, when describing the internal and external environments related to human diseases:

> Any event in the outer world which impinges on an individual modifies, however indirectly and slightly, the balance between his various organs and functions … [A]ny factor that upsets the equilibrium of [the] internal and external environments can become a determinant of diseases. As all components of both systems are interrelated, any disturbance in either of them–even though minor and not damaging in itself–can set in motion secondary effects which become destructive to the organism.[39(pp 110–111, 122)]

In the last two decades we have seen other descriptors or aspects of systems thinking, for example, as it applies to the interaction of multiple diseases within a population—*syndemics*[40], or as it applies to research frameworks that offer a "novel solutions-oriented approach to complex problems"—the *intervention-level framework*.[41] What is common across all of these perspectives is what the public health practitioner must make applicable: the ability to see how the trees make the forest, and vice-versa. For the public health practitioner who understands the dynamism and interconnectedness of the social determinants of health—so well described by Dr. Chapman and colleagues in Chapter 3—and the necessity of partnership development to address these, systems thinking is already being operationalized.

#2: Strategic Thinking

"I skate to where the puck is going to be, not where it has been."—Wayne Gretzky

Strategic thinking shares this future orientation with systems thinking; however, a fundamental aspect of strategic thinking is a consideration of the consequences of inaction. Using the examples of strategic issue identification in MAPP, "Failing to think strategically ... eventually results in the realization of an external threat, a lost opportunity, the lingering or worsening of an identified problem, and ultimately a failure to achieve the community vision."[1] At the height of the recent economic recession, Paul Kuehnert, then Director of the Kane County (Illinois) Health Department, led his agency through a realignment process that resulted in losing half of his workforce; however, failing to make the difficult strategic choices with which he was faced could have resulted in losing everything (as described further in Chapter 18).[42] Far from being overcome by the forces of change at play, Mr. Kuehnert saw that the "convergence of these severe economic conditions with the multiple challenges facing public health ... provides public health services researchers, practitioners and policy makers a unique opportunity to reinvent governmental public health in ways that truly enhance its value and assert its relevance for our society."[42(p 124)] Strategic thinking, then, is about how we view the choices before us, creating a future that is buoyed by the opportunities such choices present, not drowned by the weight of the difficulties.

#3: Communication Capacities and Capabilities

Every generation seems to lay claim to the "information generation" moniker—but it is *really* the truth for this generation! For the public health practitioner of the future, it is less, though, about the nuts and bolts of communications platforms themselves—Twitter feeds, Facebook walls, blog posts—the *how* of communications, and more about the *why*. That being said, we understand that although 91 percent of local health departments have access to smartphones, and at least basic Internet services are almost universally available, the *what* of communications remains a challenge for many, as access, for example, to research libraries or online full-length journal articles remains limited.[43] Purposeful communications must be paramount; quality must trump quantity, as it will simply not be humanly possible to either manage or digest or make use of the enormous amount of information that is already available.

#4: Entrepreneurial Orientation

Entrepreneurial orientation (EO), which has its roots in management business philosophy, may be characterized as a multidimensional construct of organizational behavior, with measures of proactiveness, innovativeness, and risk-taking.[44,45] In the health arena, this three-factor EO scale has been used in studies on not-for-profit hospitals, health care executives, health care staff, and most recently in nursing home management.[46] In many ways, EO relates to concepts that should be familiar to the public health practitioner. Proactiveness is an important element of strategic thinking, as described above. The concept of innovativeness in EO relates to similar constructs in implementation science—harkening to Everett Roger's seminal work on *Diffusion of Innovations*.[47] Risk-taking, particularly in governmental agencies which are most often risk-averse, is perhaps the most unfamiliar of the three dimensions of EO vis-à-vis public health practice. Yet, for the public health practitioner of the future, it is difficult to imagine positioning an agency in the context of the ACA without a degree of risk-taking: we simply have not been down this road quite so far. Indeed, for much of what lies ahead for public health practice across all the forces of change described earlier, all three dimensions of EO will be critical; however, the degree to which these organizational behaviors are successfully managed will be directly dependent upon how these characteristics are reflected in the people—the public health practitioners—who constitute the organizations.

#5: Transformational Ethics

It will not be enough for the public health leader to understand, facilitate, translate, and create the evidence-base for public health—every action must be amplified, ameliorated, and contextualized through a *transformational ethics*, else every positive step in population health will be met with negative repercussions for subpopulations, i.e., what will benefit the most may hurt those already most in need. Another way of framing this is simply that population health improvements may be accompanied by worsening health inequities unless the public health practitioner of the future understands public health (writ large) as social justice. Over 40 years ago, John Bryant merged the Rawlsian concept of justice with Nicholas Rescher's formulations on distributive justice to propose a principle of health care systems development: "Whatever health services are available should be equally available to all. Departures from equality of distribution are permissible only if those worst off are made better off."[48] While Dr. Bryant's conceptualization of health as social justice was in the framework of international health services development (particularly in low income/resource countries), it may serve as a model for transformational ethics in public health practice: *Whatever improvements can be made in the health of the public should be made equally to all. Departures from equality of opportunity, access, and outcomes are permissible only if health inequities are lessened.* We are past meeting the *Healthy People 2010* goal of eliminating health disparities. For the public health leader of the future, a transformational ethics can be realized through a commitment to health equity: to recast Rabbi Hillel's famous saying: if not me, whom, and if not now, when?

SUMMARY

The future of public health practice will be buffeted, pushed, and constrained by certain forces of change. The best view of the likely forces of change which will be at play is to "walk backwards into the future"—the Sumerian notion that gazing at our past reveals where our future paths will take us. Forces of change through health reform, accreditation, information technology, climate change, and demographic transitions impel us to consider the attributes that public health practitioners will need to successfully negotiate these paths: systems and strategic thinking, communication capacities, innovativeness and risk-taking, and a transformational ethics. What an exciting journey it will be to explore these visions for public health practice.

REVIEW QUESTIONS

1. What are "Forces of Change" and what do they mean in the context of public health practice?

2. Identify at least three mechanisms by which the Affordable Care Act will be a force of change for public health practice.

3. How might policy surveillance parallel other more common surveillance systems in public health practice, e.g., surveillance for influenza or other infectious diseases?

4. Define "systems thinking" and relate this concept to theories which are fundamental to public health practice.

5. What is meant by "Entrepreneurial Orientation," and how might it be used in addressing the Forces of Change?

REFERENCES

1. National Association of County and City Health Officials. Mobilizing for Action through Planning and Partnerships (MAPP). http://www.naccho.org/topics/infrastructure/mapp/index.cfm. Accessed June 27, 2012.

2. Seiler N, Malcarney M-B, Levi J. The Affordable Care Act And Public Health. In: Erwin PC, Brownson RC, eds. *Principles of Public Health Practice.* 4th ed. Stamford, CT: Cengage; 2016.

3. Berwick DM, Nolan TW, Whittington J. The triple aim: Care, health, and cost. *Health Affairs.* May 1 2008;27(3):759–769.

4. Knight MA, Kershenbaum AD, Buchanan M, Ridley J, Erwin PC. The effects of the changes in Section 317 Rules for Administration of Federally Purchased Vaccines. *Frontiers in Public Health Services and Systems Research.* 2014;3(2):Article 7.

5. Knight MA, Kershenbaum AD, Buchanan M, Ridley J, Erwin PC. The effects of the State of Tennessee Immunization Policy Change of 2011–2012 on Vaccination Uptake in East Tennessee. *Frontiers in Public Health Services and Systems Research.* 2014;3(1):Article 4.

6. Institute of Medicine, Committee on Public Health Strategies to Improve Health. *For the Public's Health: Investing in a Healthier Future.* Washington, DC. 2012.

7. Greer A, Ng V, Fisman D. Climate change and infectious diseases in North America: the road ahead. *CMAJ.* Mar 11 2008;178(6):715–722.

8. McMichael C, Barnett J, McMichael AJ. An ill wind? Climate change, migration, and health. *Environ Health Perspect.* May 2012;120(5):646–654.

9. World Health Organization. *Framework and statement: Consultation on the drafts of the "Health in All Policies Framework for Country Action" for the Conference Statement of 8th Global Conference on Health Promotion.* 2013.

10. Institute of Medicine, Committee on Public Health Strategies to Improve Health. *For the Public's Health: Revitalizing Law and Policy to Meet New Challenges.* National Academies Press; 2011.

11. Rudolph L, Caplan J, Mitchell C, Ben-Moshe K, Dillon L. *Health in All Policies: Improving Health Through Intersectoral Collaboration.* Institute of Medicine;2013.

12. National Association of County and City Health Officials. *Implementing Health in All Policies through Local Health Department Leadership.* 2012.

13. Klovdahl AS, Potterat JJ, Woodhouse DE, Muth JB, Muth SQ, Darrow WW. Social networks and infectious disease: The Colorado Springs study. *Social Science & Medicine.* 1994;38(1):79–88.

14. Liljeros F, Edling CR, Amaral LAN. Sexual networks: implications for the transmission of sexually transmitted infections. *Microbes and Infection.* 2003;5(2):189–196.

15. Harris JK, Snider D, Mueller N. Social media adoption in health departments nationwide: The state of the states. *Frontiers in Public Health Services and Systems Research.* 2013;2(1):5.

16. Harris JK, Mueller NL, Snider D. Social media adoption in local health departments nationwide. *Am J Public Health.* 2013;103(9):1700–1707.

17. Harrison C, Jorder M, Stern H, Stavinsky F, Balter S. Using online reviews by restaurant patrons to identify unreported cases of foodborne illness—New York City, 2012–2013. *Morbidity and Mortality Weekly Report (MMWR).* 2014;63(20):441–445.

18. Harris JK, Mansour R, Choucair B, et al. Health department use of social media to identify foodborne illness-Chicago, Illinois, 2013–2014. *Morbidity and Mortality Weekly Report (MMWR).* 2014;63(32):681–685.

19. Brownson RC, Bright FS. Chronic disease control in public health practice: Looking back and moving forward. *Public Health Report.* May–June 2004;119(3):230–238.

20. Zaza S, Briss PA, Harris KW, eds. *The Guide to Community Preventive Services: What Works to Promote Health?* New York: Oxford University Press; 2005.

21. U.S. Census Bureau. 2012 National Population Projections. 2014; https://www.census.gov/newsroom/releases/archives/population/cb12-243.html. Accessed November 23, 2014.

22. Cullen KA, Arguin PM. Malaria Surveillance—United States, 2011. *MMWR Surveillance Summaries. (Washington, DC: 2002).* 2013;62:1–17.

23. Gibney KB, Fischer M, Prince HE, et al. Chikungunya Fever in the United States: A Fifteen Year Review of Cases. *Clinical Infectious Diseases.* January 17, 2011.

24. McFarland JM, Baddour LM, Nelson JE, et al. Imported yellow fever in a United States citizen. *Clinical Infectious Diseases.* November 1997;25(5):1143–1147.

25. Gastañaduy PA, Redd SB, Fiebelkorn AP, et al. Measles—United States, January 1–May 23, 2014. *Morbidity and Mortality Weekly Report (MMWR).* 2014;63(22):496.

26. Oeltmann JE, Varma JK, Ortega L, et al. Multidrug-resistant tuberculosis outbreak among US-bound Hmong refugees, Thailand, 2005. *Emerging Infectious Diseases.* 2008;14(11):1715.

27. Alcindor Y. Experts: Quarantines may dissuade Ebola volunteers. *USA Today* 2014; http://www.usatoday.com/story/news/nation/2014/10/25/ebola-stricter-quarantines/17900749/. Accessed December 09, 2014

28. Kohatsu ND, Robinson JG, Torner JC. Evidence-based public health: an evolving concept. *American Journal of Preventive Medicine.* December 2004;27(5):417–421.

29. US Preventive Services Task Force. *Guide to Clinical Preventive Services: Report of the US Preventive Services Task Force.* DIANE Publishing; 1989.

30. Brownson RC, Allen P, Duggan K, Stamatakis KA, Erwin PC. Fostering more-effective public health by identifying administrative evidence-based practices: a review of the literature. *American Journal of Preventive Medicine.* September 2012;43(3):309–319.

31. Green LW, Glasgow RE, Atkins D, Stange K. Making evidence from research more relevant, useful, and actionable in policy, program planning, and practice slips "twixt cup and lip." *American Journal of Preventive Medicine.* December 2009;37 (6 Suppl 1):S187–S191.

32. Halverson PK. Performance measurement and performance standards: old wine in new bottles. *Journal of Public Health Management and Practice.* 2000;6(5):vi–x.

33. Thacker SB. Editorial: Public health surveillance and the prevention of injuries in sports: what gets measured gets done. *Journal of Athletic Training.* 2007;42(2):171.

34. Thacker SB, Berkelman RL. Public health surveillance in the United States. *Epidemiologic Reviews.* 1988;10:164–190.

35. Tobacco Education and Research Oversight Committee for California, California Department of Health. *Confronting a Relentless Adversary: A Plan for Success Toward a Tobacco-Free California 2006–2008.* 2006.

36. Biener L, Harris JE, Hamilton W. Impact of the Massachusetts tobacco control programme: Population based trend analysis. *BMJ.* 2000;321(7257):351–354.

37. Brownson RC, Chriqui JF, Stamatakis KA. Understanding evidence-based public health policy. *Am J Public Health.* 2009;99(9):1576–1583.

38. Senge PM. *The Fifth Discipline.* New York, NY: Currency Doubleday; 1990.

39. Dubos R. *Mirage of Health.* New York, NY: Harper & Brothers; 1959.

40. Singer M, Clair S. Syndemics and public health: reconceptualizing disease in bio-social context. *Medical Anthropology Quarterly.* December 2003; 17(4):423–441.

41. Johnston LM, Matteson CL, Finegood DT. Systems science and obesity policy: a novel framework for analyzing and rethinking population-level planning. *Am J Public Health.* July 2014;104(7):1270–1278.

42. Kuehnert PL, McConnaughay KS. Tough choices in tough times: enhancing public health value in an era of declining resources. *Journal of Public Health Management and Practice.* March–April 2012;18(2):115–125.

43. National Association of County and City Health Officials. 2013 National Profile of Local Health Departments 2013; http://www.naccho.org/topics/infrastructure/profile/upload/2013-National-Profile-of-Local-Health-Departments-report.pdf.

44. Miller D. The correlates of entrepreneurship in three types of firms. *Management Science.* 1983;29(7):770–791.

45. Covin JG, Slevin DP. Strategic management of small firms in hostile and benign environments. *Strategic Management Journal.* 1989;10(1):75–87.

46. Davis JA, Marino LD, Vecchiarini M. Exploring the relationship between nursing home financial performance and management entrepreneurial attributes. *Advances in Health Care Management.* 2013;14:147–165.

47. Rogers EM. *Diffusion of Innovations.* 5th ed. New York, NY: Simon and Schuster; 2010.

48. Bryant JH. Principles of justice as a basis for conceptualizing a health care system. *International Journal of Health Services.* 1977;7(4):707–719.

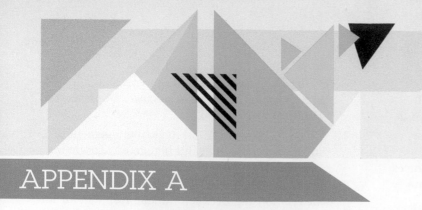

Major National Public Health Professional Associations

C. William Keck, MD, MPH • F. Douglas Scutchfield, MD

Two of the more difficult yet important challenges facing public health professionals are keeping up with developments at the state and national level that are relevant to their work and staying connected to a peer network of colleagues. Membership in professional associations can be very helpful in both these areas. Professional associations can be a mechanism for access to such useful items as relevant publications; technical and legislative updates, alerts, and summaries; issue analyses; trend forecasts; career opportunities; and policy development issues.

This appendix provides a list of some of the major national professional associations typically joined by public health practitioners. There are many other national organizations not listed here that might be of value to some in public health, and the reader is encouraged to search out and explore any group that might be professionally helpful or personally rewarding.

Public health professionals should also explore state-level professional associations in the state in which they work. Many of these associations provide the same benefits and opportunities at the state level that national associations provide at the national level. Indeed, many state associations are affiliated with national ones. Although there are too many to list here, state associations deserve consideration and support.

American Association of Public Health Dentistry (AAPHD)

3085 Stevenson Drive
Suite 200
Springfield, IL 62703
Tel: 217-529-6941
Fax: 217-529-9120
Web: http://www.aaphd.org

American Association of Public Health Physicians (AAPHP)

1605 Pebble Beach Boulevard
Green Cove Springs, Florida 32043
Tel: 1-888-447-7281
Fax: 202-333-5016
Web: http://www.aaphp.org

American College of Epidemiology (ACE)

1500 Sunday Drive, Suite 102
Raleigh, NC 27607
Tel: 919-861-5573
Fax: 919-787-4916
Web: http://acepidemiology.org/

American College of Preventive Medicine (ACPM)

455 Massachusetts Avenue, NW
Suite 200
Washington, DC 20001
Tel: 202-466-2044
Fax: 202-466-2662
Web: http://www.acpm.org

America's Health Insurance Plans (AHIP)

601 Pennsylvania Avenue, NW
South Building, Suite 500
Washington, DC 20004
Tel: 202-778-3200
Fax: 202-331-7487
Web: http://www.ahip.org

American Medical Association (AMA)

AMA Plaza
330 North Wabash Ave., Suite 39300
Chicago, IL 60611-5885
Tel: 800- 262-3211
Web: http://www.ama-assn.org

American Nurses Association (ANA)

8515 Georgia Avenue
Suite 400
Silver Spring, MD 20910
Tel: 1-800-274-4262
Web: http://www.ana.org

American Public Health Association (APHA)

800 I Street NW
Washington, DC 20001-3710
Tel: 202-777-2742
Fax: 202-777-2534
Web: http://www.apha.org

Association of Schools and Programs of Public Health (ASPPH)

1900 M Street NW, Suite 710
Washington, DC 20036
Tel: (202) 296-1099
Fax: (202) 296-1252
Web: http://www.aspph.org

Association of State and Territorial Health Officials (ASTHO)

2231 Crystal Drive
Suite 450
Arlington, VA 22202
Tel: 202-371-9090
Fax: 571-527-3189
Web: http://www.astho.org
[NOTE: There are also 20 affiliates of ASTHO, which are described in their website.]

Association for Prevention Teaching and Research (APTR)

1001 Connecticut Avenue, NW
Suite 610
Washington, DC 20036
Tel: 202-463-0550
Fax: 202-463-0555
Web: http://www.aptrweb.org

Community Campus Partnerships for Health (CCPH)

UW Box 354809
Seattle, Washington 98195-4809
Tel/Fax: 206-666-3406
Web: http://www.ccph.info/

National Association of County and City Health Officials (NACCHO)

1100 17th Street NW
Second Floor
Washington, DC 20036
Tel: 202-783-5550
Fax: 202-783-1583
Web: http://www.naccho.org

National Association of Local Boards of Health (NALBOH)

563 Carter Court, Suite B.
Kimberly Wisconsin, 54136
Tel: 920-560-5644
Fax: 920-882-3655
Web: http://www.nalboh.org

National Environmental Health Association (NEHA)

720 S. Colorado Boulevard
Suite 1000-N
Denver, CO 80246-1926
Tel: 303-756-9090
Fax: 303-691-9490
Web: http://www.neha.org

Society for Public Health Education (SOPHE)

10 G Street, NE
Suite 605
Washington, DC 20002-4242
Tel: 202-408-9804
Fax: 202-408-9815
Web: http://www.sophe.org

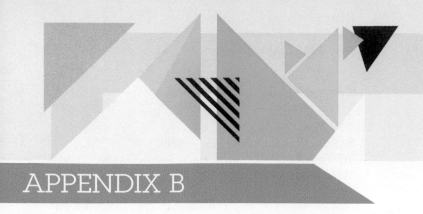

Core Competencies for Public Health Practice

Paul C. Erwin, MD, DrPH • Ross C. Brownson, PhD

INTRODUCTION

There are two sets of public health competencies that are important to the field of public health, both practice and academia. The first set of competencies—Core Competencies for Public Health Professionals—was developed by the Council on Linkages between Academia and Practice in 2001 and revised in 2010 and again in 2014.[1] These competencies will be the primary focus of this appendix, and will be described in more detail below. A second set of competencies—Core Competencies for the Master of Public Health (MPH) degree—was developed by the Association of Schools of Public Health (ASPH) in 2006.[2] These competencies include the five traditional core areas of academic public health and seven interdisciplinary/cross-cutting areas, and in general are meant to define the competencies that MPH students should achieve upon graduation (see Table B-1). Subsequent work by the Association of Schools and Programs of Public Health in its Framing the Future initiative[3] built upon these core competencies for the MPH in further defining "Key Considerations, Design Features, and Critical Content of the Core" of the MPH for the twenty-first century. To a considerable degree, the Core Competencies for the Master of Public Health have been influenced by the accrediting body for schools and programs of public health—the Council on Education for Public Health (CEPH)—which has increasingly used competency-based education standards as a part of its accreditation criteria.

In addition to the Core Competencies for the MPH, ASPH also established competencies for the Doctorate in Public Health (DrPH) degree[4], and, similar to the MPH, expanded upon these Core Competencies in 2014 through the Framing the Future initiative.[5] There are also numerous sets of core competencies for the various disciplines within public health. For example, competencies for applied epidemiology have been developed by the Centers for Disease Control and Prevention (CDC) and the Council of State and Territorial Epidemiologists for individuals working in public health practice, ranging from entry level to senior level skills.[6,7]

TABLE B-1 Domains of Core Competencies for the Master of Public Health Degree

Competency Group	Domains
Discipline-Specific	Biostatistics
	Environmental Health Sciences
	Epidemiology
	Health Policy and Management
	Social and Behavioral Sciences
Crosscutting	Communication and Informatics
	Diversity and Culture
	Leadership
	Professionalism
	Program Planning
	Public Health
	Biology
	Systems Thinking

SOURCE: Calhoun JG, Ramiah K, Weist EM, Shortell SM. Development of a Core Competency Model for the Master of Public Health Degree. *American Journal of Public Health.* 2008/09/01 2008;98(9):1598–1607.

CORE COMPETENCIES FOR PUBLIC HEALTH PROFESSIONALS

The development of core competencies by the Council on Linkages Between Academia and Public Health Practice has its roots in the Institute of Medicine's (IOM) report on *The Future of Public Health.*[8] In an effort to address the IOM's concerns that academic programs were too isolated from the practice of public health, the Johns Hopkins University School of Hygiene and Public Health established the Public Health Faculty/Agency Forum in 1990.[9] Key partners in the Forum included ASPH, American Public Health Association, Health Resources and Services Administration, and the CDC. In 1992 the Forum issued a final report titled *The Public Health Faculty/Agency Forum: Linking Graduate Education and Practice,* which provided recommendations on bridging the divide between academia and practice. The Forum also issued a list of "Universal Competencies" to help guide the education and training of public health professionals.

The momentum in addressing these fundamental challenges led to the establishment of the Council on Linkages (COL) Between Academia and Public Health Practice in 1992. The COL now includes 20 national organizations that have an interest in the education and training of public health professionals; it is funded by the CDC and staffed by the Public Health Foundation.[10] Building on the "Universal Competencies," the COL released the initial set of Core Competencies for Public Health Professionals in 2001. The Core Competencies have undergone two subsequent revisions, in 2010 and again in 2014.

The Core Competencies "reflect foundational skills desirable for professionals engaging in the practice, education, and research of public health."[11] As described on the COL's website, "The Core Competencies are organized into eight domains, reflecting skill areas within public health, and three tiers, representing career stages for public health professionals. These competencies support public health workforce development and can serve as a starting point for public health practice and academic organizations as they create workforce development plans, identify training and workforce needs, prepare for accreditation, and more."[11] The eight domains of core competencies include:

1. Analytical/Assessment Skills
2. Policy Development/Program Planning Skills
3. Communication Skills
4. Cultural Competency Skills
5. Community Dimensions of Practice Skills
6. Public Health Sciences Skills
7. Financial Planning and Management Skills
8. Leadership and Systems Thinking Skills

The three workforce tiers include public health workers in the general job categories of Front Line Staff/Entry Level (Tier 1), Program Management/Supervisory Level (Tier 2), and Senior Management/Executive Level (Tier 3). Roles and responsibilities ascribed to these three tiers include the following:[12]

Tier 1—Front Line Staff/Entry Level. Tier 1 competencies apply to public health professionals who carry out the day-to-day tasks of public health organizations and are not in management positions. Responsibilities of these professionals may include data collection and analysis, fieldwork, program planning, outreach, communications, customer service, and program support.

Tier 2—Program Management/Supervisory Level. Tier 2 competencies apply to public health professionals in program management or supervisory roles.

Responsibilities of these professionals may include developing, implementing, and evaluating programs; supervising staff; establishing and maintaining community partnerships; managing timelines and work plans; making policy recommendations; and providing technical expertise.

Tier 3—Senior Management/Executive Level. Tier 3 competencies apply to public health professionals at a senior management level and to leaders of public health organizations. These professionals typically have staff who report to them and may be responsible for overseeing major programs or operations of the organization, setting a strategy and vision for the organization, deciding on the allocation of resources, creating a culture of quality within the organization, and working with the community to improve health.

An example of the specification of core competencies across these three tiers is provided below in Table B-2.

The full set of core competencies by tier is available on the COL website (go to www.phf.org and search under "Core Competencies for Public Health Professionals.")

Among other uses, the COL has provided a crosswalk between the Core Competencies and the 10 Essential Public Health Services.[13] The COL also provides a very useful compendium of examples of the Core Competencies in use. These examples can be accessed at www.phf.org by searching under "Examples of Core Competencies Use." In addition to these examples of core competencies in use, examples of, and research on, core competencies are increasingly present in the peer-reviewed literature. Such work circles back to and reinforces the linkages between academia and public health practice, as the evidence-base for core competencies grows. Examples of the recent peer-reviewed

TABLE B-2 Examples of Core Competencies by Workforce Tier

Domain: Analytical/Assessment Skills		
Tier 1	**Tier 2**	**Tier 3**
Selects valid and reliable data	Analyzes the validity and reliability of data	Evaluates the validity and reliability of data
Domain: Policy Development/Program Planning Skills		
Contributes to implementation of organizational strategic plan	Implements organizational strategic plan	Monitors implementation of organizational strategic plan

SOURCE: Council on Linkages between Academia and Public Health Practice. Core Competencies for Public Health Professionals. 2014. Available at http://www.phf.org/resourcestools/Documents/Core_Competencies_for_Public_Health_Professionals_2014June.pdf.

literature related to the Core Competencies include a study on the construct validity of core competencies,[14] application of the core competencies model,[15] congruence with competencies for public health nursing,[16] integration with preventive medicine residencies,[17] and building a tool to track leadership competencies in maternal and child health.[18]

In the future, training programs will need to continue to move beyond simply developing competencies to answering important questions such as: Do competencies matter? How do competencies need to evolve over time? How can workforce competencies inform the further development of competencies for academic programs, and vice-versa? And, how can competencies address training and preparation for the "major forces of change" described in Chapter 32?

REFERENCES

1. Council on Linkages between Academia and Public Health Practice. Core Competencies for Public Health Professionals. 2014; http://www.phf .org/programs/corecompetencies/Pages/About_ the_Core_Competencies_for_Public_Health_ Professionals.aspx. Accessed 12/11, 2014.

2. Calhoun JG, Ramiah K, Weist EM, Shortell SM. Development of a Core Competency Model for the Master of Public Health Degree. *Am J Public Health*. 2008/09/01 2008;98(9): 1598–1607.

3. Framing the Future: The Second Hundred Years of Education for Public Health Task Force, Association of Schools and Programs of Public Health. Master of Public Health Degree for the 21st Century: Key Considerations, Design Features, and Critical Content of the Core. 2014; http://www.aspph.org/educate/models/ mph-degree-report/. Accessed 12/11, 2014.

4. Calhoun JG, McElligott JE, Weist EM, Raczynski JM. Core Competencies for Doctoral Education in Public Health. *Am J Public Health*. 2012/01/01 2011;102(1):22-29.

5. Framing the Future: The Second Hundred Years of Education for Public Health Task Force, Association of Schools and Programs of Public Health. DrPH for the 21st Century 2014.

6. Council of State and Territorial Epidemiologists. Competencies for Applied Epidemiologists in Governmental Public Health Agencies. 2014; http://www.cste.org/group/CSTECDCAEC. Accessed 10/19, 2014.

7. Birkhead GS, Davies J, Miner K, Lemmings J, Koo D. Developing competencies for applied epidemiology: from process to product. *Public Health Reports*. 2008:67–118.

8. Institute of Medicine. *The Future of Public Health*. Washington, D.C.: National Academy Press; 1988.

9. Public Health Foundation. Public Health Faculty/ Agency Forum 2014; http://www.phf.org/ programs/council/Pages/PublicHealthFaculty_ AgencyForum.aspx. Accessed 12/17, 2014.

10. Public Health Foundation. Council on Linkages Between Academia and Public Health Practice 2014; http://www.phf.org/programs/council/ Pages/default.aspx. Accessed 12/17, 2014.

11. Council on Linkages between Academia and Public Health Practice. Core Competencies for Public Health Professionals 2014; http://www.phf .org/programs/corecompetencies/Pages/About_ the_Core_Competencies_for_Public_Health_ Professionals.aspx. Accessed 12/17, 2014.

12. Council on Linkages between Academia and Public Health Practice. Core Competencies for Public Health Professionals. 2014; http://www.phf.org/ resourcestools/Documents/Core_Competencies_ for_Public_Health_Professionals_2014June.pdf. Accessed 12/20, 2014.

13. Council on Linkages between Academia and Public Health Practice. Crosswalk: Core Competencies for Public Health Professionals & the Essential Public Health Services. 2010; http://www.phf .org/resourcestools/Documents/Crosswalk_ corecompetencies_and_essential_services.pdf. Accessed 12/17, 2014.

14. Edgar M, Mayer JP, Scharff DP. Construct validity of the core competencies for public health professionals. *J Public Health Manag Pract*. Jul–Aug 2009;15(4):E7–16.

15. Stewart KE, Halverson PK, Rose AV, Walker SK. Public health workforce training: application of the Council on Linkages' core competencies. *J Public Health Manag Pract*. Sep–Oct 2010;16(5):465–469.

16. Polivka BJ, Chaudry RV, Jones A. Congruence between position descriptions for public health nursing directors and supervisors with national professional standards and competencies. *J Public Health Manag Pract*. Mar–Apr 2014;20(2):224–235.

17. Wells EV, Sarigiannis AN, Boulton ML. Assessing integration of clinical and public health skills in preventive medicine residencies: using competency mapping. *Am J Prev Med*. Jun 2012;42(6 Suppl 2):S107–116.

18. Grason H, Huebner C, Crawford AK, et al. The MCH Navigator: Tools for MCH Workforce Development and Lifelong Learning. *Matern Child Health J*. Aug 1 2014.

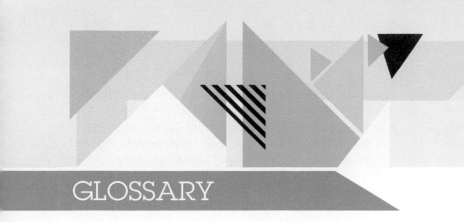

GLOSSARY

45 CFR 46 Also known as the Common Rule, this legislation established the role of institutional review boards (IRBs) for research on human subjects. See also *common rule*.

accessibility Includes availability as well as quality, affordability, variety, and cultural acceptability. For example, if healthier foods are available but are too expensive for the local consumers, then the healthier items are not accessible.

accidents An unscientific term applied to unintended events that may result in injury; the term has caused injuries to be considered by many to be unpredictable and therefore unpreventable.

accountability A means of assuring the quality and availability of public health services.

accountable care organization (ACO) An ACO is a network of doctors and hospitals that agrees to be held accountable for improving the health of its patients while reducing the rate of growth in health care spending and sharing some level of financial risk. An ACO can be held responsible not just for the health of its patients, but also for the health of the population of the community in which it operates.

accreditation A process for external, reliable, and objective validation of agency performance against a specific set of standards, and some form of reward or recognition for agencies meeting those standards.

acquired immunodeficiency syndrome (AIDS) A profound deficiency in host immunity. AIDS was first recognized in 1981 when several large U.S. cities noticed cases of *Pneumocystis* pneumonia and Kaposi's sarcoma in young gay men. HIV itself was first identified by French scientists in 1983 and verified as the cause of AIDS in 1984.

action planning The action planning process includes determining the stakeholders and public who represent the community who may have a stake in this issue, with consideration for shared ownership. This is followed by a more thorough analysis of the issue including the assets and strengths available within the community.

addiction A chronic relapsing medical condition in which a user/abuser does not have control over his or her drug or alcohol use.

administrative law The body of law created by administrative agencies through rules, regulations, orders, and decisions.

advocacy The process of supporting a particular cause or policy, which often involves the ability to advance the policy implications of public health research.

Affordable Care Act The Patient Protection and Affordable Care Act (ACA), passed in 2010, is the landmark legislation that is often referred to as "health reform" in the United States.

agendas The "list" of issues that are under active consideration for policy change or policy action. The agenda is limited by the scale and scope of the formal policy process, which is, in turn, restricted by time (e.g., the number of days in a legislative session, the election cycle), by the degree to which people can focus on a limited number of issues, and by the available resources that can be directed to a problem or issue (e.g., the budget or available income, resources, or staff).

air pollution Contamination of the air by emissions or some other form of noxious airborne agents or materials.

Amerindians Native populations in the Caribbean Islands. Amerindians originally inhabited Puerto Rico and the U.S. Virgin Islands; following Columbus's landing in 1493, these Caribbean islands became European colonies for several centuries.

analytic epidemiology The aspect of epidemiology concerned with the search for health-related causes and effects. Uses comparison groups, which provide baseline data, to quantify the association between exposures and outcomes, and test hypotheses about causal relationships.

applied ethics Prescribed actions or policies in ethical situations commonly encountered in a particular profession.

Area Health Education Centers (AHEC) Created in 1971, they enhance training of health care providers to work in underserved areas by recruiting and training minority students and students of lower socioeconomic status for health careers.

assessments A core function of public health, whereby public health agencies regularly and systematically collect, assemble, analyze, and make available information on the health of the community, including statistics on health status, community health needs, and epidemiologic and other studies of health problems.

availability Regarding healthy eating, the term refers to the proximity of food retail or food service venues to residential areas and the presence of healthier foods within these venues.

behavioral health The mental well-being of a person, with a particular focus on lifestyles that are associated with preventable and premature deaths.

behavioral risk factors Characteristics that raise the risk of behavioral health problems, including poverty, incarceration, unemployment, availability of illegal drugs, and social isolation, as well as individual level behaviors that increase health risks, such as use of tobacco, being physically inactive, and consuming excess calories.

Belmont Report A report on research ethics published in 1979 by the National Commission for the Protection of Human Subjects of Biomedical and Behavioral Research.

bioaccumulate The biological processes which result in the heightened concentration of contaminants as they proceed "up" the food chain.

bioethics To some, this term is synonymous with ethics related to all living or health-related things. Most often, it is closely aligned more narrowly with medical ethics.

Biosafety Level (BSL) In the United States, laboratory facilities are designated as BSL 1, 2, 3 or 4 according to safety practice guidelines and standards, and guidelines for air handling systems and construction. These levels are distinguished by the ability of laboratory practices and building design to control exposure to hazardous biological, chemical, and radiological agents.

built environment The human-made space in which people live, work, and recreate on a day-to-day basis. The built environment often consists of two major components: land use patterns and the transportation system.

capacity building The processes of strengthening the potential for communities, organizations, or even individuals to achieve optimal development.

Center for Medicare and Medicaid Innovation Population health initiative established under the Affordable Care Act, meant to serve as a testing ground for innovative payment and service delivery models. The goal of testing these new models of care is to reduce Medicare and Medicaid expenditures while preserving or improving the quality of care provided to beneficiaries under these publicly funded health insurance programs.

certification Completion of education or other requirements to practice a profession.

chronic disease management The combination of medical, behavioral, and mental health efforts in prevention and treatment of diseases that are long-lasting and not necessarily curable.

chronic diseases Persistent and lasting medical conditions that may be controlled rather than cured.

civic engagement The act of connecting with one's fellow citizens through (usually) community action.

climate change An atmospheric phenomenon ultimately caused by human activities that raise atmospheric carbon dioxide. It is characterized by extreme shifts in the weather, often linked to record high and low temperatures. These shifts include droughts and floods that can impact vast global regions. The change being observed is a measurable increase in the global temperature.

Clinical Laboratory Improvement Amendments Act of 1988 (CLIA '88) A federal licensure of laboratories that perform testing on human specimens.

clinical preventive services Interventions used in clinical settings intended to promote good health and prevent disease and injury. The U.S. Preventive Services Task Force provides recommendations for which clinical preventive services should be implemented and under what conditions.

coalitions Unions of people and organizations working to influence outcomes on a specific problem.

Compacts of Free Association Palau, the Marshall Islands, and the Federated States of Micronesia (comprising the districts of Pohnpei, Kosrae, Yap, and Chuuk) negotiated treaties with the United States, known as the Compacts of Free Association. These three countries are now known as the Freely Associated States (FAS). The compact agreements include protection under and hegemony by the U.S. military, free migration of citizens to and from the United States, the provision of American development "compact funding," and eligibility for many domestic, federally funded programs and technical assistance from the U.S. Department of Health and Human Services agencies.

competencies The skills, knowledge, and abilities to perform specific tasks or carry out certain functions. They form the cornerstone of efforts by schools and programs of public health, governmental public health agencies, and many public health professional groups to more systematically ensure that public health workers are equipped with the appropriate level of skills and knowledge to competently and effectively carry out their work.

common rule This federal regulation established the role of institutional review boards (IRBs) for research on human subjects. See also *45 CFR 46*.

community A group of people, for example, a neighborhood, village, or municipal or rural region, or a social group with a unifying common interest or trait, loosely organized into a recognizable unit.[1]

community development The process of people working together to affect locally determined issues/goals and the conditions that affect them.

community development workforce Sectors essential to community health development include: employers and businesses; academia; media; governmental public health agencies; the health care delivery system; nonprofit, nongovernmental, voluntary, and social entities, including ethnic and cultural groups; advocacy organizations; and the faith community.

community empowerment Enabling and supporting communities in achieving greater control over their lives.

community health The health and well-being of communities, or groups of individuals.

community needs assessment A structured process that involves identifying health issues (the needs of the community), and usually followed by searching for, developing, implementing, and evaluating interventions to address needs.

Community-Oriented Primary Care (COPC) A variation of the primary care model in which major health problems of a defined population are identified and addressed through modifications in both primary care services and other appropriate community health programs.

community water fluoridation The adjustment of the fluoride level in a public water supply that is optimal for oral health. See *fluoridation* and *water fluoridation*.

core functions (of public health) As defined by the Institute of Medicine (IOM), the three core functions are: assessment, policy development, and assurance. This is what public health must do in order to achieve its mission of assuring conditions in which people can be healthy.

cost-benefit analysis (CBA) A type of economic analysis in which all costs and benefits are converted into monetary (dollar) values and results are expressed as either the net present value or the benefits per dollars expended.

cost-effectiveness analysis (CEA) A type of economic evaluation in which all costs are related to a single, common effect. Results are usually stated as additional cost expended per additional health outcome achieved.

countermeasures Actions taken to avoid or respond to an incident.

deliberation The process of establishing intent and resolve, where a person or group explores different solutions before settling on a specific course of action.

dengue A viral illness that is transmitted by mosquitoes, usually occurring in tropical areas. Severe dengue is known as dengue hemorrhagic fever.

dental caries An infection and destructive process that results in decalcification of the enamel of teeth, which leads to destruction (cavities) of enamel and dentin and eventually the death of the tooth's nerve and blood supply, if not treated.

dental sealants A thin plastic and protective coating that is applied to the biting surfaces of the back teeth, usually the first and second permanent molars. The sealant protects the tooth from getting a cavity by shielding against bacteria and plaque.

descriptive epidemiology The study of the amount and distribution of a disease in a specified population by person, place, and time.

disasters Natural or man-made hazards that result in ecologic disruptions, or emergencies, of a severity and magnitude resulting in deaths, injuries, illness, and/or property damage that cannot be effectively managed by the application of routine procedures or resources and that result in a call for outside assistance.

disease prevention The deferral or elimination of specific illnesses and conditions by one or more interventions of proven efficacy.

Doctors of Osteopathy (DOs) Physicians whose training is similar to Medical Doctors, although osteopathic medicine emphasizes the musculoskeletal system and manipulative therapy.

early childhood decay Another term for early childhood caries.

economic globalization The growing interdependence of economies across the world through reductions in trade barriers between countries and the resulting increased flow of goods, services, and capital across countries.

economic inequality A difference in relative income experienced by a population, at either a national or local level. The term is related to the socioeconomic gradient, the steepness of which may be associated with disparities in health status.

edentulism The term used to describe complete tooth loss.

emergency management The organization of a response to disasters through multiple jurisdictions, agencies, and authorities.

emerging infectious diseases New infections resulting from changes or evolution of existing organisms, known infections spreading to new geographic areas or populations, previously unrecognized infections appearing in areas undergoing ecologic transformation, and old infections reemerging as a result of antimicrobial resistance in known agents or breakdowns in public health measures.

energy Kinetic energy (the energy of motion) is the agent of most injuries, such as lacerations and concussions; other injuries such as burns result from thermal, electrical, or chemical energy or ionizing radiation, and some result from interference with energy exchanges such as oxygen use (e.g., drowning) and thermal regulation (freezing).

enumeration A process of identifying the number and types of workers in a specific industry or professional domain. In public health, enumeration is being used to identify the numbers, demographics, and skills and training of workers currently employed in public health agencies or organizations.

environmental change An alteration to the physical environment: adding sidewalks or bike paths, building a new street or park, or adding promotional displays for healthier foods in grocery stores or restaurants.

Environmental Public Health Performance Standards (EnvPHPS) Model standards that provide measurement indicators for assessing and identifying where performance and quality improvement of Environmental Essential Public Health Services are needed.

environmental sustainability The capacity or ability to maintain the quality of the environment.

epidemiological transition A change in the pattern of disease in a country away from infectious diseases toward degenerative or chronic diseases.

epidemiological triad The interaction of the agent, the host (the individual), and the environment (the community). For some diseases (e.g., many zoonotic diseases) a fourth element—vector (e.g., ticks)—is added.

equal protection This requires that people in similar situations be treated similarly. If groups are treated differently, there must be a credible and substantive reason. The Equal Protection Clause is part of the Fourteenth Amendment to the U.S. Constitution.

essential environmental public health services (EEPHS) The Ten Essential Public Health Services as they pertain to the environment.

evaluation A process that attempts to determine as systematically and objectively as possible the relevance, effectiveness, and impact of activities in light of their objectives.

event An occurrence that may result in injury. (Events are what many people would refer to as accidents.)

evidence-based medicine (EBM) The use of evidence to drive medical decision making. The doctrine of evidence-based medicine (EBM) was formally introduced in 1992. Its origins can be traced back to the seminal work of Cochrane, who noted that many medical treatments lacked scientific effectiveness. A basic tenet of EBM is to deemphasize unsystematic clinical experience and place greater emphasis on evidence from clinical research. This approach requires new skills, such as efficient literature searching and an understanding of types of evidence in evaluating the clinical literature.

evidence-based public health (EBPH) The process of integrating science-based interventions with community preferences to improve population health. Key components of EBPH include: making decisions based on the best available, peer-reviewed evidence; using data and information systems systematically; applying program planning frameworks; engaging the community in decision making; conducting sound evaluation; and disseminating what is learned.

exposure pathways The mechanisms or routes through which exposure to infectious agents, toxins, contaminants, pollutants, etc. may occur and produce disease.

family medicine The branch of medicine that focuses on all family members, irrespective of gender and age; a large component of primary care as it is practiced in the United States.

family planning The deliberate effort by women and couples to determine the number of conceptions the woman will have and the timing of those conceptions.

federal regulation A rule or order issued by a federal executive-branch department or administrative agency, generally under authority granted by statute, which enforces or amplifies laws enacted by the legislature and has the force of law.

federal role The activities or responsibilities of the agencies and organizations within the federal government.

federalism This describes the division of power between the federal government and state governments. The basis of federalism is the Tenth Amendment to the U.S. Constitution, which states that any powers not "delegated to the United States by the Constitution, nor prohibited by it to the States, are reserved to the States respectively, or to the people."

Federally Qualified Health Centers (FQHCs) Health Centers that meet the criteria for and receive federal funding for the services they provide under Section 330 of the Public Health Services Act.

first responder Term used to describe the first medically trained responder(s) to arrive on the scene of an emergency (i.e., police, fire, EMS, and emergency management agencies).

foodborne disease (or illness) A group of diseases caused by contamination of food by disease-causing agents, typically pathogenic organisms and their toxins.[1]

forces of change Forces that have the potential to significantly impact public health practice well into the future.

foundational public health services Comprised of the Foundational Capacities and Areas; a suite of skills, programs/activities that must be available in state/local health departments system-wide.

Freely Associated States (FAS) Tropical island groups in the Pacific which include the Federated States of Micronesia, Republic of Palau, and Republic of the Marshall Islands.

Geographic Information System (GIS) GIS is a tool for capturing, managing, analyzing, and presenting geographically referenced data. A GIS facilitates the examination of spatial relationships, the identification of spatial and temporal patterns and trends, and the display of complex relationships in a more intuitive form. This can advance the understanding of complex systems, support better communication and collaboration, and improve decision-making by integrating and analyzing geo-referenced data from different sources.

global burden of diseases (GBD) An approach launched by the World Health Organization in 1991 with the aim of systematically and consistently collecting and assessing comprehensive epidemiological data on the main diseases and injuries and risks worldwide.

global health Field at the intersection of several disciplines— epidemiology, economics, demography, and sociology—that is concerned with international health issues. The term *global health*, as opposed to *international health*, implies consideration of the health needs of the people of the whole planet above the concerns of particular nations.

global health governance The formal and informal institutions, rules, and processes by states, intergovernmental organizations, and non-state actors to deal with challenges to health that require crossborder collective action to address effectively.

globalization The act of spreading across the globe; globalization is not only concerned by different flows (e.g., people, goods, money, and information) around the world but also with institutional arrangements that seek to deal with these flows.

governance Where the ultimate authority for, or control of, agency activities resides.

government-to-government relationship President Bill Clinton's Executive Order issued on April 29, 1994, directed the heads of each executive department to operate within a government-to-government relationship with federally recognized tribal governments to consult with tribes prior to taking actions that affect the tribes, to assess the impacts of federal activities on tribal trust resources, and to take steps to remove barriers that impede working directly with tribal governments.

harm reduction An action intended to reduce the potential for harm; e.g., making clean needles available to injectors via needle and syringe provision programs.

health behavior change A process which involves planning, intervention, and evaluation for the purposes of modifying a behavior to produce a different health outcome.

Health-care-acquired infections (HAIs) Infections that are acquired in a health care setting, such as in a hospital.

health disparities Differing levels of health indicators that are observed among segments of a population, discernible in the size of the health gap between the highest and lowest segment of the population.

health equity Health equity is the attainment of the highest level of health for all people. Achieving health equity requires valuing everyone equally with focused and ongoing societal efforts to address avoidable inequalities, historical and contemporary injustices, and the elimination of health and healthcare disparities.

health impact assessment (HIA) A process for assessing the impact of policies, plans, projects, or activities on health.

Health in All Policies A collaborative approach that integrates and articulates health considerations into policymaking and programming across sectors, and at all levels, to improve the health of all communities and people.

health inequities Differences related to health access, utilization, and outcomes that are unfair and unjust. This is in contrast to "health disparities," which simply indicates a difference in health that may or may not be related to fairness and justice.

Health Professional Shortage Areas (HPSAs) Primary care HPSAs are defined as having fewer than one full-time-equivalent (FTE) primary care physician for each 3,500 residents (with some variation under circumstances, e.g., poverty or language, that increase barriers to medical care).

health system transformation Fundamental changes to the inputs and processes of multiple levels of health and healthcare, for the purpose of producing improvements in outcomes.

human immunodeficiency virus (HIV) The agent that invades its human host and reproduces inside host immune system cells (*CD4 T-lymphocytes*) to produce a profound deficiency in host immunity known as acquired immunodeficiency syndrome (AIDS).

human mobility The movement of people, either voluntary or forced. It is estimated that each year more than two billion people travel on long geographic distances of which more than 1.2 billion cross national borders. This includes international tourism; migration for economic, environmental, and other reasons; and, global forced displacement including refugees, asylum-seekers, and internally displaced people.

human rights A philosophical and political view that every human being has equal dignity and worth and thus must be ensured certain resources necessary for life and protection against certain harms.

illegal use Refers to taking drugs without a prescription for some socially sanctioned purpose (e.g., using an amphetamine to work all night).

illegal recreational use Includes taking drugs without a prescription to achieve a specific mental or psychic state (e.g., taking heroin to get high).

immunization Use of a vaccine to produce humoral/antibody protection against diseases. One of the most important interventions for the control and prevention of infectious diseases. Globally, immunization has resulted in the eradication of smallpox and the near-eradication of poliomyelitis as well as preventing millions of deaths due to other diseases.

implementation The act of doing; putting into action.

Incident Command System (ICS) The standard management structure used in disaster response across the United States.

Indian health system The Indian health system, also called the "I/T/U," is inclusive of the three models for delivering health services. The "I" represents services provided by the Indian Health Services (IHS), "T" represents the programs and services operated by the tribes under the Indian Self-Determination and Education Assistance Act (ISDEAA) authorization, and "U" represents urban centers as authorized under Title V in the Indian Health Care Improvement Act.

infant mortality Deaths in the first year of life per 1,000 live births.

informatics Encompasses the many and varied aspects of managing, using, and sharing information to promote decision making in assessment, priority setting, quality and effectiveness of work activities, and evaluation. Informatics draws from computer science, information technology, engineering, social and cognitive psychology, library science, and administration because all influence the processing and use of information.

informed consent Ensuring voluntary participation in research on human subjects. Potential study participants must be informed of all the likely risks and benefits of the research before they consent to participate.

injuries Bodily damage related to acute exposure to some form of energy (kinetic, potential, or other) in amounts and at rates that exceed the individual's tolerance threshold.

injury prevention or control Intervention(s) aimed at preventing the initial event or blocking progression of the injury-producing process.

innovation New or original.

institutional review boards (IRBs) An officially sanctioned group that reviews and monitors ethical aspects of research, especially the protection of human subjects.

insular jurisdictions Island communities.

integration The act of joining, melding, or meshing.

interprofessional (IP) Between professions; e.g., interprofessional education involves educational activities that are shared or jointly experienced by different professions.

intervention Efforts taken to reduce or stop drug or alcohol use after initiation of use.

I/T/U (Indian Health Service, Tribally-Operated Programs, Urban Indian Clinics) The Indian health system, also called the "I/T/U," is inclusive of the three models for delivering health services. The "I" represents services provided by the IHS, "T" represents the programs and services operated by the tribes under ISDEAA authorization, and "U" represents urban centers as authorized under Title V in the Indian Health Care Improvement Act.

laboratory information management system (LIMS) Electronic systems which can take data directly from the instrumentation that is used for testing and, in addition to providing results, provide the quality assurance information needed to initiate results reporting and package the data for the initial laboratory analysis performed before a report is issued.

leadership Leadership is creativity in action. It is the ability to see the present in terms of the future while maintaining respect for the past. Leadership is based on respect for history and the knowledge that true growth builds on existing strengths.

Leading Health Indicators (LHI) A subset of *Healthy People 2020* objectives; primary public health concerns in the United States that were chosen based on their ability to motivate action, the availability of data to measure their progress, and their relevance as broad public health issues.

legal use Drug use that includes over-the-counter or prescription drugs.

legal recreational drug use The use of government-sanctioned psychoactive substances to achieve a specific mental or psychic state (e.g., drinking alcohol to get intoxicated).

licensure The act of obtaining a license. Some health professionals are required to obtain a state license by passing an examination in order to practice their profession. Examples common among public health workers include M.D. licenses for physicians, R.N. licenses for nurses, R.S. licenses for sanitarians, and R.D. licenses for dietitians. Maintaining licensure generally requires the worker to complete training courses to achieve a minimum number of continuing education credits within specific time intervals and then report those credits periodically to a state licensing board.

local health department An administrative or service unit of local or state government concerned with health and carrying some responsibility for the health of a jurisdiction smaller than the state.

Local Public Health System (LPHS) The consortium of agencies, institutions, and individuals whose work and activities impact community health status.

management The process of dealing with or controlling things or people.

maternal mortality Maternal deaths per 100,000 live births.

maternal mortality review (MMR) committees Formally organized groups that review all maternal deaths for the purpose of identifying potential points of intervention to prevent future deaths.

meaningful use The common term for the Centers for Medicare and Medicaid Services' Electronic Health Care Record (EHR) Incentive Programs, which incentivizes eligible hospitals, critical access hospitals, and eligible professionals to adopt, implement, and upgrade certified EHR systems to demonstrate meaningful use of these technologies. Meaningful use was enacted as a section of the American Recovery and Reinvestment Act of 2009 known as HITECH (Health Information Technology for Economic and Clinical Health).

Medicaid expansion An expansion of the Medicaid program under the ACA gives states the ability to expand Medicaid to cover *all* adults living up to 138% of the federal poverty level.

medical ethics Ethics applied to interactions between clinicians and patients. Common concerns include the autonomy of the patient and the obligation of the clinician to not knowingly harm the patient.

metabolic disease A group of diseases, including diabetes, that are characterized by abnormal metabolic processes.

models Representations of physical structures or processes and the interactions among these structures and processes that are meant more to describe and logically link phenomena together than to imply broader meanings underlying them.

modifiable Modifiable behaviors include choices about using health care services, and lifestyle habits that affect health, such as diet, physical activity, smoking, substance abuse, and sexual behavior.

morally defensible decision A decision with ethical implications that was determined by a fair process and took into account ethically important factors relevant to the situation.

multidisciplinary teams Work groups composed of or combining several usually separate fields of expertise.

National Center for Health Statistics (NCHS) NCHS is the primary federal government agency responsible for collecting, analyzing, and distributing data on health and health care. NCHS provides free downloadable public-use data files to researchers, teachers, students, and others through its Public-Use Data Files and Documentation site. NCHS also houses the Health Indicators Warehouse (HIW), which serves as a federal data hub for the U.S. Department of Health and Human Services' health data initiative.

National Prevention, Health Promotion and Public Health Council (NPC) Authorized under the ACA and chaired by the Surgeon General of the United States, the Council comprises 20 cabinet-level agencies and other offices across the federal government and is charged with incorporating a prevention perspective into the work of the member agencies.

National Prevention Strategy An ACA mandate of the National Prevention Council; released June 16, 2011, aims to guide our nation in the most effective and achievable means for improving health. Focuses on "community prevention" in ways that recognize two key points: (i) that some of the most important determinants of health are structural or "upstream," and (ii) that addressing these factors requires a cross-sector, "health in all policies" approach with a particular focus on policy and systems to create long-lasting "environmental" change.

National Public Health Performance Standards Program (NPHPSP) Launched by the Centers for Disease Control and Prevention in 2002, it includes a set of performance standards for local and state public health systems along with measures and surveillance instruments that track progress relative to these standards, focused on the 10 Essential Public Health Services.

newborn screening Screening panels characterized by the need for early postpartum detection so appropriate medical and, often dietary, treatment can be implemented to prevent serious, possibly life-threatening consequences for affected individuals.

nonmodifiable Individual characteristics that cannot be changed, such as age, race, and genotype.

nutrition assistance programs Includes the Special Supplemental Nutrition Program for Women, Infants, and Children (WIC) and the Supplemental Nutrition Assistance Program (SNAP).

objectives What one is trying to achieve; a thing aimed at or sought.

ONPRIME model A health behavior change and evaluation model that emphasizes the importance of seven process substeps: Organization, Needs/Resources Assessment, Priority Setting, Research, Interventions, Monitoring, and Evaluation.

oral health workforce Those who are engaged in the provision of oral health care, including dentists, dental hygienists, dental assistants, laboratory technicians, and office personnel.

outbreak investigation A process for identifying the cause of disease that is experienced in excess of the expected. Outbreak investigation involves seven major steps:

1. Confirm whether there truly is an epidemic.

2. Identify the illness involved.

3. Enumerate all cases and characterize them according to time, place, and person.

4. Confirm the diagnosis.

5. Formulate a hypothesis about the cause of the epidemic and the means of transmission, and test that hypothesis.

6. Take control measures to end the epidemic.

7. Prepare and disseminate a report about the epidemic.

PDSA cycle For Plan-Do-Study-Act. Describes how to test a change—by trying it, observing the consequences, and then learning from those consequences.

performance management The practice of using performance measures on an ongoing basis to improve the operation of a program, organization, or delivery system.

periodontal diseases An infection of the tissues that support the teeth, classified according to the severity of the disease. The two major stages are gingivitis and periodontitis.

police powers The power of the state to protect the health, safety, morals, and general welfare of the people. The police power is the power to restrict the liberty of individuals to protect other individuals. Communicable disease laws are enacted under the police power.

policy "All the rules" that guide behavior or people and institutions. These can be customs or they can be very specific procedure manuals or regulatory guidance based on general laws or statutes.

policy, systems, and environmental interventions Strategies to "change the context." "Policy" can include formal policies such as laws, executive orders, and regulatory measures, or informal policies such as a company's rules. "Systems" are organizations or institutions such as schools, transportation networks, parks and recreation facilities, and health care providers. "Environmental" are actions that pertain to both the built and natural environment, as well as the immediate context of an issue, and the policies that may influence such action.

policy making A "people process" of creating or establishing policy.

politics The process that decides who gets what, when, and how. Politics operates at many levels and in many places and institutions. Politics are invoked when there are things to be distributed or taken away from people and institutions.

population-based An approach that targets a population as the subject instead of the individual.

population health The health of groups or many people, usually referring to all people within a given jurisdiction, as opposed to individual-level health.

poverty A state of deprivation of those things that determine the quality of life, including food, income, clothing, shelter, and feeling in control of one's own choices.

practice-based research Research that takes place in a practice setting, e.g., in a local public health department, as opposed to a highly controlled research laboratory.

practice-based research networks (PBRNs) Partnerships between state and local public health agency practitioners and researchers. Initiated with five networks in 2008 with the support of the Robert Wood Johnson Foundation, now expanded to cover 28 states with over 1,000 state and local health departments included.

preemption Overriding of one level of authority by another; e.g., federal preemption means that federal law overrides state or local laws. The basis of "preemption" is the Supremacy Clause of the U.S. Constitution (Article VI, clause 2). Where a state and federal law conflict, the federal law preempts the state law. Generally, preemption assures national uniformity and sets a minimal standard of protection, allowing state and local governments to enact greater levels of protection of the public's health.

Pregnancy Risk Assessment Monitoring System (PRAMS) Surveillance system maintained by the states, with federal sponsorship and funding administered by the CDC.

preparedness Phase in comprehensive emergency management where officials or the public plan a response to potential disasters.

Prevention and Public Health Fund (PPHF) Created by the ACA, an allocation of reliable, mandatory funding designated specifically for public health and prevention, in addition to the funds made available through the regular appropriations process.

prevention effectiveness The systematic assessment of the impact of prevention policies, programs, and practices on health outcomes.

primary health care Social concept defined as essential health care that should be made available to everyone.

procedural due process A legal doctrine in the United States that requires government officials to follow fair procedures before depriving a person of life, liberty, or property. Required by the Due Process Clauses of the Fifth and Fourteenth Amendments to the U.S. Constitution.

professionals A person in a skilled occupation requiring formal training or education; a person who is an expert in his or her work.

public deliberation The open engagement of individuals regarding the issues that shape their public life. Public deliberation is grounded in philosophies of the social contract and bonds among individuals and institutions that shape societies' political and social life.

public health An organized activity of society to promote, protect, improve, and, when necessary, restore the health of individuals, specified groups, or the entire population. It is a combination of sciences, skills, and values that function through collective societal activities and involve programs, services, and institutions aimed at protecting and improving the health of all the people.

public health ethics Ethics applied to interactions between a public health agency and the population it serves. Common concerns are the interdependence of individuals and the tensions between the rights of individuals and the good of the community.

public health informatics The systematic application of information and computer science and technology to public health practice, research, and learning.

public health infrastructure Includes but is not limited to workforce, data and information systems, communications, partnerships, policy, and organizational competencies (e.g., leadership/governance). This is fundamental to the provision and execution of public health services at all levels; it provides the capacity to prepare for and respond to both acute (emergency) and chronic (ongoing) threats to the nation's health.

public health finance The fiscal operations and funding mechanisms of public health agencies.

public health governance The institutions, organizations, or boards that oversee the functions and activities of public health practice agencies.

public health laboratory system Includes laboratories that provide services or perform testing for biological, chemical, and radiological agents of public health significance.

public health practice The application of knowledge, skills, and competencies necessary to perform essential public health services and other activities to protect and improve the public's health.

public health services and systems research (PHSSR) A field of study that examines the organization, financing, and delivery of public health services within communities, and the impact of these services on public health.

public health system The constellation of governmental and nongovernmental organizations that contribute to the performance of essential public health services for a defined community or population.

quality assurance A system of activities and monitoring intended to provide the most accurate test result possible.

quality improvement Formal methods to improve service delivery.

quality improvement (QI) techniques Techniques that are specifically developed to help close gaps between current and desired performances of an organization.

quarantine Separating individuals who have been exposed to a communicable disease from the non-exposed (healthy) population. Such individuals have the potential to develop disease but are not (yet) symptomatic. The word comes from the Italian (seventeenth century) language *quarantena*, meaning a 40-day period.

research The application of systematic methods to discover, interpret, and advance human knowledge of our world and the universe.

response Phase in comprehensive emergency management where relief is followed by recovery, including reconstruction of the community. Emergency relief activities include saving lives, providing first aid, restoring emergency communications and transportation systems, and providing immediate care and basic needs to survivors, such as food and clothing or medical and emotional care.

Section 2713 The section of the ACA that includes specific coverage requirements for clinical preventive services.

sexually transmitted diseases (STDs) More than two dozen diseases with a variety of causal agents that are transmitted from person to person by direct contact. These pathogens reside in the genital tract and/or blood and other body fluids and are transmitted principally through sexual activities.

Siracusa Principles A set of four principles, established at a meeting in Siracusa Italy, regarding internationally recognized limitations on human rights.

social capital The collective value of relationships and networks within a community, as well as the benefits that accrue when people or organizations "do for each other" (also known as norms of reciprocity).

social class A hierarchy within society or culture that differentiates the power of individuals based on their occupation, education, income, wealth, property, ancestry, or religion.

social determinants (of health) The economic and social conditions under which people live that largely determine their health status.

social media Forms of social interaction, communication, and networking, usually through electronic devices (including cellular telephones).

social reform Movements that are organized for the purpose of improving social conditions, including housing, employment, and education.

socioeconomic factors Factors such as income, education, housing, and employment status.

stakeholders People who have a particular concern, interest, or claim a legitimate role in an activity, organization, or project.

state health agency The agency of state government that has primary responsibility for public health in the state, a term adopted by the Association of State and Territorial Health Officials (ASTHO).

substance abuse The use of a psychoactive substance for a nontherapeutic effect.

substantive due process The legal principle which allows federal courts to protect certain rights deemed fundamental from government interference under the authority of the due process clauses of the Fifth and Fourteenth Amendments to the U.S. Constitution.

Surgeon General The operational head of the U.S. Public Health Service Commissioned Corps, often referred to as "The Nation's Doctor," and considered the leading governmental public health spokesperson.

surveillance The ongoing systematic collection and timely analysis, interpretation, and communication of health information for the purpose of disease prevention and control.

supply reduction Policies in the United States that target two major approaches to reduce drug supply: law enforcement to arrest drug dealers, and border control.

synergy The combining of actions or forces which result in a product or outcome that is greater than the simple sum of the separate parts.

systematic review A review of a clearly formulated question that uses systematic and explicit methods to identify, select, and critically appraise relevant research, and to collect and analyze data from the studies that are included in the review, the goal of which is an unbiased assessment of a particular topic. Statistical methods (meta-analysis) may or may not be used to analyze and summarize the results of the included studies. It also systematically assesses the quality of identified papers (often based on the design and execution of component studies).

systems change Reforming the procedures or principles of organizations or communities regarding how they address programs, policies, and allocation of resources.

Ten Essential Services of Public Health Provides a fundamental framework for describing the public health activities that should be undertaken by public health professionals in all communities. The Core Public Health Functions Steering Committee developed the framework for the Essential Services in 1994. This Steering Committee included representatives from U.S. Public Health Service agencies and other major public health organizations.

tribal sovereignty Federal doctrine whereby each tribe is treated as a nation within a nation, the status of which is recognized either through a formal treaty or an executive order.

triple aim Defined by the federal Centers for Medicare and Medicaid Services as "better care for patients, better health for our communities, and lower costs."

trust responsibility In reference to Native Americans, a legal obligation under which the United States "has charged itself with moral obligations of the highest responsibility and trust" toward Indian tribes (*Seminole Nation v. United States*, 1942).

tuberculosis A bacterial disease caused by *Mycobacterium tuberculosis*.

Turning Point Model A foundation-funded effort to link public health agencies and their partners to other sectors of the community to better affect the underlying social causes of poor health and quality of life.

tyranny of the majority A liability or danger of utilitarianism in which a minority in the population suffers from a decision to benefit the majority.

umbrella agency A type of state-health agency with an overarching organizational structure consisting of two or more governmental functions, such as public health and social service programs or environmental quality, with a single appointed director who reports to the chief elected official such as a mayor, county commissioner, or governor.

Universal Declaration of Human Rights A United Nations statement of the minimum protection and benefits due to each human being, drafted in 1948.

utilitarianism The philosophical view that the right thing to do is that which provides the greatest good to the greatest number of people.

vehicles (or vectors) Typically transfer energy to the host, resulting in injuries. *Vehicles* are the inanimate objects that transmit the energy (e.g., cars, matches, guns), whereas *vectors* are the plants, animals, or persons that transmit the energy (e.g., biting animals, poisonous snakes, human fists).

voluntary health organizations An industry comprised of establishments engaged in raising funds for health-related research, health education, and patient services.

vulnerable individuals People who are particularly susceptible to research abuses related to constrained possibilities for informed consent. Minors, pregnant women (or fetuses), and prisoners are most commonly considered vulnerable.

war on poverty The popular name given to organized efforts during President Lyndon Johnson's administration to address the root causes of poverty and improve the conditions of those experiencing poverty.

waste management The collection, transport, treatment, and disposal of wastes, which may be land filled, incinerated, transported, stored temporarily, processed chemically to be less mobile, toxic, or reduced in volume, physically recycled or reused, injected into deep rock strata, or isolated in repositories.

water pollution Contamination of water, whether surface or groundwater, that may involve chemicals, infectious wastes, radiological wastes, or other waste products.

Women, Infants, and Children (WIC) Supplemental food program for women, infants, and children administered by the U.S. Department of Agriculture and each state.

workforce The population employed in a specified occupation.

workforce capacity The ability of the (public health) workforce to perform the necessary tasks to effectively deliver (the essential public health) services.

REFERENCES

1. Last JM. *A Dictionary of Public Health*. New York: Oxford University Press; 2007.

2. Breslow L. *Encyclopedia of Public Health*. New York: Macmillan Reference USA; 2002.

INDEX

G

O

Q

R